W9-DFE-168

MEDICAL RADIOLOGY

Diagnostic Imaging

Editors:

A. L. Baert, Leuven

M. Knauth, Göttingen

K. Sartor, Heidelberg

M. Rémy-Jardin · J. Rémy (Eds.)

Integrated Cardiothoracic Imaging with MDCT

With Contributions by

J. Aldrich · H. Alkadhi · C. R. Becker · L. Bonomo · K. Boroto · L. Boussel · E. Bouvier F. Cademartiri · C. Camus · P. Camus · A. Caulo · T. Couvreur · P. Douek · M. Dupont B. Elicker · J.-B. Faivre · J. Feignoux · D. Fleischmann · T. Flohr · P. Foucher D. Gamondès · B. Ghaye · A. B. Gorgos · A.-L. Hachulla · X. Hamoir · D. M. Hansell J. Kirsch · E. Klotz · L. La Grutta · J.–P. Laissy · A. R. Larici · F. Laurent · M. C. C. Lin G. Macis · E. Maffei · F. Maggi · B. Marincek · J. R. Mayo · L. Menchini · N. R. Mollet M. Montaudon · B. Ohnesorge · A. A. Palumbo · V. Pansini · F. Pontana M. Prokop · S. D. Qanadli · J. Rémy · M. Rémy-Jardin · D. Revel · E. Rizzo · A. Rutten J.–L. Sablayrolles · P. Stolzmann · M. L. Storto · N. Sverzellati · N. Tacelli J. M. Trautenaere · C. S. White · S. M. Yoo

Foreword by

A. L. Baert

With 247 Figures in 487 Separate Illustrations, 102 in Color and 37 Tables

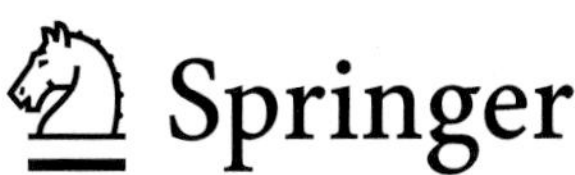

Springer

Martine Rémy-Jardin, MD, PhD
Professor, Department of Radiology
C.H.R.U. de Lille
Hôpital Calmette
Boulevard du Prof. J. Leclercq
59037 Lille Cédex
France

Jacques Rémy, MD
Professor, Department of Radiology
C.H.R.U. de Lille
Hôpital Calmette
Boulevard du Prof. J. Leclercq
59037 Lille Cédex
France

Medical Radiology · Diagnostic Imaging and Radiation Oncology
Series Editors:
A. L. Baert · L. W. Brady · H.-P. Heilmann · M. Knauth · M. Molls · C. Nieder · K. Sartor

Continuation of Handbuch der medizinischen Radiologie
Encyclopedia of Medical Radiology

ISBN 978-3-540-72386-8 e-ISBN 978-3-540-72387-5

DOI 10.1007 / 978-3-540-72387-5

Medical Radiology · Diagnostic Imaging and Radiation Oncology ISSN 0942-5373

Library of Congress Control Number: 2008924374

Cover-Design and Layout: PublishingServices Teichmann, 69256 Mauer, Germany

Printed on acid-free paper - 21/3180xq
9 8 7 6 5 4 3 2 1 0

springer.com

Foreword

This remarkable book explores yet another frontier of multidetector CT imaging, namely the widespread application of this high-performance radiological technique in the screening for cardiac and coronary artery lesions among the large group of patients at risk who undergo MDCT owing to respiratory symptoms.

The volume convincingly demonstrates the exciting new role which both general and chest radiologists can play in this medical field, as well as the many new potentially medically relevant applications of MDCT in daily radiological practice.

The editors are internationally renowned for their pioneering efforts in defining the role and scope of high resolution CT and MDCT for the study of the lung. They have published numerous articles and several highly successful handbooks on this topic. In addition, they have been able to involve many leading experts in the field as individual contributing authors to this volume.

Here, they brilliantly describe and illustrate how the fast scanning techniques and ultrahigh temporal resolution offered by state-of-the-art MDCT techniques can detect and characterise the numerous interaction processes that occur between two vital chest organs: the heart and the lungs.

I would like to congratulate both the editors and the authors for this outstanding volume, which is an excellent and timely addition to this book series.

I can highly recommend this handbook not only to all radiologists involved in chest imaging, but also to cardiologists, cardiac surgeons, pneumologists and lung surgeons as an indispensable guide for the optimal diagnostic and therapeutic management of their patients.

I am convinced that this work will rapidly find well deserved recognition and success among our readership.

Leuven

Albert L. Baert

Preface

Since its introduction into medical imaging practice in the 1980s, the major technological revolution of the scanner has focused mainly on temporal resolution. Indeed, on this basis, is it possible to classify equipment into two groups: scanners which control physiological motion and those which are subjected to physiological motion. Technical innovations have lead to an elaboration of this classification. Cardiac synchronisation is becoming an increasingly high-performance procedure, with ever less radiation exposure. Even without the use of the latter, accelerating rotation times controls motion in the slice plane and acquisition volume ever better. These physiological movements are caused by beats induced by the heart and vessels (which are quadri-dimensional) and, depending on patient condition, by oesophageal peristalsis, poorly controlled coughing, involuntary Valsalva maneuver as contrast material passes into the system, or disrupted control of apnea at full lung capacity. All anatomical structures of the thorax and their possible lesions are thus subjected to shifts. It has been shown that detection, analysis and quantification are improved by the suppression of all paracardiac motion artefacts. It can also be shown that all paracardiac gains are the result of "cardiac arrest" during acquisition. One example demonstrates this accurately: double-source technology offers temporal resolution of 83 ms without cardiac gating. It is able to acquire the entire thoracic level in 3 s, as well as the proximal coronary arteries in diastole if the cardiac frequency is at 75 bpm.

Only total immbolisation of structures and lesions suppresses motion artefacts which can have an effect not only on spatial resolution, but also on contrast resolution since shifted structures will be under-sampled. The results of this progress have an impact on CT practices. While thoracic imaging and cardiac imaging are two distinct specialties, the thoracic radiologist of today can no longer neglect examination of the heart and coronaries as he used to with earlier generations of equipment. Thus technology has opened an era of "cardiothoracic imaging" which prompts the thoracic radiologist to take a keen interest in cardiopulmonary interactions, while the cardiac radiologist needs to extend his field of analysis. These interactions are manifold: embryologic, anatomic, mechanical, physiological, physiopathological, and therapeutic. The time has come for these two specialties, thoracic imaging and cardiac imaging, to integrate the inseparable part of what was previously the domain of another specialist in their own activities.

This book is a trial of integrated cardiothoracic imaging in which a number of fields are addressed in order to alert the reader to the scale of the task, without, however, attempting to be exhaustive. The modest objective of the book is to attract the reader's attention to the cardiac effect of pulmonary vascular disease, the cardiovascular comorbidities of COPD and the cardiovascular causes and effects of their acute exacerbation, the cardiorespiratory tropism of sarcoidosis or scleroderma, as well as the management of equivocal symptoms which can be of either cardiac or respiratory origin.

The reader may find overlaps between chapters. These are certainly redundant if they express converging opinions while, in contrast, interesting if they express conflicting opinions resulting from the author's own experience and demonstrate that the use of imaging at the boundary between heart and lungs has not yet found its balance.

The reader may also encounter chapters lacking sufficient detail, such as the study of the cardio-pericardiac extent of neighbouring diseases (mediastinal, bronchopulmonary, pleural or even sub-diaphragmatic), or of therapeutic interactions between heart and lungs, a review of which alone would have merited a book of this size.

We would like to express our profound gratitude to all the authors who contributed to this book, which represents a collective work of pioneers who have just opened the door to a new specialty.

Lille

Martine Rémy-Jardin
Jacques Rémy

Contents

Part IV: Medical Applications of Integrated Cardiothoracic Imaging

Part I:

Technological Approach to Cardiothoracic Imaging

From Sixteen Slices to Nowadays – Cardiothoracic Imaging with CT

1

Thomas Flohr and Bernd Ohnesorge

CONTENTS

1.1 Introduction and Overview

The broad introduction of multi-detector row computed tomography (MDCT) into clinical practice in 1998 constituted a fundamental evolutionary step in the development and ongoing refinement of CT-imaging techniques. The first generation of MDCT systems offered simultaneous acquisition of four slices at a shortest gantry rotation time of 0.5 s and provided considerable improvement of scan speed and longitudinal (*z*-axis) resolution and better utilization of the available X-ray power compared with previous generations of single-slice CT systems (Klingenbeck et al. 1999; McCollough and Zink 1999; Hu et al. 2000). As a consequence, high-resolution imaging of larger anatomical volumes, such as the entire thorax, with a single scan acquisition and a single contrast medium injection became feasible, see Figure 1.1. The diagnosis of pulmonary embolism, already well established with single-slice CT systems at the level of segmental pulmonary arteries (Remy-Jardin et al. 1996; Remy-Jardin and Remy 1999), could be extended to the level of sub-segmental arteries thanks to the improved spatial resolution with 4×1-mm or 4×1.25-mm collimation (Schoepf et al. 2001, 2002; Remy-Jardin et al. 2002). Imaging of the heart was enabled by electro-cardiogram (ECG) synchronized data acquisition. Using optimized image reconstruction techniques, a temporal resolution of 250 ms and less was achieved with 0.5-s gantry rotation time (Kachelriess et al. 2000; Ohnesorge et al. 2000; Flohr and Ohnesorge 2001), which proved sufficient for adequate visualization of the coronary arteries at low to moderate heart rates (Achenbach et al. 2000; Becker et al. 2000; Knez et al. 2001; Nieman et al. 2001). Due to the very low table feed required for gapless volume coverage in any phase of the patient's cardiac cycle (about 3 mm/s for 4×1-mm collimation and 7.5 mm/s for 4×2.5-mm collimation), ECG-synchronized data acquisition with reasonable longitudinal resolution could not be extended to the entire thorax (about 300 mm). Hence, thoracic CT imaging with four slices was restricted to non-ECG gated acquisitions and a mere morphological assessment of the thoracic organs (d'Agostino et al. 2006).

Sixteen-slice MDCT systems (Flohr et al. 2002a, 2002b), introduced in 2001, provided simultaneous acquisition of 16 sub-millimeter slices (either 16×0.5 mm or 16×0.625 mm or 16×0.75 mm) and faster gantry rotation (rotation times down to 0.375 s). Substantial anatomical volumes could now be routinely covered with isotropic sub-millimeter spatial resolution. Due to short breath-hold times

T. Flohr, PhD
Siemens Healthcare, Computed Tomography, Siemensstrasse 1, 91301 Forchheim, Germany
B. Ohnesorge, PhD
Siemens Limited China, Healthcare, Siemens International Medical Park, 278 Zhou Zhu Road, Nanhui District, Shanghai 201318, P.R. China

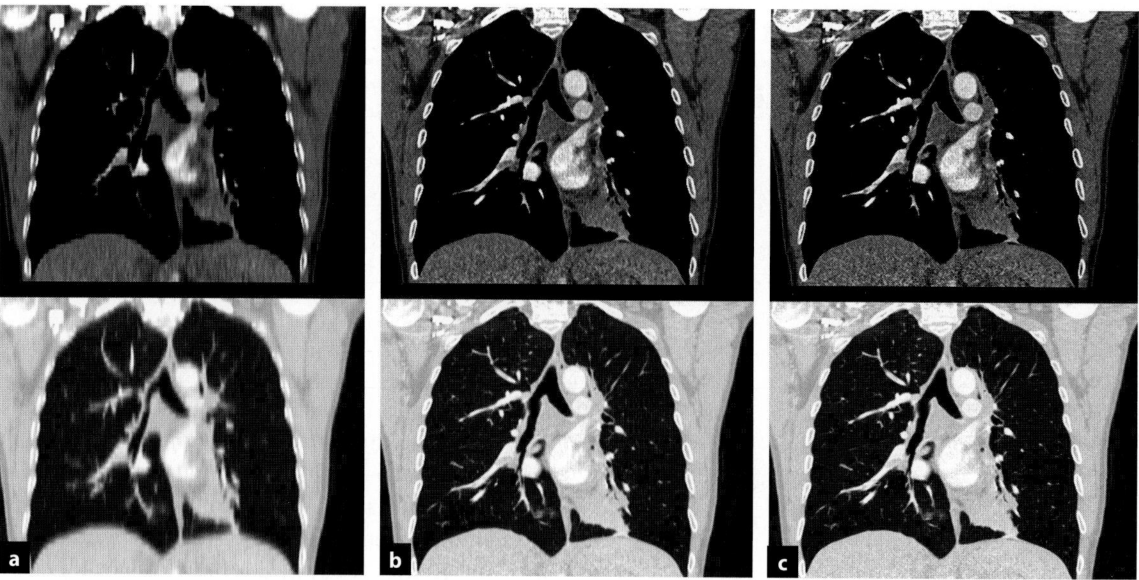

Fig. 1.1a–c. Case study (coronal MPRs) of a thorax examination in a patient with pulmonary embolism, illustrating the increased clinical performance from (**a**) single-slice CT (8-mm slices) to (**b**) 4-slice CT (1.25-mm slices), and (**c**) 64-slice CT (0.75-mm slices). Compared with single-slice CT scanners, four-slice CT systems brought about considerably improved longitudinal resolution in equivalent examination times (30 s to cover the thorax). Sixty-four-slice CT scanners provide significantly reduced examination times (5 s to cover the thorax) in combination with isotropic sub-millimeter resolution. The single-slice and 4-slice images were synthesized from the 64-slice CT data (courtesy of Profs. J. Remy and M. Remy-Jardin, Hopital Calmette, Lille, France)

of about 10 s for a CT-scan of the thorax with sub-millimeter collimation, central and peripheral pulmonary embolism could be reliably and accurately diagnosed even in dyspneic patients with a high pre-test likelihood of pulmonary embolism as the cause of their symptoms and limited ability to cooperate (Remy-Jardin et al. 2002; Schoepf et al. 2003). Furthermore, the use of MDCT for a combined assessment of pulmonary embolism and deep venous thrombosis, already introduced in 2001 (Schoepf et al. 2001), was established in clinical practice. ECG-synchronized cardiac scanning was enhanced by both, improved temporal and improved spatial resolution (Nieman et al. 2002; Ropers et al. 2003), and by considerably faster volume coverage (8 mm/s with 16×0.75-mm collimation and 16 mm/s with 16×1.5-mm collimation). Reasonable breath-hold times below 30 s to cover the entire thorax with ECG-gated acquisition protocols could be achieved by using collimation settings of 16×1.25 mm or 16×1.5 mm. While the limited longitudinal resolution hampered the detailed diagnosis of coronary arteries, motion-free visualization of the lung and the cardiothoracic vessels as well as cardiac functional evaluation became possible. Alternatively, two-phase protocols could be used to scan both the entire thorax and cardiac cavities with the highest spatial resolution. Hence, cardiac functional evaluation could be integrated into a diagnostic CT scan of the chest, providing vital information in a variety of respiration disorders, e.g., about right ventricular function and about details such as the presence of cardiomyopathy and ventricular aneurysms, plus the analysis of myocardial contractility on CT cine images (Coche et al. 2005; Delhaye et al. 2006; d'Agostino et al. 2006; Bruzzi et al. 2006a, 2006b).

In addition, first clinical studies proved the potential usefulness of ECG-synchronized imaging of the heart and the cardiothoracic vessels with one CT scan for a comprehensive diagnosis in patients with acute chest pain (Ohnesorge et al. 2005; White et al. 2005; Ghersin et al. 2006). In a sense, it is fair to say that combined cardiothoracic imaging began with the generation of 16-slice CT systems.

In 2004, all major CT manufacturers introduced MDCT systems with simultaneous acquisition of 64 slices. Two different scanner concepts were introduced by the different vendors: the "volume concept" pursued by GE, Philips and Toshiba aims at a further increase in volume coverage speed by using 64 detector rows instead of 16, thus providing 32 mm–40 mm z-coverage without changing other physical parameters of the scanner compared to the respective 16-slice version. The "resolution concept" pursued by Siemens uses 32 physical detector rows in combination with double z-sampling, a refined z-sampling technique enabled by a periodic motion of the focal spot in the z-direction, to simultaneously acquire 64 overlapping 0.6-mm slices with the goal of pitch-independent increase of longitudinal resolution and reduction of spiral artifacts (Flohr et al. 2004, 2005). With the use of 64-slice CT systems, the entire thorax can be scanned with sub-millimeter resolution in about 5 s in a non-ECG-gated mode (see Fig. 1.1), which is beneficial for the examination of emergency patients, e.g., with suspicion of acute pulmonary embolism. The improved temporal resolution due to gantry rotation times down to 0.33 s increases the clinical robustness of ECG-gated scanning at higher heart rates, thereby significantly facilitating the successful integration of CT coronary angiography into routine clinical algorithms (Leber et al. 2005; Raff et al. 2005). While image quality at higher heart rates seems to be significantly improved compared with previous generations of MDCT systems, several authors still propose the administration of beta-blockers (Leber et al. 2005; Raff et al. 2005; Mollet et al. 2005).

Sixty-four-slice CT scanners can overcome the limitations of 16-slice CT scanners with respect to combined cardiothoracic scanning, since they are able to cover the entire thorax in an ECG-gated mode with sub-millimeter collimation for a comprehensive diagnosis of morphology and cardiac function within one integrated CT examination, including high-resolution imaging of the coronary arteries (Salem et al. 2006; Bruzzi et al. 2006a, 2006b; Delhaye et al. 2007). Due to scan times usually not exceeding 20 s, sufficient contrast enhancement of the pulmonary vessels, coronary arteries and aorta can be achieved without excessive doses of contrast medium. In a study with 133 patients using ECG-gated 64-slice CT, both the underlying respiratory disease and cardiac function could be assessed from the same CT data set in 92% of the patients (Salem et al. 2006). Delhaye et al. (2007a) demonstrated that proximal and mid-coronary segments could be adequately assessed during an ECG-gated CT angiographic examination of the entire thorax without administration of beta-blockers in patients with a heart rate below 80 bpm. The authors also showed that ECG-gated 64-slice MDCT could be a clinically suitable method for screening for coronary artery disease prior to chest surgery (Delhaye et al. 2007b).

First clinical experience indicates that 64-slice CT could enable the rapid triage of patients in the emergency room who present with equivocal chest pain, non-diagnostic ECG and negative serum markers. Such patients usually undergo a period of observation with repeated assessment of ECG and cardiac markers and further workup. Inclusion of 64-slice CT into the diagnostic algorithm allows for rapid diagnosis of common causes of acute chest pain, such as pulmonary embolism, aortic dissection or aneurysm, or significant coronary artery disease. This application is often referred to as "triple rule out" (Schoepf 2007; Johnson et al. 2007a). As a downside, ECG-gated multi-slice spiral scanning of the entire thorax with high resolution can result in considerable radiation exposure, which is of particular concern in patients with low likelihood of disease, and has so far precluded the routine use of this method for the examination of patients with acute chest pain, except when there is sufficient support for the diagnosis of either aortic dissection or pulmonary embolism (Gallagher and Raff 2008). It is in any case mandatory to carefully optimize scan techniques and protocols for ECG-synchronized CT angiography of the chest according to the clinical indication. Some 64-slice CT systems are equipped with special protocols for ECG-gated examinations of the chest that utilize higher pitch values up to 0.3 for increased scan speed and reduced radiation exposure. Effective patient dose values of only 4.95 mSv were reported with the use of such protocols for low-dose ECG-gated CT angiograms of the thorax, without altering the diagnostic value of the CT scans (d'Agostino et al. 2006). Figure 1.2 shows a patient example of an ECG-gated spiral acquisition of the entire thorax with a 64-slice CT.

In 2007, a MDCT system with 128 simultaneously acquired slices was introduced based on a detector with 64×0.6-mm collimation and double z-sampling by means of a z-flying focal spot.

With the latest generation of 64- or 128-slice MDCT, the whole body can be examined with isotropic sub-millimeter resolution in very short scan times, and a further increase in the number of simultaneously acquired slices to speed up the system even more will not necessarily translate into increased clinical benefit. Instead, new developments are ongoing to solve remaining limitations of conventional MDCT scanners.

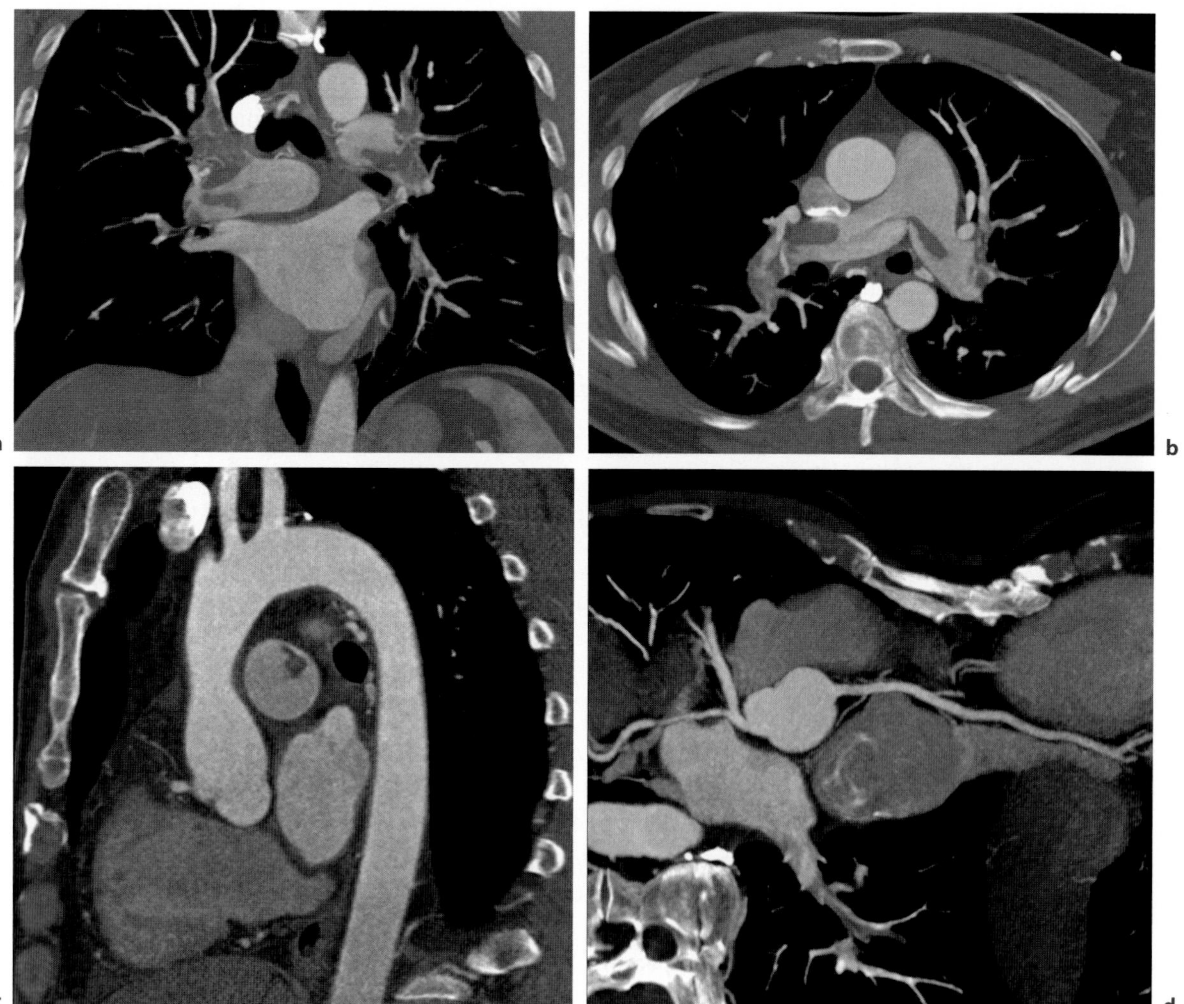

Fig. 1.2a–d. Example of a high-resolution ECG-gated chest examination using a 64-slice CT, which illustrates the potential of ECG-gated cardiothoracic scanning to assess common causes of acute chest pain, such as pulmonary embolism, aortic dissection or aneurysm, or significant coronary artery disease, in one single examination. A 49-year-old male patient with bilateral pulmonary embolism (**a**,**b**), but no evidence of disease of the thoracic aorta (**c**) and no evidence of disease of the coronary arteries (**d**) (courtesy of Hong Kong Baptist Hospital, Hong Kong, China)

Motion artifacts remain the most important challenge for integrated cardiothoracic imaging and coronary CTA even with the latest generation of MDCT. A temporal resolution of less than 100 ms at all heart rates is desirable to completely eliminate the need for heart rate control. In 2005, a dual source CT (DSCT) system, i.e., a CT system with two X-ray tubes and two corresponding detectors offset by 90°, was introduced (Flohr et al. 2006). The key benefit of DSCT for cardiothoracic scanning and coronary CTA is improved temporal resolution. A scanner of this type provides temporal resolution of a quarter of the gantry rotation time, independent of the patient's heart rate. Meanwhile, several clinical studies have demonstrated the potential of DSCT to accurately rule out significant coronary artery stenoses with little or no dependence on the patient's heart rate (Achenbach et al. 2006; Scheffel et al. 2006; Johnson et al. 2007b; Matt et al. 2007; Leber et al. 2007; Ropers et al. 2007). DSCT scanners are well suited for integrated cardiothoracic examinations, since they can overcome the restricted image quality of the coronary arteries in high heart rates, which has so far been a major limitation of these examinations in particular in acutely ill patients (Johnson et al. 2007c). In a study with 109 consecutive patients presenting with acute chest pain, the overall sensitivity for the identification of the cause of chest pain was 98% with the use of DSCT (Johnson et al. 2007c).

DSCT scanners also show promising properties for general radiology applications, such as potential dose accumulation for the examination of obese patients, or dual-energy acquisitions. Clinical applications of dual-energy CT include tissue characterization, calcium quantification and quantification of the local blood volume in contrast-enhanced scans (Johnson et al. 2007d; Primak et al. 2007; Scheffel et al. 2007; Graser et al. 2008).

Yet another challenge for CT is the visualization of dynamic processes in extended anatomical ranges, e.g., to characterize the inflow and outflow of contrast agent in the arterial and venous system in dynamic CT angiographies or to determine the enhancement characteristics of the contrast agent in volume perfusion studies. One way to solve this problem is the introduction of area detectors large enough to cover entire organs, such as the heart, the kidneys or the brain, in one axial scan (requiring 120 mm volume coverage or more). In 2007, a CT scanner with 320×0.5-mm collimation and 0.35-s gantry rotation time was introduced, which has the potential to cover the heart in one single sequential acquisition – thereby avoiding stair-step and misregistration artifacts – and to acquire dynamic volume data by repeatedly scanning the same anatomical range without table movement.

Overall, the greatest challenge of evolving CT technology is the explosion of information now available to physicians. Standardizing the display of post-processed images will be increasingly important to preserve efficient workflow and optimum patient care.

1.2 Multi-Detector Row CT (MDCT)

1.2.1 Technology

Third-generation CT scanners employ the so-called "rotate/rotate" geometry, in which both X-ray tube and detector are mounted onto a rotating gantry and rotate about the patient (Fig. 1.3). In a MDCT system, the detector comprises several rows of 700 and more detector elements that cover a scan field of view (SFOV) of usually 50 cm. The X-ray attenuation of the object is measured by the individual detector elements. All measurement values acquired at the same angular position of the measurement system are called a "projection" or "view." About 1,000 projections are typically measured during each 360° rotation. A suitable MDCT detector must provide different slice widths to adjust the optimum scan speed, longitudinal resolution and image noise for each application. Different manufacturers of MDCT scanners have introduced different detector designs: the fixed array detector consists of detector elements with equal sizes in the longitudinal (*z*-axis) direction, while the adaptive array detector comprises detector rows with different sizes in the longitudinal direction. Figure 1.4 gives an overview on the detector designs of current 16-, 64-, and 128-slice MDCT scanners.

Some MDCT scanners make use of a periodic motion of the X-ray focal spot in the longitudinal direction (z-flying focal spot, double z-sampling) to double the number of simultaneously acquired slices and to improve data sampling along the z-axis (Flohr et al. 2004, 2005). By permanent electromagnetic deflection of the electron beam in the X-ray tube, the focal spot is wobbled between two different positions on the anode plate. The amplitude of the periodic *z*-motion is adjusted in a way that two subsequent read-

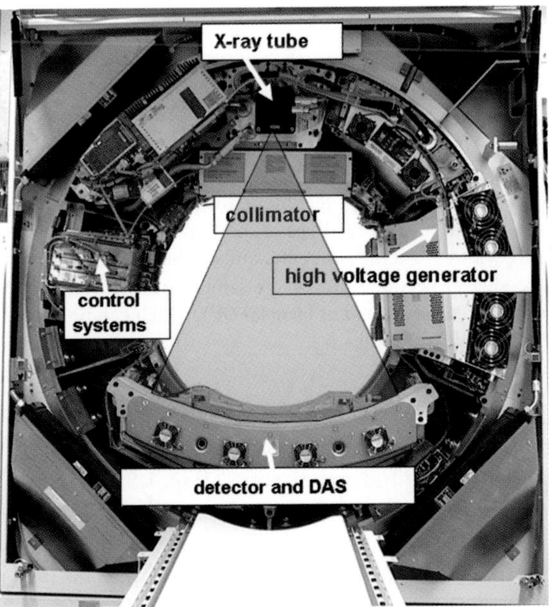

Fig. 1.3. Basic components of a modern third generation CT scanner. DAS = data acquisition system

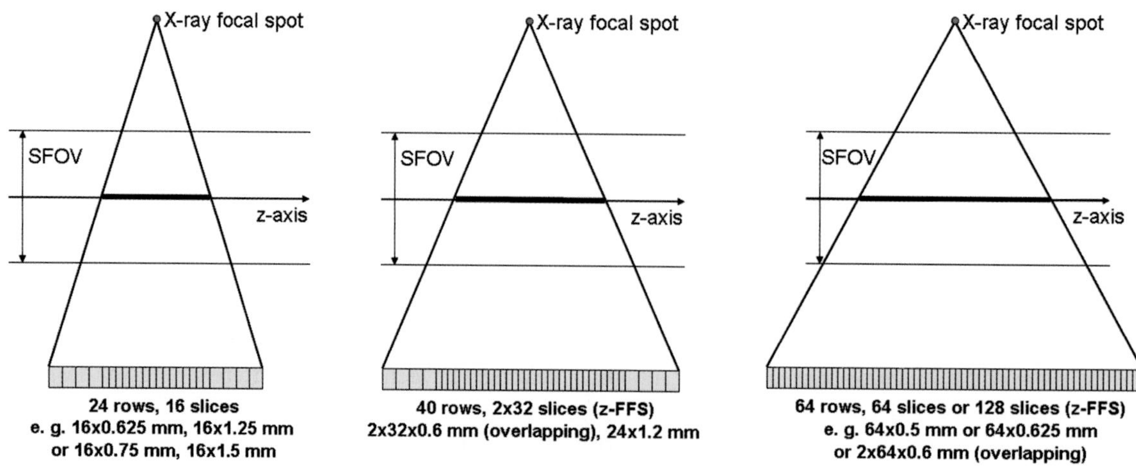

Fig. 1.4. Adaptive array detectors (comprising elements of varying size in the *z*-direction) and fixed array detectors (comprising elements of equal size in the *z*-direction) used in commercially available MDCT systems. *z-FFS* = *z*-flying focal spot

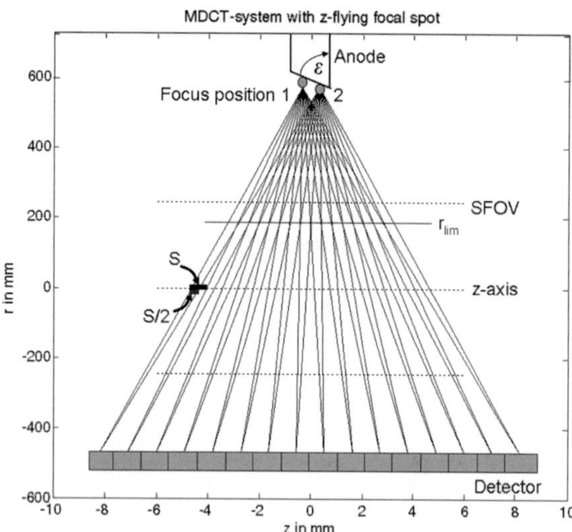

Fig. 1.5. Schematic illustration of improved *z*-sampling with the *z*-flying focal spot technique (double *z*-sampling). Two subsequent M-slice readings are shifted by half a collimated slice width S/2 at the iso-center and can be interleaved to one 2M-slice projection. Improved *z*-sampling is maintained in a range of the scan field of view (*SFOV*), which can be defined by a "limiting" radius r_{lim}

ings are shifted by half a collimated slice width in the patient's longitudinal direction (Fig. 1.5). Therefore, the measurement rays of two subsequent readings interleave in the *z*-direction, and two subsequent M-slice readings with, e.g., 0.6-mm collimated slice width are combined to one 2M-slice projection with a sampling distance of 0.3 mm at the iso-center. The clinical benefits of optimized z-sampling with the z-flying focal spot technique are improved longitudinal resolution at any pitch (Fig. 1.6) and suppression of spiral artifacts. Typical spiral artifacts result from insufficient data sampling along the z-axis and present as hyper- or hypo-dense "windmill" structures surrounding *z*-inhomogeneous high-contrast objects such as bones or contrast-filled vessels (e.g., vena cava), which rotate when scrolling through a stack of images.

Key requirement for the mechanical design of the gantry is the stability of both focal spot and detector position during rotation, in particular with regard to the rapidly decreasing rotation times of modern CT systems (from 0.75 s in 1994 to 0.3 s in 2008). Hence, the mechanical support for X-ray tube, tube collimator and data measurement system (DMS) has to be designed such as to withstand the high gravitational forces associated with fast gantry rotation. Rotation times of less than 0.25 s appear to be beyond today's mechanical limits.

1.2.2 MDCT Scan and Image Reconstruction Techniques

With the advent of MDCT, axial "step-and-shoot" scanning has remained in use for only few clinical applications, such as head scanning, high-resolution lung scanning, perfusion CT and interventional applications. Spiral/helical scanning is the method of choice for the vast majority of all MDCT examinations.

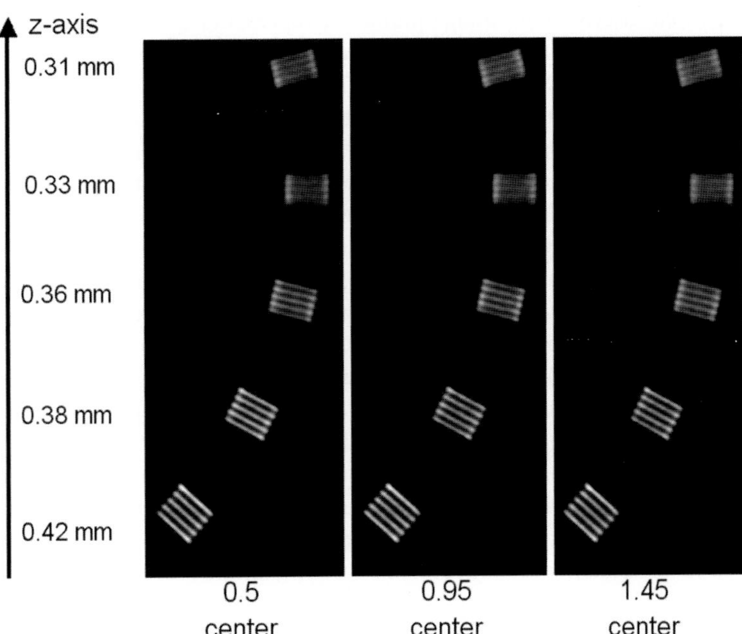

Fig. 1.6. Multi-planar reformations (*MPRs*) of a *z*-resolution phantom (high-resolution insert of the CATPHAN, the Phantom Laboratories, Salem, NY, turned by 90°). Scan data were acquired on a CT system with 32×0.6-mm collimation in a 64-slice acquisition mode using the *z*-flying focal spot and reconstructed with the narrowest slice width (nominal 0.6 mm) and a sharp body kernel. Independent of the pitch ($p=0.5$, 0.95 or 1.45), all line pair test patterns up to 16 lp/cm can be visualized. The line pair test pattern with 15 lp/cm is exactly perpendicular to the *z*-axis, corresponding to 0.33-mm longitudinal resolution

An important parameter to characterize a spiral/helical scan is the pitch. According to IEC specifications (International Electrotechnical Comission 2002) the pitch p is given by

$$p = \text{tablefeed per rotation/ total width of the collimated beam} \quad (1)$$

This definition holds for single-slice CT as well as for MDCT. It shows whether data acquisition occurs with gaps ($p > 1$) or with overlap ($p < 1$) in the longitudinal direction.

To fully exploit the potential benefits of MDCT technology, suitable scan and image reconstruction concepts had to be developed that cope with the technical challenges of MDCT imaging, such as the complicated z-sampling patterns or the cone angle problem: the measurement rays in MDCT are tilted by the so-called cone-angle with respect to a plane perpendicular to the z-axis. The cone-angle is largest for the slices at the outer edges of the detector, and it increases with increasing number of detector rows if their width is kept constant.

MDCT spiral/helical algorithms for general radiology applications have to provide acceptable image quality in terms of cone-beam artifacts and spiral "windmill" artifacts; they should allow for a certain variation of the pitch to adjust the table-feed of the scanner to clinical needs, and they should make full use of the data that are available for an image, i.e., they should not waste radiation dose. Depending on the number of slices of the respective CT system, the cone angle of the measurement rays can either be neglected – for up to about eight slices – or it has to be taken into account at least approximately – for more than eight slices. ECG-triggered and ECG-gated scan and image reconstruction techniques will be covered in the following chapter.

Pertinent spiral/helical algorithms neglecting the cone angle of the measurement rays are the 180° MLI and 360° MLI multi-slice linear interpolation approaches (Hu 1999; Hsieh 2003) or z-filter techniques (Taguchi and Aradate 1998; Schaller et al. 2000). In a *z*-filter reconstruction, all direct and complementary rays (i.e., rays in the same direction acquired half a rotation earlier or later) within a selectable distance from the image plane contribute to the image. Images with different slice widths can be retrospectively reconstructed from the same CT raw data by adjusting this distance and the corresponding weighting functions. Hence, *z*-filtering allows the user to trade off *z*-axis resolution with image noise (which directly correlates with required dose).

Commonly used reconstruction approaches accounting for the cone-beam geometry of the measurement rays are the so-called nutating slice algorithms and 3D filtered back-projection. In a nutating slice reconstruction, the 3D reconstruction task is split into a series of conventional 2D reconstructions on tilted intermediate image planes. A representative example is the adaptive multiple plane reconstruction, AMPR (Schaller et al. 2001; Flohr et al. 2003). In a 3D filtered back-projection reconstruction (Grass et al. 2000; Hein et al. 2003; Stierstorfer et al. 2004), the measurement rays are directly back-projected into a 3D volume along the lines of measurement, this way accounting for their cone-beam geometry (see Fig. 1.7).

Regardless of the specific reconstruction algorithm used in a particular CT scanner, narrow collimation scanning is generally recommended due to better suppression of partial volume artifacts, even if the pitch has to be increased for equivalent volume coverage. Similar to single-slice spiral CT, narrow collimation scanning is the key to reduce artifacts and to improve image quality. CT examinations of the chest in particular benefit from narrow collimation settings. Pitch values of 1.3–1.5 and fast gantry rotation (e.g., rotation time t_{rot} = 0.33 s) are advisable for non-ECG-gated scans of the thorax, resulting in high volume coverage speeds of up to, e.g., 90 mm/s for a CT scanner with 32 × 0.6-mm collimation and up to 180 mm/s for a CT scanner with 64 × 0.6-mm collimation.

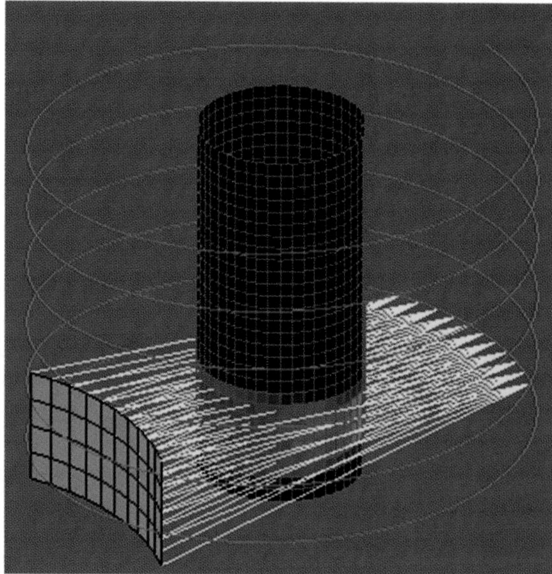

Fig. 1.7. Schematic illustration of 3D spiral/helical back-projection in parallel geometry. Each ray (*yellow*) is directly back-projected into the SFOV (*black cylinder*) along its line of measurement, thereby accounting for its cone angle. This means that each voxel in the SFOV receives contributions from those rays that pass from the X-ray source through the voxel to the detector array. The spiral/helical path is indicated in *red*. As a consequence of the rebinning procedure from fan beam geometry to parallel beam geometry, each parallel projection (the array of *yellow lines* shown in the figure) consists of rays from several fan beam projections acquired at different projection angles with different positions of the X-ray focus along the spiral path. (Illustration by courtesy of Dr. Karl Stierstorfer, Siemens Healthcare, Forchheim, Germany)

In practice, different slice widths are often reconstructed by default: thick slices for filming and initial viewing and thin slices for 3D post-processing and evaluation. The image noise in close-to-isotropic high-resolution volumes can be limited by making use of thick multi-planar reformations (MPRs) or thick maximum intensity projections (MIPs). In this way, images with the desired slice width can be obtained in arbitrary directions. As a consequence, the distinction between longitudinal and in-plane resolution has meanwhile become a historical remnant, and the traditional axial slice has lost its clinical predominance.

1.3 CT Systems with Area Detectors

An area detector is a CT detector that is wide enough to cover entire organs, such as the heart, the kidneys or the brain, in one axial scan without table movement, see Figure 1.8. Hence, a clinically useful area detector has to cover at least 120 mm in the *z*-direction. In 2007, a CT scanner with 320 × 0.5-mm collimation and 0.35-s gantry rotation time was commercially introduced by one vendor, after a long evaluation phase using prototype systems with 256 × 0.5-mm collimation and 0.5 s gantry rotation time: the CT scanner and its image reconstruction were technically evaluated (Mori et al. 2004, 2006a), phantom studies were performed (Funashabi et al. 2007), and first in-vitro studies and clinical images of pigs were presented (Funashabi et al. 2005; Mori et al. 2006b). First patient studies (Kondo et al. 2005) demonstrated the prototype's potential to visualize the cardiac anatomy and to assess cardiac function. In a preliminary clinical report (Kido et al. 2007), 90.9% of the AHA coronary segments 1, 2, 3, 5, 6, 7, 9 and 11 could be evaluated in five patients. Meanwhile, estimates for the expected radiation dose to the patient have been given (Mori et al. 2006c).

The benefits of CT scanners with area detectors for cardiothoracic scanning are two-fold: first, they

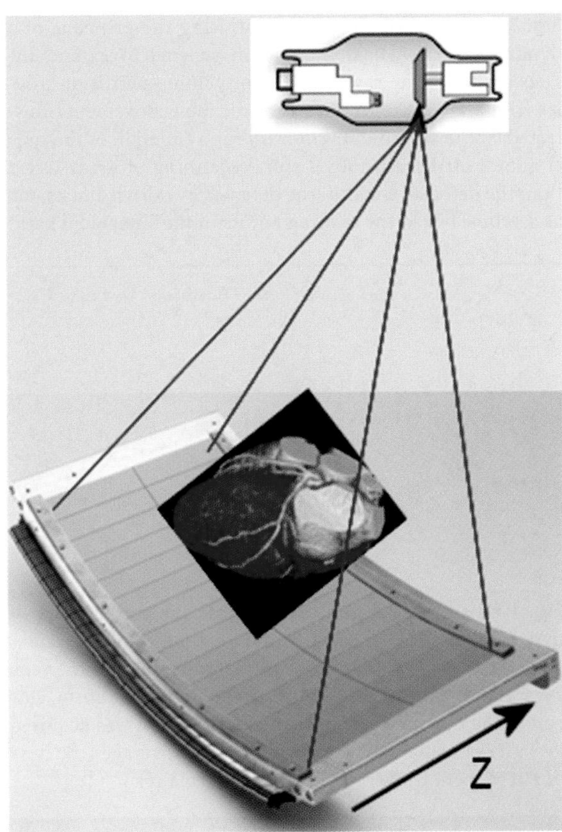

Fig. 1.8. Schematic drawing of a CT geometry with area detector large enough to cover entire organs such as the heart in a single rotation

can avoid the typical stair-step artifacts in ECG-synchronized examinations of the heart. With today's available MDCT detector z-coverage of up to 40 mm, an ECG-synchronized volume image of the heart still consists of several image slabs reconstructed from data acquired in multiple consecutive heart beats. As a consequence of insufficient temporal resolution and variations of the heart motion from one cardiac cycle to the next – in particular in case of arrhythmia – these image slabs can be blurred or shifted relative to each other, resulting in banding artifacts in MPRs or volume-rendered displays (VRTs). The width of an image slab originating from one heart beat is proportional to the detector *z*-coverage. With increasing detector *z*-coverage, the number of heart beats contributing to the volume image decreases, and so does the number of steps in case of artifacts. The diagnostic quality of a "one heart beat" cardiac examination, however, depends on the available temporal resolution. In the worst case, the entire scan will suffer from blurring and reduced image quality if it is acquired in a short RR cycle.

As a second benefit, CT systems with area detectors can acquire dynamic volume data by repeatedly scanning the same anatomical range without table movement, which is useful in dynamic CT angiographic studies or in volume perfusion studies, e.g., to distinguish hepatocellular carcinoma (HCC) from normal liver tissue (Mori et al. 2007). A prominent cardiothoracic application is the evaluation of myocardial perfusion defects, e.g., due to coronary artery narrowing. With today's MDCT technology, only limited ranges of the myocardium (3–4 cm depending on the CT scanner type and its detector *z*-coverage) can be covered with sequential ECG-controlled scan protocols without table movement to study dynamic contrast enhancement. With area detector technology, the entire myocardium can be examined. CT imaging of the myocardial perfusion is conceptually promising, yet it has to compete with other well-established modalities (in particular magnetic resonance imaging MRI), and a number of obstacles have to be overcome to prove clinical feasibility. For clinically relevant diagnostic information stress perfusion testing at elevated heart rates (e.g., after the administration of adenosine) is mandatory, which requires excellent temporal resolution – at best below 50–100 ms.

In dynamic volume studies of the entire thorax, either for perfusion evaluation or for dynamic CTA, a scan range of at least 25 cm has to be covered, which is beyond the scope of current area detector technology and requires repeated axial scans with table movement in between. In this case, dynamic spiral/helical acquisition schemes using MDCT systems with limited detector *z*-coverage may lead to similar results. Continuous periodic table movement allows for time-resolved spiral/helical scanning of areas larger than the detector *z*-width, see Figure 1.9. With an average pitch of 1 and 0.3 s gantry rotation time, a scan range of, e.g., 27 cm can be covered in 2.5 s with a 4-cm detector. Early clinical experience indicates that the temporal sampling rate is then still sufficient for perfusion evaluation of extended tumors, e.g., by means of Patlak analysis. Figure 1.10 shows a clinical example of a dynamic CTA acquisition of the thorax with a CT system with 4-cm detector, visualizing the inflow of contrast agent into the vena cava, the right heart, the left heart and the aorta. Clinical studies will be needed to identify relevant applications of such time-resolved CT angiographic studies.

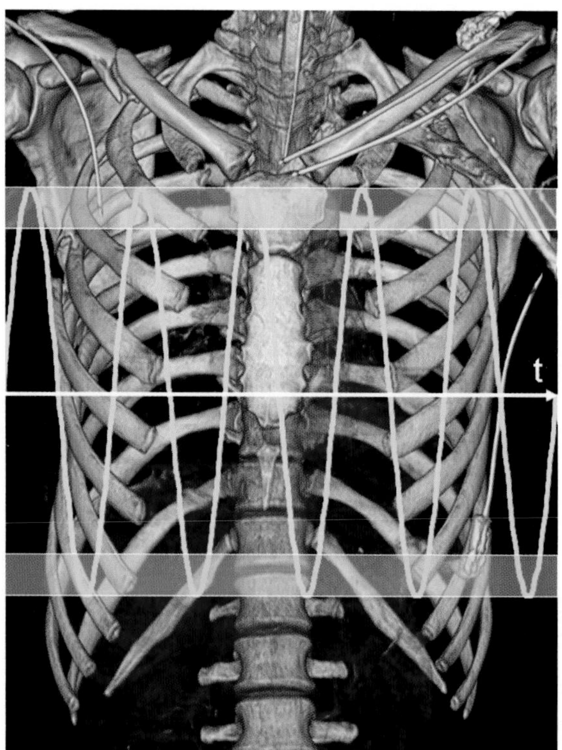

Fig. 1.9. Schematic drawing illustrating the principle of a dynamic spiral/helical acquisition scheme to extend the z-coverage in time-resolved CTA or volume-perfusion studies with MDCT. Continuous periodic table movement (illustrated by the sinusoidal *yellow line* as a function of the time t) allows for time-resolved spiral scanning of areas larger than the detector z-width (the detector z-width is illustrated as a *yellow box* at the turning points of the sinusoidal path)

Fig. 1.10. Clinical example illustrating the performance of dynamic spiral/helical acquisition for time-resolved CT angiographic studies. Inflow of contrast medium into the vena cava, the right heart, the left heart and finally the aorta. One run of the dynamic spiral (scan length 27 cm) was acquired every 2.5 s using a detector with 4 cm z-coverage (courtesy of Dr. M. Lell, University Erlangen, Germany)

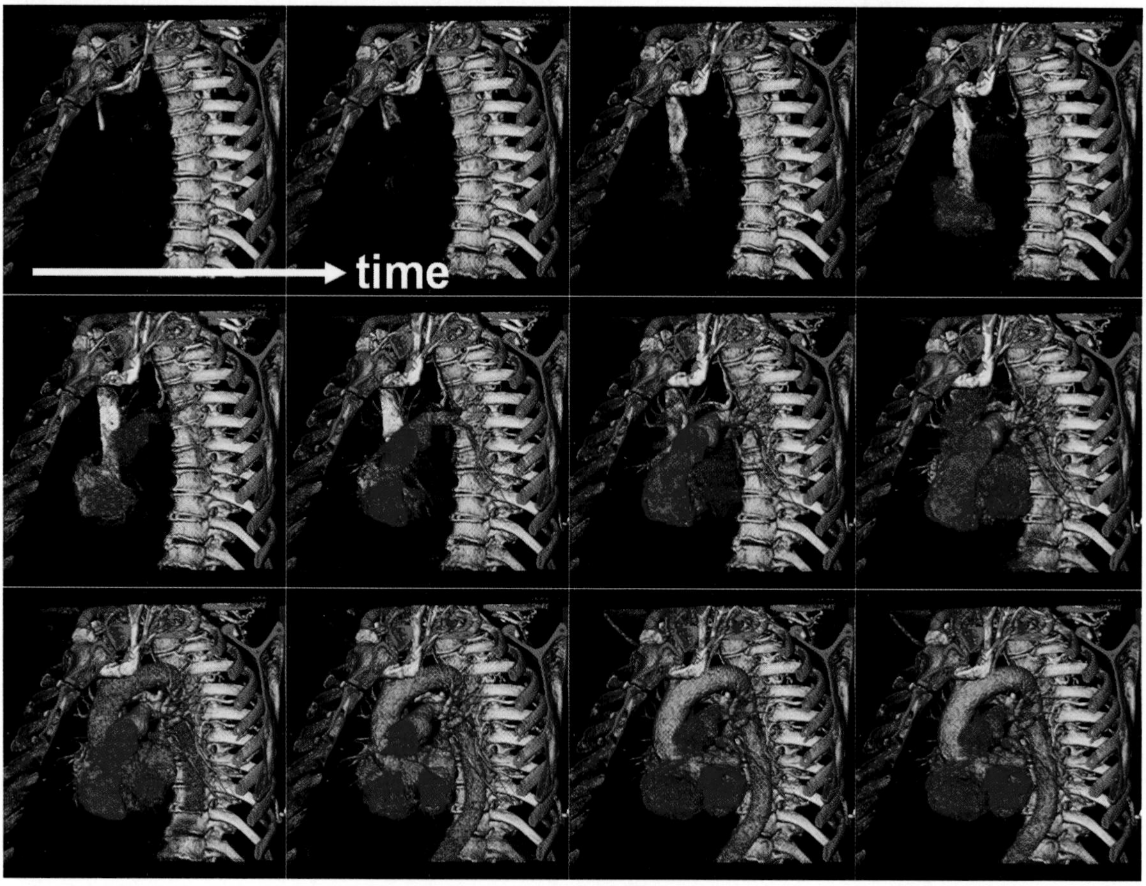

1.4 Dual-Source CT (DSCT)

Increased gantry rotation speed is a pre-requisite for clinically robust improvement of the temporal resolution with conventional third-generation MDCT systems. An alternative scanner concept that provides considerably enhanced temporal resolution but does not require faster gantry rotation is a CT with multiple tubes and corresponding detectors (Robb and Ritman 1979; Ritman et al. 1980). In 2005, a dual-source CT (DSCT) was commercially introduced. The two acquisition systems are mounted onto the rotating gantry with an angular offset of 90° (Fig. 1.11). One detector covers the entire SFOV (50 cm in diameter), while the other detector is restricted to a smaller, central field of view (26 cm). Both detectors provide simultaneous acquisition of 64 overlapping 0.6-mm slices by means of double *z*-sampling using a *z*-flying focal spot. The gantry rotation time is 0.33 s (Flohr et al. 2006). Due to the restriction of detector (B) to a 26-cm field of view, the projection data of larger objects are truncated. They have to be extrapolated in the image reconstruction process by using data acquired with detector (A) at the same view angle a quarter rotation earlier or later.

The key benefit of DSCT for cardiothoracic scanning is improved temporal resolution equivalent to a quarter of the gantry rotation time (Flohr et al. 2006). In parallel geometry, 180° of scan data (a half-scan sinogram) is necessary for ECG-synchronized image reconstruction. Due to the 90° angle between both detectors, the half-scan sinogram can be split up into two 90° data segments, which are simultaneously acquired by the two acquisition systems in the same relative phase of the patient's cardiac cycle and at the same anatomical level. With this approach, constant temporal resolution equivalent to a quarter of the gantry rotation time $t_{rot}/4$ (83 ms at 0.33 s gantry rotation) is achieved in a sufficiently centered region of the SFOV. The temporal resolution is independent of the patient's heart rate, since data from one cardiac cycle only are used to reconstruct an image (single-segment reconstruction). This is a major difference to conventional MDCT systems, which can theoretically provide similar temporal resolution by combining data from several heart cycles to an image (multi-segment reconstruction). With multi-segment approaches, temporal resolution strongly depends on the heart rate – optimal temporal resolution can only be achieved at few selected heart rates – and a stable and predictable heart rate and complete periodicity of the heart motion are required for adequate performance (see

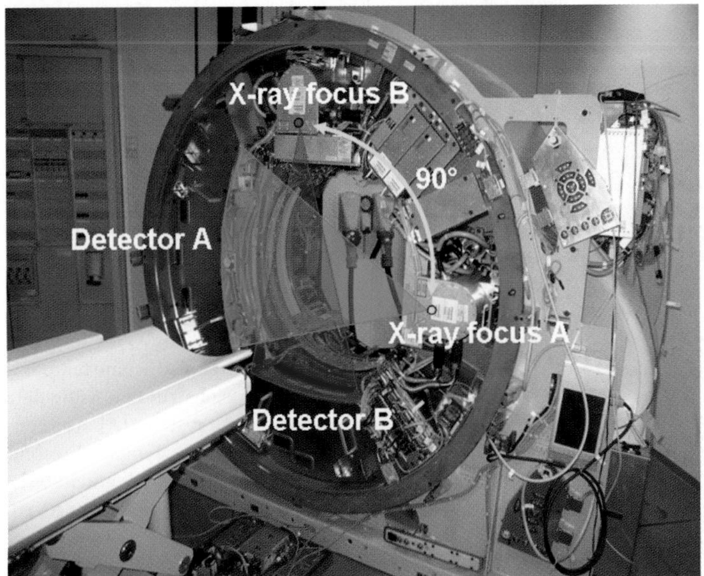

a

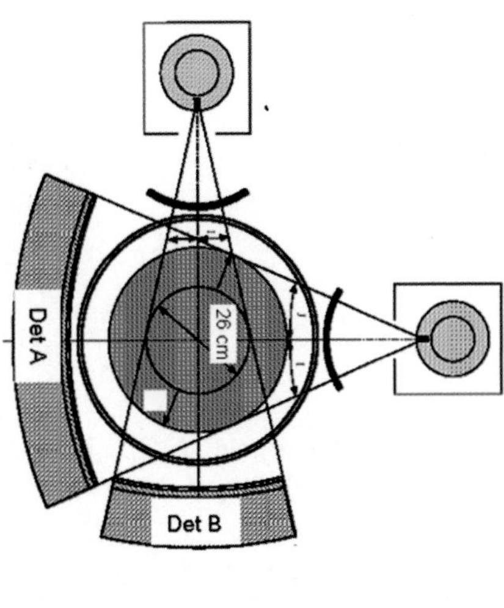

b

Fig. 1.11a,b. Picture of the open gantry of a commercially available dual source CT (*DSCT*) system using two tubes and two corresponding detectors offset by 90° (*left*). One detector (**a**) covers the entire SFOV with a diameter of 50 cm, while the other detector (**b**) is restricted to a smaller, central field of view (*right*)

Fig. 1.12 for a comparison of MDCT single-segment and multi-segment reconstruction and DSCT single-segment reconstruction for the same patient with arrhythmia).

Several clinical studies have meanwhile demonstrated that DSCT can provide diagnostic results in coronary CT angiography examinations irrespective of the patient's heart rate (Achenbach et al. 2006; Scheffel et al. 2006; Johnson et al. 2007b; Matt et al. 2007; Leber et al. 2007; Ropers et al. 2007). Very high sensitivity and negative predictive values show the strength of the technique in ruling out significant coronary artery disease (CAD) (Leber et al. 2007). While DSCT may demonstrate slightly lower per-segment evaluability for high heart rates, diagnostic accuracy for the detection of coronary artery stenoses does not decrease (Ropers et al. 2007). With DSTC, image quality is less dependent on heart rate variations than with MDCT, hence clinically robust image quality in patients with irregular heart rate during the scan can be achieved. Only heart rates that are both high and variable deteriorate image quality, but

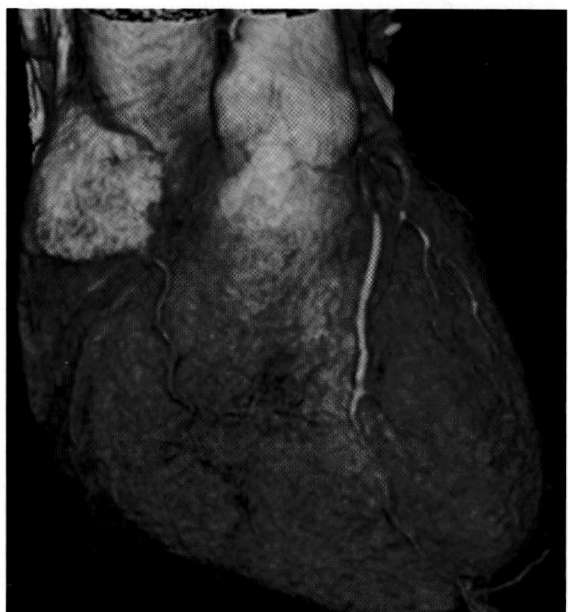

a

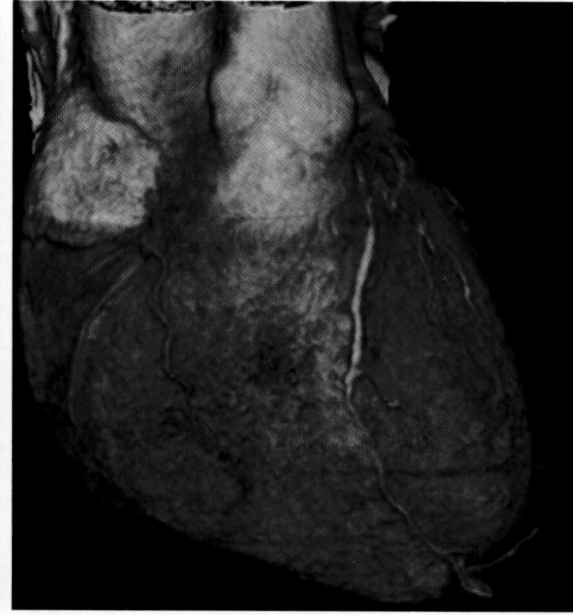

b

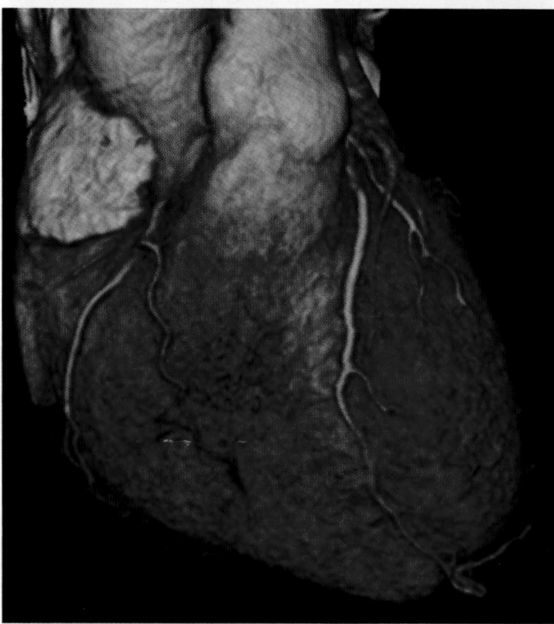

c

Fig. 1.12a–c. Volume-rendered images (*VRTs*) of a coronary CT angiographic study in a patient with severe arrhythmia (varying heart rate from 86 bpm to 122 bpm) during scan data acquisition with a DSCT system. The same rendering parameters were used for all VRTs. **a** Single-segment image reconstruction using data from only one of the two measurement systems (A). This corresponds to a scan acquired with a 64-slice single source MDCT system with 165-ms temporal resolution. Severe motion artifacts in the RCA, the LAD and the diagonal branches are caused by insufficient temporal resolution. **b** Two-segment image reconstruction using data from only one of the two measurement systems (A). As a consequence of the rapidly varying heart rate, temporal resolution is not consistently improved by the multi-segment technique. The visualization of the coronary arteries is improved, but still suffers from artifacts. **c** Single-segment image reconstruction using data from both measurement systems (A, B), resulting in 83 ms temporal resolution. The coronary arteries are now almost free of motion artifacts, despite the patient's arrhythmia (courtesy of Dr. C. Becker, University Hospital of Munich-Grosshadern, Munich, Germany)

the quality remains adequate for diagnosis (Matt et al. 2007). First clinical experience indicates that the elimination of cardiac motion due to the improved temporal resolution significantly reduces Ca blooming (Fig. 1.13), which has so far been an obstacle in the assessment of coronary artery disease in patients with significant calcifications in the coronary arteries. DSCT coronary CTA performs well in the detection of in-stent restenosis, see Figure 1.14. Although DSCT coronary CTA leads to frequent false-positive findings in small stents (≤2.75 mm), it reliably rules out in-stent restenosis irrespective of stent size (Pugliese et al. 2007). First clinical evaluations have meanwhile demonstrated promising results in the triage of patients with acute chest pain by means of DSCT (Johnson et al. 2007c; Schertler et al. 2007).

DSCT can provide high power reserves of up to 160 kW for general radiology examinations by using both X-ray tubes simultaneously, which is beneficial for long scan ranges and obese patients. Dual-energy acquisitions with both X-ray tubes operated at different kV settings have the potential to open a new era of clinical applications. The evaluation of dual-energy CT data can add functional information to the mere morphological information based on different X-ray attenuation coefficients that is usually obtained in a CT examination. Dual-energy acquisition can support the differentiation of ves-

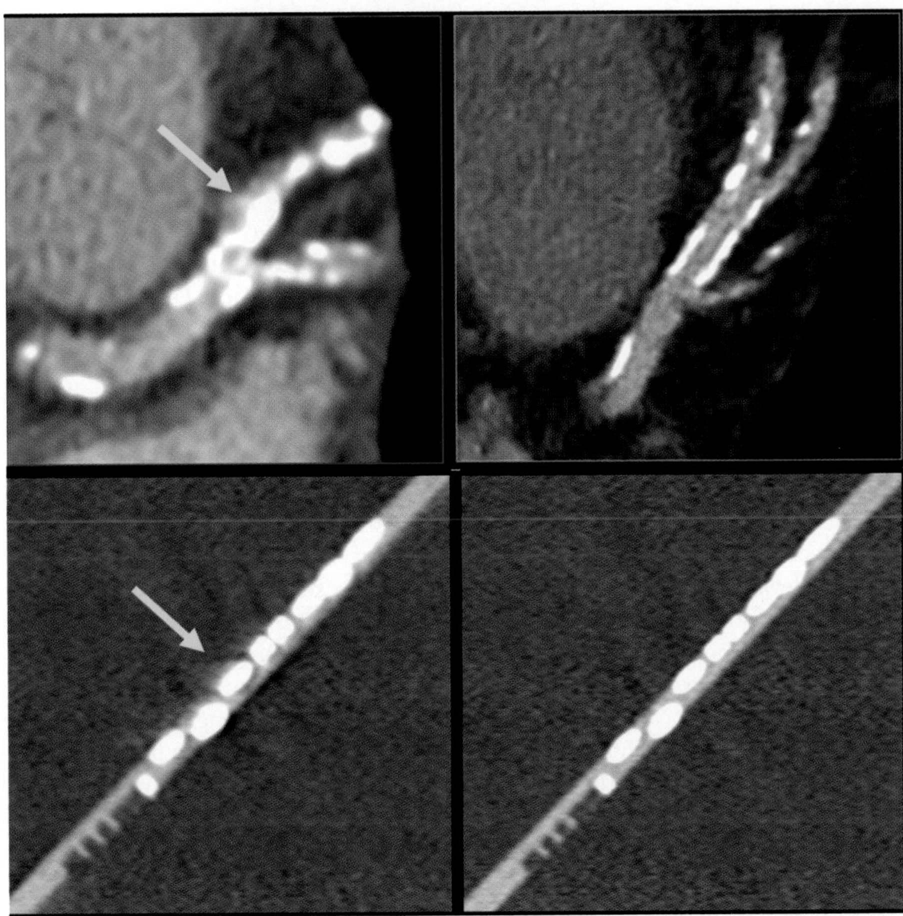

Fig. 1.13. Improved visualization of calcified plaques (reduced "blooming" artifact) at lower heart rates due to improved temporal resolution. A comparable clinical situation (calcified LAD) is shown both for a 64-slice CT system with 165 ms temporal resolution (*top left*) and a DSCT system with 83 ms temporal resolution (*top right*). The spatial resolution of both systems is similar (courtesy of Dr. S. Achenbach, Erlangen University, Germany). At least part of the blooming artifact is caused by residual coronary motion (*arrow*). This clinical result is supported by a computer simulation study of a moving coronary artery at identical spatial resolution, but different temporal resolution (165 ms, *bottom left*, versus 83 ms, *bottom right*)

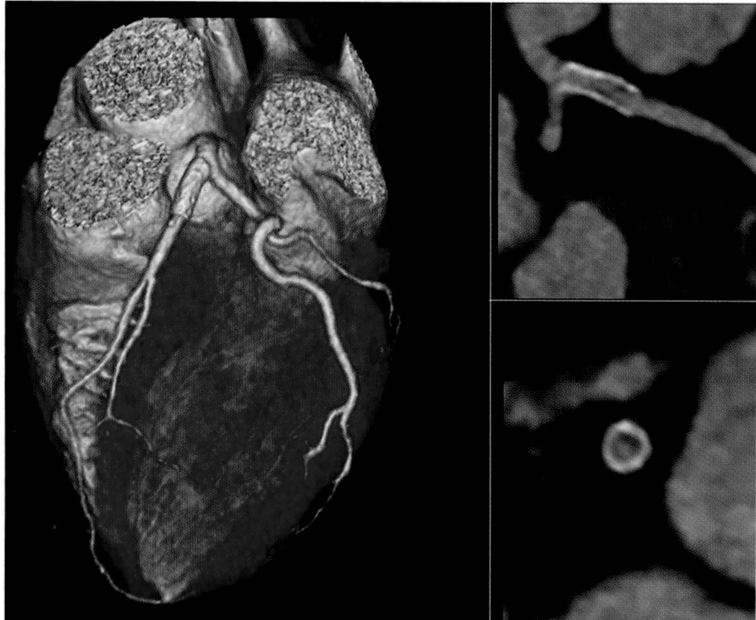

Fig. 1.14. Case study illustrating the visualization of a coronary in-stent restenosis with a DSCT system at 83 ms temporal resolution. The heart rate of the patient during examination was 70 bpm. A scan range of 148 mm was covered in 7 s (courtesy of Dr. van Wageningen, Cape Town, South Africa)

sels and bone for an automatic bone removal in CT angiographic studies, in particular in complex anatomical situations. Dual energy helps to characterize certain tissues in the human body, such as kidney stones or tendons and ligaments (Primak et al. 2007; Scheffel et al. 2007; Graser et al. 2008). With dual-energy CT techniques, uric acid, cystine, struvite and mixed renal calculi can be differentiated from other types of stones in vitro and in vivo, with accuracy ≥93% and sensitivity ≥88% depending on the scan conditions (Primak et al. 2007). This is of clinical relevance as uric acid stones may be treated pharmacologically rather than with surgical extraction or extracorporal shockwave lithotripsy. Most important, dual-energy CT is capable of visualizing and quantifying the local iodine update in tissues as a measure for the local blood supply. Potential cardiothoracic applications of this technique comprise visualization of the iodine uptake in the lung parenchyma to evaluate perfusion defects in the lung, e.g., as a consequence of pulmonary embolism (see Fig. 1.15), tumor characterization and monitoring of anti-angiogenesis tumor therapy, or quantification of myocardial enhancement to determine the myocardial blood volume (Ruzsics et al. 2008), which so far has been reserved for other modalities (see Fig. 1.16). Clinical research will be needed to fully evaluate the potential of dual-energy CT for relevant cardiothoracic applications.

1.5 Radiation Dose and Radiation Dose Reduction

In CT the average dose in the scan plane is best described by the weighted computerized tomographic dose index $CTDI_w$ (Morin et al. 2003; McCollough 2003), which is determined from measurements both in the center and at the periphery of a 16-cm lucite phantom for the head and a 32-cm lucite phantom for the body. Scan protocols for different CT scanners should always be compared on the basis of $CTDI_w$ and never on the basis of mAs, since different system geometries can lead to significant differences in the radiation dose that is applied at identical mAs. $CTDI_w$ depends on scanner geometry, slice collimation and beam pre-filtration as well as on X-ray tube voltage, tube current mA and gantry rotation time t_{rot}. To obtain a parameter characteristic for the scanner used, it is helpful to introduce a normalized $(CTDI_w)_n$ given in mGy/mAs:

$$\begin{aligned} CTDI_w &= mA \times t_{rot} \times (CTDI_w)_n \\ &= mAs \times (CTDI_w)_n \end{aligned} \qquad (2)$$

To represent the dose in a spiral/helical scan, it is essential to account for gaps or overlaps between the radiation dose profiles from consecutive rotations of the X-ray source (Morin et al. 2003). For

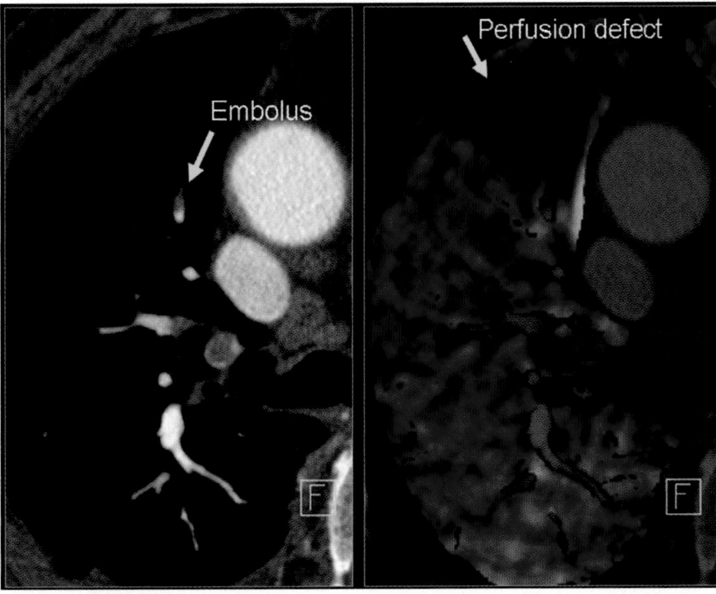

Fig. 1.15. Case study illustrating the potential of dual-energy CT to visualize the iodine uptake in the lung parenchyma as a measure for the local blood supply. Dual-energy acquisition with a DSCT results in 80 kV and 140 kV images, which are averaged for regular viewing (*left*). The *arrow* indicates a pulmonary embolus. The typical perfusion defect of the lung parenchyma resulting from the pulmonary embolus can be visualized by means of dual-energy post-processing techniques. The iodine uptake is color coded and superimposed on the regular CT image (*right*). The perfusion defect is marked by an *arrow* (courtesy of Profs. J. Remy and M. Remy-Jardin, Hopital Calmette, Lille, France)

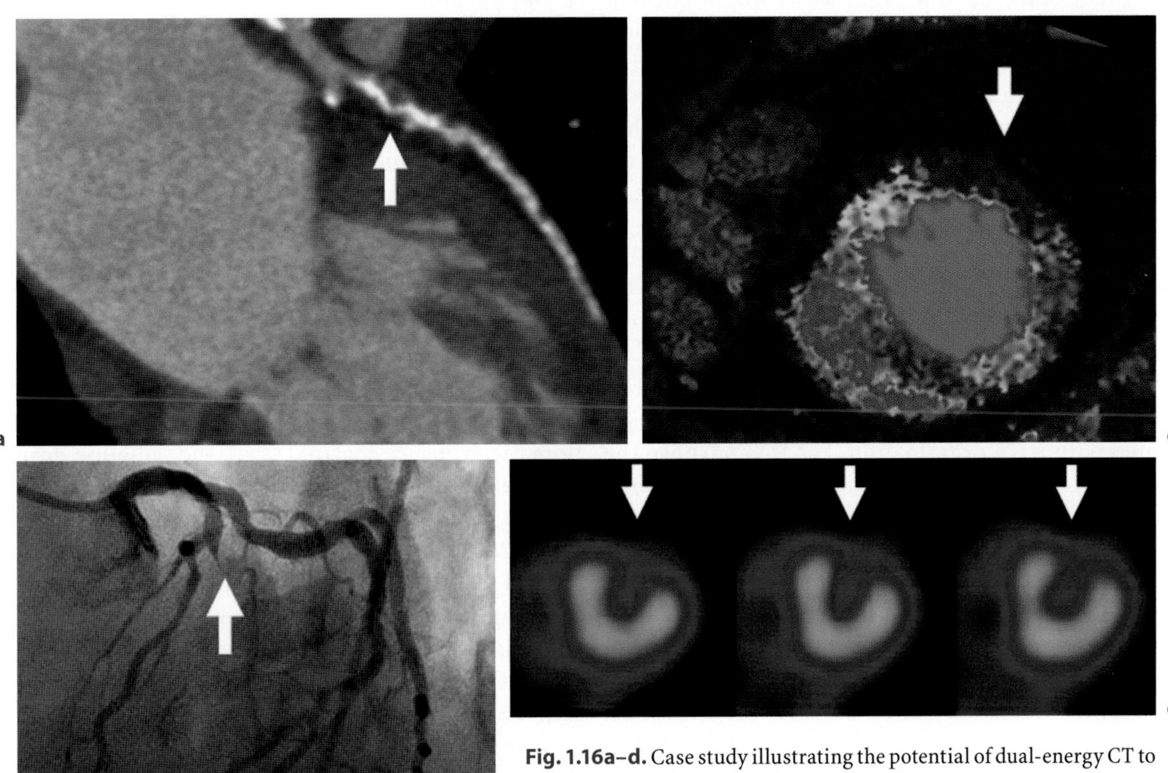

Fig. 1.16a–d. Case study illustrating the potential of dual-energy CT to visualize the iodine uptake in the myocardium in a 74-year-old woman with suspected coronary artery disease. **a** ECG-gated dual-energy spiral scan with a temporal resolution of 165 ms, depicting a subtotal stenosis (*arrow*) of the first diagonal branch, caused by extensive calcified and noncalcified plaque. **b** Correlation with coronary catheter angiography. **c** Dual-energy post-processing of the CT data reveals a myocardial blood pool deficit (*arrow*) in the first distal branch territory. The iodine uptake is color coded and superimposed on the regular CT-image. **d** Corresponding short-axis rest SPECT thallium myocardial perfusion study shows perfusion defect (*arrow*) in the same myocardial territory (courtesy of Dr. U. J. Schoepf, Medical University of South Carolina, Charleston, SC, USA)

this purpose $CTDI_{vol}$, the volume $CTDI_w$, has been introduced

$$CTDI_{vol} = 1/p \times CTDI_w \quad (3)$$

The factor $1/p$ accounts for the increasing dose accumulation with decreasing spiral pitch due to the increasing spiral overlap. Some manufacturers such as Siemens use an "effective" mAs-concept for spiral/helical MDCT scanning that includes the factor 1/p into the mAs-definition:

$$(mAs)_{eff} = mA \times t_{rot} \times 1/p = mAs \times 1/p \quad (4)$$

The dose of a spiral/helical scan is then simply given by

$$CTDI_{vol} = (mAs)_{eff} \times (CTDI_w)_n \quad (5)$$

Some other manufacturers stay with the conventional mAs definition, and the users have to perform the 1/p correction by themselves. When comparing the scan parameters for CT systems of different manufacturers, the underlying mAs definition has to be considered. The dose-length product DLP accounts for the scan range L of a CT examination. It is defined as

$$DLP = CTDI_{vol} \times L \quad (6)$$

and measured in mGy·cm.

$CTDI_{vol}$ and DLP are physical dose measures; they do not inform about the radiation risk associated with a CT examination. For this purpose the concept of "effective dose" has been introduced by the ICRP (International Commission on Radiation Protection). The effective dose is given in mSv. It is a weighted sum of the dose applied to all organs in a CT examination and includes both direct and scattered radiation. The weighting factors depend on the biological radiation sensitivities of the respective organs. Effective dose can be measured using whole body phantoms, such as the Alderson phantom, or derived from computer simulations using Monte Carlo techniques to determine scattered radiation. The effective patient dose for cardiothoracic examinations can be estimated by multiplying the DLP (in mGy·cm) with the conversion factor 0.0177 mSv/(mGy·cm). This conversion is only valid for standard-size patients. It will underestimate radiation dose for small and pediatric patients.

The most important factor for exposure reduction is an adaptation of the dose to patient size and weight (Donelly et al. 2001; Wildberger et al. 2001; Das et al. 2005), which can be achieved by reducing the mAs and selecting lower X-ray tube voltages (kV-settings).

Another means to reduce radiation dose is adaptation of the X-ray tube voltage to the intended application. In contrast-enhanced studies, such as CT angiography, the contrast-to-noise ratio for fixed patient dose increases with decreasing X-ray tube voltage, and the radiation dose to the patient can be reduced correspondingly to maintain the desired contrast-to-noise ratio. The potential for dose reduction is more significant for smaller patients. Depending on the patient size, use of 80 kV or 100 kV appears as the method of choice for CT angiography of the chest. Hohl et al. (2006) report potential dose savings of 30% when performing coronary CTA with a 100 kV protocol instead of the standard 120 kV protocol. Wintersperger et al. (2005) recommend 100 kV as the method of choice for aorto-iliac CTA, resulting in dose reduction by 30% without loss of diagnostic information.

Anatomical tube current modulation is a technique that automatically adapts the output of the X-ray tube (mA) to the patient geometry both during each rotation of the scanner to compensate for strongly varying X-ray attenuations in asymmetrical body regions, such as the shoulders, and in the longitudinal direction to maintain adequate dose when moving to different body regions, for instance from thorax to abdomen. By the use of this so-called automatic exposure control (AEC), the radiation dose can be reduced by 20–68% depending on the body region without degrading image quality (Mulkens et al. 2005; Greess et al. 2004). Automatic adaptation of the tube current to patient size prevents both over- and under-irradiation, considerably simplifies the clinical workflow for the technician and eliminates the need for look-up tables of patient weight and size for adjusting the mAs settings.

The radiation dose in ECG-gated spiral/helical examinations can be reduced by means of ECG-synchronized tube current modulation ("ECG pulsing"). During the spiral scan, the output of the X-ray tube is modulated according to the patient's ECG. The X-ray tube current is kept at its nominal value only during a user-defined phase of the cardiac cycle, in general the mid- to end-diastolic phase. During the rest of the cardiac cycle, the tube output is reduced. Clinical studies with four-slice CT systems and ECG-controlled reduction of the tube current to 20% of its nominal value demonstrated dose reduction by 30–50% depending on the patient's heart rate (Jakobs et al. 2002). Further reduction of the tube current outside the desired cardiac phases to 4% of its nominal value can reduce the radiation dose by an additional 10–15% in a standard patient population, if cardiac function need not be evaluated (Stolzmann et al. 2008). Similar to ECG-triggered axial scanning, ECG-controlled dose modulation relies on a prediction of the patient's next RR-interval length by analyzing the preceding RR intervals. So far, ECG-controlled dose modulation has provided inadequate results in patients with arrhythmia, which is a severe drawback for routine clinical use. Recently, a more versatile ECG-pulsing algorithm was introduced (Raupach et al. 2006), which estimates duration and position of the pulsing window by analyzing median, minimum and maximum RR-interval lengths, and by performing a trend analysis. This algorithm reacts flexibly to arrhythmia and ectopic beats and has the potential to considerably expand the clinical application spectrum of ECG-controlled dose modulation.

Consequent application of ECG-pulsing is mandatory for ECG-gated spiral/helical scanning of the thorax. By combining ECG-pulsing with narrow illumination window, automatic anatomical exposure control and special protocols that utilize pitch 0.3 instead of 0.2, an average effective patient dose of 4.95 mSv (d'Agostino et al. 2006; Delhaye et al. 2007) could be achieved in ECG-gated examinations of the chest with 64-slice MDCT. This value is lower than typical dose values for dedicated ECG-gated coronary CTA with 64-slice systems, since lower mAs was chosen.

DSCT systems make use of several mechanisms to reduce the radiation dose to the patient in ECG-synchronized examinations: as a consequence of the single-segment reconstruction the pitch in ECG-gated spiral/helical examinations can be significantly increased at elevated heart rates, thereby reducing the radiation dose to the patient. The pitch ranges from 0.2 at low heart rates to 0.43 at high heart rates. Integration of ECG-controlled tube current modulation with minimized length of the high-dose intervals into all ECG-gated cardiothoracic protocols can further reduce the radiation exposure. Leschka et al. (2007) recommend pulsing windows of 60–70% for heart rates <60 bpm, 60–80% for 60–70 bpm, 55–80% for 70–80 bpm and 30–80% for heart rates >80 bpm. ECG-gated spiral/helical cardiac examinations with DSCT systems result in radiation dose values that are for low heart rates similar to and for higher heart rates less than those obtained with comparable MDCT systems (McCollough et al. 2007). Stolzmann et al. (2008) reported an average effective patient dose of 7.8 mSv for ECG-gated spiral/helical coronary CTA with DSCT by utilizing the proposed techniques for dose reduction.

If the patient's heart rate is low and sufficiently stable, ECG-gated spiral/helical scans may be replaced by ECG-triggered sequential scans that lead to a further level of dose reduction. Depending on the patient size, the effective patient dose can be as low as 1.5–3 mSv for ECG-triggered coronary CTA. Scheffel et al. (2008) performed ECG-triggered coronary CTA with DSCT in 120 patients at an average radiation dose of 2.5±0.8mSv.

Further reduction of the radiation exposure will continue to be a key requirement for the design of new CT scanners. New technical developments such as, e.g., dynamic collimators, organ-specific dose modulation or fully automated kV adaptation, are on the horizon and will further minimize the radiation burden to the patient.

References

Achenbach S, Ulzheimer S, Baum U et al. (2000) Noninvasive coronary angiography by retrospectively ECG-gated multi-slice spiral CT. Circulation 102:2823–2828

d'Agostino AG, Remy-Jardin M, Khalil C, Delannoy-Deken V, Flohr T, Duhamel A, Remy J (2006) Low-dose ECG-gated 64-slices helical CT angiography of the chest: evaluation of image quality in 105 patients. Eur Radiol 16:2137–2146

Becker C, Knez A, Ohnesorge B, Schöpf U, Reiser M (2000) Imaging of non calcified coronary plaques using helical CT with retrospective EKG gating. AJR 175:423–424

Bruzzi JF, Rémy-Jardin M, Delhaye D, Teisseire A, Khalil C, Rémy J (2006a) When, why, and how to examine the heart during thoracic CT: Part 1, basic principles. AJR Am J Roentgenol 186:324–332

Bruzzi JF, Rémy-Jardin M, Delhaye D, Teisseire A, Khalil C, Rémy J (2006b) When, why, and how to examine the heart during thoracic CT: Part 2, clinical applications. AJR Am J Roentgenol 186:333–341

Coche E, Vlassenbroeck A, Roelants V, D'Hoore W, Verschuren F, Goncette L, Maldague B (2005) Evaluation of biventricular ejection fraction with ECG-gated 16-slice CT: preliminary findings in acute pulmonary embolism in comparison with radionuclide ventriculography. Eur Radiol 15:1432–1440

Das M, Mahnken AH, Mühlenbruch G, Stargardt A, Weiss C, Sennst DA, Flohr TG, Günther RW, Wildberger JE (2005) Individually adapted examination protocols for reduction of radiation exposure for 16-MDCT chest examinations. AJR Am J Roentgenol 184:1437–1443

Delhaye D, Remy-Jardin M, Teisseire A, Hossein-Foucher C, Leroy S, Duhamel A, Remy J (2006) MDCT of right ventricular function: comparison of right ventricular ejection fraction estimation and equilibrium radionuclide ventriculography, part 1. AJR Am J Roentgenol 187:1597–1604

Delhaye D, Remy-Jardin M, Salem R, Teisseire A, Khalil C, Delannoy-Deken V, Duhamel A, Remy J (2007a) Coronary imaging quality in routine ECG-gated multidetector CT examinations of the entire thorax: preliminary experience with a 64-slice CT system in 133 patients. Eur Radiol 17:902–910

Delhaye D, Remy-Jardin M, Rozel C, Dusson C, Wurtz A, Delannoy-Deken V, Duhamel A, Remy J (2007b) Coronary artery imaging during preoperative CT staging: preliminary experience with 64-slice multidetecor CT in 99 patients. Eur Radiol 17:591–602

Donelly LF, Emery KH, Brody AS et al. (2001) Minimizing radiation dose for pediatric body applications of single-detector helical CT: strategies at a large children's hospital. AJR 176:303–306

Flohr T, Ohnesorge B (2001) Heart rate adaptive optimization of spatial and temporal resolution for ECG-gated multi-slice spiral CT of the heart. JCAT 25:907–923

Flohr T, Stierstorfer K, Bruder H, Simon J, Schaller S (2002a) New technical developments in multislice CT, part 1: Approaching isotropic resolution with sub-mm 16-slice scanning. Röfo Fortschr Geb Rontgenstr Neuen Bildgeb Verfahr 174:839–845

Flohr T, Bruder H, Stierstorfer K, Simon J, Schaller S, Ohnesorge B (2002b) New technical developments in multislice CT, part 2: Sub-millimeter 16-slice scanning and increased gantry rotation speed for cardiac imaging. Röfo Fortschr Geb Rontgenstr Neuen Bildgeb Verfahr 174:1022–1027

Flohr T, Stierstorfer K, Bruder H, Simon J, Polacin A, Schaller S (2003) Image reconstruction and image quality evaluation for a 16-slice CT scanner. Med. Phys 30:832–845

Flohr T, Stierstorfer K, Raupach R, Ulzheimer S, Bruder H (2004) Performance evaluation of a 64-slice CT-system with z-flying focal spot. Röfo Fortschr Geb Rontgenstr Neuen Bildgeb Verfahr 176:1803–1810

Flohr TG, Stierstorfer K, Ulzheimer S, Bruder H, Primak AN, McCollough CH (2005) Image reconstruction and image quality evaluation for a 64-slice CT scanner with z-flying focal spot. Med Phys 32:2536–2547

Flohr TG, McCollough CH, Bruder H, Petersilka M, Gruber K, Süß C, Grasruck M, Stierstorfer K, Krauss B, Raupach R, Primak AN, Küttner A, Achenbach S, Becker C, Kopp A, Ohnesorge BM (2006) First performance evaluation of a dual-source CT (DSCT) system. Eur Radiol 16:256–268

Funabashi N, Yoshida K, Tadokoro H, Nakagawa K, Komiyama N, Odaka K, Tsunoo T, Mori S, Tanada S, Endo M, Komuro I (2005) Cardiovascular circulation and hepatic perfusion of pigs in 4-dimensional films evaluated by 256-slice cone-beam computed tomography. Circ J 69:585–589

Funabashi N, Mizuno N, Yoshida K, Tsunoo T, Mori S, Tanada S, Endo M, Komuro I (2007) Superiority of synchrony of 256-slice cone beam computed tomography for acquiring pulsating objects. Comparison with conventional multislice computed tomography. Int J Cardiol 12 118:400–405

Gallagher MJ, Raff GL (2008) Use of multislice CT for the evaluation of emergency room patients with chest pain: the so-called "triple rule-out." Catheter Cardiovasc Interv 71:92–99

Ghersin E, Litmanovich D, Dragu R, Rispler S, Lessick J, Amos O, Brook OR, Grubergc L, Beyar R, Engel A (2006) Sixteen-MDCT coronary angiography versus invasive coronary angiography in acute chest pain syndrome: A blinded prospective study. Am J Roentgenol 186:177–184

Graser A, Johnson TR, Bader M, Staehler M, Haseke N, Nikolaou K, Reiser MF, Stief CG, Becker CR (2008) Dual-energy CT characterization of urinary calculi: initial in vitro and clinical experience. Invest Radiol 43:112–119

Grass M, Köhler T, Proksa R (2000) Three-dimensional cone-beam CT reconstruction for circular trajectories. Phys Med Biol 45:329–347

Greess H, Wolf H, Suess C, Kalender WA, Bautz W, Baum U (2004) Automatic exposure control to reduce the dose in subsecond multislice spiral CT: phantom measurements and clinical results. Röfo Fortschr Geb Rontgenstr Neuen Bildgeb Verfahr 176:862–869

Hsieh J (2003) Analytical models for multi-slice helical CT performance parameters. Med Phys 30:169–178

Hein I, Taguchi K, Silver MD, Kazarna M, Mori I (2003) Feldkamp-based cone-beam reconstruction for gantry-tilted helical multislice CT. Med Phys 30:3233–3242

Hohl C, Mühlenbruch G, Wildberger JE, Leidecker C, Süss C, Schmidt T, Günther RW, Mahnken AH (2006) Estimation of radiation exposure in low-dose multislice computed tomography of the heart and comparison with a calculation program. Eur Radiol 16:1841–1846

Hu H (1999) Multi-slice helical CT: Scan and reconstruction. Med Phys 26:5–18

Hu H, He HD, Foley WD, Fox SH (2000) Four multidetector-row helical CT: Image quality and volume coverage speed. Radiology 215:55–62

Jakobs TF, Becker CR, Ohnesorge B, Flohr T, Suess C, Schoepf UJ, Reiser MF (2002) Multislice helical CT of the heart with retrospective ECG gating: reduction of radiation exposure by ECG-controlled tube current modulation. Eur Radiol 12:1081–1086

Johnson TR, Nikolaou K, Wintersperger BJ, Knez A, Boekstegers P, Reiser MF, Becker CR (2007a) ECG-gated 64-MDCT angiography in the differential diagnosis of acute chest pain. Am J Roentgenol 188:76–82

Johnson TR, Nikolaou K, Busch S, Leber AW, Becker A, Wintersperger BJ, Rist C, Knez A, Reiser MF, Becker CR (2007b) Diagnostic accuracy of dual-source computed tomography in the diagnosis of coronary artery disease. Invest Radiol 42:684–691

Johnson TR, Nikolaou K, Becker A, Leber AW, Rist C, Wintersperger BJ, Reiser MF, Becker CR (2007c) Dual-source CT for chest pain assessment. Eur Radiol Nov 22 (Epub ahead of print)

Johnson TRC, Krauß B, Sedlmair M, Grasruck M, Bruder H, Morhard D, Fink C, Weckbach S, Lenhard M, Schmidt B, Flohr T, Reiser MF, Becker C R (2007d) Material differentiation by dual energy CT: initial experience. Eur Radiol 17:1510–1517

Kachelriess M, Ulzheimer S, Kalender W (2000) ECG-correlated image reconstruction from subsecond multi-slice spiral CT scans of the heart. Med Phys 27:1881–1902

Kido T, Kurata A, Higashino H, Sugawara Y, Okayama H, Higaki J, Anno H, Katada K, Mori S, Tanada S, Endo M, Mochizuki T (2007) Cardiac imaging using 256-detector row four-dimensional CT: preliminary clinical report. Radiat Med 25:38–44

Klingenbeck-Regn K, Schaller S, Flohr T, Ohnesorge B, Kopp AF, Baum U (1999) Subsecond multi-slice computed tomography: basics and applications. EJR 31:110–124

Knez A, Becker CR, Leber A, Ohnesorge B, Becker A, White C, Haberl R, Reiser MF, Steinbeck G (2001) Usefulness of multislice spiral computed tomography angiography for determination of coronary artery stenoses. AJC 88:1191–1194

Kondo C, Mori S, Endo M, Kusakabe K, Suzuki N, Hattori A, Kusakabe M (2005) Real-time volumetric imaging of human heart without electrocardiographic gating by 256-detector row computed tomography: initial experience. J Comput Assist Tomogr 29:694–698

Leber AW, Knez A, von Ziegler F, Becker A, Nikolaou K, Paul S, Wintersperger B, Reiser M, Becker CR, Steinbeck G, Boekstegers P (2005) Quantification of obstructive and nonobstructive coronary lesions by 64-slice computed tomography. JACC 46:147–154

Leber AW, Johnson T, Becker A, von Ziegler F, Tittus J, Nikolaou K, Reiser M, Steinbeck G, Becker CR, Knez A (2007) Diagnostic accuracy of dual-source multi-slice CT-coronary angiography in patients with an intermediate pretest likelihood for coronary artery disease. Eur Heart J 28:2354–2360

Leschka S, Scheffel H, Desbiolles L, Plass A, Gaemperli O, Valenta I, Husmann L, Flohr TG, Genoni M, Marincek B, Kaufmann PA, Alkadhi H (2007) Image quality and reconstruction intervals of dual-source CT coronary angiography: recommendations for ECG-pulsing windowing. Invest Radiol 42:543–549

Matt D, Scheffel H, Leschka S, Flohr TG, Marincek B, Kaufmann PA, Alkadhi H (2007) Dual-source CT coronary angiography: image quality, mean heart rate, and heart rate variability. AJR Am J Roentgenol 189:567–573

McCollough C (2003) Patient dose in cardiac computed tomography. Herz 28:1–6

McCollough CH, Zink FE (1999) Performance evaluation of a multi-slice CT system. Med Phys 26:2223–2230

Mollet NR, Cademartiri F, van Mieghem CAG, Runza G, McFadden EP, Baks T, Serruys PW, Krestin GP, de Feyter PJ (2005) High-resolution spiral computed tomography coronary angiography in patients referred for diagnostc conventional coronary angiography. Circulation 112:2318–2323

Mori S, Endo M, Tsunoo T et al. (2004) Physical performance evaluation of a 256-slice CT scanner for four-dimensional imaging. Med Phys 31:1348–1356

Mori S, Endo M, Obata T, Tsunoo T, Susumu K, Tanada S (2006a) Properties of the prototype 256-row (cone beam) CT scanner. Eur Radiol 16:2100–2108

Mori S, Kondo C, Suzuki N, Hattori A, Kusakabe M, Endo M (2006b) Volumetric coronary angiography using the 256-detector row computed tomography scanner: comparison in vivo and in vitro with porcine models. Acta Radiol 47:186–191

Mori S, Endo M, Nishizawa K, Murase K, Fujiwara H, Tanada S (2006c) Comparison of patient doses in 256-slice CT and 16-slice CT scanners. Br J Radiol 79:56–61

Mori S, Obata T, Kato H, Kishimoto R, Kandatsu S, Tanada S, Endo M (2007) Preliminary study: color map of hepatocellular carcinoma using dynamic contrast-enhanced 256-detector row CT. Eur J Radiol 62:308–310

Morin R, Gerber T, McCollough C (2003) Radiation dose in computed tomography of the heart. Circulation 107:917–922

Mulkens TH, Bellinck P, Baeyaert M, Ghysen D, Van Dijck X, Mussen E, Venstermans C, Termote JL (2005) Use of an automatic exposure control mechanism for dose optimization in multi-detector row CT examinations: Clinical evaluation. Radiology 237:213–223

Nieman K, Oudkerk M, Rensing BJ, van Ooijen P, Munne A, van Geuns RJ, de Feyter PJ (2001) Coronary angiography with multi-slice computed tomography. Lancet 357:599–603

Nieman K, Cademartiri F, Lemos PA, Raaijmakers R, Pattynama PMT, de Feyter PJ (2002) Reliable noninvasive coronary angiography with fast submillimeter multislice spiral computed tomography. Circulation 106:2051–2054

Ohnesorge B, Flohr T, Becker C, Kopp A, Schoepf U, Baum U, Knez A, Klingenbeck Regn K, Reiser M (2000) Cardiac imaging by means of electro- cardiographically gated multisection spiral CT–Initial experience. Radiology 217:564–571

Ohnesorge BM, Hofmann LK, Flohr TG, Schöpf UJ (2005) CT for imaging coronary artery disease: defining the paradigm for its application. Int J Cardiovasc Imaging 21:85–104

Primak AN, Fletcher JG, Vrtiska TJ, Dzyubak OP, Lieske JC, Jackson ME, Williams JC Jr, McCollough CH (2007) Noninvasive differentiation of uric acid versus non-uric acid kidney stones using dual-energy CT. Acad Radiol 14:1441–1447

Pugliese F, Weustink AC, Van Mieghem C, Alberghina F, Otsuka M, Meijboom WB, Van Pelt N, Mollet NR, Cademartiri F, Krestin GP, Hunink MG, de Feyter PJ (2008) Dual-source coronary computed tomography angiography for detecting in-stent restenosis. Heart 94:848–854

Raff GL, Gallagher M J, O'Neill WW, Goldstein JA (2005) Diagnostic accuracy of noninvasive coronary angiography using 64-slice spiral computed tomography. JACC 46:552–557

Remy-Jardin M, Remy J (1999) Spiral CT angiography of the pulmonary circulation. Radiology 212:615–636

Remy-Jardin M, Remy J, Deschildre F et al. (1996) Diagnosis of pulmonary embolism with spiral CT: comparison with pulmonary angiography and scintigraphy. Radiology 200:699–706

Remy-Jardin J, Tillie-Leblond I, Szapiro D et al. (2002) CT angiography of pulmonary embolism in patents with underlying respiratory disease: impact of multislice CT on image quality and negative predictive value. Eur Radiol 12:1971–1978

Ritman E, Kinsey J, Robb R, Gilbert B, Harris L, Wood E (1980) Three-dimensional imaging of heart, lungs, and circulation. Science 210:273–280

Robb R, Ritman E (1979) High speed synchronous volume computed tomography of the heart. Radiology 133:655–661

Ropers D, Baum U, Pohle K, Anders K, Ulzheimer S, Ohnesorge B, Schlundt C, Bautz W, Daniel WG, Achenbach S (2003) Detection of coronary artery stenoses with thin-slice multi-detector row spiral computed tomography and multiplanar reconstruction. Circulation 107:664–666

Ropers U, Ropers D, Pflederer T, Anders K, Kuettner A, Stilianakis NI, Komatsu S, Kalender W, Bautz W, Daniel WG, Achenbach S (2007) Influence of heart rate on the diagnostic accuracy of dual-source computed tomography coronary angiography. J Am Coll Cardiol 50:2393–2398

Ruzsics B, Lee H, Powers ER, Flohr TG, Costello P, Schoepf UJ (2008) Myocardial ischemia diagnosed by dual-energy computed tomography. Circulation 3

Salem R, Remy-Jardin M, Delhaye D, Khalil C, Teisseire A, Delannoy-Deken V, Duhamel A, Remy J (2006) Integrated cardio-thoracic imaging with ECG-gated 64-slice multidetector-row CT: initial findings in 133 patients. Eur Radiol 16:1973–1981

Schaller S, Flohr T, Klingenbeck K, Krause J, Fuchs T, Kalender WA (2000) Spiral interpolation algorithm for multi-slice spiral CT–part I: Theory. IEEE Trans Med Imag 19:822–834

Schaller S, Stierstorfer K, Bruder H, Kachelrieß M, Flohr T (2001) Novel approximate approach for high-quality image reconstruction in helical cone beam CT at arbitrary pitch. Proc SPIE Int Symp Med Imag 4322:113–127

Scheffel H, Stolzmann P, Frauenfelder T, Schertler T, Desbiolles L, Leschka S, Marincek B, Alkadhi H (2007) Dual-energy contrast-enhanced computed tomography for the detection of urinary stone disease. Invest Radiol 42:823–829

Scheffel H, Alkadhi H, Leschka S et al. (2008) Low-dose CT coronary angiography in the step-and-shoot mode: diagnostic performance. Heart June 2 [epub ahead of print]

Schertler T, Scheffel H, Frauenfelder T, Desbiolles L, Leschka S, Stolzmann P, Seifert B, Flohr TG, Marincek B, Alkadhi H (2007) Dual-source computed tomography in patients with acute chest pain: feasibility and image quality. Eur Radiol 17:3179–3188

Schoepf UJ (2007) Cardiothoracic multi-slice CT in the emergency department. In: Ohnesorge BM, Flohr TG, Becker CR, Knez A, Reiser MF (eds) Multi-slice and dual-source CT in cardiac imaging, 2nd edn. Springer Berlin, Heidelberg, New York

Schoepf UJ, Kessler MA, Rieger CT et al. (2001) Multislice CT imaging of pulmonary embolism. Eur Radiol 11:2278–2286

Schoepf UJ, Holzknecht N, Helmberger TK et al. (2002) Subsegmental pulmonary emboli: improved detection with thin-collimation multidetector row spiral CT. Radiology 222:483–490

Schoepf UJ, Becker CR, Hofmann LK, Das M, Flohr T, Ohnesorge BM et al. (2003) Multislice CT angiography. Eur Radiol 13:1946–1961

Stierstorfer K, Rauscher A, Boese J, Bruder H, Schaller S, Flohr T (2004) Weighted FBP–a simple approximate 3D FBP algorithm for multislice spiral CT with good dose usage for arbitrary pitch. Phys Med Biol 49:2209–2218

Stolzmann P, Scheffel H, Schertler T, Frauenfelder T, Leschka S, Husmann L, Flohr TG, Marincek B, Kaufmann PA, Alkadhi H (2008) Radiation dose estimates in dual-source computed tomography coronary angiography. Eur Radiol 18:592–599

Taguchi T, Aradate H (1998) Algorithm for image reconstruction in multi-slice helical CT. Med Phys 25:550–561

White CS, Kuo D, Kelemen M, Jain V, Musk A, Zaidi E, Read K, Sliker C, Prasad R (2005) Chest pain evaluation in the emergency department: Can MDCT Provide a Comprehensive Evaluation? AJR 185:533–540

Wildberger JE, Mahnken AH, Schmitz-Rode T, Flohr T, Stargardt A, Haage P, Schaller S, Guenther RW (2001) Individually adapted examination protocols for reduction of radiation exposure in chest CT. Invest Radiol 36:604–611

Wintersperger B, Jakobs T, Herzog P, Schaller S, Nikolaou K, Suess C, Weber C, Reiser M, Becker C (2005) Aorto-iliac multidetector-row CT angiography with low kV settings: improved vessel enhancement and simultaneous reduction of radiation dose. Eur Radiol 15:334–341

Cardiac Gating

2

Thomas Flohr and Bernd Ohnesorge

CONTENTS

2.1 Introduction

Cardio-thoracic imaging with CT requires short exposure time for the acquisition of the axial slices and the corresponding dedicated scan and image reconstruction techniques to virtually freeze the cardiac motion and to avoid motion artifacts in the images. Scan and image reconstruction needs to be synchronized with the heart motion, e.g., by using information from the patient's electro-cardiogram (ECG) that is recorded in parallel to the CT scan data acquisition.

The least motion of the heart and the coronary arteries during the cardiac cycle can be observed in end-systole and mid- to end-diastole. While the duration of the end-systolic phase (approximately 100–150 ms) is more or less independent of the heart rate (and the related RR-interval time), the phase with lowest cardiac motion during diastole narrows with increasing heart rate. Hence, the mid- to end-diastolic phase and at higher heart rates also the end-systolic phase are particularly well suited for CT data acquisition (Hong et al. 2001; Kopp et al. 2001). In a study using 64-slice CT, Wintersperger et al. (2007) found out that for patients with a heart rate <65 bpm, the best image quality was predominately achieved in diastole (93%), while in patients with heart rate >75 bpm, the best image quality shifted to systole in most cases (86%).

Currently, two different ECG synchronization and data acquisition techniques are employed for multi-detector row CT (MDCT) and dual-source CT (DSCT) cardiothoracic scanning: prospective ECG triggering and retrospective ECG gating. Both will be covered in the following sections.

2.2 ECG-Triggered Axial Scanning

The simplest and most straightforward approach for ECG-synchronized CT data acquisition is prospectively ECG-triggered axial scanning, which was introduced with electron beam CT (EBCT) (Boyd and Lipton 1982; Achenbach et al. 1998; Becker et al. 2000a).

The patient's ECG-signal is monitored during the cardiac CT examination, and a series of axial scans at different z-positions (different anatomical levels) is performed with a user-defined temporal offset relative to the R-waves of subsequent heart beats. This temporal offset can be either relative (given as a certain percentage of the RR-interval time T_{RR}) or absolute (given in ms) and either forward

T. Flohr, PhD
Siemens Healthcare, Computed Tomography, Siemensstrasse 1, 91301 Forchheim, Germany
B. Ohnesorge, PhD
Siemens Limited China, Healthcare, Siemens International Medical Park, 278 Zhou Zhu Road, Nanhui District, Shanghai 201318, P.R. China

or reverse (Ohnesorge et al. 1999), see Figure 2.1. Data acquisition is therefore "triggered" by the R-waves of the patient's ECG. The principle of ECG-triggered multi-slice axial scanning is illustrated in Figure 2.2. A volume image of the heart consists of several image slabs reconstructed from axial scan data acquired in multiple consecutive heart beats. The number of axial images within an image slab corresponds to the number of active detector slices; the width of an image slab is proportional to the detector z-coverage. In between the individual axial scans the table moves to the next *z*-position; the heart volume is therefore covered by means of "step-and-shoot" scanning. Due to the time necessary for table motion, typically every second heart beat can be used for data acquisition (Fig. 2.2).

Partial scan data segments are usually acquired in ECG-triggered axial scan protocols. A partial scan consists of 180° of fan-beam data plus the total fan angle of the detector (~ 50°) plus a transition angle

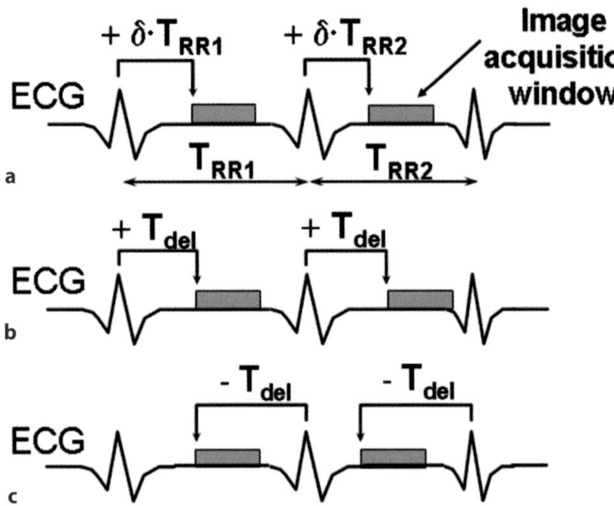

Fig. 2.1a–c. Different strategies to position the data interval for image acquisition or image reconstruction in the patient's cardiac cycle in ECG-triggered and ECG-gated CT. **a** Relative delay after an R-wave. The start of the data interval is defined at a certain fraction δ of the RR-interval time T_{RR}. **b** Absolute forward. The start of the data interval is defined at a fixed time interval T_{del} (in ms) after the previous R-wave. This approach is useful for image reconstruction in the end-systolic phase, because the T-wave occurs with an approximately constant delay after the previous R-wave. **c** Absolute reverse. The start of the data interval is defined at a fixed time interval T_{del} (in ms) prior to an R-wave. This approach allows for consistent imaging in the end-diastolic phase

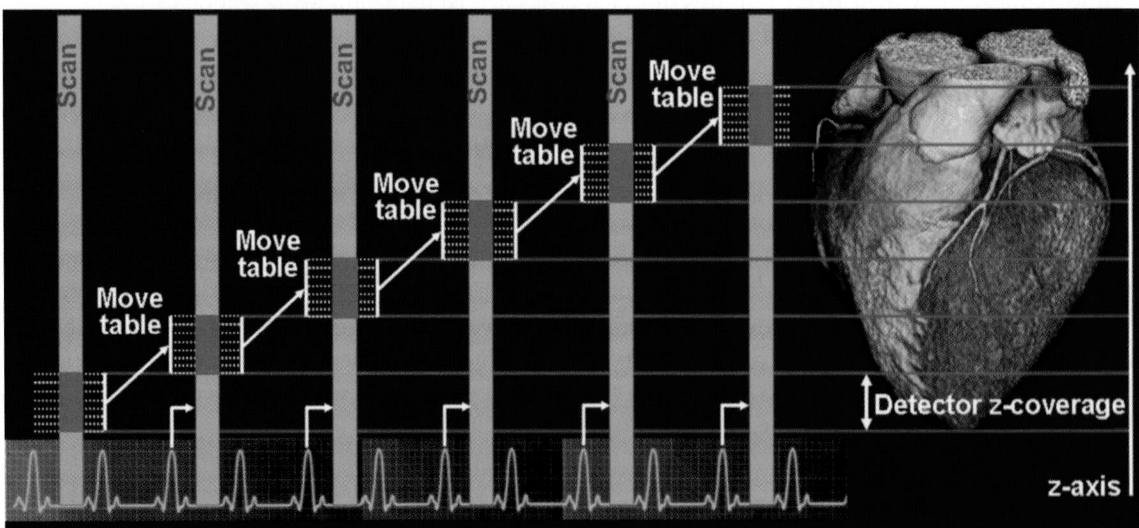

Fig. 2.2. Principle of ECG-triggered multi-slice axial scanning. The patient's ECG is schematically shown as a function of time on the horizontal axis. The *z*-positions of the detector slices relative to the patient (eight slices in this example) are indicated by the *dashed white lines*. Usually, partial scan data intervals (which are marked as *red boxes*) are acquired at a user-defined temporal offset to the R-waves. An ECG-triggered volume image of the heart consists of several image slabs acquired in multiple consecutive heart beats. The width of an image slab corresponds to the *z*-width of the detector

for smooth data weighting, in total 240–260° of fan-beam data. This is the minimum data interval that is sufficient for image reconstruction throughout the entire scan field of view (SFOV) of usually 50-cm diameter. The temporal resolution at a certain point in the SFOV is determined by the acquisition time window of the data contributing to the reconstruction of that particular image point. In a conventional approach, the entire partial scan data segment is used for image reconstruction in any point of the SFOV. Redundant data are weighted using algorithms such as the one described by PARKER (1982). The resulting temporal resolution is about 0.22–0.24 s for 0.33-s gantry rotation time. To improve temporal resolution, modified reconstruction approaches for partial scan data have been proposed (OHNESORGE et al. 2000; FLOHR and OHNESORGE 2001), which are best explained in parallel geometry. A modern CT scanner acquires data in fan-beam geometry. Each measurement ray is characterized by the projection (view) angle α and by its fan angle β within the projection. Each ray can also be denoted by coordinates θ and b in parallel geometry. θ is the azimuthal angle, and b denotes the distance of a ray from the iso-center, see Figure 2.3. A simple coordinate transformation relates the two sets of variables

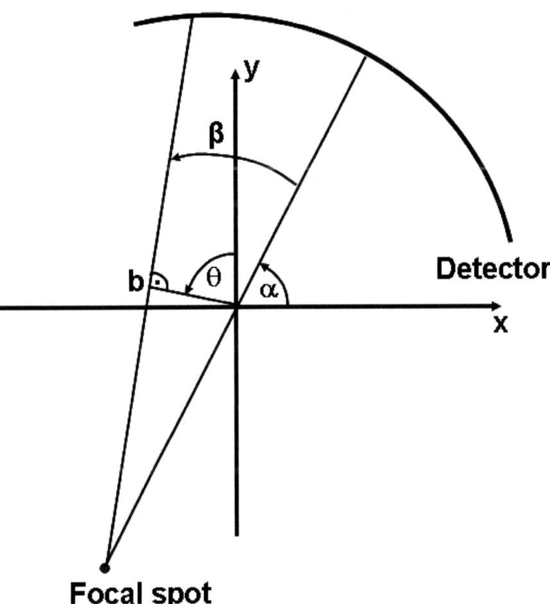

Fig. 2.3. Geometry of CT-data acquisition. A modern CT scanner acquires data in "fan beam geometry," characterized by the projection angle α and by the fan angle β within a projection. Another set of variables serving the same purpose is θ and b. b denotes the distance of a ray from the iso-center. θ and b are the coordinates of a ray in "parallel geometry"

$$\theta = \alpha + \beta,\ b = R_F \sin \beta \tag{1}$$

R_F is the distance from the focus to the iso-center. Using this equation, the measured fan-beam data can be transformed to parallel data, a procedure called "rebinning". In parallel geometry, 180° of scan data, a half-scan segment, is necessary for image reconstruction. As a consequence of data acquisition in fan-beam geometry, a partial scan interval of 180° plus the detector fan angle is necessary to provide a half-scan segment in parallel geometry. At the iso-center of the scanner, for $\beta = 0$, 180° of the acquired fan-beam data is sufficient to provide 180° of parallel data, see Equation (1). If all redundant data are neglected, the temporal resolution at the iso-center can be as good as 180°/360° times the gantry rotation time (half the gantry rotation time, e.g., 165 ms for 0.33 s gantry rotation time).

With DSCT systems, the required half-scan segment in parallel geometry can be split into two quarter-scan segments (FLOHR et al. 2006), which are simultaneously acquired by the two measurement systems in the same cardiac phase and at the same anatomical level, see Figure 2.4. Hence, the temporal resolution for ECG-triggered axial scanning with DSCT is a quarter of the gantry rotation time (83 ms for 0.33 s gantry rotation time) in a sufficiently centered region of interest.

The extracted half-scan segment in parallel geometry is used as an input to a convolution back-projection reconstruction. In the convolution step, the measurement rays undergo a filter-operation that controls image sharpness and image noise. In the back-projection step, the filtered CT data are projected into the image space to create the CT image. For CT systems with up to 16 slices, the cone angle of the measurement rays, that is the angle between a ray and a plane perpendicular to the z-axis, is usually neglected (FLOHR et al. 2003). The rays are treated as if they were perpendicular to the *z*-axis, which is of course only an approximation in particular for the outer rows of a multi-row detector, where the cone angle is largest. Two-dimensional back-projection algorithms are applied to the data to produce one axial image for each individual detector slice. Hence, the number of axial images per axial scan corresponds to the number of active detector slices. With wider detectors and increasing number of detector rows, 3D back-projection becomes mandatory. Using this approach, the measurement rays are back-projected into a 3D volume along the lines of measurement, this way accounting for their cone-

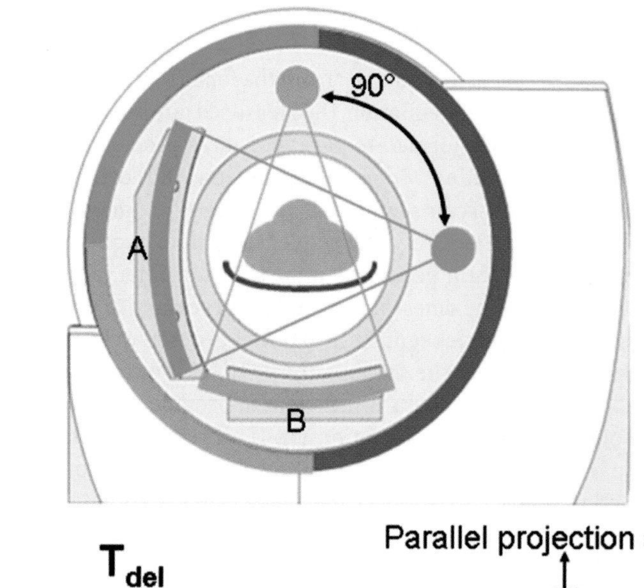

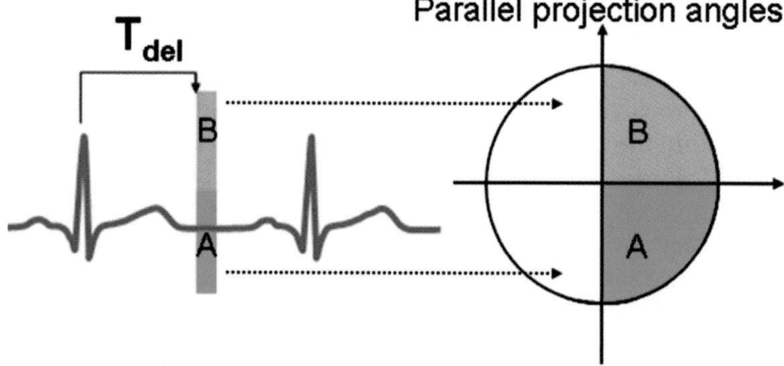

Fig. 2.4. Schematic illustration of a dual source CT (DSCT) using two tubes and two corresponding detectors offset by 90°. The 180° half-scan segment in parallel geometry necessary to reconstruct an image at a certain phase within the patient's cardiac cycle (e.g., at a time T_{del} after the R-peak) is split into two 90° data segments (indicated *green* and *orange*) that are acquired by both measurement systems simultaneously at the same anatomical level. A scanner of this type provides temporal resolution equivalent to a quarter of the gantry rotation time, independent of the patient's heart rate

beam geometry. With 3D back-projection, a 3D image volume is obtained for each axial scan, and images at arbitrary *z*-positions z_{ima} within this volume can be generated by *z*-reformation (Stierstorfer et al. 2004).

Prospective ECG-triggering combined with "step-and-shoot" acquisition of axial slices is the most dose-efficient way of ECG-synchronized CT scanning as only the very minimum of scan data needed for image reconstruction is acquired in the previously selected heart phase. As a drawback, reconstruction of images in different phases of the cardiac cycle for functional evaluation is not possible, and the method encounters its limitations for patients with severe arrhythmia, since ECG-triggered axial scanning depends on a reliable prediction of the patient's next RR interval by using the mean or median durations of the preceding RR intervals. "Mis-triggering" due to arrhythmia or ectopic beats causes image blurring, or image slabs from subsequent cardiac cycles may be shifted relative to each other, resulting in stair-step artifacts in MPRs, see Figure 2.5.

While ECG-triggered axial scanning was abandoned for coronary CT angiography with 4-slice, 8-slice and 16-slice CT systems due to long acquisition times with thin slices, the method has recently been re-introduced for 64-slice CT systems (Hsieh et al. 2006). With ECG-triggered 64-slice CT, the entire heart can be covered with sub-millimeter slices within a reasonable breath-hold time at very low radiation dose to the patient, see Figure 2.6. A recently introduced CT system equipped with a 320 × 0.5-mm detector has the potential to cover the heart with one single ECG-triggered axial scan. The diagnostic quality of this one shot examination, however, depends on the available temporal resolution and the stability of the patient's heart rate. In the worst case, the entire scan can be non-diagnostic, if it is acquired during an ectopic beat or in a period of arrhythmia.

Currently, ECG-triggered axial scanning is restricted to patients with low and regular heart rates, and evaluation of functional parameters of the heart is not possible. Developments are ongoing to

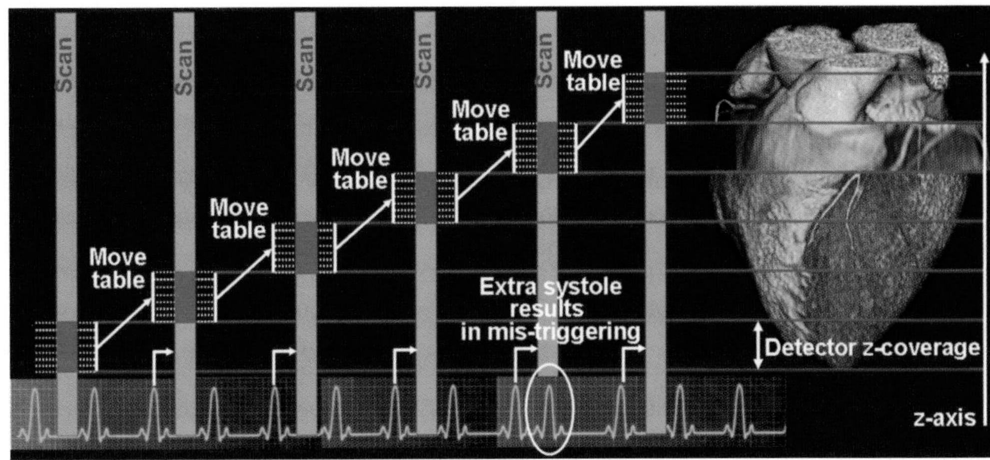

Fig. 2.5. Limits of ECG-triggered multi-slice axial scanning. In a conventional approach, the length of the patient's next RR-interval is estimated from the mean duration of the preceding RR-intervals. In case of arrhythmia and ectopic beats, mis-triggering occurs, and scan data are acquired in the wrong phase of the patient's cardiac cycle. As a consequence, the image quality of the corresponding image slab will be compromised. In currently investigated, modified approaches, the scan is automatically repeated at the same z-position if an ectopic beat or an extra-systole has occurred

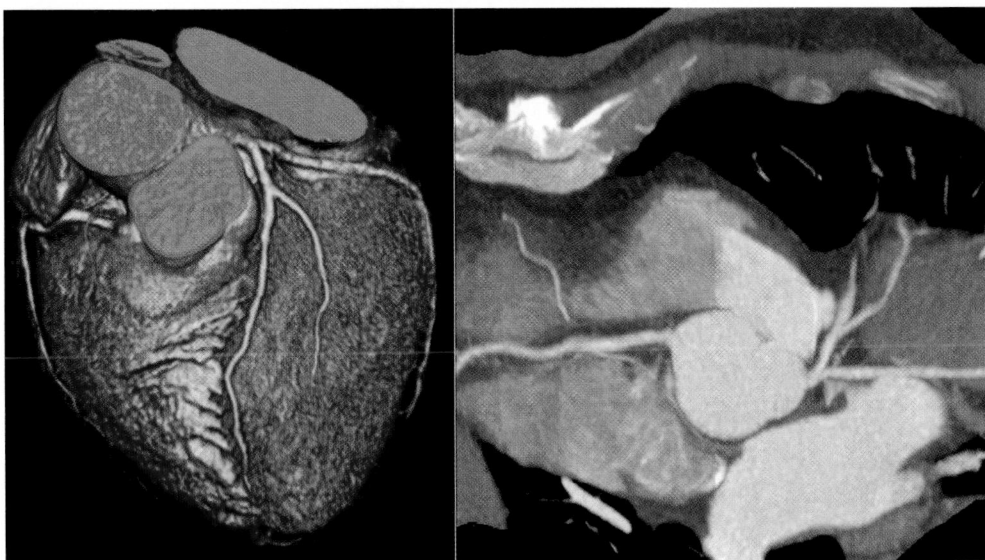

Fig. 2.6. Case study illustrating the performance of ECG-triggered sequential acquisition ("step and shoot" scanning) for coronary CTA using a DSCT system with 83-ms temporal resolution. ECG-triggered sequential acquisition is a means to reduce radiation dose to the patient, provided the heart rate is stable enough (courtesy of Dr. J. Hausleiter, German Heart Center, Munich, Germany)

enhance the application spectrum of ECG-triggered axial CT, e.g., by introducing more versatile triggering concepts. With refined approaches, the scan can be automatically repeated at the current table position to reliably avoid stair-step artifacts in case of ectopic beats, and an optional padded scan data range, i.e., the acquisition of data intervals longer than a partial scan, allows for retrospective optimization of the reconstruction phase similar to spiral examinations. In combination with the improved temporal resolution of modern MDCT and in particular DCST systems, these new techniques may lead to a revival of ECG-triggered axial scanning in clinical routine.

2.3 ECG-Gated Spiral/Helical Scanning

The heart volume is covered by a spiral/helical scan in retrospectively ECG-gated examinations, while the patient's ECG is recorded simultaneously to allow for a retrospective selection of the data segments used for image reconstruction. ECG-gated spiral scanning had already been introduced for single-slice CT (Bahner et al. 1999; Kachelriess and Kalender 1998). The results, however, were not convincing due to poor temporal resolution and insufficient volume coverage with thin slices. The introduction of four-slice CT systems in 1999, which provided faster volume coverage and improved temporal resolution, was the first step for ECG-gated spiral CT on its way to clinical routine use (Achenbach et al. 2001; Becker et al. 2000b; Knez et al. 2001; Nieman et al. 2001). The principle of retrospectively ECG-gated MDCT spiral/helical scanning is schematically shown in Figure 2.7. The table moves continuously, and continuous spiral/helical scan data of the heart volume are acquired. Only scan data measured in a pre-defined cardiac phase, usually the mid- to end-diastolic or the end-systolic phase, are used for image reconstruction (Ohnesorge et al. 2000; Flohr and Ohnesorge 2001). Images can be reconstructed in every heart beat; hence faster volume coverage than with prospectively ECG-triggered axial scanning is possible.

A variety of dedicated image reconstruction approaches for ECG-gated multi-slice spiral/helical CT have meanwhile been proposed (e.g., Kachelriess et al. 2000; Taguchi and Anno 2000; Ohnesorge 2000; Flohr and Ohnesorge 2001, Flohr et al. 2003; Bruder et al. 2001; Grass et al. 2003). Depending on the number of active detector slices, 2D or 3D filtered back-projection is used. For CT systems with up to 16 slices, adequate image quality was demonstrated with 2D back-projection neglecting the cone angle of the measurement rays (Flohr et al. 2003). In this case, the reconstruction of ECG-gated multi-slice spiral/helical data aims at the generation of individual axial images – comparable to ECG-triggered axial scanning – and requires a two-step approach: spiral/helical interpolation of the multi-slice scan data in the desired cardiac phases (the red boxes in Fig. 2.7) to compensate for the continuous table

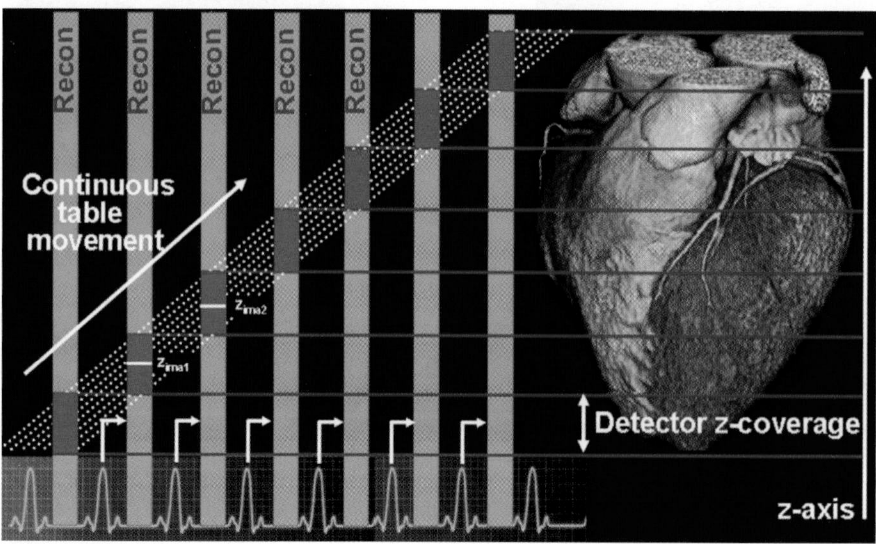

Fig. 2.7. Principle of retrospectively ECG-gated MDCT spiral/helical scanning using single-segment reconstruction. The patient's ECG is schematically shown as a function of time on the *horizontal axis*. The *z*-positions of the detector slices (eight slices in this example) relative to the patient are indicated by the *dashed white lines*. The table moves continuously, and continuous spiral/helical scan data of the heart volume are acquired. Only scan data acquired in a predefined cardiac phase, usually the diastolic phase, are used for image reconstruction (marked as *red boxes*). The *white horizontal lines* represent axial images at two *z*-positions, z_{ima1} and z_{ima2}. Since no axial scan data are available, spiral/helical interpolation to the desired *z*-positions is needed for 2D reconstruction approaches. To ensure gapless volume coverage of the heart, the spiral pitch has to be adapted to the patient's heart rate. Typically, very low pitch values (0.2–0.25) are required. With increasing heart rate, the table feed can be increased

movement and to produce axial half-scan segments at the desired image z-positions, followed by a partial scan reconstruction of the half-scan segments similar to ECG-triggered axial reconstruction. For CT systems with 64 and more slices, the cone angle of the measurement rays can no longer be neglected; 3D back-projection has to be used, which aims at the generation of a 3D image volume (Grass et al. 2003; Stierstorfer et al. 2004). Hence, no spiral interpolation to axial image planes as an intermediate step is performed. Instead, the multi-slice scan data segments in the desired cardiac phases (the red boxes in Fig. 2.7) are filtered to control image sharpness and noise, and the measurement rays are then directly back-projected into the 3D volume along the lines of measurement. Each voxel receives contributions from those rays that pass from the X-ray source through the voxel to the detector array. Axial images or images on arbitrarily tilted planes are obtained by a z-reformation of the 3D image volume.

In DSCT systems the required half-scan segments are composed of quarter-scan segments simultaneously acquired by both detectors in the desired relative phases of the patient's cardiac cycle. The quarter-scan segments undergo a filter operation, followed by 3D back-projection into the 3D image volume. By using appropriate data weighting, the quarter-scan segments complement to a half-scan segment.

For ECG-gated spiral/helical CT, both single-segment and multi-segment reconstruction have been introduced into clinical practice (Kachelriess et al. 2000; Taguchi and Anno 2000; Flohr and Ohnesorge 2001). In a single-segment approach, each image is reconstructed from a half-scan data segment that is acquired in one heart period (this situation is illustrated in Fig. 2.7). The temporal resolution is constant and equals half the gantry rotation time for MDCT-systems (165 ms for 0.33 s rotation time) or a quarter of the gantry rotation time for DSCT systems (83 ms for 0.33 s rotation time).

The temporal resolution of MDCT scanners can be improved by dividing the half-scan data segment into $N = 2–4$ sub-segments acquired in subsequent cardiac cycles, see Figure 2.8. Note that in this case each image is reconstructed from data sub-segments with temporal gaps in between. For DSCT scanners, both measurement systems can be treated independently, and each quarter-scan segment is

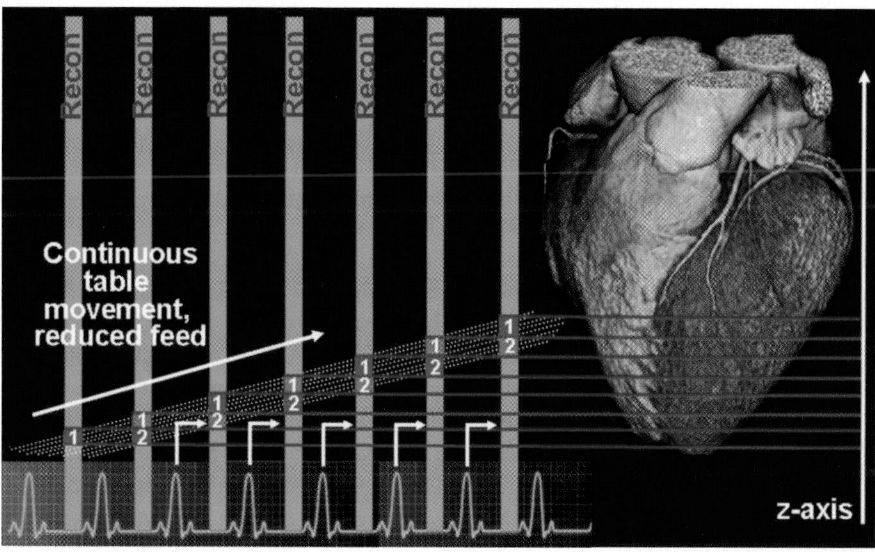

Fig. 2.8. Principle of retrospectively ECG-gated MDCT spiral/helical scanning using $N = 2$ sub-segments of multi-slice data from consecutive heart periods (marked as "1" and "2") for image reconstruction. Both sub-segments are acquired in the same relative phase of the patient's cardiac cycle, and they fit together to make up the half-scan segment required for image reconstruction. Ideally, each sub-segment is shorter than a half-scan, thereby improving temporal resolution (see the *red boxes*, which are less wide than in Fig. 2.7). Compared with single-segment reconstruction (Fig. 2.7), the pitch has to be considerably reduced to ensure gapless volume coverage: each z-position of the heart has to be seen by a detector slice during two cardiac cycles

divided into $N = 2$–4 sub-segments. When using multi-segment reconstruction, the patient's heart rate and the gantry rotation time of the scanner have to be de-synchronized to enable improved temporal resolution. Two requirements have to be met: first, the sub-segments have to fit together in projection space to build up a full half-scan interval. As a consequence, the start projections of subsequent sub-segments have to be shifted relative to each other. For two-segment reconstruction as an example, the start-projection angle of the second sub-segment must correspond to the end-projection angle of the first sub-segment or vice versa. Second, all sub-segments have to be acquired in the same relative phase of the patient's heart cycle to reduce the "exposure time" per image. If the patient's heart beat and the rotation of the scanner are completely synchronous, the two requirements are contradictory. This is best illustrated by an example. If a patient with a constant heart rate of 60 bpm is examined by using a MDCT scanner with 0.5 s gantry rotation time, the same heart phase always corresponds to the same projection angle, and a half-scan segment cannot be divided into smaller sub-segments acquired in successive heart periods. In this case, the temporal resolution cannot be improved beyond single-segment reconstruction. In the best case, when the patient's heart beat and the rotation of the MDCT scanner are optimally de-synchronized, the half-scan segment can be divided into N sub-segments of equal lengths, each of which requires an acquisition time of $1/(2N)$ times the gantry rotation time within the same relative heart phase. Generally, depending on the relation of rotation time and patient's heart rate, temporal resolution is not constant, but varies between one half and $1/(2N)$ times the gantry rotation time for MDCT. There are "sweet spots," heart rates with optimum temporal resolution, and heart rates where temporal resolution cannot be improved beyond half the gantry rotation time. Similarly, temporal resolution varies between one quarter and $1/(4N)$ times the gantry rotation time for DSCT. Figure 2.9 shows the temporal resolution of MDCT and DSCT systems at 0.33 s gantry rotation, both for single-segment reconstruction and for two-segment reconstruction.

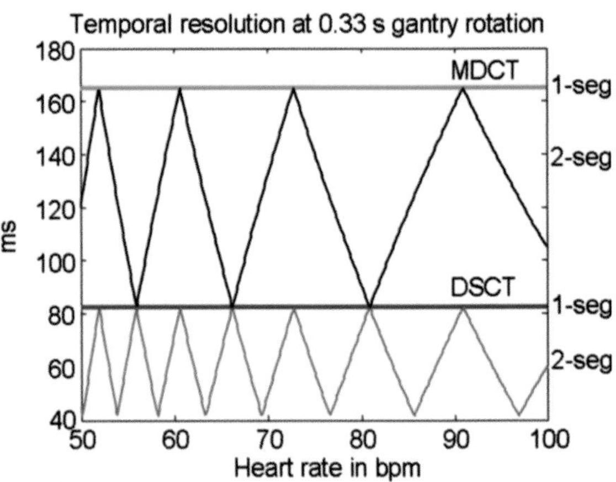

Fig. 2.9. Temporal resolution for ECG-gated spiral/helical scanning with MDCT and DSCT systems at 0.33-s gantry rotation time, both for single-segment reconstruction and for two-segment reconstruction. The DSCT system provides 83-ms temporal resolution independent of the patient's heart rate by means of single-segment reconstruction

Continuous volume coverage in retrospectively ECG-gated multi-slice spiral CT of the heart requires limitation of the spiral pitch p[1] depending on the patient's heart rate. If N-segment reconstruction is applied, every z-position of the heart needs to be scanned by a detector slice at every time during the N heart cycles. For the sake of simplicity, we assume constant RR-cycle time T_{RR}. In a time interval of N cardiac cycles $N \cdot T_{RR}$, the table can travel one full detector z-width. This leads to the following simple equation for the maximum pitch

$$p \leq \frac{T_{rot}}{N \cdot T_{RR}} \tag{2}$$

T_{rot} is the gantry rotation time of the scanner. The use of N-segment reconstruction requires significantly reduced volume coverage speed in particular at lower heart rates: the larger N and T_{RR} are, the more the spiral pitch has to be reduced, resulting in increased examination times and increased radiation dose to the patient. If the pitch is too high, certain z-positions will not be sampled by a detector slice in the desired phase of the cardiac cycle (Fig. 2.10). To obtain images at these z-positions, far-reaching interpolations are needed, which degrade image quality and reduce spatial resolution in the z-direction (Fig. 2.11).

Multi-segment reconstruction approaches rely on a complete periodicity of the heart motion, and they encounter their limitations for patients with arrhythmia (Fig. 2.12). It has been demonstrated that

[1] p is the table feed per rotation divided by the total collimated z-width of the detector

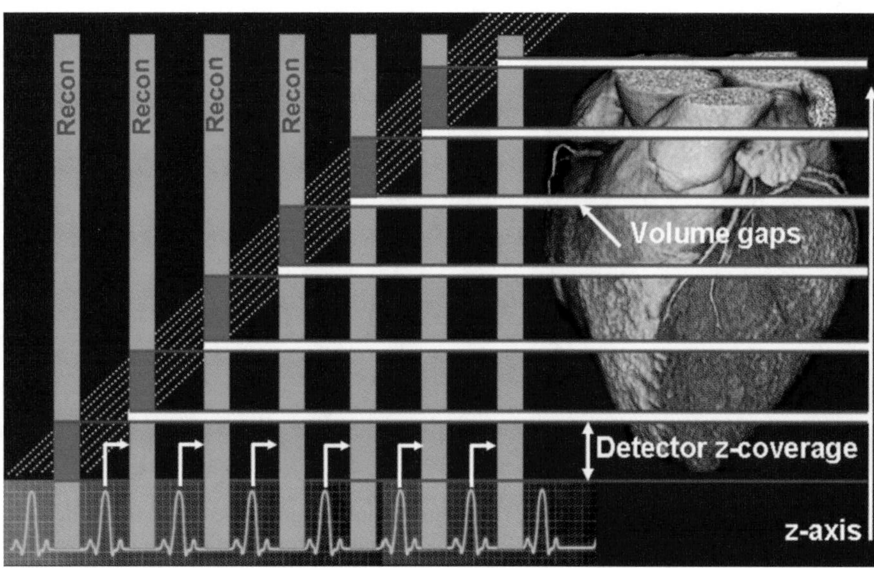

Fig. 2.10. Illustration of retrospectively ECG-gated MDCT spiral/helical scanning using single-segment reconstruction with inadequate spiral pitch (compare to Fig. 2.7). The pitch is not properly adapted to the patient's heart rate: the table moves too fast, and certain *z*-positions are not covered by a detector slice in the desired phase of the cardiac cycle. The reconstruction of images in these volume gaps requires far-reaching interpolations, which degrade longitudinal resolution

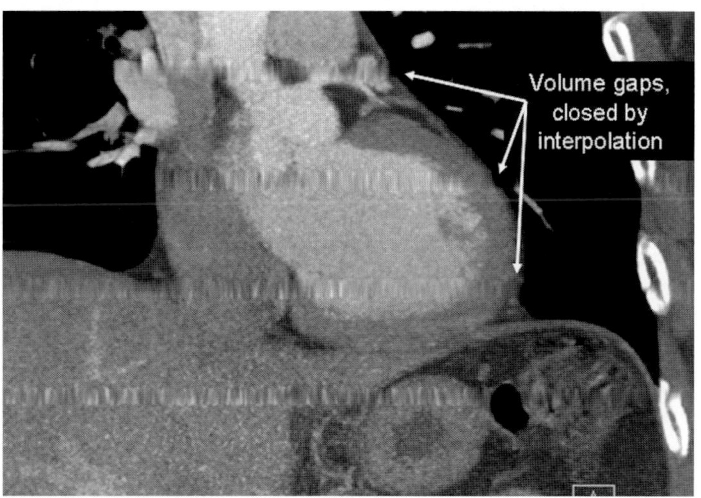

Fig. 2.11. Example of a retrospectively ECG-gated spiral/helical cardiac scan with *z*-interpolation artifacts. Volume gaps as a consequence of inadequately high pitch (see Fig. 2.10) had to be closed by far-reaching interpolations, which degrade image quality

multi-segment reconstruction for imaging of cardiac and coronary anatomy is clinically most useful when only two segments are used (Greuter et al. 2007). In some MDCT scanners, the partial scan data segment is automatically divided into one or two sub-segments depending on the patient's heart rate during examination [Adaptive Cardio Volume ACV algorithm (Flohr and Ohnesorge 2001)]. At low heart rates below a certain threshold, one sub-segment of consecutive multi-slice spiral data from the same heart period is used. At higher heart rates, two sub-segments from subsequent heart cycles contribute to the half-scan data segment. In some other MDCT scanners, the single-segment half-scan images are reconstructed prospectively as base-line images, followed by a two-segment reconstruction

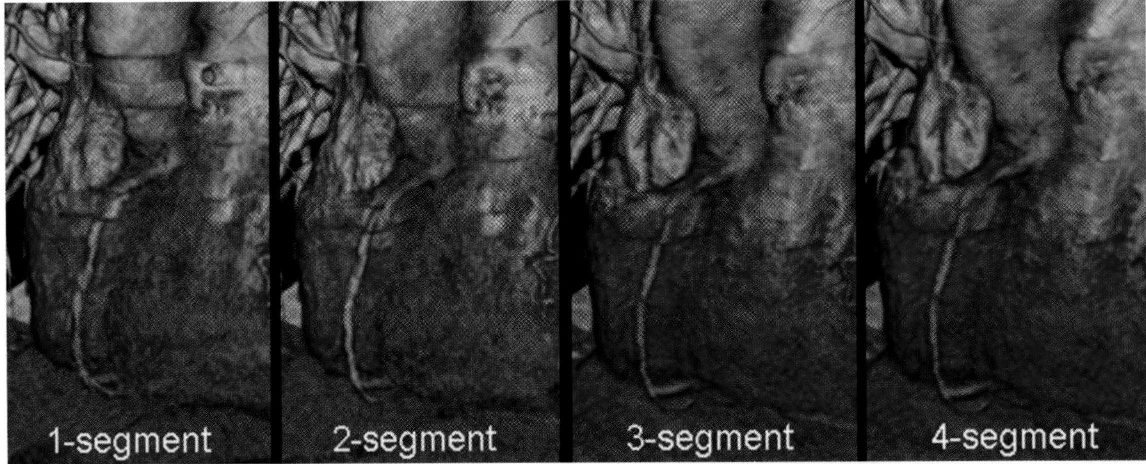

Fig. 2.12. Clinical example illustrating the limits of multi-segment reconstruction. The right coronary artery (RCA) of a patient with rapidly varying heart rate (70 bpm–126 bpm) during examination is shown. Scan data were acquired using a 64-slice CT scanner at 0.33-s gantry rotation time. The images were reconstructed at 45% of the cardiac cycle. Image quality improves significantly when performing two- or three-segment reconstruction instead of single-segment reconstruction. Nevertheless, the images remain non-diagnostic for certain segments of the RCA even with four-segment reconstruction due to the rapidly varying heart rate (courtesy of Dr. C. Becker, Klinikum Großhadern, Munich, Germany)

retrospectively for a potential gain of temporal resolution at higher heart rates. Another approach is to prospectively adjust the rotation time of the scanner to the heart rate of the patient to obtain the best possible temporal resolution for a multi-segment reconstruction. Prospectively adapting the rotation time of the scanner and exploiting multi-segment reconstruction requires a stable and predictable heart rate during examination and complete periodicity of the heart motion. Large and rapid variations of the patient's heart rate are a severe limitation for ECG-synchronized cardiac CT even with 64-slice CT scanners at 0.33 s gantry rotation (Leschka et al. 2006).

With DSCT systems, data from one cardiac cycle only are typically used to reconstruct an image (single-segment reconstruction), and constant temporal resolution equivalent to a quarter of the gantry rotation time $T_{rot}/4$ is achieved in a centered region of the scan field of view that is covered by both acquisition systems. For T_{rot}= 0.33 s, the temporal resolution is 83 ms, independent of the patient's heart rate. This is a major difference to MDCT, which can provide similar temporal resolution only by using multi-segment reconstruction with the above-mentioned disadvantages. In contrast to MDCT scanners, DSCT systems can handle both high heart rates and high heart rate variability with little influence on the image quality (Matt et al. 2007). Following Equation 2 with $N = 1$, the table feed in DSCT systems can be efficiently adapted to the patient's heart rate and significantly increased at elevated heart rates, thereby reducing the examination time and the radiation dose to the patient. In single source CT, one can usually not increase the pitch at higher heart rates, because multi-segment reconstruction must be used to improve temporal resolution.

By means of ECG-gated spiral/helical data acquisition, image reconstruction during different heart phases is feasible by shifting the start points of the data segments used for image reconstruction relative to the R-waves. This allows for a retrospective selection of reconstruction phases that provide best image quality in an individual patient (Hong et al. 2001; Kopp et al. 2001; Wintersperger et al. 2007). Besides the morphological information that is in many cases derived from images reconstructed in mid- to end-diastole, additional reconstructions of the same scan data in other phases of the cardiac cycle enable analysis of cardiac function parameters, such as end-diastolic volume, end-systolic volume and ejection fraction. In case of arrhythmia and premature beats, retrospective ECG editing can help to still achieve diagnostic image quality by discarding certain RR intervals for image reconstruction or by individually shifting the reconstruction phases in different heart cycles (Cademartiri et al. 2006), while such techniques are not yet fully available for ECG-triggered axial acquisitions.

As a drawback, relatively high radiation exposure is involved with retrospectively ECG-gated spiral imaging of the heart due to continuous X-ray exposure and overlapping data acquisition at low table feed. To maintain the benefits of ECG-gated spiral CT but reduce patient dose, ECG-controlled dose modulation ("ECG-pulsing") has been developed (Jakobs et al. 2002). A detailed description may be found in Chapter 1, together with other techniques to reduce the radiation exposure.

2.4 Alternative Scan and Reconstruction Techniques

2.4.1 ECG Gating with Increased Pitch

ECG-gated spiral/helical scanning requires substantially lower table feed than conventional multi-slice spiral/helical scanning without ECG gating. Hence, coverage of the entire chest with thin slices within a short breath-hold was not possible with 4-slice and 16-slice CT scanners. For these systems, a modified ECG-gated spiral acquisition technique was proposed that enables the use of higher pitch values than conventional ECG gating (Flohr et al. 2002). Instead of restricting the data ranges for image reconstruction to narrow, user-selected time intervals at the same relative time points within the patient's cardiac cycles, which requires very low pitch, the alternative method allows image reconstruction at multiple time points within the cardiac cycles; only scan data acquired in the systolic phase with strongest heart motion are excluded from image reconstruction. The alternative ECG-gating method does not prescribe image reconstruction in pre-defined cardiac phases, but rather exclusion of data within a user-selectable temporal window of width ΔT, see Figure 2.13. By the use of this method the pitch can be substantially increased to values between 0.5 and 0.6, which is sufficient to cover the entire thorax with thin slices within a single breath-hold even with 4-slice and 16-slice CT systems. While the patient example (dissection of the thoracic aorta) in Figure 2.14 demonstrates substantial reduction of motion artifacts in axial slices compared to the

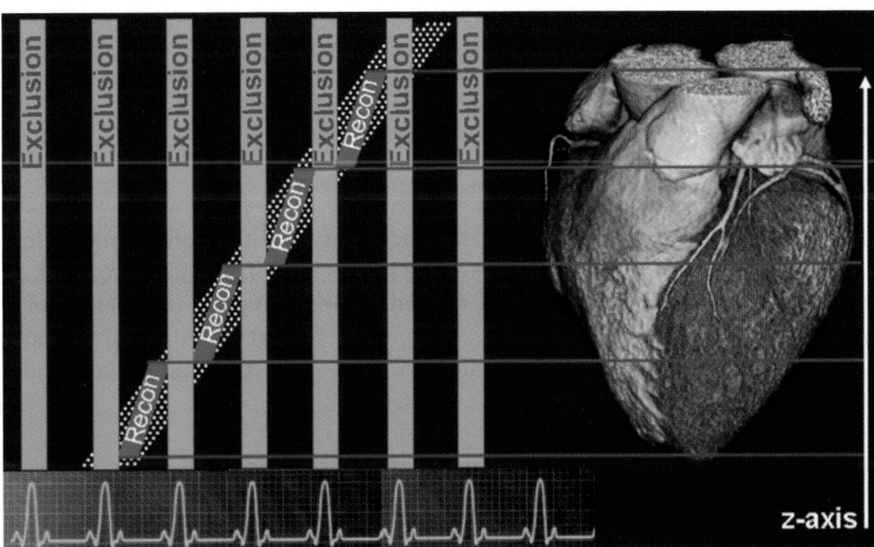

Fig. 2.13. Principle of retrospectively ECG-gated MDCT spiral/helical scanning with extended volume coverage, using relaxed gating to increase the pitch. The patient's ECG is schematically shown as a function of time on the *horizontal axis*. The *z*-positions of the detector slices (eight slices in this example) relative to the patient are indicated by the *dashed white lines*. The table moves continuously, and continuous spiral/helical scan data of the heart volume are acquired. Scan data acquired in a pre-defined cardiac phase, usually the systolic phase, are excluded from image reconstruction. Images are reconstructed from half-scan data segments starting at variable time points in the allowed phases of the patient's cardiac cycles (the *red parallelograms*)

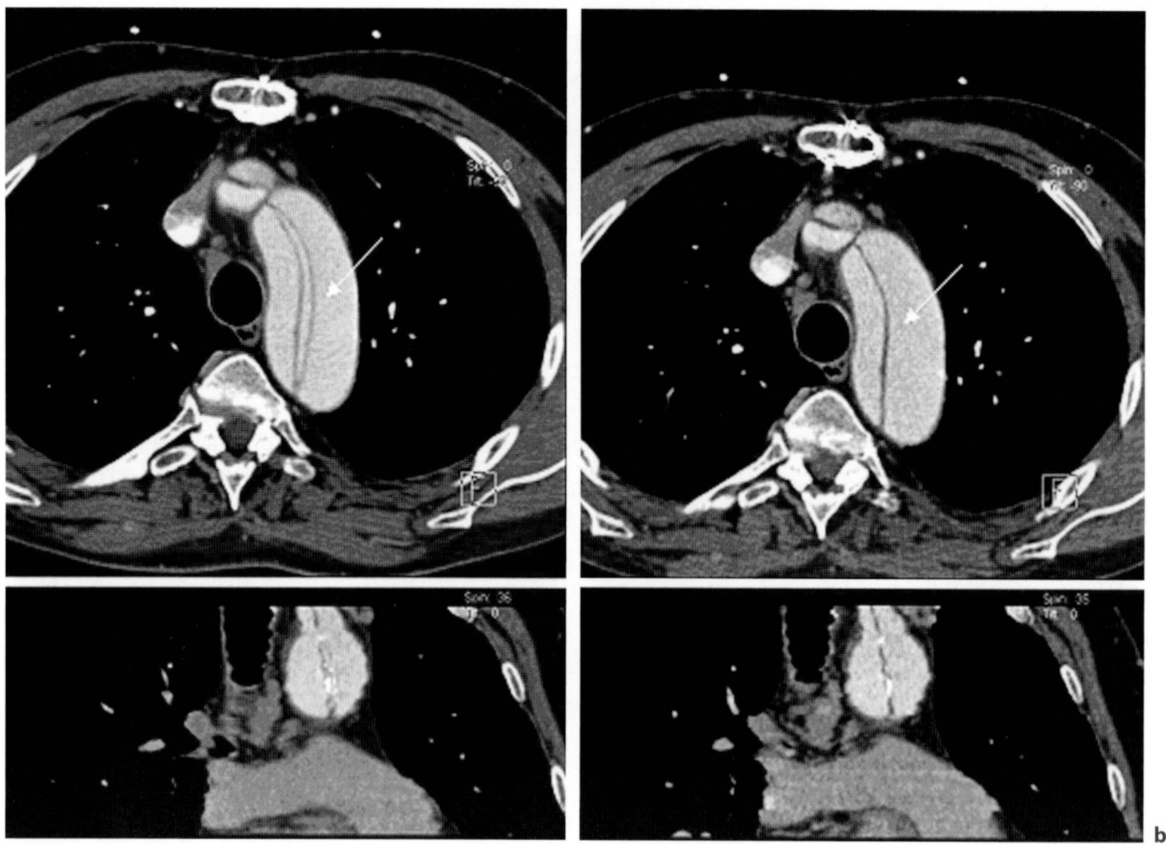

Fig. 2.14a,b. Case study showing ECG-gated spiral/helical reconstruction with extended volume coverage for evaluation of the ascending and descending aorta in comparison to multi-slice spiral reconstruction with a standard algorithm. Scan data were acquired using a four-slice CT system with 4×1 mm collimation. With standard reconstruction (**a**) considerable pulsation artifacts are visible that produce a double contour (*arrow*). The intimal flap of the type-A dissection can be evaluated free of pulsation artifacts on corresponding sections (**b**) using ECG-gated spiral reconstruction with extended volume coverage (courtesy of Cleveland Clinic Foundation, Cleveland, OH)

non-gated reconstruction, step and displacement artifacts in multiplanar reformations (MPRs) cannot be completely avoided due to the relaxed ECG-gating conditions.

With the advent of 32- and 64-slice CT scanners, the method was abandoned, since ECG-gated examinations of the entire thorax with thin slices were now feasible with regular ECG-gated acquisition protocols. Using a typical pitch of 0.2 that is required for gapless volume coverage down to heart rates of 40 bpm, a 250-mm scan range can be covered within 12–23-s breath-hold time. For patients with heart rates of at least 60 bpm during the scan, dedicated cardiothoracic examination protocols have been proposed that do not allow multi-segment reconstruction at higher heart rates and increase the pitch to values of about 0.3, thus providing 50% increased volume coverage speed and correspondingly reduced radiation dose to the patient (Johnson et al. 2007; d'Agostino et al. 2006). Due to the efficient automatic adaptation of the pitch to the patient's heart rate, DSCT systems are well suited for ECG-gated cardiothoracic examinations.

2.4.2 Alternative Synchronization of Data Acquisition and Cardiac Motion

The reconstruction phase in ECG-synchronized CT scans is commonly selected by using the R-waves as reference time points. The R-waves can be easily detected in the patient's ECG due to their high signal amplitude. Cardiac image reconstruction is frequently performed during end-systole and mid- to end-diastole, which have to be estimated by means of appropriate phase parameters relative to the R-wave. More advanced ECG-gating techniques are currently investigated that determine the location of the end-systolic phase based on the detection of the T-wave and the location of the end-diastolic phase based on the detection of the P-wave. In a clinical study, Sato et al. (2003) reported superior results for end-diastolic reconstruction based on P-wave-gating compared with the conventional method using a relative delay to the R-wave.

Despite its widespread use for phase consistent cardiac imaging, the patient's ECG only represents an indirect measure of cardiac motion. In some cases the electrical stimulation does not directly correspond to the contraction of the heart, such as in patients with atrial fibrillation or with extra-systoles. Therefore, motion detection algorithms have been investigated that aim at a direct evaluation of cardiac motion from the measured scan data.

One approach (Ohnesorge et al. 1999) compares complementary parallel projections (i.e., projections that are half a rotation apart), which should be identical for non-moving objects. The degree of deviation is a measure for cardiac motion. However, the accuracy and consistency of the signal for reproducible detection of equivalent phases in consecutive cardiac cycles are limited. A more recent approach, the so-called Kymogram algorithm (Kachelriess et al. 2002), uses the variation of the center of mass from projection to projection as a measure for cardiac motion. The authors reported that peaks of this so-called Kymogram function often correlate with the positions of the R-waves in the corresponding ECGs, and that Kymogram gated image reconstruction can produce results comparable to ECG-gated image reconstruction. A clinical study, however, demonstrated problematic outcomes when using Kymogram-gated image reconstruction in particular for patients with irregular heart rates (Fischbach 2004).

Currently, ECG-correlated data acquisition and image reconstruction remains the method of choice to synchronize CT scanning with the cardiac motion. P-wave and T-wave gating appear as promising alternatives to the established R-wave gating, if accurate automated P-wave and T-wave detection algorithms become available. Approaches to detect cardiac motion from CT scan data cannot yet provide sufficient robustness in clinical routine. To date, the use of such algorithms is restricted to a back-up role for the ECG, e.g., in case of bad signal detection, R-wave mis-registration or failure of the ECG.

References

Achenbach S, Moshage W, Ropers D, Nössen J, Daniel WG (1998) Value of electron-beam computed tomography for the non-invasive detection of high-grade coronary artery stenoses and occlusions. N Engl J Med 339:1964–1971

Achenbach S, Giesler T, Ropers D, Ulzheimer S, Derlien H, Schulte C, Wenkel E, Moshage W, Bautz W, Daniel WG, Kalender WA, Baum U (2001) Contrast-enhanced, retrospectively electrocardiographically-gated, multislice spiral computed tomography. Circulation 103:2535–2538

d'Agostino AG, Remy-Jardin M, Khalil C, Delannoy-Deken V, Flohr T, Duhamel A, Remy J (2006) Low-dose ECG-gated 64-slices helical CT angiography of the chest: evaluation of image quality in 105 patients. Eur Radiol 16:2137–2146

Bahner ML, Böse J, Lutz A, Wallschläger H, Regn J, van Kaick G (1999) Retrospectively ECG-gated spiral CT of the heart and lung. Eur Radiol 9:106–109

Becker CR, Jakobs TF, Aydemir S, Becker A, Knez A, Schöpf UJ, Brüning R, Haberl R, Reiser MF (2000a) Helical and single-slice conventional CT versus electron beam CT for the quantification of coronary artery calcification. AJR 174:543–547

Becker CR, Knez A, Ohnesorge B, Schoepf UJ, Reiser MF (2000b) Imaging of noncalcified coronary plaques using helical CT with retrospective ECG-gating. Am J Roentgenol 175:423–444

Bruder H, Stierstorfer K, Ohnesorge B, Schaller S, Flohr T (2001) Segmented cardiac volume reconstruction – A novel reconstruction scheme for multi-slice cardiac CT. The Sixth International Meeting on Fully Three-Dimensional Image Reconstruction in Radiology and Nuclear Medicine, Pacific Grove, 161–164

Boyd DP, Lipton MJ (1982) Cardiac computed tomography. Proc IEEE 71:298–307

Cademartiri F, Mollet NR, Runza G, Baks T, Midiro M, McFadden EP, Flohr TG, Ohnesorge B, de Feyter PJ, Krestin GP (2006) Improving diagnostic accuracy of MDCT coronary angiography in patients with mild heart rhythm irregularities using ECG editing. AJR 186:634–638

Fischbach R (2004) Clinical evaluation of Kymogram-gated cardiac image reconstruction with 16-slice CT (abstract). Radiology 231(P)

Flohr T, Ohnesorge B (2001) Heart rate adaptive optimization of spatial and temporal resolution for ECG-gated multi-slice spiral CT of the heart. JCAT 25:907–923

Flohr T, Prokop M, Schöpf, Kopp A, Becker C, Schaller S, White R, Ohnesorge B (2002) A new ECG-gated multi-slice spiral CT scan and reconstruction technique with extended volume coverage for cardio-thoracic applications. Eur Radiol 12:1527–1532

Flohr T, Ohnesorge B, Bruder H, Stierstorfer K, Simon J, Suess C, Schaller S (2003) Image reconstruction and performance evaluation for ECG-gated spiral scanning with a 16-slice CT system. Med Phys 30:2650–2662

Flohr TG, McCollough CH, Bruder H, Petersilka M, Gruber K, Süß C, Grasruck M, Stierstorfer K, Krauss B, Raupach R, Primak AN, Küttner A, Achenbach S, Becker C, Kopp A, Ohnesorge BM (2006) First performance evaluation of a dual-source CT (DSCT) system. Eur Radiol 16:256–268

Grass M, Manzke R, Nielsen T, Koken P, Proksa R, Natanzon M, Shechter G (2003) Helical cardiac cone beam reconstruction using retrospective ECG gating. Phys Med Biol 48:3069–3084

Greuter MJW, Flohr T, van Ooijen PMA, Oudkerk M (2007) A model for temporal resolution of multidetector computed tomography of coronary arteries in relation to rotation time, heart rate and reconstruction algorithm. Eur Radiol 17:784–812

Hong C, Becker CR, Huber A, Schöpf UJ, Ohnesorge B, Knez A, Brüning R, Reiser MF (2001) ECG-gated reconstructed multi-detector row CT coronary angiography: Effect of varying trigger delay on image quality. Radiology 220:712–717

Hsieh J, Londt J, Vass M, Li J, Tang X, Okerlund D (2006) Step-and-shoot data acquisition and reconstruction for cardiac X-ray computed tomography. Med Phys 33:4236–4248

Jakobs TF, Becker CR, Ohnesorge B, Flohr T, Suess C, Schoepf UJ, Reiser MF (2002) Multislice helical CT of the heart with retrospective ECG gating: reduction of radiation exposure by ECG-controlled tube current modulation. Eur Radiol 12:1081–1086

Johnson TR, Nikolaou K, Becker A, Leber AW, Rist C, Wintersperger BJ, Reiser MF, Becker CR (2007c) Dual-source CT for chest pain assessment. Eur Radiol Nov 22 [Epub ahead of print]

Kachelrieß M, Kalender WA (1998) Electrocardiogram-correlated image reconstruction from subsecond spiral computed tomography scans of the heart. Med Phys 25:2417–2431

Kachelrieß M, Ulzheimer S, Kalender WA (2000) Electrocardiogram-correlated image reconstruction from subsecond multi-row spiral CT scans of the heart. Med Phys 27:1881–1902

Kachelrieß M, Sennst DA, Maxlmoser W, Kalender WA (2002) Kymogram detection and Kymogram-correlated image reconstruction from subsecond spiral computed tomography scans of the heart. Med Phys 29:1489–1503

Knez A, Becker CR, Leber A, Ohnesorge B, Becker A, White C, Haberl R, Reiser MF, Steinbeck G (2001) Usefulness of multislice spiral computed tomography angiography for determination of coronary artery stenoses. Am J Cardiol 88:1191–1194

Kopp AF, Schröder S, Küttner A, Heuschmid M, Georg C, Ohnesorge B, Kuzo R, Claussen CD (2001) Coronary arteries: Retrospectively ECG-gated multi-detector row CT angiography with selective optimization of the reconstruction window. Radiology 22:683–688

Leschka S, Wildermuth S, Boehm T, Desbiolles L, Husmann L, Plass A, Koepfli P, Schepis T, Marincek B, Kaufmann PA, Alkadhi H (2006) Noninvasive coronary angiography with 64-section CT: effect of average heart rate and heart rate variability on image quality. Radiology 241:378–385

Matt D, Scheffel H, Leschka S, Flohr TG, Marincek B, Kaufmann PA, Alkadhi H (2007) Dual-source CT coronary angiography: image quality, mean heart rate, and heart rate variability. AJR Am J Roentgenol 189:567–573

Niemann K, Oudkerk M, Rensing BJ, van Ooijen P, Munne A, van Geuns RJ, de Feyter P (2001) Coronary angiography with multi-slice computed tomography. Lancet 357:599–603

Ohnesorge B, Flohr T, Schaller S, Klingenbeck-Regn K, Becker CR, Schöpf UJ, Brüning R, Reiser MF (1999) Technische Grundlagen und Anwendungen der Mehrschicht CT. Radiologe 39:923–931

Ohnesorge B, Flohr T, Becker CR, Kopp AF, Knez A, Baum U, Klingenbeck-Regn K, Reiser MF (2000) Cardiac imaging by means of electrocardiographically gated multisection spiral CT: Initial experience. Radiology 217:564–571

Parker D (1982) Optimal short scan convolution reconstruction for fan-beam CT. Med Phys 9:254–257

Sato Y, Kanmatsuse K, Inoue F, Horie T, Kato M, Kusama J, Yoshimura A, Imazeki T, Furuhashi S, Takahashi M (2003) Noninvasive coronary artery imaging by multislice spiral computed tomography – A novel approach for a retrospectively ECG-gated reconstruction technique. Circ J 67:107–111

Stierstorfer K, Rauscher A, Boese J, Bruder H, Schaller S, Flohr T (2004) Weighted FBP – a simple approximate 3D FBP algorithm for multislice spiral CT with good dose usage for arbitrary pitch. Phys Med Biol 49:2209–2218

Taguchi K, Anno H (2000) High temporal resolution for multi-slice helical computed tomography. Med Phys 27:861–872

Wintersperger BJ, Nikolaou K, von Ziegler F, Johnson T, Rist C, Leber A, Flohr T, Knez A, Reiser MF, Becker CR (2006) Image quality, motion artifacts, and reconstruction timing of 64-slice coronary computed tomography angiography with 0.33-second rotation speed. Invest Radiol 41:436–442

Cardiothoracic Image Postprocessing

3

Thomas Flohr and Bernd Ohnesorge

CONTENTS

3.1 Introduction

Image postprocessing is the use of imaging techniques either to derive additional information from the original axial images of a CT scan or to hide unwanted information that distracts from the clinical findings. The basis for image postprocessing is a three-dimensional image volume, which in most cases consists of a stack of individual axial images. The fundamental three-dimensional unit in this volume is called a "voxel." Ideally, the spatial resolution of volume image data is high and isotropic, i.e., each voxel is of equal dimensions in all three spatial axes. Isotropic sub-millimeter resolution is the basis for image display in arbitrarily oriented imaging planes and advanced image postprocessing techniques. With the advent of multi-detector row CT (MDCT) and its ongoing refinement, isotropic sub-millimeter voxels can be obtained for the majority of clinical examinations, improving the diagnostic quality of image postprocessing and turning it into a vital component of medical imaging today, in particular for CT angiography (Prokop et al. 1997; Rankin 1999; Addis et al. 2001; Lawler et al. 2002).

The axial source images contain the basic information of a CT scan; they can be supplemented by multiplanar reformations (MPRs), curved MPRs, maximum intensity projections (MIPs), curved MIPs, shaded surface display (SSD), and direct volume-rendering techniques (VTRs), which are commonly available on most clinical workstations. Information on the use of these imaging techniques for cardiac CT can be found, for example, in Vogl et al. (2002), van Ooijen et al. (2003), de Feyter and Krestin (2005), and Ferencik et al. (2007).

3.2 Axial Images

Axial images are the basic outcome of a CT scan. They include all information that has been acquired. The review of thin axial slices is the method of choice for the diagnosis of acute pulmonary embolism (Marten et al. 2003) and for the quick morphological assessment of the cardiothoracic vasculature, including the coronary arteries.

The matrix size for axial images in CT is generally 512 × 512 picture elements (pixels). Considered as a part of a three-dimensional image volume, an axial image is a layer of 512 × 512 voxels

T. Flohr, PhD
Siemens Healthcare, Computed Tomography, Siemensstrasse 1, 91301 Forchheim, Germany
B. Ohnesorge, PhD
Siemens Limited China, Healthcare, Siemens International Medical Park, 278 Zhou Zhu Road, Nanhui District, Shanghai 201318, P.R. China

within that volume. The size of the voxel in the image plane (in the x-y direction, in-plane voxel size) is determined by the field of view (FOV); perpendicular to it (in the z-direction, through-plane voxel size), it is given by the reconstruction slice width. The FOV of an axial image is the diameter of the area that is depicted in the image. The in-plane voxel size can be calculated as FOV/matrix size. Typically, a FOV of 300–350 mm is chosen for image reconstruction in thoracic examinations, resulting in 0.59–0.68-mm in-plane voxel size. For a detailed reconstruction of the heart and the coronary arteries, the FOV is reduced to 150-180 mm, with a corresponding reduction of the in-plane voxel size to 0.29–0.35 mm. The in-plane voxel size is not necessarily equivalent to the in-plane resolution of a CT image, since the choice of the convolution kernel (filter) for image reconstruction plays a major role in determining the in-plane resolution. Typical convolution kernels used for coronary CTA provide a maximum resolution of 8–12 lp/cm, corresponding to 0.4–0.6 mm object size that can be differentiated. Hence, for a FOV of 150–180 mm, the convolution kernel limits the resolution – and not the matrix size of the image. Further reducing the FOV for image reconstruction will not improve image resolution in this case, despite the further reduced in-plane voxel size. In-plane resolution is only limited by the in-plane voxel size for high-resolution thorax imaging with a large FOV of 300–350 mm.

As an example, Figure 3.1 shows axial images at different anatomical levels of a coronary CTA examination in a patient with a stenosis in the right coronary artery (RCA) acquired with a 64-slice CT scanner.

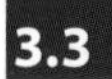

3.3 Multiplanar Reformations (MPRs)

Multi-planar reformations (MPRs) are a straightforward extension of axial images. In a MPR, a plane is defined in a three-dimensional image volume, and all voxels on that plane are visualized in a planar image. Axial images can be considered as MPRs that cut the volume image in the x-y direction. In thoracic imaging, they are often complemented by sagittal and coronal MPRs, which cut the volume image in the y-z direction and in the x-z direction. Axial images, sagittal and coronal MPRs are orthogonal to each other (Fig. 3.2). Thin axial images combined with coronal MPRs show excellent diagnostic accuracy in the diagnosis of acute pulmonary embolism (Marten et al. 2003). Sagittal and coronal MPRs are of limited use in coronary artery imaging due the complex course of the coronary arteries – in this case, oblique MPRs are more helpful. Two stacks of oblique planes are of particular interest: the planes parallel to a line along the left anterior descending artery (LAD) and the planes parallel to a line connecting the right coronary artery (RCA) and circumflex artery (CX). Representative images are shown in Figure 3.3, together with the corresponding MIP reconstructions (see below). Scrolling through the first set of planes will allow following the tortuous course of the LAD; scrolling through the second set of planes will display the anatomy of RCA and CX. It has been demonstrated that the evaluation of MDCT coronary angiography with interactive oblique MPRs permits significantly higher diagnostic accuracy than evaluation of prerendered images (Ferencik et al. 2007). In cardiothoracic imaging,

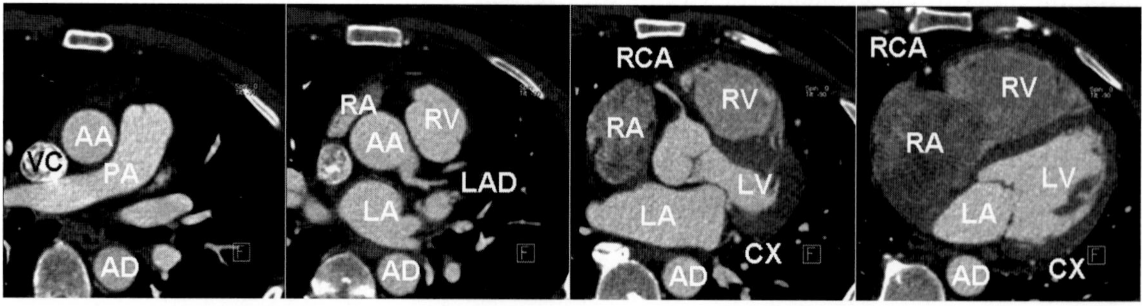

Fig. 3.1. Axial images at different anatomical levels (in the cranio-caudal direction) of a coronary CTA examination in a patient with a stenosis in the right coronary artery. Axial images include all information that has been acquired in a CT scan and should be reviewed in any case. *AA* = ascending aorta, *PA* = pulmonary artery, *AD* = descending aorta, *VC* = vena cava, *RA* = right atrium, *RV* = right ventricle, *LA* = left atrium, *LV* = left ventricle, *LAD* = left ascending coronary artery, *RCA* = right coronary artery, *CX* = circumflex artery (case courtesy of Dr. S. Achenbach, Erlangen University, Germany)

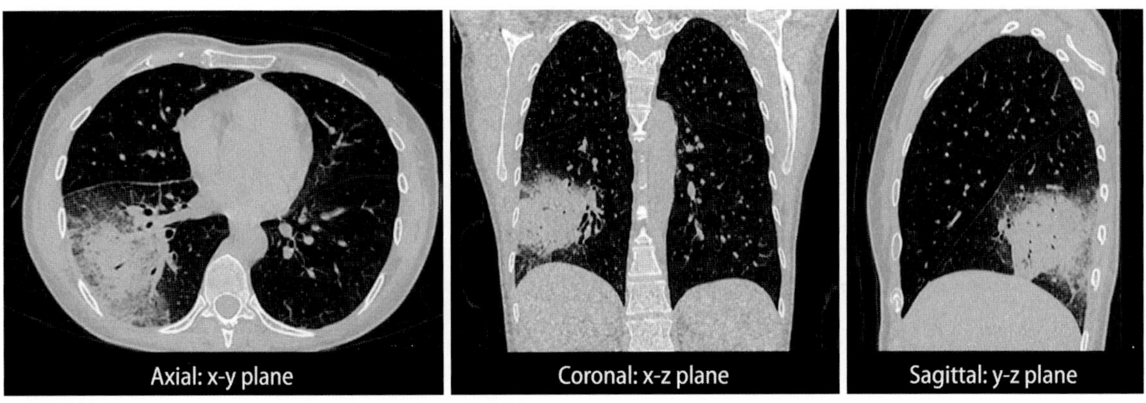

Fig. 3.2. Axial image, coronal and sagittal multiplanar reconstruction (MPR) of a CT thorax examination in a 44-year-old female patient with leukemia, who suffered from breathing difficulties. The CT scan revealed aspergiliosis in the lower lobe of the right lung. Axial images, coronal and sagittal MPRs are perpendicular to each other and frequently used in cardiothoracic imaging (courtesy of Dr. C. Becker/ Dr. K. Nikolaou, Klinikum Großhadern, Munich, Germany)

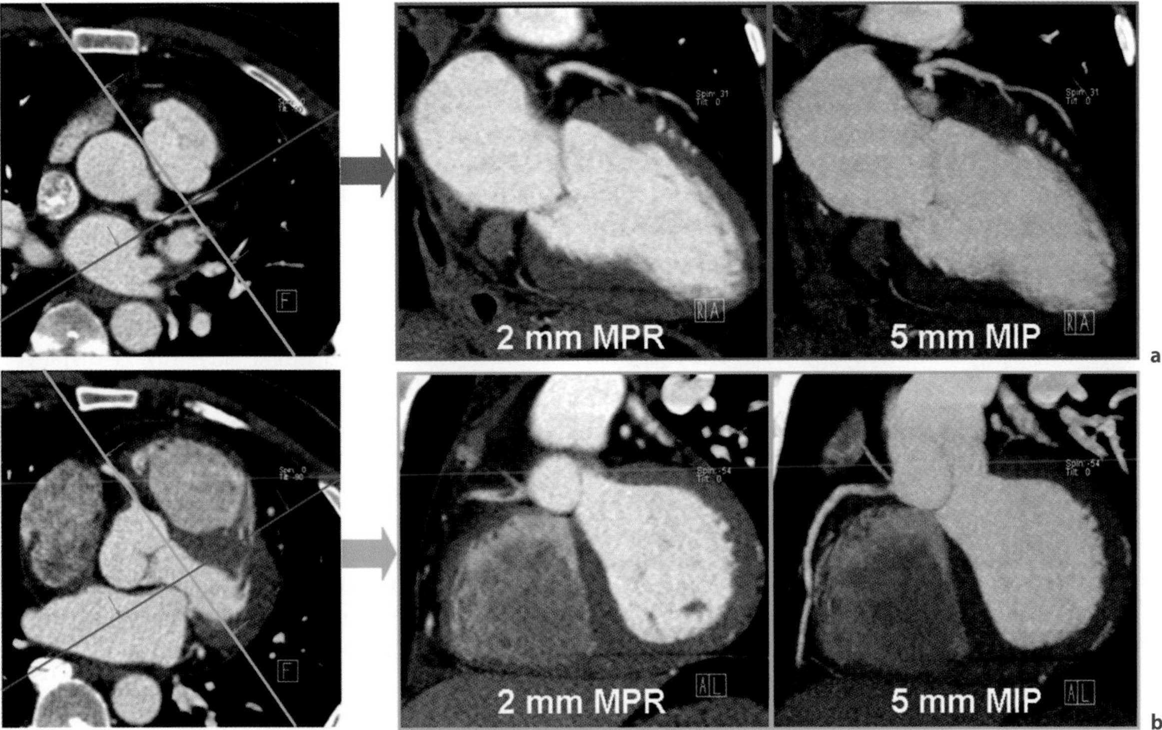

Fig. 3.3a,b. Multiplanar reconstructions (MPRs) and thin-slab maximum intensity projections (MIPs) for the case shown in Fig. 3.1. The *green* and *red* lines in the axial images indicate the orientations of the MPRs and MIPs. *Red* (**a**): plane along the left anterior descending artery (*LAD*). *Green* (**b**): Plane along the right coronary artery (*RCA*). Stacks of MPRs and MIPs in pre-defined directions are the basis for a standardized routine evaluation workflow

the use of oblique MPRs, in particular radial MPRs, may significantly improve the recognition of subsegmental pulmonary embolism (Pech et al. 2004).

The resolution of a MPR depends on both the in-plane resolution of the original axial images, which is mainly determined by the convolution kernel (filter), and the through-plane resolution (z-axis resolution), which is a function of reconstruction slice width and image increment. For spiral CT, through-plane resolution can be improved by reconstructing overlapping images with an increment of 0.5-0.7 times the reconstruction slice width. In this way, objects with a size down to 0.7-0.9 times the reconstruction slice width can be resolved in the longitudinal (z-) direction. Depending on the orientation of the MPR, the relative influence of in-plane and through-plane (z-axis) resolution varies, and so does the resulting MPR resolution, in particular for non-isotropic image data. Considering the typical in-plane resolution of 0.5–0.6 mm in cardiothoracic examinations, it is obvious that one should reconstruct the axial source images with sub-millimeter slice width to optimize MPR image quality. The 64-slice CT systems can provide up to 0.33-mm z-axis resolution using overlapping images with a reconstruction slice width of 0.6 mm (Flohr et al. 2004, 2005). The resolution of MPRs is then homogeneous irrespective of the orientation of the MPR image planes.

To trade-off image resolution and image noise, the slab thickness of a MPR can be modified. Then all voxels along the viewing ray within a given distance orthogonal to the MPR plane are averaged, and a so-called slab MPR is created (Fig. 3.4). Slab MPRs, e.g., with 2–5-mm slab thickness, are useful to reduce image noise and to visualize larger parts of tortuous vessels.

Curved MPRs are defined on curved planes, which are straightened for display. They are useful to follow the course of a tortuous vessel along its entire length (Fig. 3.5). Curved MPRs can be generated manually as in the example shown in Figure 3.5. The user then places multiple seed points along the vessel, and the software connects them by an interpolated curve. Alternatively, advanced postprocessing software is available that provides automatic calculation of the centerline of a vessel, which defines the curved visualization plane (Fig. 3.6). A more detailed description of advanced vessel analysis will be given in Sect. 3.6.

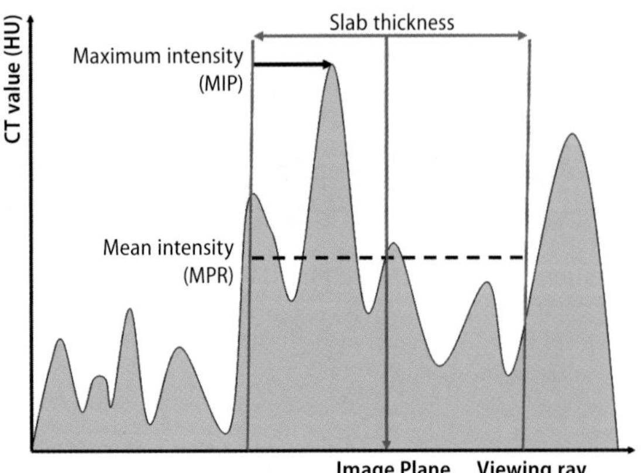

Fig. 3.4. Illustration of slab MPR and slab MIP reconstruction. For a slab MPR, the CT values within a user-selectable slab thickness along the viewing ray are averaged. The mean intensity is displayed. For a slab MIP, the maximum CT number along the ray within the selected slab is chosen

MPRs are readily available, and they do not require extensive user interaction, e.g., to segment potentially overlapping structures as in other postprocessing approaches. This is why MPRs can be used in routine clinical evaluation algorithms. MPRs maintain the full information of the axial CT images, in particular CT density values (CT numbers, HU values). On the other hand, they are operator dependent, and improper positioning may introduce false-negative and false-positive stenoses, or give a wrong estimation of the degree of stenosis (Fig. 3.7). Interactive viewing of overlapping stacks of MPRs, at best from multiple viewing angles, is therefore recommended (Ferencik et al. 2007).

3.4 Maximum Intensity Projections (MIPs)

In maximum intensity projections (MIPs), parallel rays in the viewing direction are cast through the 3D image volume, and only the maximum CT number encountered along each ray is displayed in the resulting two-dimensional MIP image. MIPs preserve the grey scale of the original axial images, and they reduce the visually perceived image noise without compromising the visually perceived image sharpness. The differentiation between contrast-enhanced vascular structures and background is good, and calcifications are clearly depicted. MIPs do not provide any depth information, which is a drawback for the visualization of complex anatomy, such as the thoracic vessels, but does not play a major role for coronary artery imaging. MIPs are projection images; high-density structures, such as the contrast-filled cavities of the heart, may therefore overlap the coronary arteries in the projection direction and obscure structures of interest. For the same reason, hypo-attenuating intraluminal lesions may not be identified, unless they are adjacent to the vessel wall and the proper viewing direction has been chosen.

To avoid these shortcomings, thin-slab MIPs (Napel et al. 1993) have been introduced. In a thin-slab MIP, the maximum CT number along the viewing ray within a user-selectable distance orthogonal to the MIP plane (the slab thickness) is displayed

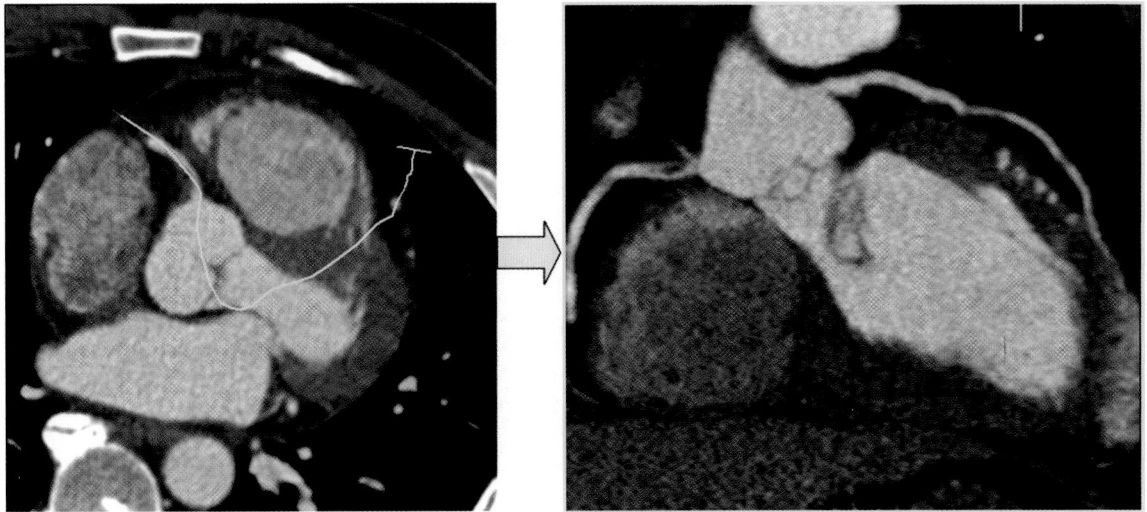

Fig. 3.5. Curved MPR for the case shown in Figure 3.1. Note the stenosis in the RCA. The *yellow line* in the axial image indicates the curved image plane of the MPR, which has been generated manually. Curved MPRs can be used to follow the course of a tortuous vessel along its entire length

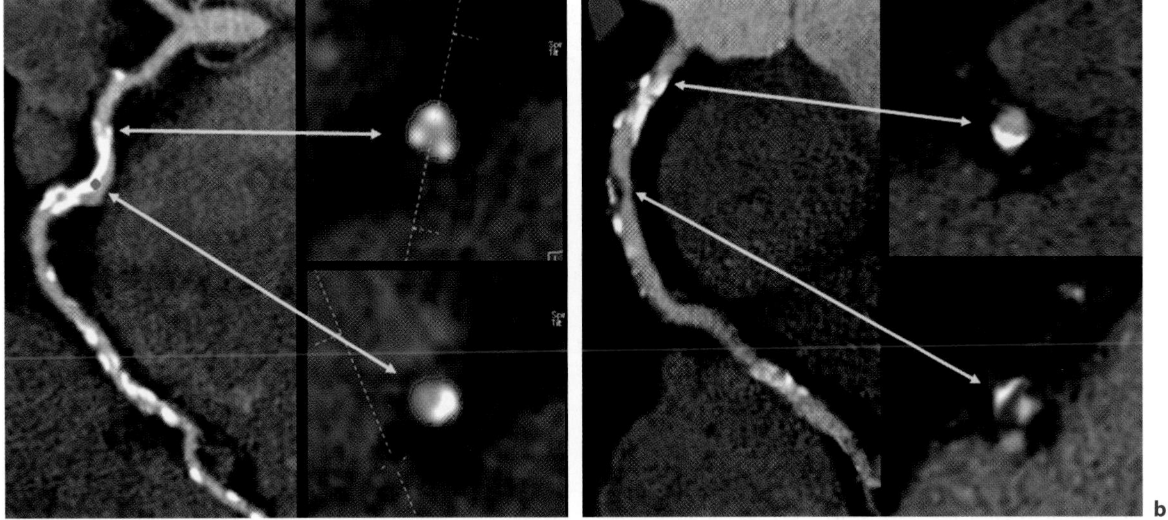

Fig. 3.6a,b. Curved MPRs along the RCA and cross sections perpendicular to the centerline of the RCA for two patients with severe three-vessel disease. The *yellow arrows* mark the positions of the cross sections on the vessel. Curved MPRs and the corresponding perpendicular cross sections–in this case automatically generated by an advanced postprocessing software package–are helpful tools for an analysis of the coronary arteries [courtesy of (**a**) Dr. J. Jacobs, New York University, NY, and (**b**) Dr. J. Breen, Mayo Clinic Rochester, MN]

(Fig. 3.4). For an evaluation of coronary arteries, the thickness of the slab has to be adjusted to the size and the course of the artery. Typical slab thicknesses range from 3 to 10 mm. In a standardized approach, reconstructing series of thin-slab MIP images with an increment smaller than the slab thickness (e.g., 1-mm increment for 3-mm slab thickness) is recommended. For cardiac imaging, one should consider the same planes as discussed for slab MPRs, in particular planes parallel to a line connecting the RCA and CX, and planes parallel to a line along the LAD. Thin-slab MIPs with 5-mm slab thickness along the RCA and LAD are shown in Figure 3.3 and can be directly compared to the corresponding MPR reconstructions. In more interactive evaluation approaches, thin-slab MIPs can be scrolled through

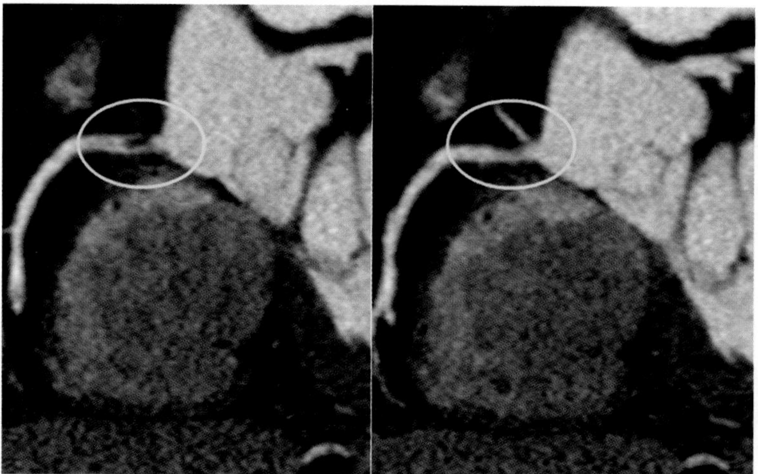

Fig. 3.7. Two MPRs on slightly shifted image planes along the RCA for the case shown in Figure 3.1. While the left MPR correctly reveals significant stenosis, the right MPR underestimates the degree of stenosis. MPRs are operator dependent, and improper positioning may introduce false-negative and false-positive stenoses or give a wrong estimation of the degree of stenosis. MPRs from different viewing angles–at best interactively manipulated–are therefore recommended for vascular evaluation

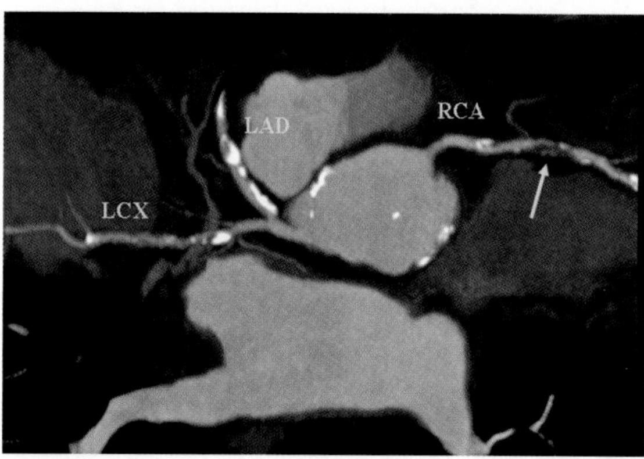

Fig. 3.8. Coronary CT angiography examination of a patient with chest pain. A curved thin-slab MIP reconstruction visualizes the main coronary artery segments in one image and reveals multiple calcified, non-calcified, and mixed lesions. The non-calcified stenosis (*arrow*) in the *RCA* can be readily assessed. Curved thin-slab MIPs may include multiple vessels in a single image, thereby improving reading efficiency (courtesy of Dr. U. J. Schoepf, Medical University of South Carolina, Charleston, SC)

the volume (sliding thin-slab MIPs). By carefully adjusting both the thickness and the orientation of the MIP plane, each coronary artery can be displayed in its entire length in many cases.

In analogy to curved MPRs, curved thin-slab MIPs have been introduced (Raman et al. 2003). Curved thin-slab MIPs may include multiple vessels in a single image, thereby improving interpretation efficiency by reducing the number of images required to assess vasculature with MIPs. Figure 3.8 shows an example of a curved thin-slab MIP reconstruction of a coronary CTA data set, which visualizes the main coronary artery segments in one image.

Similar to MPRs, MIPs are fast and easily available. In many institutions, they are the basis for a standardized routine evaluation workflow of the coronary arteries. When the slab thickness is properly selected, the visualization of non-calcified and mixed plaques is excellent. On the other hand, MIPs use only a part of the available data, thus discarding information that is included in the original axial images. Relevant anatomical details may be obscured by overlapping structures, and stenoses may be under- or overestimated (van Ooijen et al. 2003). MIPs are not recommended for the visualization of stents, since the in-stent lumen will be obscured due to the principle of the MIP projection. For the same reason, clods in pulmonary arteries cannot be adequately displayed. MIPs are therefore not suited for the diagnosis of pulmonary embolism (Marten et al. 2003).

3.5 Volume-Rendering Techniques (VRT)

Direct volume-rendering techniques (VRTs) are advanced 3D postprocessing methods that have meanwhile entered clinical routine thanks to continuous improvement of both computer hardware and software. VRTs use all available data in the volume image. A voxel-intensity histogram, i.e., a histogram of CT numbers, is generated, and several parameters are assigned to each voxel according to its CT number (HU value), such as color, brightness, and opacity. Similar to MIP projections, rays are cast through the 3D image volume in the viewing direction. Deviating from MIPs, however, all voxels along a ray contribute to the resulting pixel in the VRT image. Sometimes the term "compositing" is used to specify how each traversed voxel contributes to the final image. By means of a so-called transfer function, T, the user assigns an opacity to each voxel according to its CT number (HU value), which describes the absorption of light by this voxel. The opacities of all voxels along the viewing ray are summed up using weighting factors. Assume we walk along the ray from voxel 1 to voxel (n–1) and finally voxel n. The CT density Sum_n of the resulting pixel in the VRT image can be calculated in a recursive manner according to

$$Sum_n = Op_n \cdot CT_n + (1- Op_n) \cdot Sum_{n-1} \quad (3.1)$$

Op_n is the opacity of voxel n; CT_n is its CT number (HU value). An opacity of 0 ($Op_n = 0$) means that the corresponding voxel is completely transparent; it does not contribute to the resulting VRT image. An opacity of 1 ($Op_n = 1$) means that the corresponding voxel is completely opaque (non-transparent). Values between 0 and 1 characterize different degrees of transparency. It is obvious from Equation 3.1 that when a pixel n with opacity $Op_n = 1$ is traversed, the contribution of all preceding voxels will be set to 0, since $(1–Op_n) = 0$. In other words, as soon as a completely opaque voxel has been traversed, only this voxel will be shown in the resulting image, and all previously traversed voxels will be hidden. Assigning different opacities to different ranges of CT values by means of a transfer function, T, enables the user to control the contribution of voxels within these CT density ranges to the resulting VRT image: he can make these voxels more or less transparent, thus hiding or showing the corresponding anatomical details and adjusting 3D depth, contrast, and transparency of the VRT image. The relevant anatomical structures in cardiothoracic images are fat with a CT density of approximately –100 HU, soft tissue with a CT density of approximately 50 HU, contrast-filled vessels with a CT density of approximately 200–300 HU, and calcifications and bony structures with a CT density > 100–150 HU. Usually, linear, triangular or trapezoidal transfer functions, T, are used to assign opacity to a certain range of CT numbers (HU values). Figure 3.9 shows a grey-scale VRT reconstruction of a heart. At the bottom, the

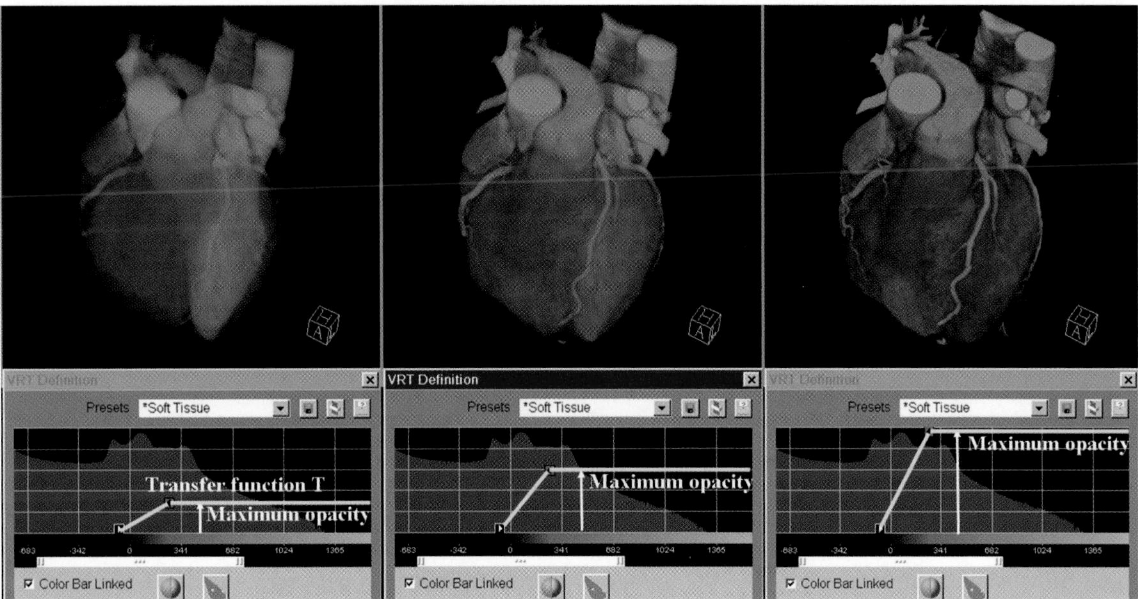

Fig. 3.9. Volume-rendered images (VRTs) demonstrating the influence of opacity. By means of a so-called transfer function, T, an opacity value is assigned to each voxel according to its CT number in order to make the voxel more or less transparent. The diagrams on the *bottom* indicate the histogram of the CT values and the respective transfer functions (*yellow lines*). *Left*: low maximum opacity. The image looks transparent and has a large 3D depth, but it lacks contrast. LAD and CX are barely visible. *Center*: medium maximum opacity. 3D depth decreases, and contrast increases. *Right*: high maximum opacity. Only the surface of the heart is visible, but the coronary arteries are much better and more sharply delineated; see the side branches of the RCA

histogram of the CT numbers is shown together with the transfer function T (yellow line). The opacity for all voxels with a CT number less than –80 HU is set to zero: these voxels are not displayed in the resulting VRT. The opacity increases linearly in the range –80 HU to 250 HU, and constant maximum opacity is assigned to all voxels with a CT number >250 HU. With these settings, soft tissue (at about 50 HU) is relatively transparent, and contrast-filled vessels–the structures of interest–are relatively opaque. The visibility of the contrast-filled coronary arteries is therefore enhanced. Figure 3.9 demonstrates the effect of increasing maximum opacity levels: on the left, the maximum opacity is low. The resulting VRT image looks transparent; it is characterized by large 3D depth, but low contrast. In the center, the maximum opacity is at a medium level; on the right it is high: the 3D depth of the resulting VRT images decreases until only the surface of the heart is visible. On the other hand, contrast for objects in the foreground increases, and the coronary arteries are much better and more sharply delineated; see in particular the side branches of the RCA.

Instead of grey values, colors can be attributed to the voxels according to their CT numbers; see Figure 3.10. Each voxel n with a certain CT number (HU value) CT_n is assigned a color $RGB(CT_n)$. Although the choice of colors is arbitrary, a brownish red is most commonly used for soft tissue, and lighter colors are used for the visualization of contrast-filled vessels.

To improve the visibility of boundaries between different tissue types and the delineation of anatomical structures, gradient transfer functions are used in more elaborate VRT approaches. For this purpose, the opacity is modulated according to the local CT density gradients. In homogenous areas with small density changes (small gradients), the opacity is reduced; these areas will therefore be visualized more transparently. In areas with abrupt density changes, the opacity is increased. The visualization of boundaries between tissues will therefore be enhanced. Furthermore, shading and local illumination techniques can be used to improve the three-dimensional impression of the VRT images. Local illumination models introduce additional light sources that illuminate the object from a predefined direction. They allow the approximation of the light intensity reflected from each point on the surface of an object, usually by calculating the sum of ambient light, diffuse reflection, and specular reflection in the viewing direction.

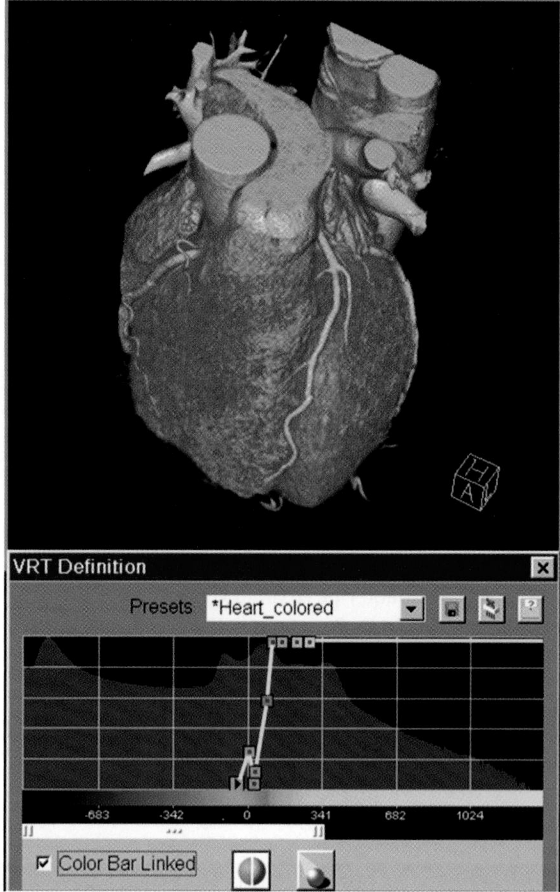

Fig. 3.10. In a VRT, colors instead of grey values can be attributed to the voxels according to their CT numbers and their opacities. In this example, soft tissue is assigned a *brownish red*, whereas a *lighter brown* is used for the contrast-filled coronary arteries with higher CT numbers (compare to Figure 3.9, *right*)

Similar to MPRs and MIPs, oblique slab VRTs are available for an interactive evaluation of anatomical details.

VRTs require extensive user interaction for adequate imaging results. In most cases, the segmentation of overlapping structures is required, e.g., to remove the rib cage and the pulmonary vessels for a VRT visualization of the heart. With advanced cardiac evaluation packages, the heart can be automatically isolated. VRTs depend on a multitude of user-definable parameters. They are helpful for a visualization of results, in particular to non-radiologists, but they are of limited value for primary diagnosis in cardiac and cardiothoracic CT examinations. The variety of parameters and settings and the lack of standardization impair the ability of VRTs to correctly assess coronary diameters and coronary artery stenoses (Mahnken et al. 2003). On the other hand, VRTs provide good insight into the three-dimensional relationship of anatomical structures. This is why they are helpful in the evaluation of aberrant cardiothoracic anatomy, such as anomalous coronary arteries, and bypass grafts (Fig. 3.11).

3.6 Advanced Cardiothoracic Image Postprocessing

In addition to the on-going refinement of CT acquisition technology with the goal of integrating cardiac and cardiothoracic imaging into routine clinical protocols, advanced visualization and evaluation tools have been developed. They provide the user with optimized clinical workflow solutions, e.g., for vessel segmentation and vessel analysis, for evaluation of cardiac function parameters and detailed reporting functionality. These advanced application packages make use of all available 3D postprocessing techniques, such as MPRs, MIPs, and VRTs, to simplify and streamline the clinical workflow.

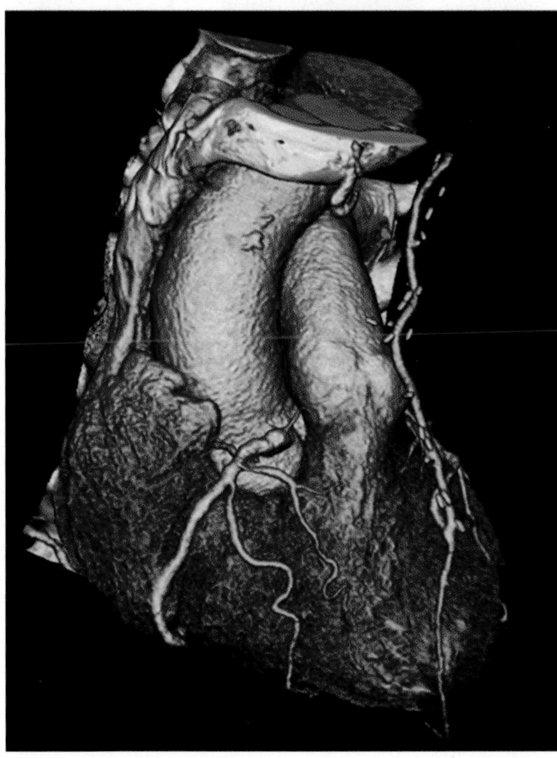

Fig. 3.11. VRTs are mainly useful for a demonstration of the diagnosis. They provide good insight into the three-dimensional relationship of anatomical structures, e.g., in the case of anomalous coronary arteries or bypass grafts. In this example, the heart of a patient with LIMA bypass graft is shown. The images were acquired on a dual source CT (courtesy of Dr. S. Achenbach, Erlangen University, Germany)

3.6.1 Advanced Cardiac Evaluation

In a typical software package for advanced cardiac postprocessing, MPRs and VRTs of a coronary CTA image data set are shown for a first orientation, with the rib cage automatically removed ("heart isolation") so that only the heart is visible. The coronary arteries are then automatically segmented to calculate curved MPRs or curved MIPs along the respective center lines. Two different types of vessel segmentation are currently used. In a vessel probe approach, the user places a marker (mouse click) in the vessel of interest. A centerline extending on both sides of the marker is calculated, and the corresponding vessel segment is displayed as a curved MPR. In a vessel segmentation approach, the entire coronary artery tree is segmented as a first step. In some software packages, the segmentation of the coronary artery tree is automatically performed as a pre-processing step, so that the segmented coronary arteries are already available when the user starts the evaluation. Arteries or branches that are not initially recognized by the segmentation algorithm can usually be appended by marking them with a mouse click. The user can then define centerlines on the coronary artery tree–e.g., by a mouseclick–to produce curved MPRs along the respective coronary arteries as a basis for further evaluation.

MPRs on straight planes perpendicular to the centerline of the vessel are usually displayed in addition to curved MPRs to facilitate the comprehensive evaluation of coronary artery stenosis and plaques. In some application packages, the degree of a stenosis has to be manually measured (e.g., by a length measurement using an electronic ruler); in some others, it is automatically determined by calculating area ratios or maximum diameter ratios of the vessel's cross sections. A scoring system for lumen narrowing (Schmermund et al. 1998) can be used to describe different grades of coronary artery stenosis: A = angiographically normal segment (0% stenosis), B = non-obstructive disease (1–49% lumen diameter narrowing), C = significant stenosis (50–74%),

D = high-grade stenosis (75–99%), and E = total occlusion (100% stenosis). Figure 3.12 shows a screenshot of comprehensive cardiac evaluation software (syngo Circulation, Siemens Healthcare, Forchheim, Germany). The bottom right image represents a VRT of the segmented coronary artery tree with a centerline (indicated in red) along the RCA. Three markers indicate a high-grade stenosis of the RCA. The top right image shows a curved MPR along this centerline. The top left image shows a cross section perpendicular to the centerline at the position indicated by the red dot in the top right image.

Clinical studies have demonstrated the potential of MDCT not only to detect, but also to some degree to characterize non-calcified and calcified plaques in the coronary arteries based on their CT number (Schroeder et al. 2001a,b; Becker et al. 2003; Caussin et al. 2004; Leber et al. 2003, 2006; Carrascosa et al. 2006; Pohle et al. 2007). Meanwhile, the development of advanced evaluation tools that help visualize and quantify plaques in the coronary arteries is on-going. Figure 3.13 shows a curved MPR along the RCA and a cross-sectional image perpendicular to the centerline for the same patient as in Figure. 3.12. Using a plaque-evaluation tool, the voxels belonging to four different ranges of CT numbers, which may represent different types of plaques, are color-coded. The volume of the compartments can be calculated, and an individual "plaque burden" can be derived for the patient. Clinical studies are needed

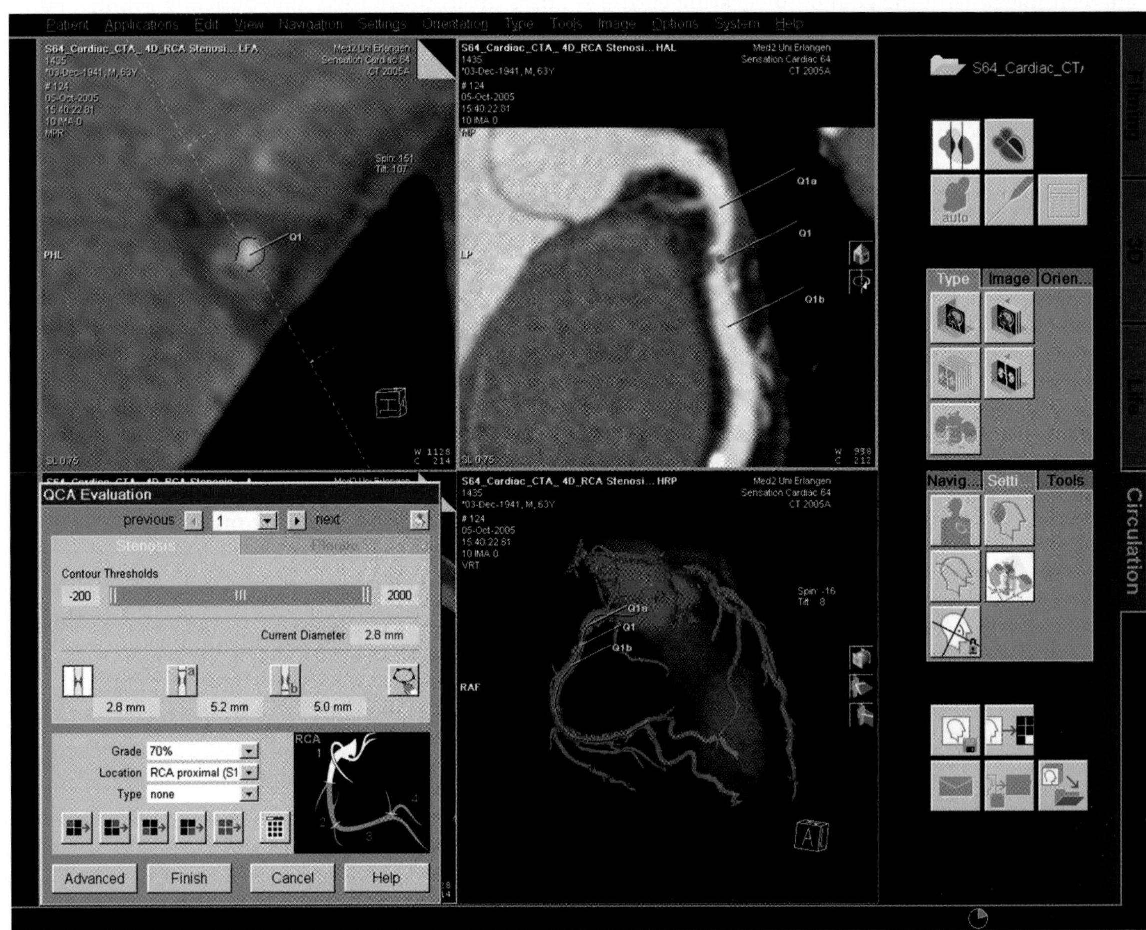

Fig. 3.12. Case study demonstrating advanced cardiac vessel analysis for a patient with significant stenosis of the RCA (courtesy of Dr. S. Achenbach, Erlangen University, Germany). The images are processed using an advanced cardiac evaluation software (syngo Circulation, Siemens Healthcare, Forchheim, Germany). Segmented coronary artery tree with a centerline along the RCA and three markers indicating the high-grade stenosis (*bottom right*), curved MPR along the RCA following the centerline (*top right*), and cross section perpendicular to the centerline of the RCA (*top left*). The *red dot* marks the position of the cross-sectional image. Cross sections perpendicular to the centerline of a vessel are helpful for an evaluation of the vessel, in this case for the grading of the stenosis

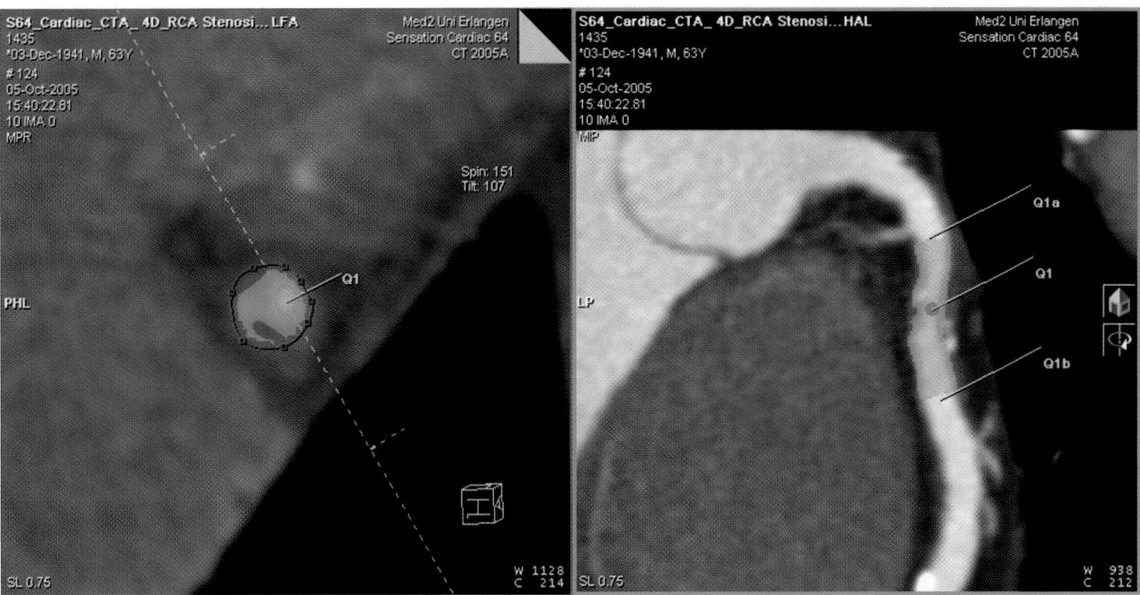

Fig. 3.13. Plaque evaluation tool, assigning different colors to voxels within different ranges of CT numbers. In this example, a stenosis in the RCA is evaluated (same case as in Figure 3.12). *Dark green* is used for voxels with CT numbers between -25 HU and 50 HU (potential "lipid" plaques), *light green* is used for voxels with CT-numbers between 50 HU and 150 HU (potential "fibrous" plaques), *orange* is used for voxels between 150 HU and 500 HU (contrast-filled lumen), and *pink* is used for voxels with CT numbers >500 HU (calcifications)

to evaluate the potential and the clinical relevance of these plaque quantification tools. Ideally, they could, for example, be used to monitor the therapy response of patients undergoing medical treatment aimed at reducing their total plaque burden.

Any contrast-enhanced retrospectively ECG-gated MDCT data set that has been acquired to visualize the cardiac anatomy can be re-used for the assessment of cardiac function (Juergens et al. 2002, 2004; Heuschmid et al. 2003, 2006; Kopp et al. 2005; Mahnken et al. 2007; Brodoefel et al. 2007). Measurement of global cardiac function and of some regional function parameters by MDCT is possible through image reconstruction of the heart in different phases of the cardiac cycle. Global cardiac function is represented by end-diastolic volume, end-systolic volume, ejection fraction, and left ventricular stroke volume, which can be derived from reconstructions of the left ventricle in the end-diastolic and end-systolic phase of the cardiac cycle. These reconstructions can also serve for the determination of regional function parameters such as wall thickness and systolic wall thickening. Image reconstruction at multiple equidistant time points throughout the cardiac cycle can reveal additional information about regional wall motion, in particular when the images are displayed as a cine-loop. In addition, measurements of right ventricular volume and function can provide important information for the diagnosis, treatment, follow-up, and prognosis of various cardiac and pulmonary diseases (Delhaye et al. 2006; Remy-Jardin et al. 2006).

To streamline and simplify analysis of cardiac function, advanced postprocessing tools are available that enable a fully or semi-automated volumetric segmentation of the contrast-enhanced cardiac chambers, the calculation of global cardiac function parameters, such as end-diastolic volume, end-systolic volume, ejection fraction, or stroke volume, and the visualization of wall thickening or wall motion. It has been demonstrated that automated threshold-based 3D segmentation enables accurate and reproducible CT assessment of left ventricular volume and function with excellent correlation with results of manual 2D short-axis analysis (Juergens et al. 2008). Figure 3.14 shows a screenshot of a comprehensive cardiac evaluation software (syngo Circulation, Siemens Healthcare, Forchheim, Germany), demonstrating the automated 3D segmentation of the left ventricle and the determination of epicardial and endocardial contours. Figure 3.15 shows a polar map representation ("bull's eye plot") of systolic wall thickening with a projection of the coronary arteries for the same patient as in Figures 3.12 and 3.13.

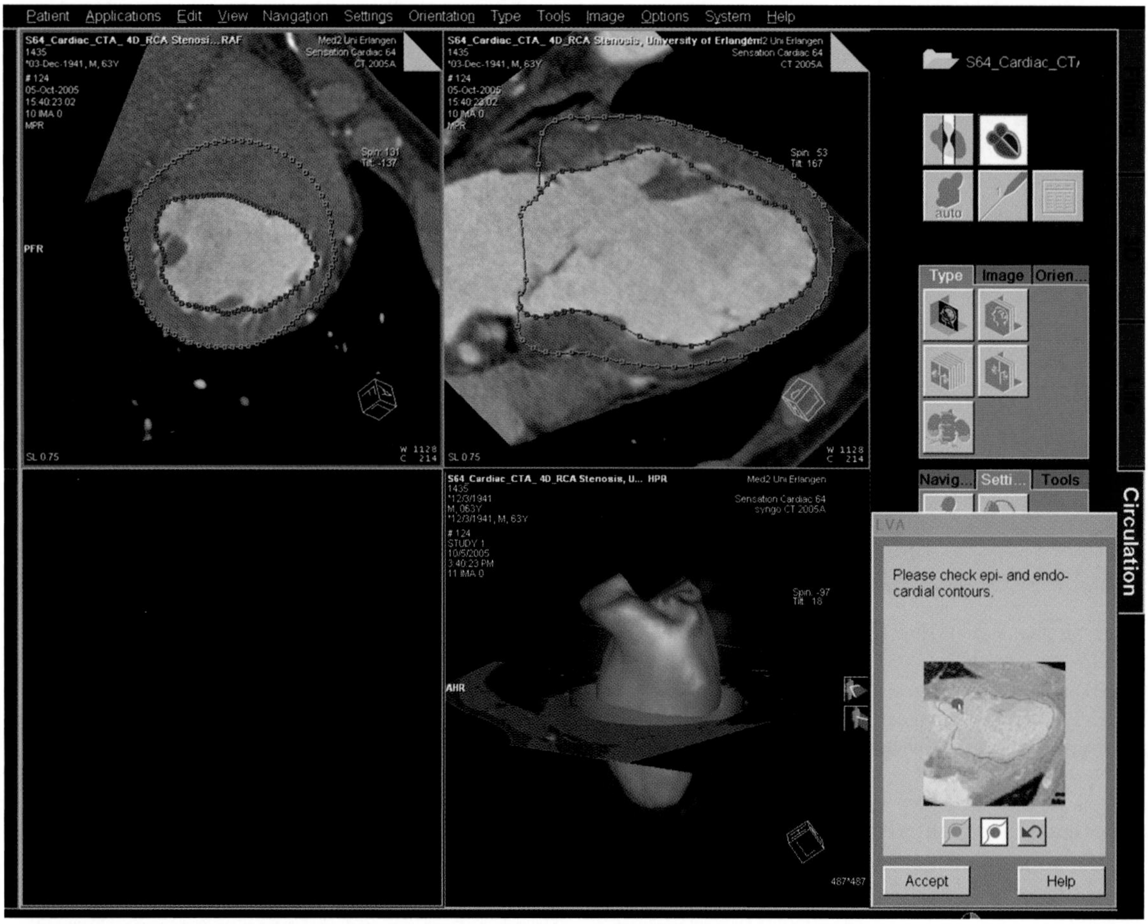

Fig. 3.14. Case study demonstrating advanced cardiac function analysis for a patient with significant stenosis of the RCA (same case as in Figure 3.12). The images are processed using an advanced cardiac evaluation software (syngo Circulation, Siemens Healthcare, Forchheim, Germany). Short axis (*top left*) and long axis visualization (*top right*) of the left ventricle with automatically determined epicardial and endocardial contours as a basis for the calculation of global and regional function parameters

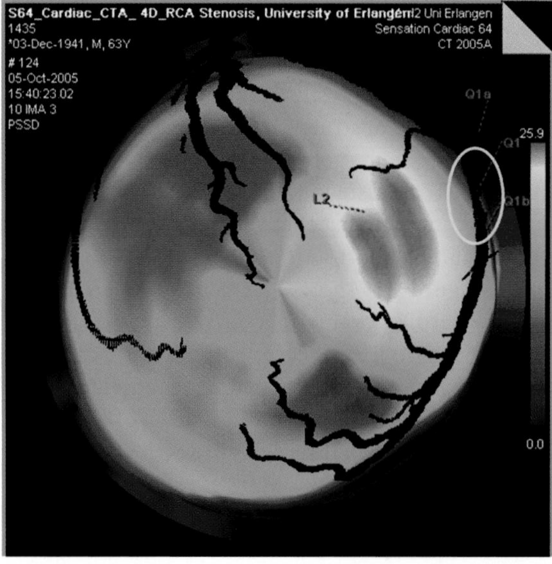

Fig. 3.15. Polar map ("bull's eye plot") visualizing wall thickening with a projection of the coronary arteries for the same patient as in Figure 3.12. A wall-thickening abnormality (*red*) can be observed in the territory that is supplied by the stenotic segment of the RCA (*yellow circle*)

A wall-thickening abnormality can be observed in the territory that is supplied by the stenotic segment of the RCA.

Some other 3D postprocessing techniques can be used for cardiac CT, such as virtual endoscopy, which is known from CT colonoscopy. Virtual endoscopy can provide a spectacular visualization of the inner surface of contrast-filled coronary arteries; its clinical use in cardiac imaging, however, is doubtful.

3.6.2
Advanced Cardiothoracic Evaluation

As a consequence of the on-going technical refinement, inclusion of MDCT into the diagnostic algorithm allows for comprehensive evaluation of cardiothoracic diseases and for rapid diagnosis of common causes of acute chest pain, such as pulmonary embolism, aortic dissection, or aneurysm, or significant coronary artery disease. Advanced visualization and evaluation tools may help to optimize the clinical workflow also for the assessment of non-cardiac findings.

For general vascular analysis, vessel probe approaches are most helpful. Similar to coronary artery evaluation, the user places one or more markers (mouse clicks) into the vessel of interest. A centerline is then calculated, and the corresponding vessel segment is automatically displayed as a curved MPR, together with orthogonal cross sections (Fig. 3.16). A variety of measurement tools is usually available to further evaluate stenoses, aneurysms, or dissections.

Computer-aided diagnosis (CAD) tools have been proposed to facilitate the diagnosis of pulmonary embolism. In a clinical evaluation of a CAD prototype (Buhmann et al. 2007), the CAD software showed a sensitivity comparable to that of the general radiologists, but with more false positives. CAD detection of findings incremental to the radiologist suggests benefit when used as a second reader. Particularly inexperienced readers benefit from consensus with CAD data, thereby greatly improving detection of segmental and subsegmental emboli (Engelke et al. 2008; Das et al. 2008). As a drawback, some CAD systems show high false-negative results that demand technologic improvement (Maizlin et al. 2007). Overall, application of CAD tools may improve the diagnostic accuracy and decrease the interpretation time of CT angiography for the detection of pulmonary emboli in the peripheral arterial tree and further enhance the acceptance of this test as the first line diagnostic modality for suspected PE (Schoepf et al. 2007).

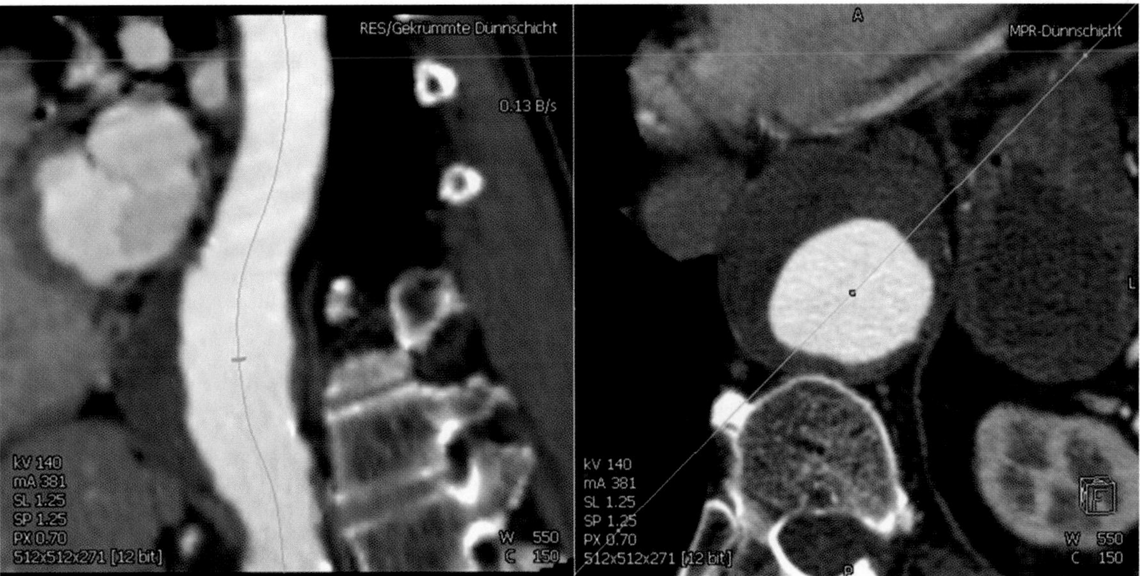

Fig. 3.16. Curved MPR along the aorta and cross section perpendicular to the centerline for a patient with aortic aneurysm. Automated vessel analysis tools can facilitate the assessment of non-cardiac findings in cardiothoracic examinations (courtesy of Dr. C. Becker, Klinikum Großhadern, Munich, Germany)

References

Addis KA, Hopper KD, Iyriboz TA, Liu Y, Wise SW, Kasales CJ, Blebea JS, Mauger DT (2001) CT angiography: In vitro comparison of five reconstruction methods. Am J Radiol 177:1171–1176

Becker CR, Nikolaou K, Muders M, Babaryka G, Crispin A, Schoepf UJ, Loehrs U, Reiser MF (2003) Ex vivo coronary atherosclerotic plaque characterization with multi-detector-row CT. Eur Radiol 13(9):2094–2098

Brodoefel H, Kramer U, Reimann A, Burgstahler C, Schroeder S, Kopp A, Heuschmid M (2007) Dual-source CT with improved temporal resolution in assessment of left ventricular function: a pilot study. AJR Am J Roentgenol 189(5):1064–1070

Buhmann S, Herzog P, Liang J, Wolf M, Salganicoff M, Kirchhoff C, Reiser M, Becker CH (2007) Clinical evaluation of a computer-aided diagnosis (CAD) prototype for the detection of pulmonary embolism. Acad Radiol 14(6):651–658

Carrascosa PM, Capunay CM, Garcia-Merletti P, Carrascosa J, Garcia MF (2006) Characterization of coronary atherosclerotic plaques by multidetector computed tomography. Am J Cardiol 97:598–602

Caussin C, Ohanessian A, Ghostine S, Jacq L, Lancelin B, Dambrin G, Sigal-Cinqualbre A, Angel CY, Paul JF (2004) Characterization of vulnerable nonstenotic plaque with 16-slice computed tomography compared with intravascular ultrasound. Am J Cardiol 94:99–100

Das M, Mühlenbruch G, Helm A, Bakai A, Salganicoff M, Stanzel S, Liang J, Wolf M, Günther RW, Wildberger JE (2008) Computer-aided detection of pulmonary embolism: Influence on radiologists' detection performance with respect to vessel segments. Eur Radiol 2008 Feb 22 [Epub ahead of print]

de Feyter PJ, Krestin GP (2005) Computed tomography of the coronary arteries, Chap. 2: Image post-processing. Taylor and Francis, London

Delhaye D, Remy-Jardin M, Teisseire A, Hossein-Foucher C, Leroy S, Duhamel A, Remy J (2006) MDCT of right ventricular function: comparison of right ventricular ejection fraction estimation and equilibrium radionuclide ventriculography, part 1. AJR Am J Roentgenol 187(6):1597–1604

Engelke C, Schmidt S, Bakai A, Auer F, Marten K (2008) Computer-assisted detection of pulmonary embolism: performance evaluation in consensus with experienced and inexperienced chest radiologists. Eur Radiol 18(2):298–307

Ferencik M, Ropers D, Abbara S, Cury RC, Hoffmann U, Nieman K, Brady TJ, Moselewski F, Daniel WG, Achenbach S (2007) Diagnostic accuracy of image postprocessing methods for the detection of coronary artery stenoses by using multidetector CT. Radiology 243(3):696–702

Flohr T, Stierstorfer K, Raupach R, Ulzheimer S, Bruder H (2004) Performance evaluation of a 64-slice CT-system with z-flying focal spot. Röfo Fortschr Geb Rontgenstr Neuen Bildgeb Verfahr 176:1803–1810

Flohr TG, Stierstorfer K, Ulzheimer S, Bruder H, Primak AN, McCollough CH (2005) Image reconstruction and image quality evaluation for a 64-slice CT scanner with z-flying focal spot. Med Phys 32(8):2536–2547

Heuschmid M, Küttner A, Schröder S, Trebar B, Burgstahler C, Mahnken A, Niethammer M, Trabold T, Kopp AF, Claussen CD (2003) Left ventricular functional parameters using ECG-gated multidetector spiral CT in comparison with invasive ventriculography. Röfo Fortschr Geb Rontgenstr Neuen Bildgeb Verfahr 175:1349–1354

Heuschmid M, Rothfuss JK, Schröder S, Fenchel M, Stauder N, Burgstahler C, Franow A, Kuzo RS, Küttner A, Miller S, Claussen CD, Kopp AF (2006) Assessment of left ventricular myocardial function using 16-slice multidetector-row computed tomography: comparison with magnetic resonance imaging and echocardiography. Eur Radiol 16(3):551–559

Jürgens KU, Grude M, Fallenberg EM, Opitz C, Wichter T, Heindel W, Fischbach R (2002) Using ECG-gated multidetector CT to evaluate global left ventricular myocardial function in patients with coronary artery disease. Am J Roentgenol 2002, 179:1545–1550

Jürgens KU, Maintz D, Grude M et al (2004) Semiautomated analysis of left ventricular function using 16-slice multidetector-row computed tomography (MDCT) of the heart in comparison to steady-state-free-precession (SSFP) cardiac magnetic resonance imaging. Eur Radiol 2004, 14:S2–272

Jürgens KU, Seifarth H, Range F, Wienbeck S, Wenker M, Heindel W, Fischbach R (2008) Automated threshold-based 3D segmentation versus short-axis planimetry for assessment of global left ventricular function with dual-source MDCT. AJR Am J Roentgenol 190(2):308–314

Kopp AF, Heuschmid M, Reinmann A, Küttner A, Beck T, Ohmer M, Burgstahler C, Brodoefel H, Claussen CD, Schröder S (2005) Evaluation of cardiac function and myocardial viability with 16- and 64-slice multidetector computed tomography. Eur Radiol 15 [Suppl 4]:D15–D20

Lawler LP, Corl FM, Fishman EK (2002) Multi-detector row and volume-rendered CT of the normal and accessory flow pathways of the thoracic systemic and pulmonary veins. Radiographics 22:S45–60

Leber AW, Knez A, White CW, Becker A, von Ziegler F, Muehling O, Becker C, Reiser M, Steinbeck G, Boekstegers P (2003) Composition of coronary atherosclerotic plaques in patients with acute myocardial infarction and stable angina pectoris determined by contrast-enhanced multislice computed tomography. Am J Cardiol 91(6):714–718

Leber AW, Becker A, Knez A, von Ziegler F, Sirol M, Nikolaou K, Ohnesorge B, Fayad ZA, Becker CR, Reiser M, Steinbeck G, Boekstegers P (2006) Accuracy of 64-slice computed tomography to classify and quantify plaque volumes in the proximal coronary system: a comparative study using intravascular ultrasound. J Am Coll Cardiol 47:672–677

Mahnken AH, Wildberger JE, Sinha AM, Dedden K, Stanzel S, Hoffmann R, Schmitz-Rode T, Günther RW (2003) Value of 3D-volume rendering in the assessment of coronary arteries with retrospectively ECG-gated multislice spiral CT. Acta Radiologica 44(3):302–309

Mahnken AH, Bruder H, Suess C, Muhlenbruch G, Bruners P, Hohl C, Guenther RW, Wildberger JE (2007) Dual-source computed tomography for assessing cardiac function: a phantom study. Invest Radiol 42(7):491–498

Maizlin ZV, Vos PM, Godoy MB, Cooperberg PL (2007) Computer-aided detection of pulmonary embolism on CT angiography: initial experience. J Thorac Imaging 22(4):324–329

Marten K, Funke M, Obenauer S, Baum F, Grabbe E (2003) The contribution of different postprocessing methods for multislice spiral CT in acute pulmonary embolism. Röfo Fortschr Geb Rontgenstr Neuen Bildgeb Verfahr 175(5):635–639

Napel S, Rubin GD, Jeffrey RB Jr (1993) STS-MIP: a new reconstruction technique for CT of the chest. J Comput Assist Tomogr 17(5):832–838

Pech M, Wieners G, Lopez-Hänninen E, Röttgen R, Bittner R, Engert U, Ricke J (2004) The diagnostic value of radial multiplanar reformatting (MPR) in the CT-diagnosis of pulmonary embolism. Röfo Fortschr Geb Rontgenstr Neuen Bildgeb Verfahr 176(11):1576–1581

Pohle K, Achenbach S, MacNeill B, Ropers D, Ferencik M, Moselewski F, Hoffmann U, Brady TJ, Jang IK, Daniel WG (2007) Characterization of non-calcified coronary atherosclerotic plaque by multi-detector row CT: comparison to IVUS. Atherosclerosis 190:174–180

Prokop M, Shin HO, Schanz A, Schaefer-Prokop CM (1997) Use of maximum intensity projections in CT angiography: a basic review. Radiographics 17(2):433–451

Raman R, Napel S, Rubin GD (2003) Curved-slab maximum intensity projection: method and evaluation. Radiology 229(1):255–260

Rankin CS (1999) CT angiography (Review). Eur Radiol 9:297–310

Remy-Jardin M, Delhaye D, Teisseire A, Hossein-Foucher C, Duhamel A, Remy J (2006) MDCT of right ventricular function: impact of methodologic approach in estimation of right ventricular ejection fraction, part 2. AJR Am J Roentgenol 187(6):1605–1609

Schmermund A, Rensing BJ, Sheedy PF, Bell MR, Rumberger JA (1998) Intravenous electron-beam computed tomographic coronary angiography for segmental analysis of coronary artery stenosis. Am J Cardiol 31:1547–1554

Schoepf UJ, Schneider AC, Das M, Wood SA, Cheema JI, Costello P (2007) Pulmonary embolism: computer-aided detection at multidetector row spiral computed tomography. J Thorac Imaging 22(4):319–323

Schroeder S, Kopp A, Baumbach A, Meisner C, Kuettner A, Georg C, Ohnesorge B, Herdeg C, Claussen C, Karsch K (2001a) Noninvasive detection and evaluation of atherosclerotic coronary plaques with multi-slice computed tomography. JACC 37(5):1430–1435

Schroeder S, Flohr T, Kopp AF, Meisner C, Kuettner A, Herdeg C, Baumbach A, Ohnesorge B (2001b) Accuracy of density measurements within plaques located in artificial coronary arteries by X-ray multislice CT: Results of a phantom study. JCAT 25(6):900–906

van Ooijen PM, Ho KY, Dorgelo J, Oudkerk M (2003) Coronary Artery Imaging with Multidetector CT: Visualization Issues. Radiographics 23:e16

Vogl TJ, Nasreddin DA, Diebold T, Engelmann K, Ay M, Dogan S, Wimmer-Greinecker G, Moritz A, Herzog C (2002) Techniques for the detection of coronary atherosclerosis: Multi-detector row CT coronary angiography. Radiology 223:212–220

4 Contrast Medium Utilization

Dominik Fleischmann and Margaret C. C. Lin

CONTENTS

D. Fleischmann, MD
Associate Professor of Radiology, Cardiovascular and Thoracic Imaging Sections, Department of Radiology, Stanford University Medical Center, 300 Pasteur Drive, Room S-068B, Stanford CA 94305-5105, USA
M. C. C. Lin, MD
Assistant Professor of Radiology, Thoracic Imaging Section, Department of Radiology, Stanford University Medical Center, 300 Pasteur Drive, Room S-068B, Stanford CA 94305-5105, USA

4.1 Introduction

Contrast medium (CM) administration remains an integral part of thoracic and cardiovascular CT. While simple, empiric injection protocols (fixed volume and fixed scanning delay) are sufficient for non-vascular CM-enhanced thoracic CT, cardiac and CT angiographic applications require more sophistication. The goal is to achieve strong enhancement of the vascular territory (or territories) of interest synchronized with CT data acquisition, which requires integrating knowledge of arterial enhancement dynamics with the technical capabilities and acquisition parameters of the CT scanner. The increasing breadth of cardiovascular CT applications, ranging from pulmonary CTA over left atrial mapping, coronary and thoracic CTA, to complex applications aiming at simultaneous opacification of systemic and pulmonary circulations with minimal artifacts, make this a challenging task. CT scanner technology is continuously evolving, with scan times becoming shorter with every new CT scanner generation. The long-term merit of providing detailed scanning and injection protocols for a given scanner generation is therefore short-lived and of limited value. Understanding the basic principles of arterial enhancement dynamics in the chest, on the other hand, and learning how vascular enhancement can be controlled by user-selectable parameters is of great benefit to everyone involved in the design and execution of current and future scanning and injection protocols for cardiovascular CT.

The purpose of this chapter is therefore to first review the physiologic and pharmacokinetic principles of vascular enhancement ('key-rules' of arterial enhancement) and explain how these principles apply to different vascular territories in the thorax. The remainder of this chapter reviews the techniques to synchronize vascular enhancement with CT data acquisition and explains basic cardiovascular CT injection protocols.

4.2 Physiologic and Pharmacokinetic Principles

The key to contrast medium delivery for cardiovascular CT applications is to understand the relationship between intravenously injected CM and subsequent vascular enhancement. The first step is to realize the fundamental difference between vascular (arterial) enhancement and tissue (organ) enhancement. For non-vascular CT (e.g., imaging of the liver during a parenchymal phase), the degree of organ opacification correlates closely with the volume of CM administered, and it is also inversely related to a patient's body weight. This is easy to understand since all iodinated X-ray contrast agents are extracellular fluid markers, and extracellular space correlates with body weight (Dawson and Blomley 1996). Arterial enhancement, on the other hand, is not immediately related to CM volume. Arterial enhancement is controlled by two key factors – or 'key rules' as summarized in Table 4.1 (Fleischmann 2002): (1) the amount of iodinated CM delivered per unit of time, which – for a given iodine concentration – is simply the injection flow rate (mL/s) and (2) the injection duration of such a contrast medium injection in seconds (s). Of course, the injection flow rate multiplied by the injection duration equals the CM volume, so CM volume does indirectly play a role, notably since most power injectors require that a planned CM injection is keyed into the injector interface as CM volume and flow rate. However, as will become more apparent later, it is substantially more useful to consider injection protocols for cardiovascular CT as injection flow rate times injection duration. For example, an intravenous CM injection described as '100 ml @ 5 ml/s' should be understood as '5 ml/s for 20 s,' because the latter can be more intuitively translated into the expected strength and length of a desired vascular enhancement phase. The importance of thinking about injection protocols as injection flow rate multiplied by the injection duration cannot be overemphasized. It is the most important learning objective of this chapter and is also reflected in the first two 'key rules' listed in Table 4.1.

4.2.1 Early Arterial Contrast Medium Dynamics

Time attenuation responses to intravenously injected CM vary between vascular territories and even more so between different individuals, but they all share the same basic principles. Figure 4.1 schematically illustrates the early arterial contrast medium dynamics as observed in the aorta: When a 16-ml test bolus of CM is injected intravenously, it causes an arterial enhancement response in the aorta after a certain time interval. This time interval needed for the CM to arrive in the arterial territory of interest is referred to as the contrast medium transit time (t_{CMT}), an important landmark for scan timing. The arterial time attenuation response itself consists of two phases. The first peak of the time attenuation response is referred to as the "first pass" effect. This

Table 4.1. Key rules of early arterial contrast medium dynamics for CT angiography and their consequences

Key rules of arterial enhancement
§1 Arterial enhancement is proportional to the iodine administration rate
Arterial opacification can be increased by increasing the injection flow rate and/or by increasing the iodine concentration of the contrast medium.
§2 Arterial enhancement increases with the injection duration
Longer CM injections have a cumulative effect on arterial enhancement A minimum injection duration of approximately 10 s is always needed to achieve adequate arterial enhancement
§3 Individual enhancement is controlled by cardiac output
Cardiac output is inversely proportional to arterial opacification (i.e., high cardiac output results in decreased arterial enhancement, and vice versa). Cardiac output correlates with body weight Increasing or decreasing both the injection rate and the injection volumes to body weight, at least for large (>90 kg) and small (<60 kg) individuals, respectively, reduces the interindividual variability of arterial enhancement

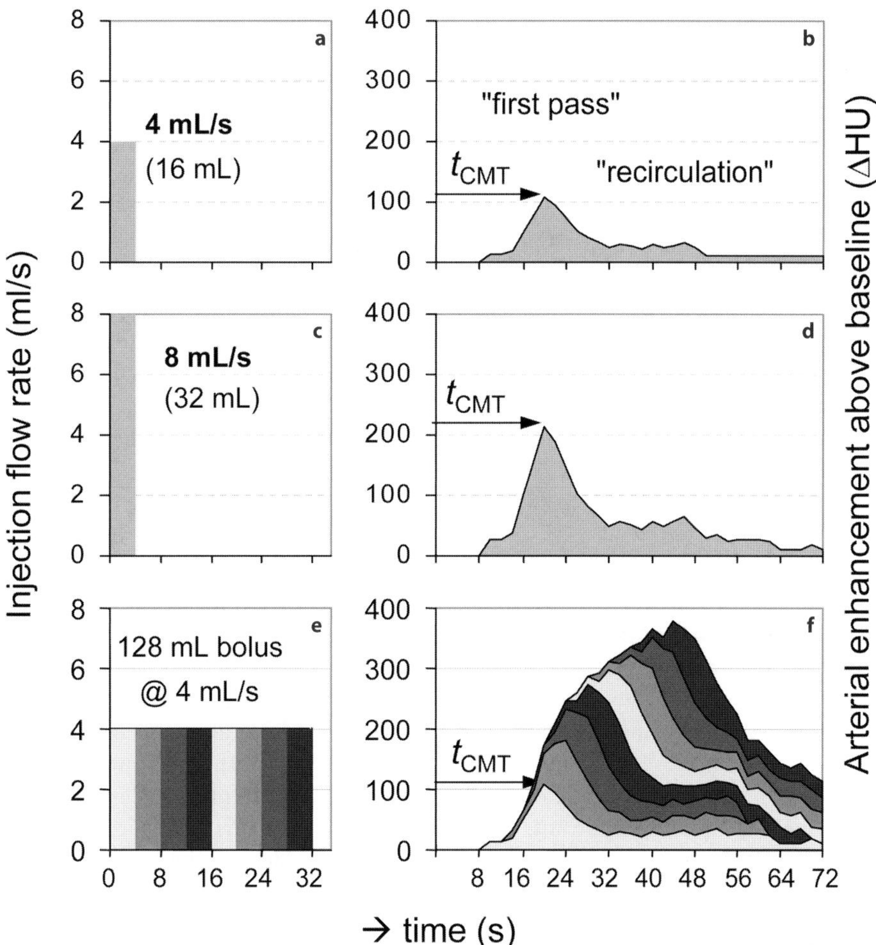

Fig. 4.1a–f. Simple "additive model" illustrating the effects of injection flow rate and injection duration on arterial enhancement. Intravenous contrast medium (*CM*) injection (**a**) causes an arterial enhancement response (**b**), which consists of an early "first pass" peak and a lower "recirculation" effect. Doubling the injection flow rate (doubling the iodine administration rate) (**c**) results in approximately twice the arterial enhancement (**d**). The effect of the injection duration (**e**) can be regarded as the sum (time integral) of several enhancement responses (**f**). Note that due to the asymmetric shape of the test-enhancement curve and due to recirculation effects, arterial enhancement following an injection of 128 ml (the time integral of 8 consecutive 16 ml) increases continuously over time [adopted from (Fleischmann 2002), with permission]

is followed by the 'recirculation' phase, characterized by the fact that the tail of the time-attenuation curve does not return to zero after the first-pass, but undulates above the baseline. This tail is only in part caused by true recirculation of opacified blood from highly perfused organs such as the brain and the kidney. Early on, it is mostly a consequence of bolus broadening, but detailed knowledge of the cause of the 'recirculation' phase is not essential for our purposes. It is very important, however, to acknowledge its existence, because it explains the effect of the injection duration on vascular enhancement.

4.2.1.1 Effect of Injection Flow Rate on Arterial Enhancement (§1)

For a given patient and vascular territory, the degree of arterial enhancement is directly proportional to the iodine administration rate. Figure 4.1 shows that when the injection rate is doubled from 4 ml/s to 8 ml/s, or more precisely, if the iodine administration rate is increased from 1.2 g to 2.4 g of iodine per second (if a 300 mg I/ml CM is used), the corresponding enhancement response is twice as strong. Note that changing the iodine concentration of the contrast agent has the same proportional effect on arterial enhancement as changing the injection flow rate has.

There are physiologic and practical limitations to increasing the injection flow rates, however. Injection flow rates of 8 ml/s or greater have been shown to not directly translate into stronger enhancement (Claussen et al. 1984), possibly because of pooling in the central venous system with reflux into the inferior vena cava – a phenomenon that can be observed with even moderate and low flow rates in patients with significantly decreased cardiac output. High injection flow rates are also limited by the size of the intravenous cannula, most of which would not allow injection rates greater than 6 ml/s for an 18-G cannula, even if warmed (and thus less viscous) contrast agents are used.

4.2.1.2 Effect of Injection Duration on Arterial Enhancement (§2)

The effect of increasing (or shortening) the injection duration is more difficult to understand than the direct relationship of the iodine administration rate, but it is equally important. One intuitive way to think about the effect of the injection duration is shown in Figure 4.1. A longer injection duration of, e.g., 32 s (128 ml total volume) can be regarded as the sum of eight subsequent injections of small "test boluses" of 4-s duration (16 ml each). Each of these eight "test boluses" has its own effect on arterial enhancement, in terms of first pass and recirculation, respectively. Under the assumption of a time-invariant linear system (Fleischmann and Hittmair 1999), the cumulative enhancement response to the entire 128 ml injection equals the sum (time integral) of each enhancement response to their respective eight test boluses (Fleischmann 2002). Note that the 'recirculation' effects of the earlier test boluses overlap (and thus sum up) with the first pass effects of later test boluses, resulting in the typical continuous increase of arterial enhancement over time.

4.2.1.3 Physiologic Parameters Affecting Vascular Enhancement (§3)

The degree of arterial enhancement following the same intravenous contrast medium injection is highly variable between individuals. Even in patients considered to have normal cardiac output, mid-aortic enhancement may range from 140 HU to 440 HU (a factor of three) between patients (Sheiman et al. 1996). If body weight is taken into account, the average aortic enhancement ranges from 92 to 196 HU/ml/kg (a factor of two) (Hittmair and Fleischmann 2001). Adjusting the contrast medium injection rates (and volumes) to body weight will therefore reduce interindividual differences of arterial enhancement, but it will not completely eliminate them. Body-weight adjustment of injections is nevertheless recommended for patients with small (< 60 kg) and large (> 90 kg) body size.

The fundamental physiologic parameter affecting arterial enhancement is cardiac output and, to a lesser degree, central blood volume. Cardiac output is inversely related to the degree of arterial enhancement, particularly in first pass dynamics (Bae et al. 1998). This can be understood intuitively when thinking about a CM injection as 'flow of iodine' (iodine molecules per second), injected into a larger 'flow of blood' (ml of blood per second). The relative amount of 'flow of iodine' into the 'flow of blood' will determine the iodine concentration in the blood, and thus its CT attenuation. Arterial enhancement is therefore lower in patients with high cardiac output, but it is stronger in patients with low cardiac output (despite the delayed t_{CMT} in the latter).

4.2.2 Early Contrast Medium Dynamics in the Chest

Equipped with good understanding of early arterial enhancement dynamics, we will now look at the relative time attenuation dynamics of central venous, pulmonary and systemic arterial enhancement within the chest, because of their relevance for scan timing, for avoiding streak artifacts, for avoiding or maintaining right ventricular opacification during cardiac CT, and for simultaneous pulmonary and systemic opacification.

The sequence of early vascular enhancement effects in the thorax following intravenous administration of CM is illustrated in Figure. 4.2, which shows a series of non-incremental dynamic images obtained every 2 s at the level of the pulmonary artery following the injection of a small test bolus. CM appears immediately after the beginning of the injection, relatively undiluted and incompletely mixed, in the superior vena cava [which collects approximately one third (~ 25 ml/s) of the cardiac output (~ 85 ml/s)]. This causes not only bright en-

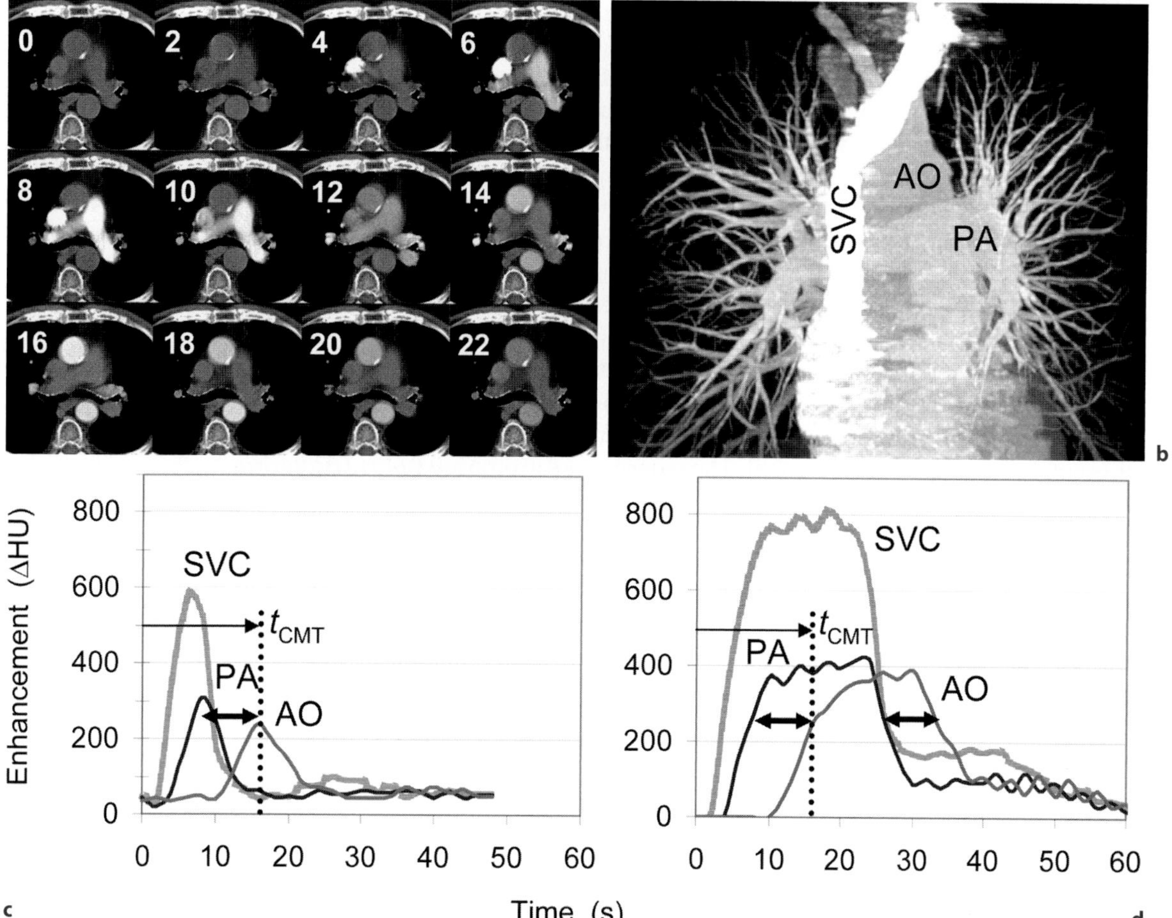

Fig. 4.2a–d. Early contrast medium dynamics in the chest. **a** Sequence of vascular enhancement observed in a non-incremental dynamic CT acquisition following the intravenous injection of a small test bolus are shown (see text for details). **b** Maximum intensity projection of a MDCT pulmonary angiogram shows extensive opacification of the left brachicephalic vein and SVC. As densely opacified blood is mixed with unenhanced blood from the inferior vena cava in the right atrium and ventricle, the pulmonary arterial enhancement is substantially smaller than the enhancement in the SVC. Aortic enhancement is again slightly less than PA enhancement. Analysis of the time attenuation curves from a 4-s test injection (**c**) allows predicting the time attenuation curves for a prolonged, 20-s injection (**d**). *SVC* superior vena cava; *PA* pulmonary artery; *AO* thoracic aorta; t_{CMT} contrast medium transit time for the aorta; *double-headed arrows* in (**c**) and (**d**) indicate pulmonary transit time. Adapted from (Fleischmann 2003), with permission

hancement, but also perivenous streak artifacts. The subsequent enhancement of the pulmonary arteries and the thoracic aorta is less strong, because it has mixed in the right atrium and ventricle with blood from the inferior vena cava (~60 ml/s). The time-attenuation curves for each vascular territory are plotted in Figure 4.2c. Note, that pulmonary arterial enhancement begins immediately (2 s) after enhancement of the superior vena cava. This is an important observation, because it explains why it is currently impossible to completely avoid perivenous streak artifacts in pulmonary CT angiograms. The transit time from the SVC to the pulmonary circulation is just too short for current scanners even with scan times in the range of 5 s.

The bolus is delayed and broadened in the pulmonary circulation and left heart chambers, and finally appears in the thoracic aorta after another 6–8 s or so. The 'pulmonary transit time', i.e., the time it takes for the bolus to travel from the right ventricle to the systemic circulation, is thus much longer than the SVC-to-pulmonary transit time, and it is also more variable between individuals. The pulmonary transit time is important for some cardiac imaging protocols, because it determines the temporal relationship of right and left ventricular enhancement.

Figure 4.2d integrates the relative enhancement effects (in Δ HU, above baseline) for a prolonged injection of 20 s for each vessel, respectively. Note, that the enhancement events now show a much greater overlap in time. However, the order and the absolute onset-times of the respective time-attenuation events are maintained: pulmonary enhancement again begins again immediately after SVC opacification, and it takes again another 6–8 s for the aorta to enhance. Similarly, pulmonary opacification decreases immediately after CM is flushed from the SVC, but is maintained in the systemic circulation for another 6–8 s in this particular example before it decreases as well. The sequence of events can also be seen on a MIP of a thoracic CT angiogram (Fig. 4.2b), where the craniocaudal direction corresponds to the time axis shared by all vascular territories (SVC, right heart and pulmonary, left heart and systemic arteries). Short acquisition times with fast scanners allow scanning at specific time windows of enhancement if timed correctly.

4.3 Synchronizing CM Enhancement with CT Data Acquisition

A fixed scanning delay cannot be recommended for cardiac or vascular CT, because the arterial contrast medium transit time (t_{CMT}) is prohibitively variable between individual patients – ranging from as short as 8 to as long as 40 s in patients with cardiovascular diseases. The scanning delay (the time interval between the beginning of a CM injection and the initiation of CT data acquisition) needs to be timed relative to the t_{CMT} of the vascular territory of interest. It is important to realize that with fast MDCT acquisitions, the t_{CMT} itself does not necessarily serve as the scanning delay, but rather as a landmark relative to which the scanning delay can be individualized. Depending on the vessels of interest, an additional delay relative to the t_{CMT} can be selected. In CTA, this additional delay may be as short as 2 s ("t_{CMT} + 2 s"), but often additional delays of 5 or 8 s are used ("t_{CMT} + 8 s"). The notation "t_{CMT} + 8 s" means that the scan is initiated 8 s after the CM has arrived in the target vasculature. Transit times can be easily determined using either a test-bolus injection or an automatic bolus triggering technique.

4.3.1 Test Bolus

The injection of a small test bolus (15–20 ml) while acquiring a low-dose dynamic (non-incremental) CT acquisition is a reliable means to determine the t_{CMT} from the intravenous injection site to the arterial territory of interest (Van Hoe et al. 1995). The t_{CMT} equals the time-to-peak enhancement interval measured in a region-of-interest (ROI) placed within a reference vessel (Fig. 4.1).

4.3.2 Automated Bolus Triggering

For bolus triggering, a circular region of interest (ROI) is placed into the target vessel on a non-enhanced image. While CM is injected, a series of low-dose non-incremental scans are obtained, and the attenuation within the ROI is monitored. The t_{CMT} equals the time when a predefined enhancement threshold ("trigger level") is reached (e.g., 100 ΔHU). Because of technical reasons, however, the CT acquisition cannot begin immediately. Automated bolus triggering thus inherently causes a slight delay relative to the t_{CMT}, the "trigger delay." The trigger delay depends on the scanner model and on the longitudinal distance between the monitoring series and the starting position of the scan. Also, if a pre-recorded breath-holding command is programmed into the CT acquisition, this increases the minimal "trigger delay" before a scan can be initiated as well. The minimal trigger delay is usually 2 s, which can be ignored when designing an injection protocol. If a longer trigger delay is necessary or intentionally chosen, e.g., 8 s ("t_{CMT} + 8s"), the injection duration needs to be increased accordingly. Bolus triggering is a very robust and practical technique for routine use and has the advantage that it does not require an additional test-bolus injection.

4.3.3 Right Ventricular Opacification in Cardiac CT

With fast enough CT scanners, it is possible to achieve bright systemic arterial enhancement without perivenous artifacts (notably if saline flushing is used), and it is also possible to achieve bright systemic enhancement when CM has been

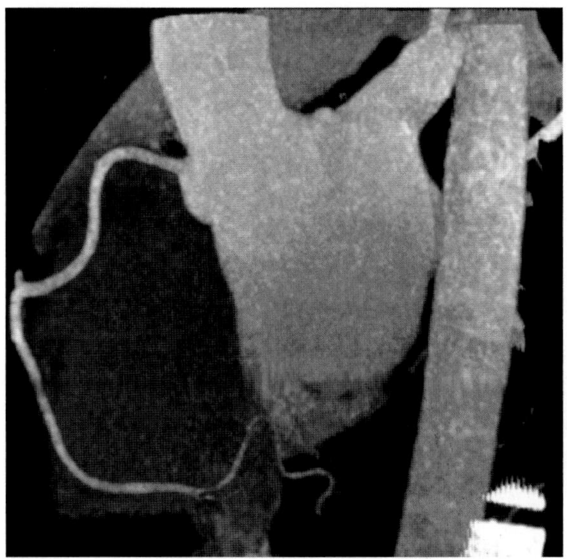

Fig. 4.3. 'Levocardiogram' effect. Coronary CT angiogram with saline flushing. Thin-slab MIP image through the right coronary artery shows complete flushing of contrast medium out of the right ventricle, resulting in exquisite, artifact-free visualization of the right coronary artery. (Image courtesy of C. Becker, Munich)

cleared (nearly) completely out of the right atrium and ventricle. This effect leads to a very nice depiction of the right coronary artery in MIP or volume-rendered coronary CTA images (Fig. 4.3), because it is no longer obscured by artifacts and bright opacification of the right atrium and ventricle (the 'levo-cardiogram' effect). This effect – which by the way was not necessarily planned intentionally, but rather observed coincidentally – is not consistently achievable, however, if an individual's pulmonary transit time is short (at least with current retrospectively ECG-gated helical data acquisition).

Complete flushing of the right ventricle may also be a disadvantage, however, if delineation of the right ventricular cavity (and thus the RV border of the interventricular septum) is diagnostically desirable (Fig. 4.4a–c), such as for the assessment of left ventricular function and mass. This limitation can been overcome by the injection of diluted contrast medium (10–20%) rather than normal saline following the main bolus. Alternatively, a long injection duration and a long scanning delay also result in good right chamber enhancement due to recirculation of opacified blood from the brain and the kidneys (Fig. 4.4d–f).

4.3.4 Simultaneous Pulmonary and Systemic Arterial Enhancement

If bright opacification of both the pulmonary and the systemic arteries is desired, for example, to evaluate for both pulmonary embolism and thoracic aortic dissection, the injection duration needs to additionally include the pulmonary transit time. The simplest way to do this is to use a thoracic aortic CTA protocol and empirically add another 10 s to the injection duration. The scanning delay remains unchanged relative to the aortic t_{CMT}. The same effect can be achieved by using a pulmonary CTA protocol and adding 10 s to both the injection duration and the scanning delay relative to the pulmonary t_{CMT}. Both strategies will opacify both the pulmonary and the systemic arteries in the majority of patients, i.e., in patients with pulmonary transit times less than 10 s.

In situations where the pulmonary transit time can be expected to be particularly long or hard to predict, such as in patients with severe right heart failure, or patients with surgically repaired congenital heart diseases, it is advisable to obtain a test bolus injection and plan the protocol individually based on the specific time-attenuation curves seen in the pulmonary and systemic arterial systems. Alternatively, one can also obtain two scans, one early and one delayed.

4.4 CM Injection Strategies for Cardiovascular CT

The traditional paradigm of injection protocol design aims at choosing an injection flow rate and injection duration that matches the scan time. Scan times for CTA vary widely, however, and may range from more than 30 s for a thoracoabdominal CTA using a 4-channel MDCT to as short as 4 s for an abdominal CTA using a 64-channel MDCT. Even shorter scan times will become possible in the near future. No single strategy of CM injection for cardiovascular CT can therefore be applied. Since the introduction of 64-channel MDCT, we have observed a paradigm shift, where for the first time, injection protocols are not designed to match the scan time, but instead the CT acquisition protocol is designed to match the injection protocol.

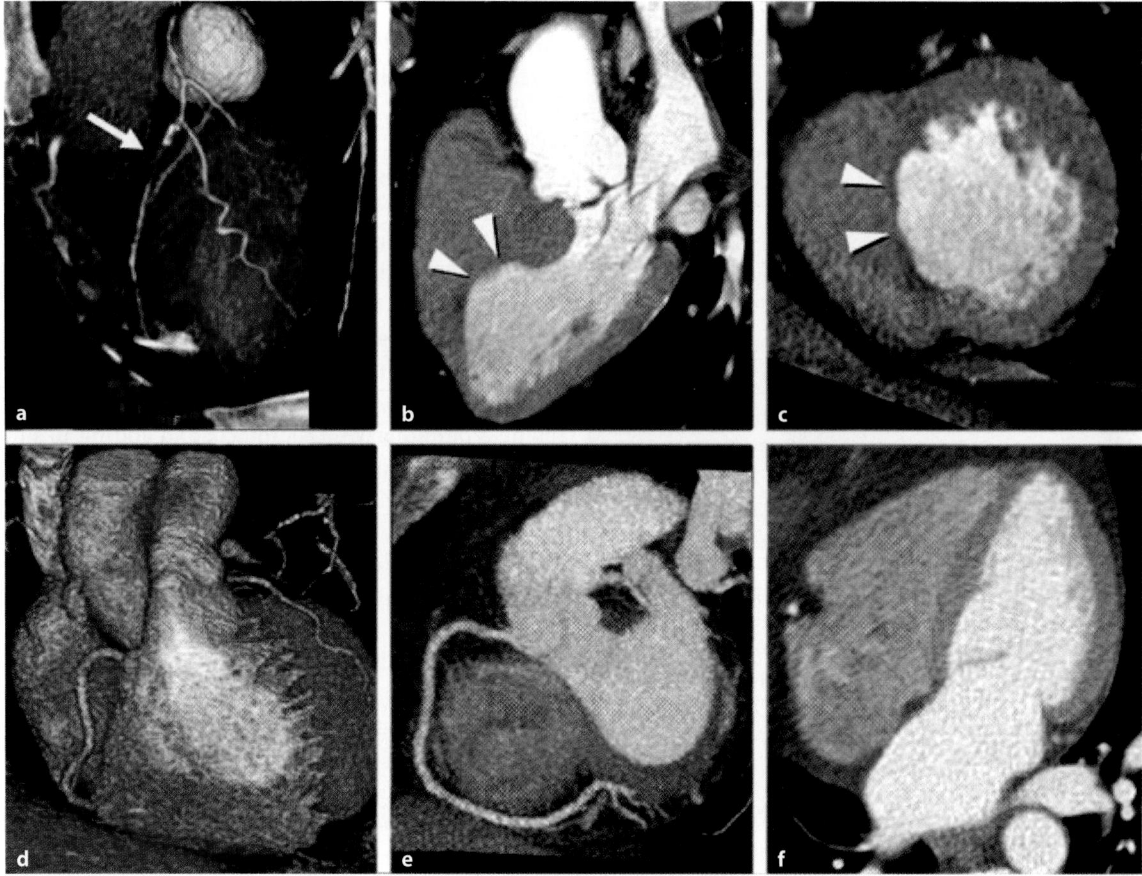

Fig. 4.4a–f. Right ventricular opacification in cardiac CT. Volume-rendered image (**a**), three-chamber view (**b**) and short-axis view (**c**) in a 68-year-old man with a short LAD occlusion [*arrow* in (**a**)]. Note that the thickness of the akinetic anterior septal wall (*arrowheads*) cannot be assessed due to the lack of right ventricular opacification. Coronary CT angiogram in an obese woman before gastric bypass surgery (**d–f**) and limited venous access (20-G cannula) shows good opacification of the left ventricle and the right coronary artery without major artifacts from right heart chambers (**e**,**f**). Adequate enhancement of the right heart chambers was achieved by using a comparably slow injection rate (4 ml/s) but a long injection duration (30 s) and long scanning delay relative to the aortic contrast medium transit time (t_{CMT} + 15). Recirculating contrast medium enhanced venous blood maintains right atrial and ventricular enhancement after the end of the main bolus

4.4.1 Basic Strategy: Injection Time Equals Scan Time

The traditional injection strategy for CTA – derived in the era of single-slice CT – was to inject CM for a duration that is equal to the scan time. Thus, for a 40-s abdominal CTA acquisition, the injection duration would also be 40 s, resulting in a fairly large CM dose of 160 ml if a typical injection flow rate of 4 ml/s was used. Scan timing was determined either by using a test bolus or by bolus tracking.

This basic strategy is still useful for many CTA applications as well as for cardiac CT whenever scan times are in the range of 10–20 s. Over the years of CT evolution with increasingly shorter scan times, the injection flow rates have also increased from 4 ml/s to 5 ml/s and even 6 ml/s. At the same time, the iodine concentration of the CM used has also increased from the traditional 300 mg I/ml to 350, 370, or 400 mg I/ml at most institutions. This is not at all surprising, because the lower opacification from shorter injections (a consequence of *Rule §2*) has to be compensated for by increasing the iodine flux (see *Rule §1*) (Fig. 4.5). By increasing the injection flow rate from 4 to 5 ml/s and using a contrast agent with, e.g., 350 rather than 300 mg I/ml concentration, the iodine flux and thus arterial enhancement is increased by 45%.

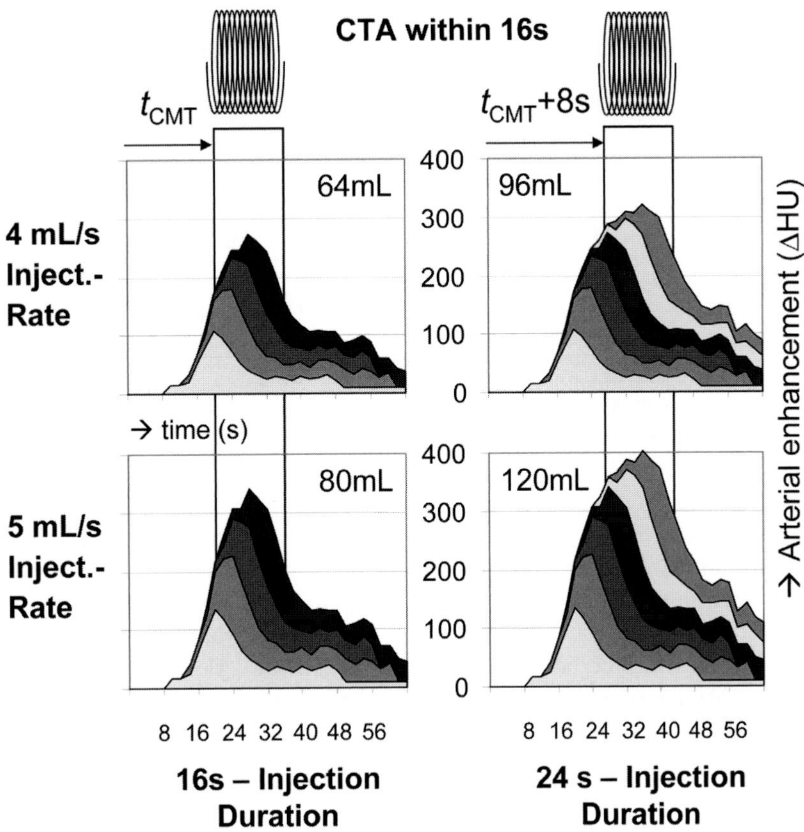

Fig. 4.5. Strategies to improve arterial enhancement with fast CT acquisitions. Two strategies to increase arterial enhancement compared to what can be achieved from a 16-s injection at 4 ml/s (*upper left panel*) can be employed – either alone or in combination: Increasing the injection rate from 4 to 5 ml/s increases the enhancement approximately 20% (*lower left panel*). Alternatively, one can also increase the injection duration and the scanning delay – taking advantage of the fact that enhancement increases with longer injection durations (*right upper panel*). Maximum enhancement can be achieved when both the injection rate (and/or the iodine concentration) as well as the injection duration are increased (*right lower panel*) simultaneously. From reference (Fleischmann 2005), with permission).

4.4.2 Basic Strategy with Additionally Increased Scanning Delay

With even faster scanners it became readily apparent that the basic strategy (injection duration equals scan time) alone is not applicable for scan times well below 10 s. It is not possible to achieve adequate arterial enhancement from, e.g., a 4-s injection duration to match a 4-s scan time. The injection flow rates that might allow this would simply be too high to be practical (15 ml/s), and scan timing would be even less forgiving. The obvious solution is simply to increase the injection duration and to increase the scanning delay accordingly – in other words, make use of *Rule §2*. Note that with this second approach, the injection duration is no longer equal to but rather longer than the scan time, and the scanning delay is not equal to but rather longer than the t_{CMT} (Fig. 4.5).

We use such a protocol for all 8- and 16-channel CT angiograms, and also for 64-channel coronary CTAs (Table 4.2): We use an injection rate of 5 ml/s (range: 4–6 ml/s) using 370 mg I/ml contrast agent. The injection duration is 8 s longer than the scan time (e.g., for a 12-s acquisition, we inject 5 ml/s for 20 s, resulting in a total volume of 100 ml). Automated bolus triggering is used to individualize the scanning delay such that the acquisition will start approximately 8 s after the CM arrives in the target vasculature ('t_{CMT}+8s').

Table 4.2. Injection protocol for 64-channel coronary CTA

Scan time injection duration: (scan time + 8 s)		10 s 18 s (10 s + 8 s)	12 s 20 s (12 s + 8 s)	14 s 22 s (14 s + 8 s)
Body weight	CM flow rate	CM volume	CM volume	CM volume
<55 kg	4.0 ml/s	72 ml	80 ml	88 ml
56–65 kg	4.5 ml/s	81 ml	90 ml	99 ml
66–85 kg	5.0 ml/s	90 ml	100 ml	110 ml
86–95 kg	5.5 ml/s	99 ml	110 ml	121 ml
>95 kg	6.0 ml/s	108 ml	120 ml	132 ml

CM: contrast medium (370 mg I/ml concentration)

4.4.3 Strategies for 64-Channel CT and Beyond: The Paradigm Shift

Short scan times certainly have advantages in the setting of CTA, such as shorter breath-holding, fewer motion artifacts, and – to some extent – less total volume of CM. However, fast CTA acquisitions also have disadvantages and using maximum scan speed may even be detrimental, because very fast acquisitions may not allow complete and sufficient opacification of a diseased arterial tree, even if timed correctly. This has been observed in mesenteric CTA, in aortic aneurysms, and most notably in lower extremity CT angiograms. Another difficulty with CTA injection protocols is that they are difficult to standardize across different patients and vascular territories because the acquisition times may be quite different, even within the same application.

So instead of the traditional paradigm, where the injection duration is chosen to match the scan time, the technical capabilities of modern 64-channel scanners allow us to reverse this paradigm, and now select the scan time, based on the injection protocol. The injection protocol is chosen such that it allows good opacification with reasonable injection flow rates for a wide range of patients.

Our current integrated acquisition and CM injection strategy for 64-channel CTA is therefore to deliberately slow down the CT acquisition and – importantly – use the same scan time for a given vascular territory for every patient (the pitch thus varies between patients). Automated tube-current modulation is used not only to avoid increasing the radiation dose to the patient, but also to control image noise. The user is thus able to set the desired image noise for a given CT application, which will then be constant within individuals and vary only mildly across individuals. When the same scan time is used for all patients, one can always use the same injection duration as well. For example, we have chosen a scan time of 10 s for abdominal CTA, with an injection duration of 18 s and a scanning delay of t_{CMT} + 8 s, as determined by bolus triggering (Table 4.3). This strategy allows breath-holding for virtually all patients. It results in reliably strong arterial enhancement because of both high iodine flux and increased scanning delay relative to the t_{CMT}, while avoiding excessive injection flow rates. Image noise is constant within and across individuals by using automated tube current modulation. The final advantage of always using the same injection duration is that now injection flow rates (and volumes) can easily be adjusted to body weight.

4.5 Conclusion

CM delivery remains an integral part of cardiovascular CT. While CT technology continues to evolve, the physiologic and pharmacokinetic principles of arterial enhancement will remain unchanged in the foreseeable future. A basic understanding of early contrast medium dynamics thus provides the foundation for the design of current and future CM injection protocols. With these tools in hand, CM utilization can be optimized for various clinical applications of CT and optimized for each patient. This ensures optimal CM utilization while exploiting the full capabilities of continuously evolving MDCT technology.

Table 4.3. Integrated 64-channel MDCT acquisition and injection protocol for abdominal CTA

Acquisition	64×0.6 mm (number of channels × channel width); automated tube current modulation (250 quality reference mAs)		
Pitch	Variable (depends on volume coverage, usually <1.0)		
Scan time	FIXED to 10 s (in all patients)		
Injection duration	FIXED to 18 s (in all patients)		
Scanning delay	t_{CMT}+8 s (scan starts 8 s after CM arrives in the aorta, as established with automated bolus triggering)		
Contrast medium	High concentration (370 mgI/ml)		
Injection flow rates and volumes	Individualized to body weight		
	Body weight	CM flow rate	CM volume
	<55 kg	4.0 ml/s	72 ml
	56–65 kg	4.5 ml/s	81 ml
	66–85 kg	5.0 ml/s	90 ml
	86–95 kg	5.5 ml/s	99 ml
	>95 kg	6.0 ml/s	108 ml

CM: contrast medium; t_{CMT} : contrast medium transit time

References

Bae KT, Heiken JP, Brink JA (1998) Aortic and hepatic contrast medium enhancement at CT. Part II. Effect of reduced cardiac output in a porcine model. Radiology 207:657–662

Claussen CD, Banzer D, Pfretzschner C, Kalender WA, Schorner W (1984) Bolus geometry and dynamics after intravenous contrast-medium injection. Radiology 153:365–368

Dawson P, Blomley MJ (1996) Contrast agent pharmacokinetics revisited: I. Reformulation. Acad Radiol 3 (Suppl 2):S261–263

Fleischmann D (2002) Present and future trends in multiple detector-row CT applications: CT angiography. Eur Radiol 12:S11–S16

Fleischmann D (2003) Techniques for contrast media injections. In: Schoepf UJ (ed) Multidetector-row CT of the thorax. Springer, Berlin Heidelberg New York, pp 47–59

Fleischmann D (2005) Contrast-medium administration. In: Catalano C, Passariello R (eds) Multidetector-row CT angiography. Springer, Berlin Heidelberg New York, pp 41–54

Fleischmann D, Hittmair K (1999) Mathematical analysis of arterial enhancement and optimization of bolus geometry for CT angiography using the discrete fourier transform. J Comput Assist Tomogr 23:474–484

Hittmair K, Fleischmann D (2001) Accuracy of predicting and controlling time-dependent aortic enhancement from a test bolus injection. J Comput Assist Tomogr 25:287–294

Sheiman RG, Raptopoulos V, Caruso P, Vrachliotis T, Pearlman J (1996) Comparison of tailored and empiric scan delays for CT angiography of the abdomen. Am J Roentgenol 167:725–729

Van Hoe L, Marchal G, Baert AL, Gryspeerdt S, Mertens L (1995) Determination of scan delay time in spiral CT angiography: utility of a test bolus injection. J Comput Assist Tomogr 19:216–220

Dose Reduction in Chest CT

5

JOHN R. MAYO and JOHN ALDRICH

CONTENTS

5.1 Introduction

The invention and rapid development of computerized tomography is one of the major medical advances of our time. Current multidetector CT scanners can image the entire chest in 2–5 s, producing up to 1,000 slices, each composed of sub-millimeter isometric voxels. These high signal-to-noise ratio, large field-of-view images provide non-invasive anatomic evaluation of the chest with similar information content to that achievable at autopsy. In vivo physiologic functional information regarding the pulmonary vasculature, systemic vasculature or airways can be obtained by acquiring CT images while administering intravenous contrast media or performing breathing maneuvers, respectively. Expert radiological interpretation of these volume data sets can differentiate diseases that are clinically indistinguishable, but demonstrate unique changes at the gross anatomic level.

For example, a previously well patient presenting to the emergency room with acute shortness of breath, pleuritic chest pain and a normal chest physical examination has clinical findings consistent with pulmonary embolism, early pneumonia or a small pneumothorax. The chest radiograph cannot differentiate these possibilities with confidence. However, contrast-enhanced chest CT can simultaneously examine the pulmonary vasculature, lung parenchyma and pleural space with high accuracy in a single 5-min examination, facilitating rapid and confident triage and treatment for this common emergency room problem.

This unique diagnostic power makes CT the first choice examination for many adult and pediatric clinical presentations and accounts for the explosive growth in of CT examinations in the last 20 years. Multiple studies have documented this dramatic increase in CT utilization in industrialized countries over the last 20 years. In a study performed at an academic institution in the US, METTLER et al. (2000) found that CT accounted for 6.1% of radiological examinations in 1990, increasing to 11.1% by 1999. Similar findings have been reported in studies from the UK (SHRIMPTON and EDYVEAN 1998) and Canada (ALDRICH et al. 2006).

However, the increased utilization of CT comes with a price, increased population radiation exposure. In most cases adding CT to diagnostic imaging algorithms has substantially increased patient X-ray radiation exposure. For example, a chest CT (3–6 mSv) has 60 to 120 times the radiation dose of the postero-anterior (PA) chest radiograph (0.05 mSv). In addition, since CT is so available and easy to perform, it is liberally applied to ex-

J. R. MAYO, MD, Professor of Radiology and Cardiology
J. ALDRICH, PhD, Professor of Radiology
Department of Radiology, University of British Columbia, 899 W 12th Avenue, Vancouver BC V5Z 1M9, Canada

clude potentially serious, but statistically unlikely diagnoses, often solely to reassure anxious patients and clinicians. The net result is greatly increased CT utilization and resulting population radiation dose. It is noted that in some situations, CT has replaced radiological examinations with higher dose (e.g., bronchography, nuclear medicine ventilation perfusion scintigraphy followed by pulmonary angiography) while providing equivalent or superior diagnostic information, but these situations are in the minority.

The increased radiation dose of chest CT compared to the PA chest radiograph arises from two properties of the CT technique (Sprawls 1992). First, unlike analogue film radiography in which the image acquisition and display are both reliant on the film, CT is a digital technique in which image acquisition and display can be independently manipulated. Therefore, when CT dose is excessive, the image does not become too dark (as it does in film radiography), but instead improves because of decreased image noise (Rothenberg and Pentlow 1992). Second, visualization of image noise is enhanced by the ability to map the entire visible gray scale onto a selected segment of the CT number scale. As a result, image degradation due to quantum noise (mottle) is easily visible and may interfere with image interpretation. As a result of these two effects and the overwhelming drive of radiologists for the very best image quality to support high levels of diagnostic accuracy and confidence, CT images are often obtained using high radiation exposure to the patient. Studies in many countries have shown wide variation in the level of radiation used for equivalent CT examinations among institutions (Shrimpton and Edyvean 1998; Aldrich et al. 2006). In addition, studies have shown radiologists, referring clinicians and patients may be unaware of the high level of radiation exposure associated with CT examinations, further contributing to its use in low-yield situations (Lee et al. 2004). It is noted excessive radiation exposure can occur with plain radiographic digital imaging modalities such as computed radiography (CR) and digital radiography (DR), but the base level of exposure in these modalities is much lower.

In the early 1990s concern was raised regarding radiation dose in chest CT (Di Marco and Briones 1993; Naidich et al. 1994; Di Marco and Renston 1994). The authors of these studies concluded that these CT data demonstrated that greater consideration needed to be given to optimizing CT exposures. In spite of these early warnings, the development of multidetector row CT scanner, the increase in the number of CT scanners and the development of new high-radiation dose CT chest techniques (e.g., cardiac CT) have increased the magnitude of the problem.

The purpose of this chapter is to outline (1) evidence indicating the detrimental effect of radiation dose at the level administered in chest CT examinations, (2) parameters that affect CT radiation dose, (3) advances in dose reduction in the chest CT and (4) the interaction between CT radiation dose and diagnostic accuracy. A complete review of radiation dosimetry and bioeffects is beyond the scope of this chapter.

5.2 Radiation Bioeffects

There has been considerable debate within the medical community regarding the risk of low-level radiation exposure from CT. The reason for this debate arises from the complexity of the data supporting the detrimental effect of ionizing radiation on humans. In broad overview the detrimental effects of ionizing radiation can be divided into two major categories, deterministic and stochastic effects.

Deterministic effects, skin erythema, skin necrosis and hair loss only occur above a threshold dose that lies well above those administered in diagnostic chest CT examinations. Radiation exposure at deterministic dose levels is usually only seen in complex interventional cases and will not be discussed further in this chapter. By comparison, stochastic effects are believed to have no radiation dose threshold and can occur at the low doses delivered in chest CT. Mechanistically, stochastic effects are believed to be mediated by chemical damage to the DNA molecule and clinically manifest as an increased risk of cancer and genetic defects. Stochastic effects occur randomly and the risk of occurrence is dependent on the type of ionizing radiation administered, the tissue receiving the radiation and the age of the subject at the time of exposure. It is believed that dose fractionation, a substantial modifier of detrimental effect for deterministic radiation doses, does not substantially modify the stochastic risk (Ullrich et al. 1987).

Subjects exposed to the atomic bomb explosions in 1945 are the most extensively studied radiation exposure cohort. This group is unique since it is large, covers all ages, has been extensively studied over 60 years and was not selected on the basis of underlying disease. It is estimated that a substantial subgroup of the 25,000 survivors received less than 50 mSv, a low level of exposure, approximating the dose range delivered by multiple chest CT exams. The major observed effect in the group that received low doses of radiation (5 to 150 mSv) has been an increase in the risk of cancer over the past 60 years. It is noted that the effect has been an increase in the number of cancers, not an earlier presentation of cancers. However, these data must be extrapolated to even lower dose levels to predict the cancer risk associated with radiation exposure from a single chest CT, and the nature of this extrapolation has proven to be highly controversial.

Disagreement among experts has been based on three non-resolvable issues: uncertainty in the actual radiation exposure received by individuals exposed to nuclear explosion since on-site radiation dose measurements were not obtained, differences in the natural cancer risk of the Japanese population compared to other populations and the different quality of the radiation imparted by atomic bombs compared to X-ray-based medical imaging. As a result of these controversies, learned societies have come to varying conclusions on the risk attributable to radiation exposure at the levels found in chest CT. The International Commission on Radiological Protection, or ICRP, used a linear no-threshold extrapolation of nuclear explosion data and estimated 50 additional fatal cancers induced per million people exposed to 1 mSv of medical radiation (ICRP-60 1991). In contrast the French Academy of Science concluded there was not sufficient evidence to support an increased cancer risk associated with radiation exposures less that 20 mSv (Tubiana et al. 2005), a level above that delivered in chest CT examinations (<6 mSv). Further conflicting evidence on the impact of low-level radiation exposure is found in tissue culture experimental studies that have shown induction of free radical detoxification mechanisms with low-level radiation exposure (Strzelczyk et al. 2007). This has led some to suggest that low-level radiation exposure, at the same level as that used in chest CT, may be beneficial, an effect known as radiation hermesis.

In 2007 additional important data were added to the debate regarding the cancer induction effect of low-level radiation (Cardis et al. 2007). The 15-country study reported on the cancer induction effect of low-level radiation exposure in 407,000 radiation workers who were followed for over 20 years, providing 5.2 million person-years of follow-up. This study is unique as it reports on the largest cohort to date, has accurate dosimetry and investigated multiethnic workers. Ninety percent of the subjects received a dose less than 50 mSv, and on average each worker received a dose of 19 mSv. Therefore, this study is reporting on low-level doses close to those received during a single chest CT examination (3–6 mSv). This study found an excess relative risk (ERR) for all-cause mortality of 0.42 per Sievert (0.00042 per mSv) with a statistically significant increasing excess relative risk with increasing radiation dose ($P < 0.02$), indicating a dose-response effect. The increased risk in all-cause mortality was mainly due to an increase in mortality from all cancers.

A sub-analysis stratified by dose categories (less than 400, 200, 150 and 100 mSv) showed that the risk estimates were not driven by cancers seen in the highest dose categories. Therefore, this study, which is the largest study of low-dose protracted exposure to ionizing radiation to date, supports the concept that there is a small cancer risk from the low dose of ionizing radiation delivered in CT examinations. These new data add supportive evidence to the concern over radiation dose delivered in chest CT examinations and support the use of the ALARA principle (As Low As Reasonably Achievable) for these exams. It is noted that only workers were studied; thus, there is no information on children, and since 90% of the workers were men who received over 98% of the cumulative dose, limited information is available on the effect in women.

The influence of age at exposure and of sex has been studied in the nuclear explosion cohort, showing that radiation risk is modified by these subject factors (Pierce et al. 1996; Brenner et al. 2001). The increased radiation sensitivity of children is felt to arise from two biologic facts: they have more time to express the cancer-inducing effect of radiation and they have more rapidly dividing cells than adults that are inherently more radiation sensitive.

It has been found that women have approximately twice the risk compared to males for the same level of radiation exposure. Increased female risk is heightened in chest CT by the presence of radiosensitive breast tissue in the radiated field. Radiation dose to breast tissue has been calculated (Parker et al. 2005) and directly measured (Hurwitz et al. 2006;

MILNE 2006) with a wide variation in reported average values, ranging from 10 to 70 mGy. The variation in values is related to CT parameter settings, differences in size and configuration of breast tissue, and methods to calculate or directly measure radiation dose. Clearly, all CT-associated breast radiation dose values reported are substantial when compared with the average glandular dose of 3 mGy for standard two-view screening mammography. It is noted that there is a strong effect of age at exposure for breast tissue, with lower risk for subjects (BRENNER 2004) above the age of 40. These factors must be taken into account in setting chest CT radiation dose parameters in CT chest examinations for women. Breast shields, thyroid shields (FRICKE et al. 2003; HOPPER et al. 1997) and X-ray tube current modulation techniques have been employed to decrease radiation dose to these superficial and radiosensitive tissues within the chest. These techniques have been shown to decrease breast radiation exposure delivered in chest CT scans. However, these dose-modifying techniques must be used with due consideration of their impact on image diagnostic quality.

5.3 Radiation Dose Measurement

There are many methods currently in use for quantifying ionizing radiations (Table 5.1) (HUDA 1997). The fact that several methods exist attests to the complexity of this issue. In our opinion the most simple radiation dose measure is effective dose, a parameter that allows easy comparison of the detrimental effect of radiation exposure among different radiological examinations on different body parts.

Effective dose is a measurement that estimates the whole body dose that would be required to produce the same stochastic risk as the partial body dose that was actually delivered in a localized CT scan. It is useful because it allows comparison of CT dose to other types of radiation exposure such as whole body radiation exposure secondary to natural background radiation. Effective dose is calculated by summing the absorbed doses to individual organs weighted for their radiation sensitivity (ICRP-60 1991). The measurement unit is the sievert (Sv) or milli-sievert (mSv). Since an effective dose requires determination of absorbed dose to each body organ multiplied by their radiation sensitivity, the distribution of radiation dose in the body must be determined. Chest CT has a markedly asymmetric dose distribution, with higher dose found peripherally and lower dose centrally due to the shielding effects of body tissue. This makes it difficult to calculate the exact effective dose for each patient. Instead, a simpler calculation is performed (Fig. 5.1). Scanner manufacturers use dose data derived from measurements made in head and body phantoms to determine a weighted CT dose index (CTDI) for each CT scanner model at all available selections of tube voltage (kVp), tube current (mA) and rotation time (s). The selected pitch value is then incorporated to produce a CT exposure index, the $CTDI_{VOL}$. Once the scan length is determined from the topogram, the appropriate $CTDI_{VOL}$ is combined with the actual length scanned in the patient to calculate the dose length product (DLP). Since the administered radiation dose is linearly related to the length scanned in the patient, the scanned volume should be tightly

Table 5.1. Methods of quantifying ionizing radiation. Reprinted with permission from MAYO et al. Radiology 2003; 228: p 16, Table 5.1

Method	Conventional units	International System of Units, or SI
Radiation exposure	roentgens (R)	coulombs per kilogram (C/kg)
Absorbed dose	rads (rad)	grays (Gy) [b]
Equivalent dose	rems	sieverts (Sv) [c]
Effective dose	Effective dose equivalent (Sv) [a]	

Note–Abbreviations of the units of measure are in parentheses.
[a] 1977 tissue-weighting factors.
[b] D multiplied by ICRP radiation weighting factor WR. The WR for X-rays is 1.
[c] 1990 tissue-weighting factors.

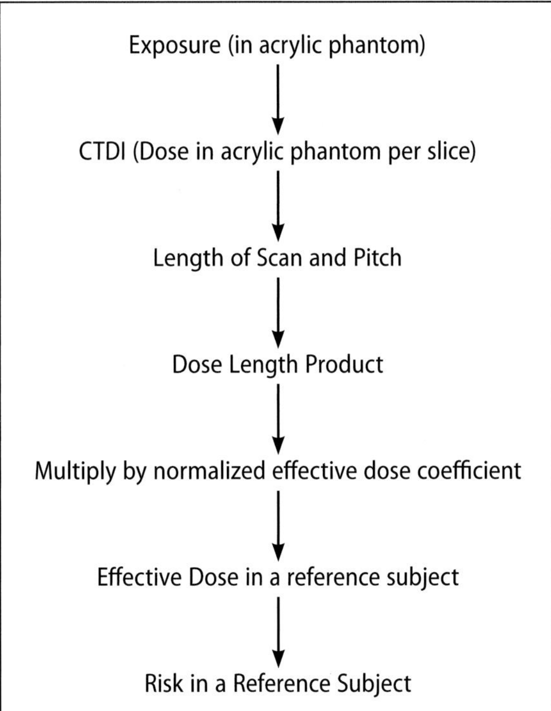

Fig. 5.1. Diagram shows algorithm for the estimation of radiation exposure risk from CT

confined to the region of interest. Inadequate anatomic training of technicians can lead to expanded scanned volumes, which can substantially increase radiation dose.

The DLP is a measure of the radiation dose delivered to that patient during the scan. An estimated effective dose for that scan can then be calculated by multiplying the DLP value by the normalized effective dose coefficients (Table 5.2) for the scanned body part. This normalized effective dose coefficient accounts for the radiation sensitivity of the body region scanned based on its composition. The DLP value is shown on the current the CT scanner displays once the topogram has been obtained and the region to be scanned prescribed. In chest CT, multiplying the DLP by 0.017 allows the radiologist or technologist to easily calculate the estimated effective dose of the examination prior to scan acquisition. The DLP value can also be archived in the picture archiving and communication system (PACS) by storing the protocol page. Newer DICOM standards for CT enable the storage of dose data in the DICOM header of each examination. Use of the DLP value provides a convenient and quick tool to assess CT effective dose values and compare to established standards.

Table 5.2. Dose length product (DLP) to effective dose (E) conversion coefficients

Study	E/DLP (mSv/mGy cm)
Head	0.0023
Chest	0.017
Abdomen	0.015
Abdomen-plevis	0.017
Pelvis	0.019

Radiation dose surveys have noted wide variations in DLP settings for identical examinations between institutions (Shrimpton and Edyvean 1998; Aldrich et al. 2006; Panzer et al. 1989; Nishizawa et al. 1991). To decrease this variation and protect the public from inadvertent overexposure, the European Community (2000) has published suggested reference dose values for chest CT examinations, with a DLP value of 650 mGy·cm. This reference dose value was obtained by surveying a large number of institutions in Europe and adopting the 75th percentile of responses as the reference dose values. This value serves as a guide to acceptable practice in any institution.

5.4 Scanner Radiation Efficiency

Several physical aspects of CT scanners result in wasted radiation dose. These include the shielding effect of the collimator between the patient and the detector (post patient collimator), imperfect collimation of the X-ray beam and movement of the X-ray focal spot. The sum of all these effects is measured by the geometric efficiency of the CT scanner.

Single-detector-row CT scanners with their wide detectors typically have higher geometric efficiency than multi-detector row scanners. The decreased geometric efficiency of multi-detector row CT scanners arises from three major factors: the gaps between detector elements in the array, the effect of focal spot penumbra and the motion of the focal spot. Since the focal spot of the X-ray tube is not a point, the collimator cannot perfectly collimate the beam. Therefore, the edge of the beam, or penumbra, has spatially varying X-ray intensity. In single-detector-row helical CT scanners, this portion of the beam can be detected and used in the reconstruction process. With multi-detector row CT scanners, however, use of the penumbra would result in different readings from detectors in this region compared with those in the central, or umbra, portion of the beam. Therefore, the active detectors in multi-detector row CT scanners measure only the umbra or non-varying part of the X-ray beam. Radiation in the penumbra falls on inactive detectors or off the edge of the detector array and is discarded, although it contributes to patient radiation dose. In addition, thermal and mechanical stresses within the X-ray tube cause the focal spot to move. As a result, the X-ray beam wanders slightly across the detector array during CT data acquisition. Widening the X-ray beam to compensate for the penumbra and focal spot motion leads to a decrease in the geometric efficiency and an increase in the radiation dose. Because the penumbra is a fixed size, its effect is greatest on four-section CT scanners operating with thin-section collimation. The effect is progressively less severe with 8-, 16-, 32- and 64-section multi-detector row CT scanners. Manufacturers have devised beam-tracking systems to stabilize the position of the X-ray beam and thereby minimize the radiation-wasting effect of focal spot motion (Toth et al. 2000).

CT scanners require a minimum of 180 degrees of raw scan data (projections) to reconstruct an image. This requirement, coupled with helical scan acquisition, results in wasted radiation dose to the patient at the top and the bottom of the scanned volume. This effect is proportionally most substantial when small volumes are scanned and is most pronounced in children. In the chest this effect can increase radiation dose by up to 36 percent (Tzedakis et al. 2005). Z over-scanning can be minimized by modifying the motion of the collimators at the beginning and the end of the scan.

Scattered radiation is formed by the interaction of the primary beam with the body of the patient. Scattered radiation exits the body in all directions, and if detected it reduces contrast and may generate artifacts. Because of scatter and imperfect collimation, the radiation intensity profile does not fall to zero at the edge of the nominal section width. It has been shown by using a single-section CT scanner that contiguous sections generate a peak radiation dose approximately 50% greater than that of a single CT section (10-mm collimation, 10-mm table increment, measured at the surface of a 15-cm head phantom) (Pentlow et al. 1977). Helical CT scanning with a pitch of 1 results in a dose distribution that is essentially equivalent to that of contiguous single-detector row CT imaging (McGee and Humphreys 1994).

CT detectors vary in their efficiency. Ideally, a detector should count all incident beam X-ray photons. Depending on the technology used, however, detectors will record only 60% (high-pressure xenon detectors) to 95% (solid-state detectors) of the incident X-ray photons. All multi-detector row scanners use solid state detectors. The accuracy of conversion of the absorbed X-ray signal into an electrical signal is known as the conversion efficiency. The overall dose efficiency of the scanner is the product of the geometric efficiency, the quantum detection efficiency and the conversion efficiency (Cunningham 1995). The overall dose efficiency can vary substantially between scanners. Noise is also introduced by the electronics of the data acquisition system of the scanner. The sum of quantum noise and electronic noise results in differences in image quality between scanners at the same radiation dose.

CT is similar to other radiological techniques in that the primary X-ray beam is filtered to eliminate low-energy photons, which would be preferentially absorbed relative to high-energy photons and contribute to radiation dose. With CT, additional spatially varying filtration is often placed in the primary X-ray beam. These filters reduce (1) the necessary dynamic range of the detector system in the periphery of the detector array and (2) the radiation dose for larger fields of view. They are often referred to as bow-tie filters because of their shape, and they create variations in entrance radiation exposure depending on both the size of the object and its position in the field of view. For some CT scanners, multiple filters of varying shapes are moved into place based on the specified field of view of the scan. In other scanners these filters are permanently positioned. These filters substantially reduce radiation dose of CT scans in adult patients, but they are less effective in pediatric patients. These filters can interact with radiation dose reduction systems if patients are incorrectly centered within the CT scanner bore leading to increased radiation dose (Li et al. 2007). Technologists must be aware of this effect and carefully center patients within the CT gantry.

5.5 Radiation Dose Reduction at the CT Scanner Level

Reduction in radiation dose results in increased image noise and decreased image quality. Studies assessing the subjective evaluation of chest CT scans have demonstrated that radiologists consistently gave higher image-quality scores to images obtained with a higher radiation dose (HAAGA et al. 1991; MAYO et al. 1995). Image noise is easily measured by placing a region of interest (> 100 pixels) in an area of uniform density in the body (e.g., the thoracic aorta) (SPRAWLS 1992). The standard deviation of the pixel values represents image noise. It is noted that the choice of reconstruction algorithm greatly influences the resultant image noise, and higher noise is obtained by using high-spatial-frequency reconstruction algorithms (e.g., bone or lung algorithms) rather than low-spatial-frequency algorithms (e.g., standard, soft-tissue algorithm). High-spatial-frequency reconstruction algorithms are most commonly used when one is searching for fine structures within bones or lung tissue. The increase in image noise associated with the high-spatial-frequency algorithm is not a problem in these applications, because of the high radiographic contrast of these tissues.

Radiation dose and image noise can be modified by adjusting the tube current, scan time and tube voltage. In practice, the tube current is most frequently adjusted to change the radiation dose and image noise. In most CT scanners, the tube current is adjustable in steps from 20 mA to approximately 400 mA. The radiation dose can also be linearly affected by scan time, but the time is usually minimized in imaging of the chest to reduce the effect of patient motion. Increasing the tube voltage increases the output of the X-ray tube. If the tube current and scan times are not changed, decreasing the tube voltage will decrease the radiation dose to the patient. Changes in tube voltage also affect CT tissue attenuation values, which can change tissue contrast in a complex fashion. Tube voltage may be reduced when scanning smaller patients, especially if intravenous contrast media is administered. The lower tube current will increase the subject contrast provided by the contrast media and provide diagnostic scans at reduced radiation dose. It is noted that the radiation exposure delivered at a given tube voltage and current setting will vary greatly between CT scanners of different models and manufacturers because of differences in scanner geometry (X-ray tube-to-patient separation) and X-ray tube filtration.

Helical CT scanners introduced a new parameter: pitch. For single-detector row helical CT scanners, pitch is defined as the table travel per 360° X-ray tube rotation divided by the beam collimation (POLACIN et al. 1992). In many cases the table feed (e.g., 5 mm per X-ray tube rotation) and beam collimation (e.g., 5 mm) are identical, and the resultant pitch is 1. This yields one helical turn per section thickness and a radiation exposure essentially equal to that of contiguous transverse sections. However, the table can be made to feed more rapidly (e.g., 10 mm per X-ray tube rotation) without changing the beam collimation (5 mm). This results in a pitch of 2. Examinations with pitch values greater than 1 cover larger volumes in shorter times, which provides either reduced motion artifact or a larger area of coverage. On single-slice scanners, examinations obtained with elevated pitch have lower image quality because the section profile is broadened. However, the radiation dose delivered by the examination is decreased by the value of the pitch (e.g., one-half of the radiation exposure for a pitch of 2) if the tube voltage and current are kept constant. It should be noted that in many multi-detector row scanners, the tube current is automatically increased to compensate for increased noise at higher pitch values, which eliminates the reduction in radiation dose. Some manufacturers report the mA value as effective mA (eff mA), the actual tube current (mA) divided by the pitch value to directly account for the relative change in tube current with the change in the pitch value. Multi-detector row scanners have a complex relationship among detector configuration, reconstructed slice thickness, reconstruction algorithm and resultant spatial resolution, contrast resolution and image noise. As a result the selection of specific acquisition parameters may require some experimentation to obtain a favorable trade off between acquisition parameters, image quality and radiation dose. A medical physicist may be helpful in exploring this complex data space.

Overlapping sections or helical CT scanning with a pitch of less than 1 results in increased radiation dose. In cardiac-gated CT, the reconstruction must be synchronized to the cardiac cycle to eliminate heart motion. For heart rates between 50 and 80 beats per minute using a single-tube scanner (Siemens Sensation 64 Cardiac, Siemens Medical Solutions, Erlangan, Germany) with a gantry rotation time of approximately 350 ms, a pitch of 0.2 must be used to ensure that there is a complete set of projection data available for every location at all points in the cardiac cycle. This low pitch value creates a radiation dose build-up effect known as helical overscan. Using a pitch of 0.2 increases the radiation dose of a cardiac-gated scan by a factor of 7 over a non-cardiac-gated scan (pitch 1.4) using equivalent kVp and mA values. This effect accounts for the very high dose (15–20 mSv) of these single-tube retrospectively gated cardiac acquisitions. Using a dual-tube cardiac-gated CT scanner, the data acquisition rate is twice that of a single tube scanner, allowing an increase in the pitch value from 0.2 to 0.5 as heart rates increase from below 50 to above 100 beats per minute. This provides a corresponding decrease in the radiation dose of the examination as the heart rate increases. All retrospective helical examinations are also susceptible to step artifacts if the patient breaths or the heart rate is irregular during the examination.

Modulating the tube current (mA) according to the phase of the cardiac cycle is another approach to reduce the dose of cardiac-gated CT examinations. In most cases the coronary arteries are best viewed during late diastole (65–85% of the R to R interval) when the heart is relatively motionless. This is especially true for those vessels that run in the atrioventricular groove, the right and circumflex coronary arteries. Optimal imaging of coronary vessels is achieved using a high spatial resolution acquisition at high dose in late diastole. Using ECG pulsing the tube current is decreased by 80% or 96% in the remainder of the cardiac cycle providing a radiation dose reduction of approximately 50% (8 mSv) or 70% (5 mSv) over the non-ECG pulsed exam (16 mSv). Reducing the tube current by 70% provides noisy but diagnostic images of the left ventricular chamber and valves (Fig. 5.2). If the tube current is reduced by 94%, images are cannot be reconstructed, and no functional information of the left ventricular chamber or valves is provided.

Another approach dose reduction in cardiac CT is the elimination of helical overscan through the use of a cardiac-gated step and shoot technique. This acquisition scheme provides a non-helical scan gated to the relatively motion-free 65% to 85% portion of the R-to-R interval. Depending on the width of the detector, rapidity of table movement and the overlap between adjacent slice clusters, cardiac scan times of 5 to 10 s can be achieved. The dose savings are substantial, with complete coronary artery evalua-

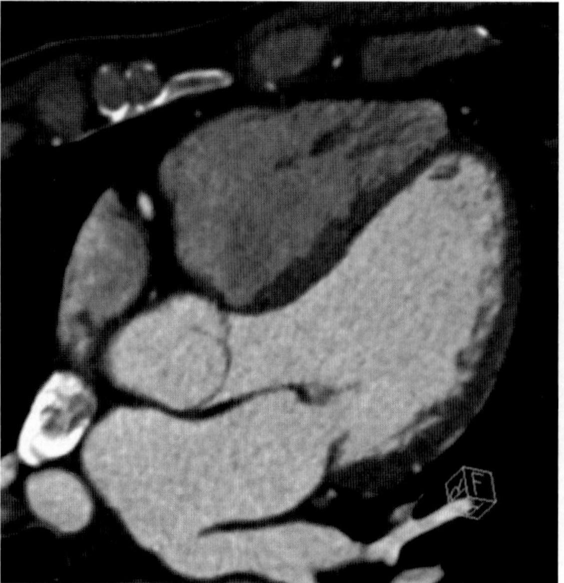

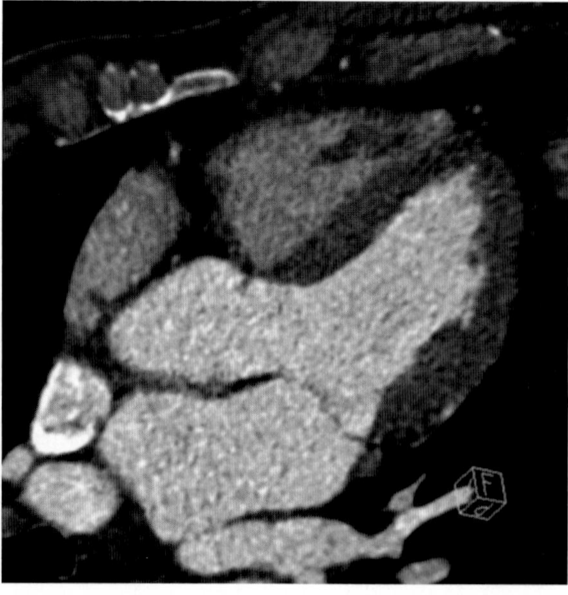

Fig. 5.2a,b. Helical retrospectively cardiac-gated chest CT scan in a 48-year-old male with atypical chest pain showing the effects of ECG tube current modulation. **a** Image obtained in mid diastole (75% of the R-to-R interval) reconstructed using 1-mm slice thickness at 1-mm spacing at high tube current shows a low noise three-chamber image with associated high radiation dose. **b** Image obtained in mid systole (30% of the R-to-R interval) reconstructed using 1-mm slice thickness at 1-mm spacing shows higher noise image obtained at low radiation dose, adequate for assessment of left ventricular regional wall thickness and in cine mode, regional wall motion

tion using 1.5 to 4 mSv. Similar to the highest levels of ECG tube current modulation in retrospective helical acquisitions, no functional information regarding left ventricular motion or valve motion is available. The multiple table steps required by 32- and 64-detector-row scanners make this technique as susceptible to breathing artifacts and heart rate variations as the retrospective helical technique.

A low-dose cardiac acquisition can be acquired using a shoot-only technique using the recently released scanner equipped with a 320-row detector array and a cone beam reconstruction. The advantage of this approach is the elimination of artifacts secondary to breathing and heart rate variation since the entire cardiac volume is acquired in one heartbeat. A non-helically acquired multiphase cardiac acquisition is also possible using this large detector, which with tube current modulation should provide anatomic views of the coronary arteries and functional information with dose similar to the retrospective helical acquisition. Although conceptually promising, further experience is required with this large detector array scanner to establish its clinical utility.

In the past, the tube current of CT scanners was uniform at all angles around the patient and for the full longitudinal (cranial caudal) extent of the scan. However, the chest is an elliptical object that has higher attenuation from left to right than from anterior to posterior. Attenuation also varies as the chest is scanned longitudinally from cranial to caudal. CT image quality is disproportionately degraded by views with few photons (photon starvation) compared to the image quality improvement associated with views with high photon counts. To address this issue, manufacturers have introduced programs that adjust the tube current depending on the attenuation of the object in both the transverse (x, y) and longitudinal (z) directions to minimize either photon-starved or photon-rich projections, maximizing image quality while minimizing radiation dose. This tube current modulation technique has been shown to produce a substantial reduction in radiation dose (Kalender et al. 1999a,b; Greess et al. 2000) with minimal degradation of image quality. Routine use of dose modulation systems is recommended as they compensate for asymmetry in the size and density of the body section being scanned, resulting in a signal-to-noise ratio that is adequate for diagnosis but is not excessive (Tack et al. 2003). However, these dose modulation systems may interact with the patient positioning and intrinsic beam filtering, producing increased radiation dose in patients who are incorrectly centered with the bore of the CT scanner. Algorithms to automatically center patients in the CT scanner bore are being developed (Li et al. 2007). In the interim, technologist's attention to patient position is an important component of radiation dose reduction. Tube current modulation schemes in association with novel reconstruction techniques have also been developed to reduce radiation dose to superficial radiation-sensitive tissues in the chest, most notably the breast and thyroid. Further experience with these new radiation dose modulation systems is required before they can be widely employed.

Repeated scanning of the same region (e.g., unenhanced and contrast-material enhanced) increases the radiation dose in a linear fashion. Therefore, if unenhanced CT is routinely performed prior to the contrast-enhanced CT with both using the same technical parameters, the radiation dose is doubled. This dose build-up effect can be reduced if the unenhanced CT is a reduced tube current low-dose acquisition or a gapped high-resolution study (e.g., 1-mm collimation at 10-mm spacing), for which the radiation dose is 10% of that of contiguous conventional CT or helical CT with a pitch of 1.

Finally, in addition to optimal patient centering, technologists can act as major contributors to patient radiation dose reduction by limiting the scanned volume to the region of interest and adjustment of the tube current based on the patient's size (Aldrich et al. 2006). Optimal dose reduction strategies require close communication and cooperation between the radiologist, technologist and medical physicist.

5.6 Dose Reduction in Chest CT

The concept of reduced tube current for conventional 10-mm collimation chest CT was introduced in 1990 by Naidich et al., who demonstrated acceptable image quality for assessment of lung parenchyma with low tube current settings (20 mAs). While these images were adequate for assessing lung parenchyma, they had a considerable increase in noise, which resulted in marked degradation of image quality with mediastinal windows. For this reason the authors noted that such low-dose techniques were most suited for assessment of children and possibly for screening the lung parenchyma of patients at high risk for lung cancer. These recommendations have been implemented and further studied in lung cancer screening programs (Henschke et al. 1999; Itoh et al. 2000; Swensen et al. 2002) (Fig. 5.3).

Similar dose reduction strategies have been applied to thin-section CT (also known as high-resolution CT) of the chest performed on single-section CT scanners. In these images, no significant difference in lung parenchymal structures was seen between low-dose (40 mAs) and high-dose (400 mAs) thin-section CT images (Zwirewich et al. 1991). Although differences were not statistically significant, changes in ground-glass opacity were difficult to assess on low-dose images because of the increased image noise. Therefore, it was recommended that 200 mAs should be used for initial thin-section CT and lower doses (i.e., 40–100 mAs) should be used for follow-up CT examinations. These findings, made on single-slice CT scanners, would be expected to translate to thin-section images obtained on multidetector CT scanners.

The relationship between radiation exposure and image quality with both mediastinal and lung windows has been evaluated on conventional 10-mm collimation chest CT images (Mayo et al. 1995) on a single-slice CT scanner. Although findings of this study showed a consistent increase in mean image quality with higher radiation exposure, they did not show a significant difference in the detection of mediastinal or lung parenchymal abnormalities from 20 to 400 mAs. The authors concluded that with the CT scanner model they used, adequate image quality could be consistently obtained in average-sized patients by using tube currents of 100–200 mAs. This study was limited by the small number of patients (n=30), the specific CT scanner factors (geometry, filtration, tube voltage) and the experimental design, which limited low-dose sections to two levels that often were not those with clinically relevant findings. The authors noted that to evaluate further the effect of reduced radiation dose on diagnostic accuracy in chest CT, comparison of complete chest CT studies at a variety of radiation exposures in a large number of patients would be required. However, they noted that such a study could not be performed in patients because of the unacceptable radiation dose that would result from multiple CT examinations at differing radiation exposures. Additionally, the variable effect of motion artifacts in repeated chest CT scans would make comparison of diagnostic findings difficult.

A practical method for evaluating the effect of reduced radiation dose on image quality is computer simulation (Mayo et al. 1997). The technique consists of obtaining a diagnostic scan with standard dose and then modifying the raw scan data by adding Gaussian-distributed random noise to simulate the increased noise associated with reduced radiation exposure. The raw scan data are then reconstructed using the same field of view and reconstruction algorithm as the high-dose reference scan. In a validation trial, experienced chest radiologists were unable to distinguish simulated reduced-dose CT images from real reduced-dose CT images (Mayo et

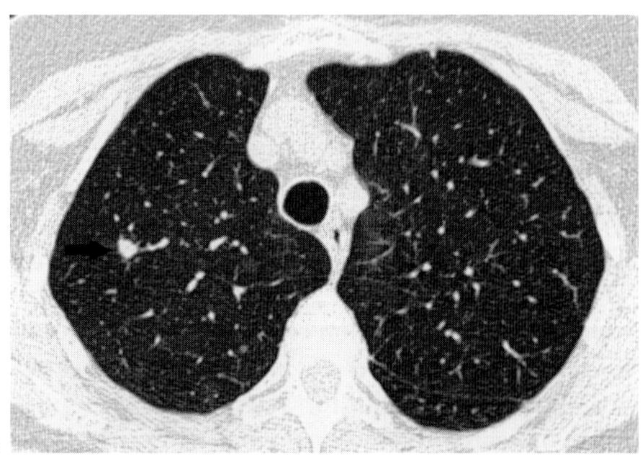

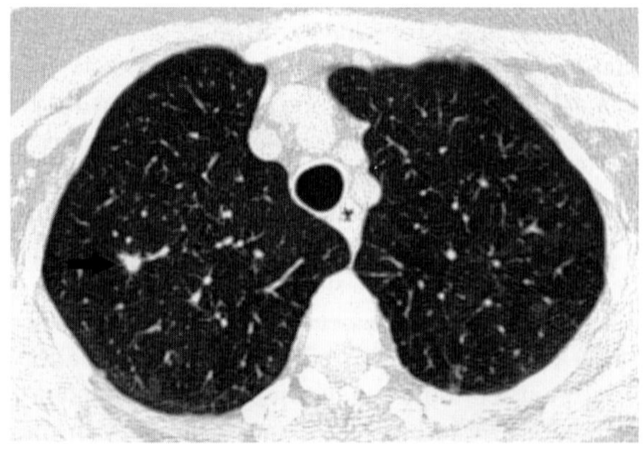

Fig. 5.3a,b. Transverse 1-mm collimation non-contrast-enhanced chest CT scan viewed at lung parenchymal settings (window 1,500 HU, level -700 HU) in a 63-year-old female with a 30-pack/year smoking history. The 7 × 5-mm stage-1A pathologically proven adenocarcinoma (*arrow*) in the apical segment of the right upper lobe is seen equivalently on the low-dose screening exam (40 mAs, DLP 116 mGy·cm, 2 mSv effective dose) (**a**) compared to the high-dose CT exam for fuzzy wire placement (130 mAs, DLP 377 mGy·cm, 6.5 mSv) (**b**)

al. 1997). Computer simulation allows investigators to determine the effect of dose reduction on diagnostic accuracy without exposing patients to radiation unnecessarily. In addition, the simulated images are in exact registration with the original images, eliminating artifacts that would be seen with repeated scanning. This technique has been used to evaluate the diagnostic effect of radiation dose reduction in pediatric abdominal CT (Frush et al. 2002), undifferentiated chest CT (Mayo et al. 2004) and CT pulmonary angiography (Tack et al. 2005; MacKenzie et al. 2007).

The largest chest CT simulated reduced-dose study (Mayo et al. 2004) involved use of a validated computer simulation technique to generate simulated 100- and 40-mA reduced tube current scans from 150 clinically indicated conventional tube current chest CT examinations. The only difference between the conventional and the reduced tube current images generated with this technique was the level of random noise in the images, which increased as the simulated tube current was reduced. The authors used a novel experimental design to compensate for the lack of a gold standard in the experiment. They measured the effect of reduced tube current on reader evaluation of 14 mediastinal structures and lung findings using the first evaluation of the high-dose CT scan as the gold standard. They found that as the simulated tube current was reduced, overall agreement between interpretations of the reduced tube current scans compared to the gold standard was reduced compared to repeated interpretation of the high-dose gold standard examination ($P< 0.05$). This study indicated that reduced tube current CT examinations can result in inferior interpretation of diagnostically significant findings. These data support the widely observed resistance of radiologists to substantial radiation exposure reduction due to the negative impact on image quality and their reduced diagnostic confidence.

However, this study has several limitations that all arise from the absence of an external gold standard. In the absence of an external gold standard for the presence of abnormalities, the authors used the first interpretation of the high-dose examination as the reference standard and then compared the reproducibility of repeated interpretation of the high-dose scan and the interpretation of the reduced dose scans. They postulated that if the reduced tube current scans provide the same information as the high-dose scan, and if observers were consistent in identifying and recording abnormal findings, there should be no significant difference in terms of the level of agreement between the initial and repeated high-dose scan interpretation and the level of agreement between the high-dose scan interpretation and the reduced-dose scan interpretation. For the purpose of the study, intraobserver agreement required consistent classification of a total of 14 mediastinal and lung abnormalities (including subgroup classifications) rather than agreement as to the final diagnosis. The order in which the conventional tube current, 100-mA, and 40-mA scans were read was not recorded, making it impossible to assess the effect of reading order on the data. The authors simply relied on the sheer volume of interpretations to minimize the effect of observer memory on the results. This may have created a learning bias in which the observers became familiar with abnormalities as the scans were repeatedly interpreted. In addition, images in this study were acquired by using single-section helical CT scanners and interpreted on film at a fixed window and level setting. Therefore, this study cannot directly address the current practice of interpreting images acquired with multi-detector row CT scanners on workstations using operator-controlled window width and level settings. Finally, the observers were used to working in a high-dose environment, which may have led to inferior reading skills on reduced dose examinations.

In summary, the results of this study suggest that there may be a lower limit to dose reduction in chest CT when interpreting both mediastinal and lung images. These data suggest that this limit appears to lie between 100 and 200 mA using the currently available reconstruction algorithms. It is also noted that although the impact on imaging findings was assessed, the impact on clinically relevant diagnostic accuracy was not assessed.

Two studies of simulated radiation dose reduction have been performed in subjects receiving CT pulmonary angiography (CTPA) examinations. Dose reduction in CTPA examinations is important as it is estimated that 20% are performed in young female patients (Musset et al. 2002), a particularly susceptible cohort to the effects of radiation dose. One study measured detection of intraluminal filling defects consistent with pulmonary embolism in 21 subjects (Tack et al. 2005). This study found no difference in frequencies of positive and inconclusive results (P=0.21 and 0.08, respectively), positive and negative consistent values (P=0.19 and 0.34, respectively) and the branching order of the most distal artery with a filling defect (P=0.41) depending on the radiation dose. However, all subjects harbored at least one pulmonary embolism. The absence of a control population of negative studies imposes a substantial difference from the clinical setting for the evaluation of pulmonary embolism where the majority of studies are negative. The second study assessed 18 patients with PE and 20 control subjects without PE (MacKenzie et al. 2007). This study found significant reductions in diagnostic certainty ($P<0.02$) and image quality ($P<0.02$) and an increase in perceived technical limitations ($P<0.01$) as the simulated radiation dose was decreased. Clearly, further research with larger study cohorts is required to definitively determine the effect of dose reduction on PE studies.

In the absence of further data, the sum of all these radiation dose reduction trials suggests that strategies for further chest CT radiation dose reduction should be directed toward techniques that reduce radiation exposure without substantially increasing image noise. Adaptive reconstruction algorithm techniques are an example of such an approach (Kachelriess et al. 2001). Finally, it is noted that radiation exposure can be eliminated completely if the chest CT examination is not performed. It is incumbent on radiologists to educate referring clinicians on the radiation dose administered in chest CT, to suggest alternative non-X-ray based imaging for more radiation sensitive subjects (children, young adults, pregnancy) and screen requests on the basis of clinical indication.

5.7 Conclusion

The introduction of helical and multi-detector row CT scanners has resulted in an increase in the number of indications for and the diagnostic accuracy of chest CT examinations. However, despite increasing education and awareness, the current level of radiation exposure from CT remains high. The 15-country study has added further information to support the linear, no threshold approach to the detrimental effects of radiation dose in the range below 20 mSv, similar to that received in chest CT scans (3–6 mSv). Current radiation dose surveys continue to indicate that there is large variation in the technical factors employed by radiologists (Aldrich et al. 2006), and there is a resultant large variation in the radiation dose to patients between institutions. Reference dose values for chest CT have been developed and published. Radiologists need to monitor the radiation dose delivered in examinations within their institutions, adopt and adhere to national radiation-dose guidelines and investigate further dose-reduction strategies within their own practices. Further research into the complex relationship between radiation exposure, image noise and diagnostic accuracy should be encouraged to scientifically establish the minimum radiation doses that provide adequate diagnostic information for standard clinical questions. Once these minimum levels of image quality are determined and validated, automatic exposure controls for CT scanners should be programmed to ensure that all patients undergo CT with techniques that conform to the ALARA (As Low As Reasonably Achievable) principle. Finally, new approaches to image reconstruction should be addressed to maximize the relationship between dose and image quality.

As dispensers of this known carcinogen, radiologists must take the lead in promoting all of these measures for patient protection. Since children, young adults, women and pregnancy have been shown to increase radiation sensitivity, the most strident dose reduction efforts should be focused on these groups. Finally, it is noted that the complexity of CT requires a close collaboration between radiologists and medical physicists to successfully reduce radiation dose while maintaining diagnostic accuracy.

Reference

Aldrich JE, Bilawich AM, Mayo JR (2006a) Radiation doses to patients receiving computed tomography examinations in British Columbia. Can Assoc Radiol J 57:79–85

Aldrich JE, Chang SD, Bilawich AM, Mayo JR (2006b) Radiation dose in abdominal computed tomography: the role of patient size and the selection of tube current. Can Assoc Radiol J 57:152–158

Brenner D (2004) Radiation risks potentially associated with low dose CT screening of adult smokers for lung cancer. Radiology 231:440–445

Brenner DJ, Elliston CD, Hall EJ, Berdon WE (2001) Estimated risks of radiation-induced fatal cancer from pediatric CT. Am J Roentgenol 176:289–296

Cardis E, Vrijheid M, Blettner M et al. (2007) The 15 country collaborative study of cancer risk among radiation workers in the nuclear industry: Estimates of radiation related cancer risks. Radiat Res 167:396–416

Cunningham IA (1995) Computed tomography: instrumentation. In: Bronzino JE (ed) The biomedical engineering handbook.CRC Press, Boca Raton, pp 990–1002

Di Marco AF, Briones B (1993) Is chest CT performed too often? Chest 103:985–986

Di Marco AF, Renston JP (1994) In search of the appropriate use of chest computed tomography. Chest 106:332–333

European Community (2000) European guidelines on quality criteria for computer tomography. EUR 16262EN. Office for Official Publication of the European Communities, Luxemberg

Fricke B, Donnelly L, Frush D et al. (2003) In plane bismuth breast shields for pediatric CT: Effects on radiation dose and image quality using experimental and clinical data. AJR Am J Roentgenol 180:407–411

Frush DP, Slack C, Hollingsworth HH et al. (2002) Computer simulated radiation dose reduction for abdominal multidetector CT of pediatric patients. AJR Am J Roentgenol 179:1107–1113

Greess H, Wolf H, Baum U et al. (2000) Dose reduction in computed tomography by attenuation-based on-line modulation of tube current: evaluation of six anatomical regions. Eur Radiol 10:391–394

Haaga JR, Miraldi F, MacIntyre W, LiPuma JP, Bryan PJ, Wiesen E (1981) The effect of mAs variation upon computed tomography image quality as evaluated by in vivo and in vitro studies. Radiology 138:449–454

Henschke CI, McCauley DI, Yankelevitz DF et al. (1999) Early lung cancer action project: overall design and findings from baseline screening. Lancet 354:99–105

Hopper KD, King S, Lobell M, TenHave T, Weaver J (1997) The breast: In-plane X-ray protection during diagnostic thoracic CT-shielding with bismuth radioprotective garments. Radiology 205:853–858

Huda W (1997) Radiation dosimetry in diagnostic radiology. Am J Roentgenol 169:1487–1488

Hurwitz L, Yoshizumi T, Reiman R et al. (2006) Radiation dose to the female breast from 16 MDCT protocols. AJR Am J Roentgenol 186:1718–1722

ICRP-60 (1991) Recommendations of the International Commission on Radiological Protection. Pergamon Press, Oxford

Itoh H, Ikeda M, Arahata S et al. (2000) Lung cancer screening: minimum tube current reqired for helical CT. Radiology 215:175–183

Kachelrieß M, Watzke O, Kalender W (2001) Generalized multi-dimensional adaptive filtering for conventional and spiral single-slice, multi-slice, and cone-beam CT. Med Physics 28:475–490

Kalender WA, Wolf H, Suess C, Gies M, Greess H, Bautz WA (1999a) Dose reduction in CT by on-line tube current control: principles and validation on phantoms and cadavers. Eur Radiol 9:323–328

Kalender WA, Wolf H, Suess C (1999b) Dose reduction in CT by anatomically adapted tube current modulation. II. Phantom measurements. Med Physics 26:2248–2253

Lee C, Haims A, Monico E, Brink J, Forman H (2004) Diagnostic CT scans: assessment of patient physician and radiologist awareness of radiation dose and possible risks. Radiology 231:393–398

Li J, Udayasankar UK, Toth TL, Seamans J, Small WC, Kalra MK (2007) Automatic patient centering for MDCT: effect on radiation dose. Am J Roentgenol 188:547–552

MacKenzie J, Nazario-Larrieu J, Cai T et al. (2007) Reduced-dose CT: Effect on reader evaluation in detection of pulmonary embolism. AJR Am J Roentgenol 189:1371–1379

Mayo JR, Hartman TE, Lee KS, Primack SL, Vedal S, Müller NL (1995) CT of the chest: minimal tube current required for good image quality with the least radiation dose. Am J Roentgenol 164:603–607

Mayo JR, Whittall KP, Leung AN et al. (1997) Simulated dose reduction in conventional chest CT: validation study. Radiology 202:453–457

Mayo JR, Kim KI, MacDonald S et al. (2004) Reduced radiation dose helical chest CT: effect on reader evaluation of structures and lung findings. Radiology 232:749–756

McGee PL, Humphreys S (1994) Radiation dose associated with spiral computed tomography. Can Assoc Radiol J 45:124–129

Mettler FA Jr, Wiest PW, Locken JA, Kelsey CA (2000) CT scanning: patterns of use and dose. J Radiol Prot 20:353–359

Milne E (2006) Female breast radiation exposure (letter). AJR Am J Roentgenol 186:E24

Musset D, Parent F, Meyer G et al. (2002) Diagnostic strategy for patients with suspected pulmonary embolism: a prospective multicentre outcome study. Lancet 360:1914–1920

Naidich DP, Marshall CH, Gribbin C, Arams RS, McCauley DI (1990) Low-dose CT of the lungs: preliminary observations. Radiology 175:729–731

Naidich DP, Pizzarello D, Garay SM, Müller NL (1994) Is thoracic CT performed often enough? Chest 106:331–332

Nishizawa K, Maruyama T, Takayama M, Okada M, Hachiya J, Furuya Y (1991) Determinations of organ doses and effective dose equivalents from computed tomographic examination. Br J Radiol 64:20–28

Panzer W, Scheurer C, Zankl M (1989) Dose to patients in computed tomography examinations: results and consequences from a field study in the Federal Republic of Germany. In: Moores BM, Wall BF, Eriskat H, Schibilla H (eds) Optimization of image quality and patient exposure in diagnostic radiology. British Institute of Radiology Report 20, London

Parker MS, Hui FK, Camacho MA, Chung JK, Broga DW, Sethi NN (2005) Female breast radiation exposure during CT pulmonary angiography. Am J Roentgenol 185:1228–1233

Pentlow KS, Beattie JW, Laughlin JS (1977) Parameters and design considerations for tomographic transmission scanners. In: Ter-Pogossian MM, Phelps ME, (eds) Reconstructive tomography in diagnostic radiology and nuclear medicine. University Park Press, Baltimore, pp 267–279

Pierce D, Shimizu Y, Preston D et al. (1996) Studies of the mortality of atomic bomb survivors. Report 12, part 1. Cancer: 1950–1990. Radiat Res 146:1–27

Polacin A, Kalender WA, Marchal G (1992) Evaluation of section sensitivity profiles and image noise in spiral CT. Radiology 185:29–35

Rothenberg LN, Pentlow KS (1992) Radiation dose in CT. RadioGraphics 12:1225–1243

Shrimpton PC, Edyvean S (1998) CT scanner dosimetry. Br J Radiol 71:1–3

Sprawls P Jr (1992) AAPM tutorial. CT image detail and noise. RadioGraphics 12:1041–1046

Strzelczyk J, Damilakis J, Marx M, Macura K (2007) Facts and controversies about radiation exposure, Part 2: Low level exposures and cancer risk. J Am Coll Radiol 4:32–39

Swensen SJ, Jett JR, Sloan JA et al. (2002) Screening for lung cancer with low-dose spiral computed tomography. Am J Resp Crit Care Med 165:508–513

Tack D, De Maertelaer V, Gevenois PA (2003) Dose reduction in multidetector CT using attenuation-based online tube current modulation. AJR Am J Roentgenol 181:331–334

Tack D, De Maertelaer V, Petit W et al. (2005) Multi-detector row CT pulmonary angiography: Comparison of standard-dose and simulated low-dose techniques. Radiology 236:318–325

Toth TL, Bromberg NB, Pan TS et al. (2000) A dose reduction X-ray beam positioning system for high-speed multislice CT scanners. Med Physics 27:2659–2668

Tubiana M, Aurengo A, Averbeck D et al. (2005) Dose effect relationships and estimation of the carcinogenic effect of low doses of ionizing radiation. Academie des Sciences and Academie Nationale de Medicine, Paris

Tzedakis A, Damilakis J, Perisinakis K, Stratakis J (2005) The effect of z overscanning on patient effective dose from multidetector helical computed tomography examinations. Med Physics 32:1621–1629

Ullrich R, Jernigan M, LC S, Bowles N (1987) Radiation carcinogenesis: time-dose relationships. Radiat Res 111:179–184

Zwirewich CV, Mayo JR, Müller NL (1991) Low-dose high-resolution CT of lung parenchyma. Radiology 180:413–417

Acquisition Protocols

6

Jacques Kirsch, Michaël Dupont, and Xavier Hamoir

CONTENTS

6.1 Introduction

Cardiac CT imaging is a rapidly evolving technique. It benefits from the latest technical improvements in computed tomography, particularly concerning the rotation times, the detector coverage and the reconstruction speed. The major challenge in cardiac CT coronarography is to overcome some specific problems such as cardiac movements and rhythm, the small size of the coronaries and the coverage of the whole heart in one breath-hold. Moreover, this exam must be conducted with the lowest possible radiation dose. These particularities lead to the development of new machines and new concepts every year.

J. Kirsch, MD
Department of Radiology, Clinique Notre Dame, Avenue Delmée 9, 7500 Tournai, Belgium
M. Dupont, MD
Department of Radiology, UCL Cliniques Universitaires Saint Luc, Avenue Hippocrate 10, 1200 Brussels, Belgium
X. Hamoir, MD
Department of Radiology, Clinique Notre Dame, Avenue Delmée 9, 7500 Tournai, Belgium

6.2 Patient and ECG Leads Positioning

Patients must be properly informed of the procedure, and particularly about what they may feel as the contrast is injected. The breath-hold necessary to conduct the exam must be explained and tested several times just before image acquisition. Patients are positioned on the CT examination table head first in the supine position, arms above the head. They should be as comfortable as possible. An adequate ECG tracing is important for prospective or retrospective ECG gating. Three ECG leads are attached to obtain an adequate, noise-free, ECG tracing showing a recognizable QRS complex. Conductive gel and shaving hairy attachment sites can help get a better signal.

6.3 Heart Rate Control

6.3.1 Goal

For several reasons, slow heart rates favor good image quality. Most of the cardiac contraction and motion occurs during systole, and the heart remains nearly motionless during diastole. Systole duration does not vary significantly depending on the heart rate. With higher heart rates, diastole shortens, and the interval desirable for image acquisition is reduced. For this reason, heart rates below 65 bpm are desirable for examinations performed with CT scanners with 64 or fewer sections

With low heart rates, it becomes possible to work with single segment reconstruction that allows image reconstruction in a single heart beat without the need to average the data from two to five heart beats. This improves image quality and reduces radiation dose by the use of higher pitches. However, new dual-source CT (Siemens Definition) achieves a significantly better temporal resolution (83 ms) and therefore allows the scanning of patients with heart rates up to 120–140 bpm.

6.3.2 Means

A proper explanation of the examination and reassurance of the patient reduces stress and associated higher heart rates. Inspiration during breath-hold decreases heart rate by four to six beats per minute. To further reduce cardiac heart rate, β-blockers such as metoprolol can be used. IV administration is preferred by most teams, as it can be injected immediately before the exam. Metoprolol tartrate (Lopressor, Novartis) is a β1-adrenoreceptor antagonist, and the most commonly used IV β-blocker. Other β-blockers are likely to have similar effects on heart rate.

Main contraindications to β-blockers are a heart rhythm of less than 60 bpm (but β-blockers are not needed in these cases), systolic blood pressure of less than 100 mmHg, second or third degree atrioventricular block, sick sinus syndrome, chronic obstructive pulmonary disease, severe cardiac insufficiency, asthma, or allergy to the medication or its constituents.

In the absence of contraindication, an initial bolus of 5 mg IV metoprolol tartrate (or alternatively 2.5 mg over 1 min followed by a second injection of 2.5 mg over 1 min given 5 min later) is injected over 1 min to the patient lying on the scanner table. If the heart rate is insufficiently reduced (over 70 bpm), a second injection of 5 mg (over 1 min) can be administered. A third injection can be given up to the maximum total dose of 15 mg of metoprolol tartrate.

Some teams use Esmolol (Brevibloc, Baxter) in place of metoprolol tartrate. It is also a cardioselective β-blocker, but with a plasma half-life of 4 to 9 min instead of 3 to 7 h for metoprolol tartrate. It has the theoretical advantage to minimize the secondary effects to a few minutes only.

Oral administration of metoprolol is an alternative to the IV form, but should ideally be commenced the night before the examination, with an initial dose of 50–100 mg of metoprolol tartrate. One hour before scanning, another oral dose is given (a third dose can be given in the absence of sufficient heart rate control, but delays the CT exam of 1 h). If there are contraindications to the use of β-blockers, calcium channel blockers are an alternative. Nevertheless, some contraindications of these medications are common, notably second or third degree atrioventricular block. Diltiazem (Cardizem, Hoechst Marion Roussel) can be administered intravenously at the dose of 0.25 mg/kg of body weight (up to 25 mg total) or in an oral regimen of 30 mg of regular-release diltiazem.

6.3.3 A Note on Nitroglycerin

The use of sublingual nitroglycerin (Nitro-Quick, Ethex) has increased in CT coronarography in the last few years. It is not a heart rhythm control drug, but allows for a better visualization of the coronary tree by increasing the lumen area (mostly in normal arteries, less in the diseased coronary artery segments). It has the drawback of overestimating the degree of stenosis. Tablets or sprays administered sublingually (0.4 mg) are the most commonly used forms. Contraindications to nitroglycerin are mainly hypotension and right myocardial infarction. The most frequently encountered secondary effects are headaches and hypotension.

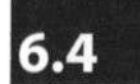

6.4 Acquisition Parameters

6.4.1 Rotation Speed and Collimation

Coronaries are very small, with a diameter of 4 mm proximally to 1 mm and less in the distality, with a complex course along the heart. Clinically, it is important to be able to assess the lumen of the coronary tree down to 1.5 mm. The spatial resolution must be as good as possible, using the thinnest possible collimation. The collimation varies from 0.625 to 0.5 mm in actual CTs. The z-flying focal spot concept allows a practical collimation of 0.3 mm with detectors of 0.6 mm. The coronary tree is constantly moving rapidly. To minimize movement's artifacts, the best monosegment temporal resolution is mandatory. The fastest gantry rotation time should be chosen to achieve the best possible image quality. Depending on the constructor, the rotation time varies from 0.3 s/rotation to 0.4 s/rotation. The dual-source CT cuts rotation time by two thanks to its two tubes (0.165 ms for a gantry rotation time of 0.33 s/rotation). The corresponding temporal resolution is the rotation time divided by 2, because 180° data acquisition is sufficient to reconstruct one image. (Figs. 6.1, 6.2; Tables 6.1, 6.2)

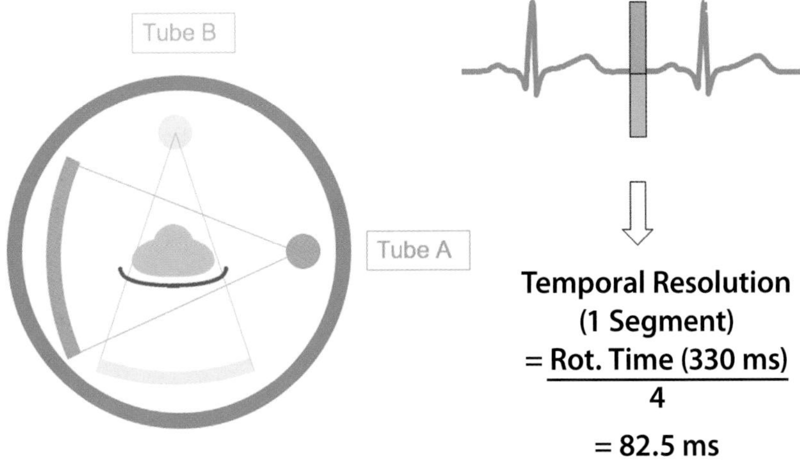

Fig. 6.1. In DSCT, the two X-ray sources and detectors are positioned at 90-degree angles and the temporal resolution reaches 82.5 ms (rotation time divided by four)

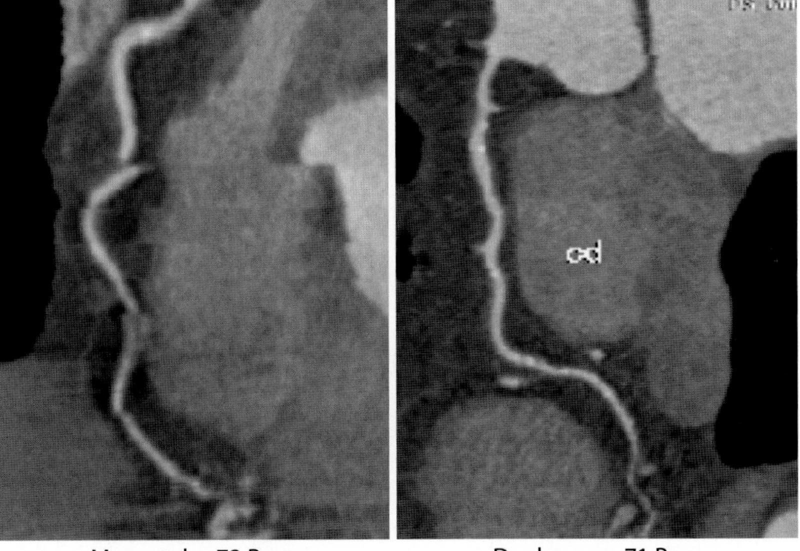

Fig. 6.2. Curved MPR reconstruction of right coronary artery (same patient with similar heart rate) explored with single source CT (*left panel*) and dual-source CT (*right panel*). DSCT allows for significant reduction of cardiac motion artifacts

Table 6.1. Cardiac CTA acquisition parameters recommended by constructers for currently available scanners

Scanner	Philips Brilliance 64	GE 64 VCT	Toshiba Aquilion 64	Siemens Sensation 64	Siemens Definition (DSCT)
Colimation	64×0.625	64×0.625	64×0.5	32×0.625	32×0.6 (X2)
z focal flying spot	No	No	No	Yes	Yes (X2)
Number of slices/rotation	64	64	64	64	64 (X2)
Recon thickness	0.6–0.9	0,6	0.5	0.6 or 0.75	0.6 or 0.75
Recon increment	50%	0.6	0.3	0.4 or 0.5	0.4 or 0.5
Pitch factor	0.2	0.2–0.26	0.138–0.623	0.2	Auto (0.2 to 0.5)
Rotation time	0.4 s	0.35 s	0.35–0.6 s HR dependent	0.33 s	0.33 s
KV	120–140	100–120	100–120–135	100–120	120
mAs/rotation	290–378	260	105–157	256	320
mAs	700–900	400–750	466–700	770	750–800
Matrix	512	512	512	512	512
FOV	Max 500	160–170	320 (scan) 200 (recon)	Max 700	Max 300
Length	120–150	120–140	120–160	120–150	120–150
Scan time	8–10 s	5 s	6–8 s	12 s	Depending on pitch: 6–12 s
Bypass grafts	15 s (25 cm)	6.5 s	15.5 s (25 cm)	17 s	Depending on pitch: 12–17 s
True temporal resolution	210 ms	175 ms	175 ms	165 ms	83 ms
Multisegment recon	Yes	Yes	Yes (down to 35 ms)	Yes	Yes
Filter (stent)	CD	detail	FC05	B46f	B46f
(Stand.)	XCC	std	FC43	B25f	B25f
(Obese)	XCB	std		B36f	B36f
ECG auto current variation	Yes: down to 20%	Yes: down to 20%	Yes: from 100% to 10%	Yes: down to 20%	Yes: down to 20% or 4%
Anatomic dose modulation	Yes: dose right, except in ECG-gated scans	Yes (auto mA)	Yes: sure exposure (for cardiac ECG modulation)	Yes (care dose)	Yes (care dose)
Prospective gating	Yes	"Snapshot pulse"	Yes (with spiral CT)	Yes	"Adaptative cardio seq"

6.4.2 Tube Current and Voltage

Usual tube voltage setting is 120 kV, but can be reduced depending from the morphotype of the patient. Substantial dose saving can be obtained by lowering the tube voltage to 100 kV in slim adults and adolescents. Eighty kV can be used in the pediatric population without use of ECG gating technology. Increasing the tube voltage to 140 kV is generally not recommended because of the lesser iodine absorption of X-rays at higher kV. Tube current varies around 800 mAs. Two systems must be activated in order to reduce the patient's exposure to radiation: the ECG auto current variation (ECG pulsing) and anatomic dose modulation.

With ECG auto current dose variation the tube current in systole is divided by 5 (20%) to 25 (4%) in comparison with the current in diastole. This system is only useful with patients with slow and

Table 6.2. Cardiac CTA acquisition parameters for future CTs presented at RSNA 2007

Scanner	Philips iCT *	Toshiba Aquilion ONE*	Siemens Definition AS+*	GE (HD CT ?)**
Collimation	128×0.625	12–16 cm 0.5 mm	64×0.6	
z focal flying spot	Yes	No	Yes	
Number of slices/rotation	256	320	128	
Recon thickness	0.6–0.9	0.5	0.6	
Recon increment	50%	0.25	0.3	
Pitch factor	0.14	NA: sequential	0.15	
Rotation time	0.27 s	0.35–0.45 HR dependent	0.3	
KV	120–140	100–120–135	120–140	
mAs/rotation	189–243	123–203	160	
mAs	700–900	123–203	800	
Matrix	512	512	512	
FOV	Max 500	320 (scan) 200 (recon)	Max 500	
Length	120–150	120–160	120–150	
Scan time	5 s–6.5 s	0.35–1.4 s	4–5	
Bypass grafts	11 s (25 cm)	3 s	6–8 s	
True temporal resolution	135 ms 1-cycle recon	175 ms 1-cycle recon	150 ms 1-cycle recon	
Multisegment recon	Yes	Yes (down to 41 ms)	Yes	
Filter (stent)	CD	FC05	B46f	
(Stand)	XCC	FC43	B25f	
(Obese)	XCB		B36f	
ECG auto current variation	Yes: down to 20%	Yes: 100% to 0%	Yes: 20%–4%	
Anatomic dose modulation	Yes: dose right, except in ECG-gated scans	Yes: sure exposure (for cardiac ECG modulation)	Yes (care dose)	

*Scanner specs from constructors January 2008
**Not available in January 2008

steady heart rates in whom the optimal window for image reconstruction predictably occurs during diastole. At higher heart rates, the optimal reconstruction window is more difficult to predict and can correspond to the end systolic phase. The ECG pulsing can become a disadvantage at high heart rates by lowering tube current during the useful phase. The anatomic dose modulation adapts the tube current to the morphotype and region that is explored.

6.4.3 Prospective ECG Gating

All of these previous concepts concern retrospective ECG gating helical coronary CTA. An old technique used in the beginning of CTA with prospective ECG gated reconstruction comes to new life with the new multi-dector CT with large or very large coverage (64, 128, 256 or 320 images per rotation). This prospective ECG gating acquisition is an axial, step-

and-shoot technique that benefits from the large or very large detector coverage to image the entire heart in only a few X-ray exposures [in 1 (320 rows) to 3 or 4 rotations (64 to 128 rows)]. Therefore, the dose is significantly reduced compared to the helical mode.

6.5 Reconstruction Parameters

6.5.1 Field of View and Spiral Length

A small field of view (16–20 cm) that encompasses only the heart is commonly used for coronary CTA evaluation in order to maximize the spatial resolution. For the assessment of extra cardiac findings, the field of view must be enlarged to 35–40 cm with 3-mm-thick slices. The length of the spiral is usually limited to the heart, with an acquisition beginning at the level of the carina and extending to the diaphragm. Exceptions are coronary artery bypass graft and triple rule out (simultaneous evaluation of the coronary tree, aorta and pulmonary arteries) examination that needs whole thorax coverage.

If the length of the acquisition encompasses only the heart, the upper third of the thorax is not included, and extra cardiac findings can be missed. Therefore, some teams add a second low-dose short acquisition on the missing part of the thorax. Other teams prefer to perform a whole thorax low-dose ECG gated acquisition first and to use it to evaluate the calcium scoring and the extra cardiac findings.

6.5.2 Reconstruction Thickness

Images are usually reconstructed with a slice thickness of 0.5 to 0.75 mm, with a reconstruction increment ranging from 0.3 to 0.5 mm (30% overlapping). Some advise to use a reconstruction slice thickness that is slightly wider than the collimated slice thickness. The pixel matrix is the classical 512 × 512 pixels for all constructors.

6.5.3 Reconstruction Kernel

All constructors offer a specific reconstruction filter (or kernel) for cardiac CTA reconstructions. These kernels typically are of a medium smooth type, being a compromise between edge enhancement to provide a good spatial resolution and a smoothening to reduce image noise as much as possible. For the evaluation of coronary artery stents, a kernel with stronger edge enhancement is recommended to better delineate the edge of the stent and to optimize the differentiation between beam-hardening artifacts and intimal hyperplasia. Additionally, such a kernel can also be used in case of heavy calcifications in coronary arteries (Fig. 6.3).

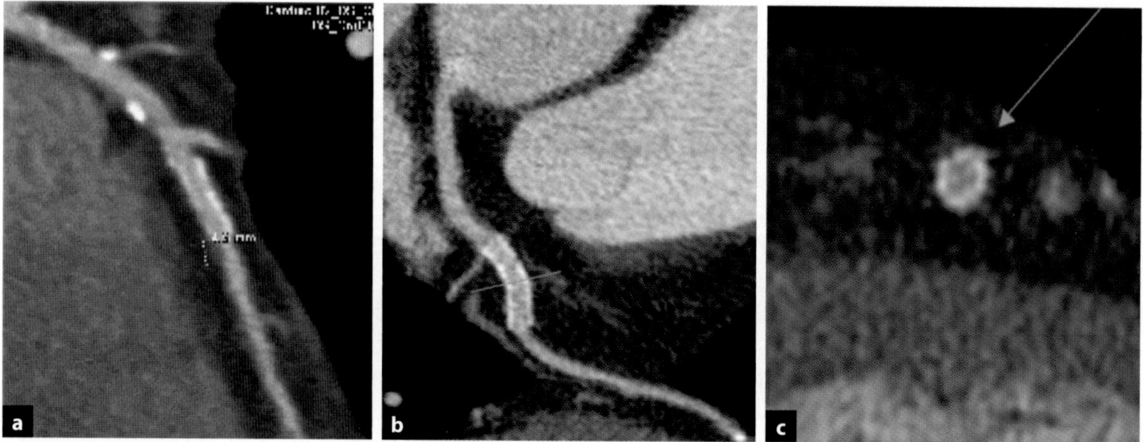

Fig. 6.3a–c. Curved MPR reconstruction of the LAD in the left anterior descending artery: **a** shows the stent with the routine CT angiography kernel and **b,c** show the stent with the sharp cardiac dedicated kernel

Reference

Achenbach S, Ropers D, Kuettner A et al. (2006) Contrast-enhanced coronary artery visualization by dual-source computed tomography: initial experience. Eur J Radiol 57:331–335

Achenbach S, Ulzheimer S, Baum U et al. (2000) Noninvasive coronary angiography by retrospectively ECG-gated multislice spiral CT. Circulation 102:2823–2828

Andrus MR, Holloway KP, Clark DB (2004) Use of β-blockers in patients with COPD. Ann Pharmacother 38:142–145

Becker CR, Knez A, Leber A et al. (2002) Detection of coronary artery stenoses with multislice helical CT angiography. J Comput Assist Tomogr 26: 750–755

Bley TA, Ghanem NA, Foell D et al. (2005) Computed tomography coronary angiography with 370-millisecond gantry rotation time: evaluation of the best image reconstruction interval. J Comput Assist Tomogr 29:1–5

Ferencik M, Moselewski F, Ropers D et al. (2003) Quantitative parameters of image quality in multidetector spiral computed tomographic coronary imaging with submillimeter collimation. Am J Cardiol 92:1257–1262

Flohr T, Bruder H, Stierstorfer K, Simon J, Schaller S, Ohnesorge B (2002) New technical developments in multislice CT, part 2: sub-millimeter 16-slice scanning and increased gantry rotation speed for cardiac imaging. Rofo Fortschr Geb Rontgenstr Neuen Bildgeb Verfahr 174:1022–1027

Flohr T, Ohnesorge B (2001) Heart rate adaptive optimization of spatial and temporal resolution for electrocardiogram-gated multislice spiral CT of the heart. J Comput Assist Tomogr 25:907–923

Flohr T, Stierstorfer K, Bruder H, Simon J, Schaller S (2002) New technical developments in multislice CT – Part 1: Approaching isotropic resolution with sub-millimeter 16-slice scanning. Rofo Fortschr Geb Rontgenstr Neuen Bildgeb Verfahr 174:839–845

Flohr TG, McCollough CH, Bruder H et al. (2006) First performance evaluation of a dualsource CT (DSCT) system. Eur Radiol 16:256–268

Flohr TG, Schaller S, Stierstorfer K, Bruder H, Ohnesorge BM, Schoepf UJ (2005) Multi-detector row CT systems and image-reconstruction techniques. Radiology 235:756–773

Gerber TC, Kuzo RS, Karstaedt N et al. (2002) Current results and new developments of coronary angiography with use of contrast-enhanced computed tomography of the heart. Mayo Clin Proc 77:55–71

Gerber TC, Kuzo RS, Lane GE et al. (2003) Image quality in a standardized algorithm for minimally invasive coronary angiography with multislice spiral computed tomography. J Comput Assist Tomogr 27:62–69

Giesler T, Baum U, Ropers D et al. (2002) Noninvasive visualization of coronary arteries using contrast-enhanced multidetector CT: influence of heart rate on image quality and stenosis detection. AJR 179:911–91

Hamoir X, Salovic D, Bouziane T, Kirsch J (2007) Dual source CT: Cardio-pulmonary applications. JBR-BTR 90:77–79

Herzog C, Abolmaali N, Balzer JO et al. (2002) Heart-rate-adapted image reconstruction in multidetector-row cardiac CT: influence of physiological and technical prerequisite on image quality. Eur Radiol 12:2670–2678

Herzog C, Arning-Erb M, Zangos S et al. (2006) Multi-detector row CT coronary angiography: influence of reconstruction technique and heart rate on image quality. Radiology 238:75–86

Herzog C, Nguyen SA, Savino G et al. (2007) Does two-segment image reconstruction at 64-section CT coronary angiography improve image quality and diagnostic accuracy? Radiology 244:121–129

Hoffmann MH, Shi H, Schmitz BL et al. (2005) Noninvasive coronary angiography with multislice computed tomography. JAMA 293:2471–2478

Hong C, Becker CR, Huber A et al. (2001) ECG-gated reconstructed multi-detector row CT coronary angiography: effect of varying trigger delay on image quality. Radiology 220:712–717

Jakobs TF, Becker CR, Ohnesorge B et al. (2002) Multislice helical CT of the heart with retrospective ECG gating: reduction of radiation exposure by ECG-controlled tube current modulation. Eur Radiol 12:1081–1086

Johnson TR, Nikolaou K, Wintersperger BJ et al. (2006) Dual-source CT cardiac imaging: initial experience. Eur Radiol 16:1409–1415

Kopp AF, Schroeder S, Kuettner A et al. (2001) Coronary arteries: retrospectively ECG-gated multidetector row CT angiography with selective optimization of the image reconstruction window. Radiology 221:683–688

Kopp AF, Schroeder S, Kuettner A et al. (2002) Noninvasive coronary angiography with high-resolution multidetector-row computed tomography: results in 102 patients. Eur Heart J 23: 1714–1725

Leschka S, Alkadhi H, Plass A et al. (2005) Accuracy of MSCT coronary angiography with 64-slice technology: first experience. Eur Heart J 26:1482–1487

Leschka S, Husmann L, Desbiolles LM et al. (2006) Optimal image reconstruction intervals for non-invasive coronary angiography with 64-slice CT. Eur Radiol 16:1964–1972

Maintz D, Seifarth H, Raupach R et al. (2006) Sixty-four-slice multidetector coronary CT angiography: in vitro evaluation of 68 different stents. Eur Radiol 16:818–826

Matt D, Scheffel H, Leschka S et al. (2007) Dual-source CT coronary angiography: image quality, mean heart rate, and heart rate variability. AJR 189:567–573

Nieman K, Cademartiri F, Lemos PA, Raaijmakers R, Pattynama PM, de Feyter PJ (2002) Reliable noninvasivecoronary angiography with fast submillimeter multislice spiral computed tomography. Circulation 106:2051–2054

Nieman K, Rensing BJ, van Geuns RJ et al. (2002) Noninvasive coronary angiography with multislice spiral computed tomography: impact of heart rate. Heart 88:470–474

Ohnesorge B, Becker C, Flohr T, Reiser MF (2002) Multislice CT in cardiac imaging: technical principles, clinical application and future developments. Springer, Berlin Heidelberg New York, pp 3–109

Ohnesorge B, Flohr T, Becker C et al. (2000) Cardiac imaging by means of electrocardiographically gated multisection spiral CT: initial experience. Radiology 217:564–571

Pannu HK, Alvarez W Jr, Fishman EK (2006) β-blockers for cardiac CT: a primer for the radiologist. AJR 186 (6 Suppl):S341–S345

Salpeter SR, Ormiston TM, Salpeter EE, Poole PJ, Cates CJ (2003) Cardioselective beta-blockers for chronic obstructive pulmonary disease: a meta-analysis. Respir Med 97:1094–1101

Scheffel H, Alkadhi H, Plass A et al. (2006) Accuracy of dual-source CT coronary angiography: first experience in a high pre-test probability population without heart rate control. Eur Radiol 16:2739–2747

Schoepf J, Zwerner P, Savino G et al. (2007) Coronary CT-angiography. Radiology 244:48–63

Schoepf J, Becker CR, Ohnesorge BM, Yucel EK (2004) CT of coronary artery disease. Radiology 232:18–37

Schroeder S, Kopp AF, Kuettner A et al. (2002) Influence of heart rate on vessel visibility in noninvasive coronary angiography using new multislice computed tomography: experience in 94 patients. Clin Imaging 26:106–111

Seifarth H, Wienbeck S, Juergens KU et al. (2007) Optimal systolic and diastolic reconstruction windows for coronary CT angiography using dual-source CT. AJR 189:1317–1321

Shim SS, Kim Y, Lim SM (2005) Improvement of image quality with beta-blocker premedication on ECG-gated 16-MDCT coronary angiography. AJR 184:649–654

Part II:

Anatomical and Physiological Approach to Cardiothoracic Imaging

Cardiac and Coronary Artery Anatomy and Physiology

7

Jean-Louis Sablayrolles, Erik Bouvier, Jean Marc Trautenaere, and Jacques Feignoux

CONTENTS

J.-L. Sablayrolles, MD
E. Bouvier, MD
J. M. Trautenaere, MD
J. Feignoux, MD
Centre Cardiologique du Nord, 32–36 Avenue des Moulins Gémeaux, 93200 Saint Denis, France

7.1 Anatomical Basis

In imagery based on slices, whether CT or MRI, the analysis of cardiac structures, and particularly the coronary arteries, differs from that applied in classical techniques such as coronary angiography. A review of cardiac anatomy will provide necessary landmarks for this new imaging technology. The heart volume to be explored is a cube of 15×15×15 cm. The heart can be considered as a regular ovoid lodged in the thorax (Fig. 7.1). This ovoid is divided into four chambers: the two atria and the two ventricles. The aorta has its origin in the left ventricle, the pulmonary artery in the right ventricle. These chambers have their own walls, and the whole structure is surrounded by the pericardial sac.

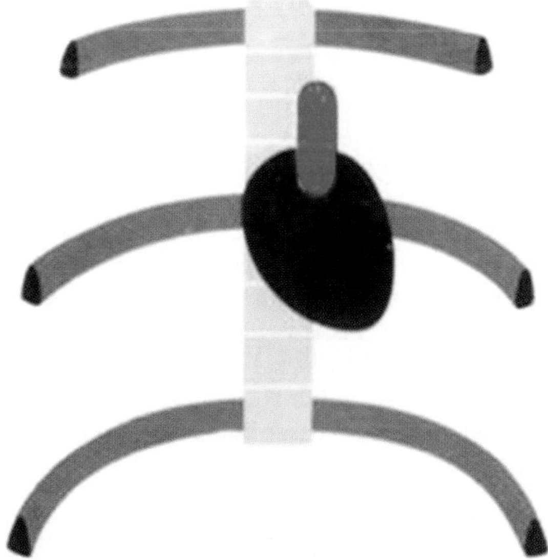

Fig. 7.1. The heart can be considered as a regular ovoid lodged in the thorax

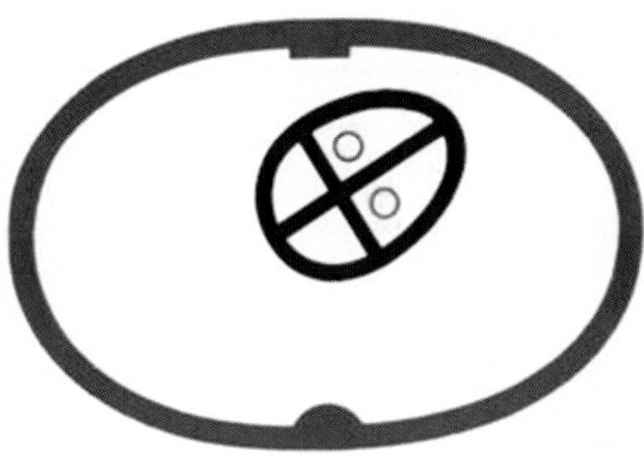

Fig. 7.2. Heart chamber positions in the thorax

Due to the oblique position of the heart in the thorax, the chambers are positioned as follows (Fig. 7.2).

- the left atrium is the most posterior of the chambers;
- the right atrium and the left ventricle in a median position;
- the right ventricle is the most anterior;
- the pulmonary artery is therefore situated anterior to the aorta, which is slightly further to the left.

7.1.1 Heart Chamber Anatomy

The heart chambers, the origin of the aorta and the pulmonary artery are covered by the pericardium.

7.1.1.1 The Pericardium

The pericardium is divided into the serous and the fibrous pericardium:

- the innermost serous pericardium is separated from the subepicardial myocardium by the epicardial adipose through which the coronary arteries pass. This is a virtual cavity delimited by two layers, the visceral and the parietal.
- the fibrous pericardium is a thickening of mediastinal conjunctive tissue lining the parietal layer of the serious pericardium.

Areas of reflection between the visceral layer and the parietal layer located at the base of the heart and at the root of the aorta and the trunk of the pulmonary artery are formed of recesses, the largest of which is the transverse sinus located behind the ascending aorta and the pulmonary artery and above the right atrium and the left atrium. In fact, either the circumflex artery in case of abnormal attachment or a right internal mammary bypass may be found here. It is in tight contact with the valvular aortic plane.

Presently, imaging techniques do not enable to separate the various structures of the pericardium. This results in a fine, regular line of tissue density underscored by the hyopodense epicardial and mediastinal adipose. Its usual thickness is less than 2 mm (Fig. 7.3).

7.1.1.2 Interauricular and Interventricular Walls

The heart chambers are distinguished by right chambers and left chambers (Fig. 7.4).

The right chambers, i.e., the right atrium and ventricle, are separated from the left chambers, the left atrium and ventricle by interauricular and interventricular walls. The interventricular wall, or septum, presents a muscular component in most cases. Its average thickness is approximately 10 mm. The membranous component or membranous septum is more and smaller in size. It is located in the vicinity of the interauricular wall with respect to the aortic orifice. Its thickness does not exceed 2 mm. The inter auricular wall or septum is a thin membrane that separates the atriums (Fig. 7.4).

7.1.1.3 The Right Atrium

The right atrium is a chamber with a large vertical axis receiving the superior vena cava and the inferior vena cava. The triangle-shaped left auricle is located on the front of the orifice of the superior vena cava (Fig. 7.5).

The inferior vena cava terminates in the lower side of the atrial chamber. Its origin is bordered in front by the valvula of the inferior vena cava (the Eustachian valve). The orifice of the coronary sinus that allows drainage of the venous myocardial blood is located between the interatricular septum and the orifice of the inferior vena cava.

7.1.1.4 The Right Ventricle

The right ventricle is triangle-shaped. Its wall is rather thin, approximately 0.5 mm. It presents nu-

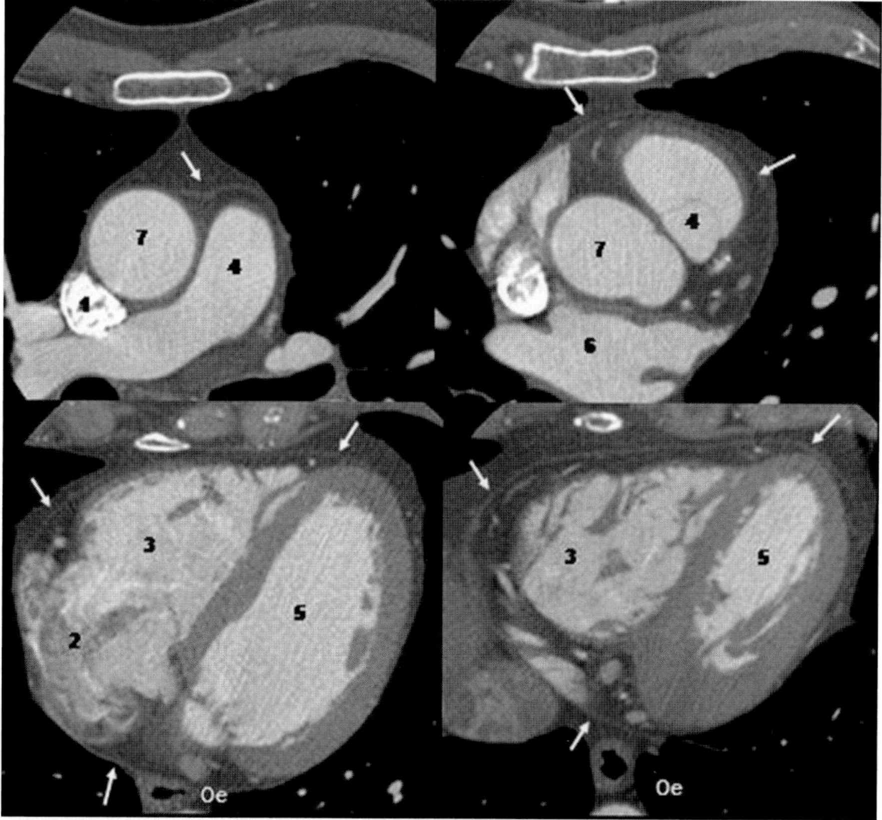

Fig. 7.3. Axial view – pericardium (*arrows*): (*2*) right atrium, (*3*) right ventricle, (*4*) pulmonary artery, (*5*) left ventricle, (*6*) left atrium, (*7*) ascending aorta

merous trabeculae, in particular the ansiform band that extends to the anterior side of the ventricle at its inferior extremity to the internal wall of the ventricle below and in front of the infandibulum (Fig. 7.6).

On the internal wall of the right ventricle, papillary muscles attaching chords holding the cuspids of the tricuspid valve are visible. In the ventricular chamber, two chambers are distinguished, composing the postero-inferior inflow chamber and the outflow chamber or the pulmonary infandibulum. The pulmonary ostium is located at the top of this outflow chamber.

7.1.1.5 The Left Atrium

The left atrium is oval-shaped. Its posterior side receives the pulmonary veins. In front of the superior pulmonary vein is the left auricle (Fig. 7.7).

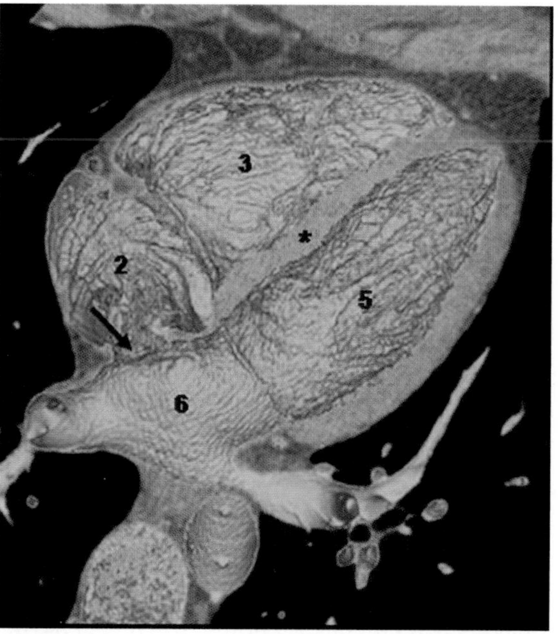

Fig. 7.4. Heart chambers: (*2*) right atrium, (*3*) right ventricle, (*5*) left ventricle, (*6*) left atrium, (*) inter-ventricular septum, (*arrow*) inter-atrium septum

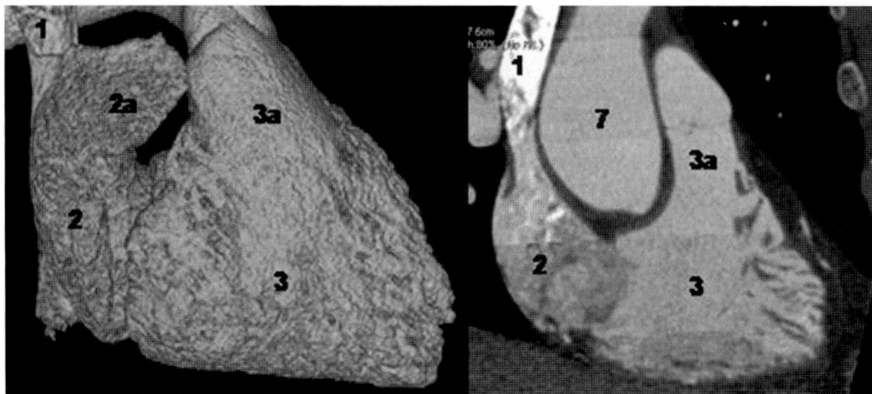

Fig. 7.5. 3D and 2D coronal view. Right heart chambers: (*1*) Superior vena cava, (*2*) right atrium, (*2a*) right auricle, (*3*) right ventricle (RV): (*3a*) RV inflow portion, (*3b*) RV infandibulum

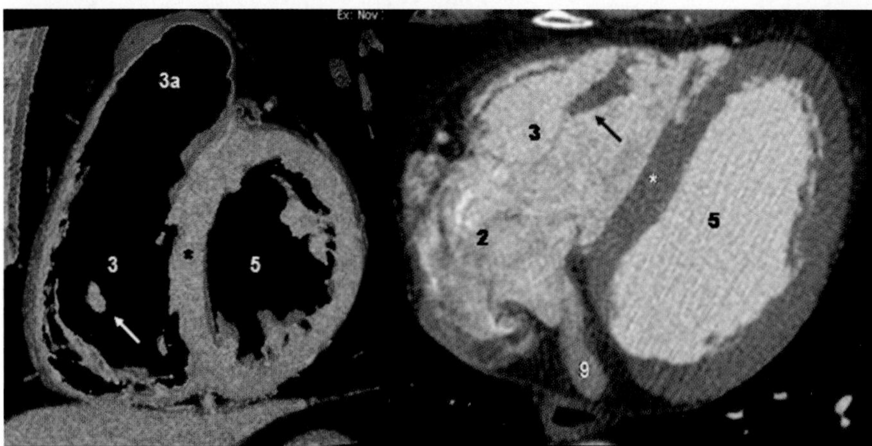

Fig. 7.6. 3D and 2D view. Right ventricle: (*3*) inflow portion, (*3a*) infandibulum, (*5*) left ventricle, (*9*) coronary sinus, papillary muscle (*arrow*), interventricular septum (*), 5- LV

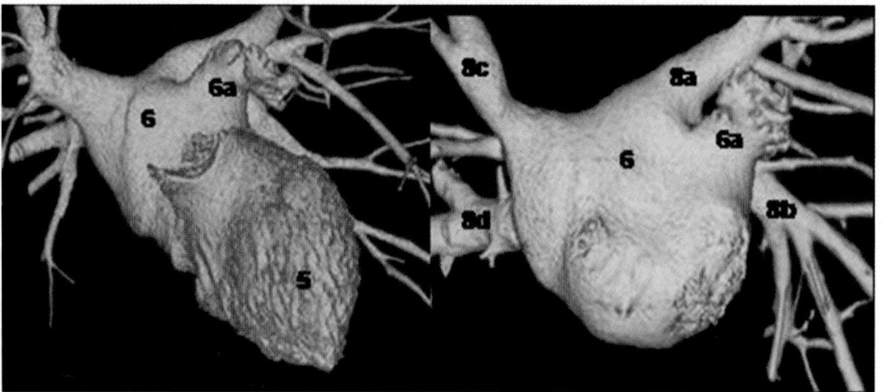

Fig. 7.7. 3D view. *5* LV, (*6*) left atrium, (*6a*) left auricle, (*8a*) left superior pulmonary veins (PV), *8b* left inferior PV, *8c* right superior PV, *8d* right inferior PV

7.1.1.6
The Left Ventricle

The left ventricle is an oval-shaped chamber with thick walls approximately 10 mm in diameter during diastole. The papillary muscles or pillars attach to the walls by intermediary of the chordae tendineae and maintain the valves of the mitral apparatus. Anterior papillary muscles are discernable at approximately the middle third of the anterior side, and the posterior papillary muscle is located more apically. The chamber is divided into two chambers separated by the anterior cusp of the mitral valve and the chordae: the inflow chamber and the outflow chamber are in contact with the aortic valvular orifice (Fig. 7.8).

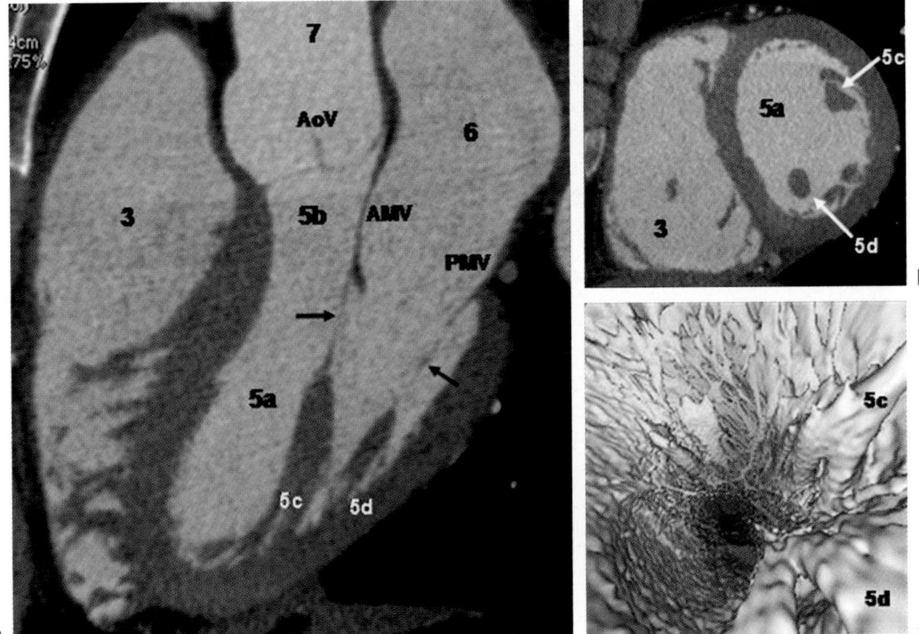

Fig. 7.8a–c. 2D three chambers (**a**) and short axis views (**b**), navigator to apex (**c**), (*3*) Right ventricle, left ventricle: (*5a*) inflow portion, (*5b*) outflow portion, anterior (*5c*) and posterior (*5d*) papillary muscles, (*6*) left atrium (LA), (*7*) ascending aorta (Ao), chordae (*arrow*), anterior (*AMV*) and posterior (*PMV*) valves, aortic valves (*AoV*)

7.1.2 Heart Valve Anatomy

7.1.2.1 Aortic Valves and Aorta

The fibrous skeleton of the heart includes the aortic ring and the mitral ring. The aortic valve inserts in the aortic ring and is comprised of two anterior cusps and a posterior cusp. Its diameter is from 23 to 29 mm in men and from 20 to 26 mm in women. The illuminated surface of valves open during systole is greater than 200 mm^2 (Figs. 7.9, 7.10).

The initial segment of the aorta (segment 0) extends from the aortic valve to the sino-tubular junction and is dilated in three sinuses:

- the right anterior sinus of Vasalva (RASV) or right coronary sinus turns into the the right coronary artery;
- the left anterior sinus of Vasalva (LASV) or left coronary sinus turns into the common trunk;
- the posterior sinus of Vasalva (PSV) or non-coronary sinus.

The diameter of segment 0 is from 31 to 37 mm in men and from 27 to 33 mm in women. The ascending aorta (segment 1) extends from the sino-tubular to the brachio-cephalic arterial trunk. Its diameter is from 23 to 29 mm in men and from 20 to 26 mm in women.

7.1.2.2 Mitral Valves

The mitral valve is located between the left atrium and the left ventricle. It inserts in the mitral ring that is part of the fibrous skeleton of the heart, continuous with the aortic ring. It comprises the anterior large cusp (LC) and the posterior small cusp (SC). During ventricular systole, occlusion of the mitral orifice occurs in front of the mitral ring. Its diameter is from 30 to 35 mm (Figs. 7.11, 7.12).

7.1.2.3 Pulmonary Valves and the Pulmonary Artery

The pulmonary valve is comprised of three cusps (Fig. 7.13):

- two posterior cusps
- one anterior cusp

The pulmonary ring has a diameter of 20 to 22 mm. The trunk of the pulmonary artery is almost entirely intra pericardial. Its diameter is 35 mm.

7.1.2.4 Tricuspid Valves

The tricuspid valve inserts in the tricuspid ring. It is composed of three cusps: anterior, posterior and septal. Its diameter is from 35 to 38 mm (Fig. 7.14).

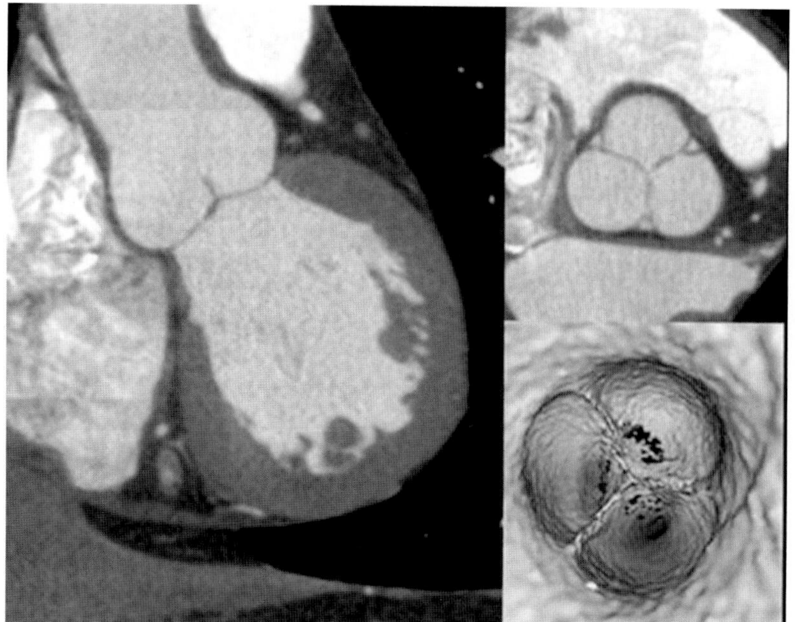

Fig. 7.9. 2D and navigator of the aortic valves in diastole (80% of the cardiac cycle)

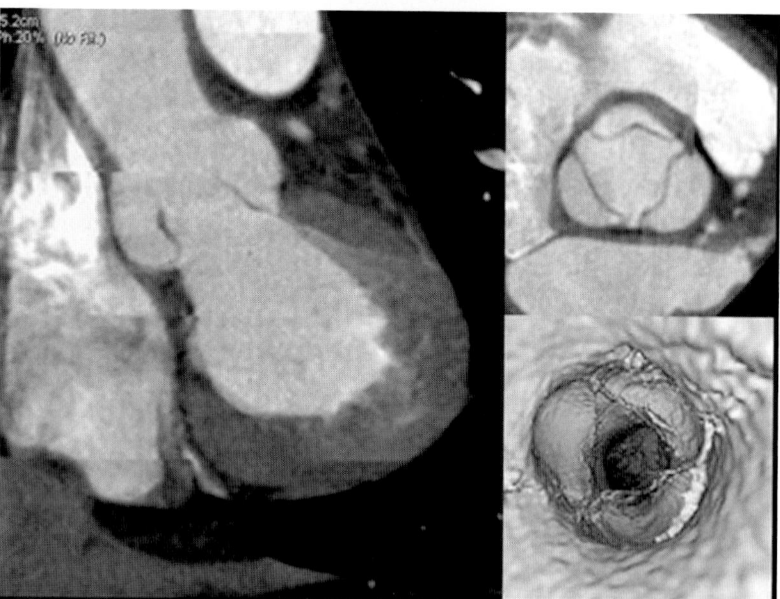

Fig. 7.10. 2D and navigator of the aortic valves in systole (20% of the cardiac cycle)

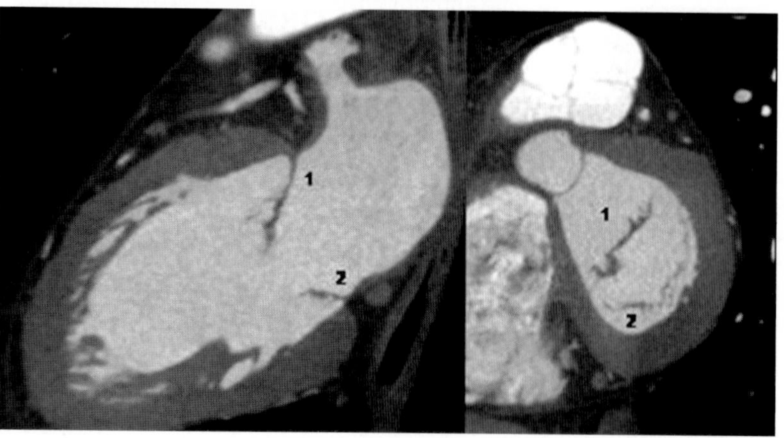

Fig. 7.11. 2D large (*1*) and short (*2*) axis: mitral valves open during diastole (80% of cardiac cycle)

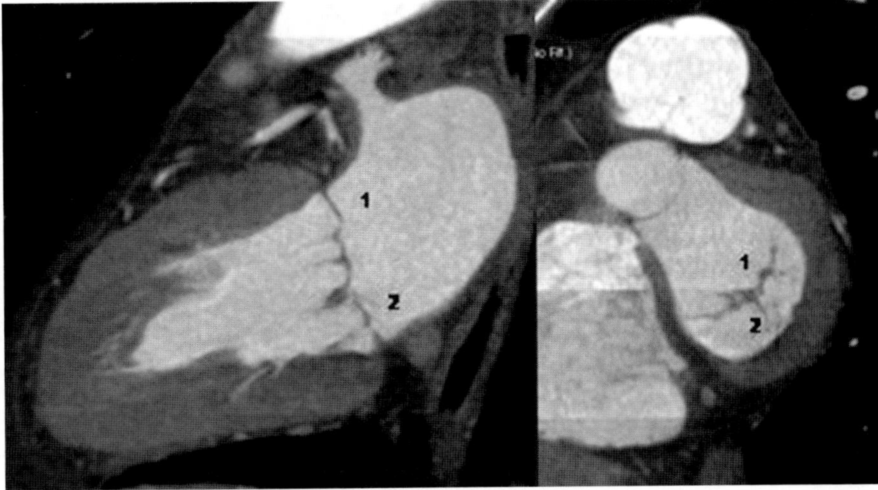

Fig. 7.12. 2D large (*1*) and short (*2*) axis: mitral valves closed during systole (20% of cardiac cycle)

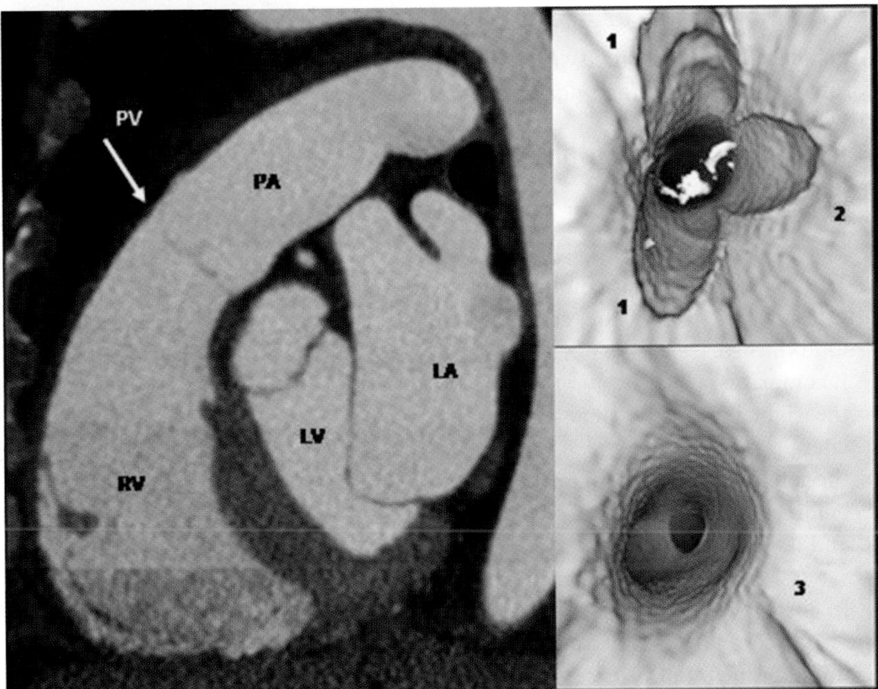

Fig. 7.13. 2D and navigator – pulmonary valves (*arrow*), *1* posterior cusps, *2* anterior cusp, *3* PA trunk

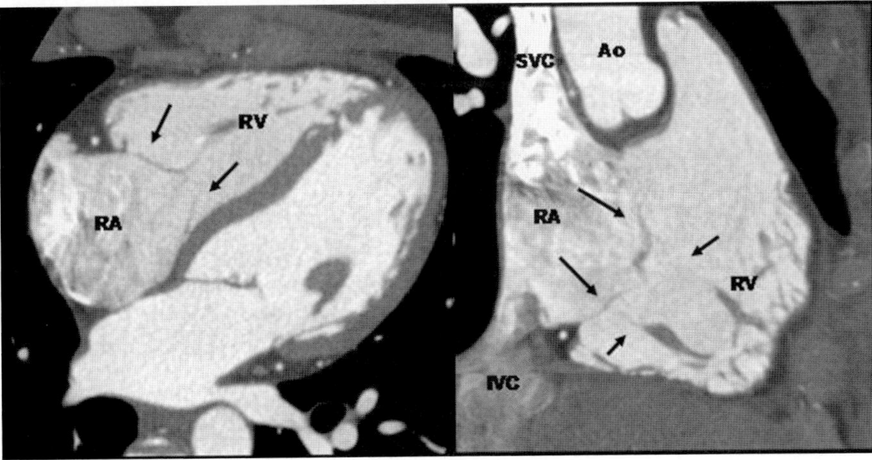

Fig. 7.14. 2D – tricuspid valves, cordae and papillary muscles of the right ventricle (*arrow*)

7.1.3 Coronary Artery Anatomy

7.1.3.1 The Coronary Ostia

The coronary arteries arise from the aorta and run around this ovoid structure in a deep position. The right coronary artery arises from the right anterior part of the aortic sinus and runs forward to join the right coronary sulcus. The left coronary artery arises from the left anterior aortic sinus and runs backwards and then forwards again around the pulmonary artery (Fig. 7.15).

7.1.3.2 Division of Coronary Arteries

At this level it divides into two main branches. The coronary arteries, as their name suggests, form a crown around the heart.

It is in fact possible to distinguish (Fig. 7.16):

- a posterior crown,
- an anterior loop.

The posterior crown is composed of the coronary arteries, which follow the coronary sulcus right around the heart.

It comprises:

- the right coronary artery and its left postero-lateral artery
- the left coronary: the main trunk of the artery before division, then the left circumflex artery and its terminal part.

In 80% of cases the posterior circle is formed by the right coronary artery and its retro-ventricular terminal branch. In this case, the right coronary artery is dominant.

The anterior loop that passes over the apex is formed by branches of the right and left coronary arteries. This loop arises on the upper surface of the heart from the left coronary artery of which it forms the anterior interventricular branch or left anterior descending artery (LAD). This joins the interventricular sulcus, crosses the apex and rises beyond, tending to join up on the diaphragmatic surface of the heart with the diaphragmatic branch of the loop, i.e., the rear interventricular branch of the right coronary artery.

The ring and the loop have many connections by anastomosis between the terminal and collateral branches.

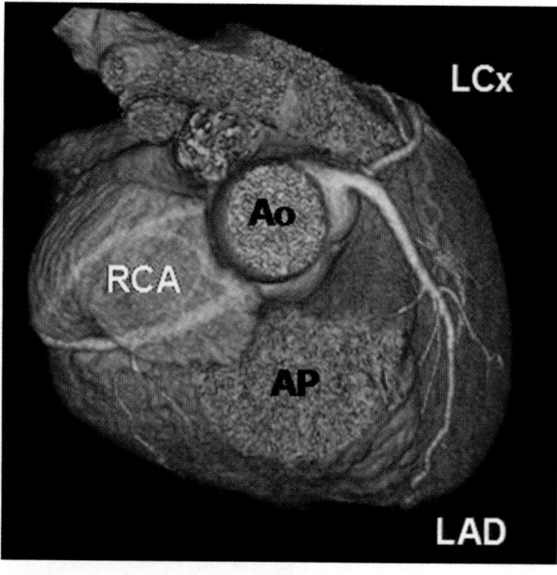

Fig. 7.15. 3D spider view (*superior view*), coronary ostia

The posterior crown comprises:

- The right coronary artery (RCA) and
- its left postero lateral artery (PLA);
- the left coronary artery system (LCA),
- with its main trunk (MT), then the left
- circumflex artery and its terminal
- branch (LCx)

The anterior loop comprises:

- The left anterior descending artery
- (LAD)
- The right posterior descending artery
- (PDA)

Collaterals: three types can be distinguished:

1. Anterior branches:
- anterior ventricular arteries
- right marginal branches (RMG)
- diagonal branches (Diag.)
- left marginal branches (LMB)

2. Septal branches:
- interventricular septal branches of LAD
- interventricular septal branches of RCA
- AV node branches

3. Posterior branches:
- the atrial branches

The posterior crown, the anterior loop, the anterior collaterals and the septal branches create a net-

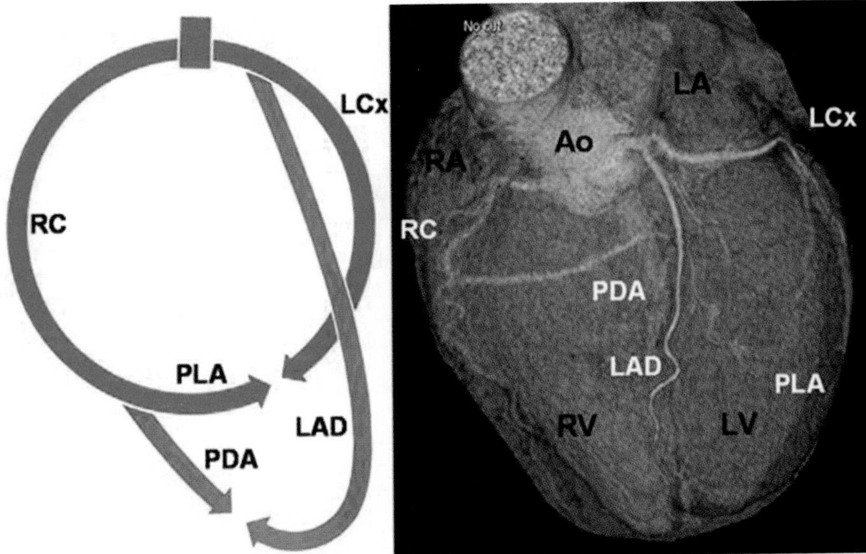

Fig. 7.16. Division of the coronary arteries

work that completely enmeshes the heart (Fig. 7.17). All parts of the mesh can communicate as required by the opening up of shunts.

There are some variations:

- The LCx will usually rise to one or several marginal branches.
- In case of left dominance, the LCx can supply a PDA.
- On rare occasions, a diagonal branch can be larger than the LAD.
- If a third branch arises from the LMT, between the LAD and LCx, that branch is called the intermediate branch, ramus intermedius or ramus.

7.1.3.3 Identification of Coronary Arteries in 3D Imaging (MIP or Angiographic View) and 2D Imaging

See Figures 7.18 to 7.20.

7.1.3.4 Segmentation of Coronary Arteries in 3D Imaging (MIP or Angiographic View and Volume Rendering)

In the classification system for coronary artery segments according to the American College of Cardiology/American Heart Association Guidelines for Coronary Angiography, the number of segments is 27 coronary segments. In our routine, we use a simplified artery segment model of 18 coronary segments to compare coronary CTA and coronary angiography.

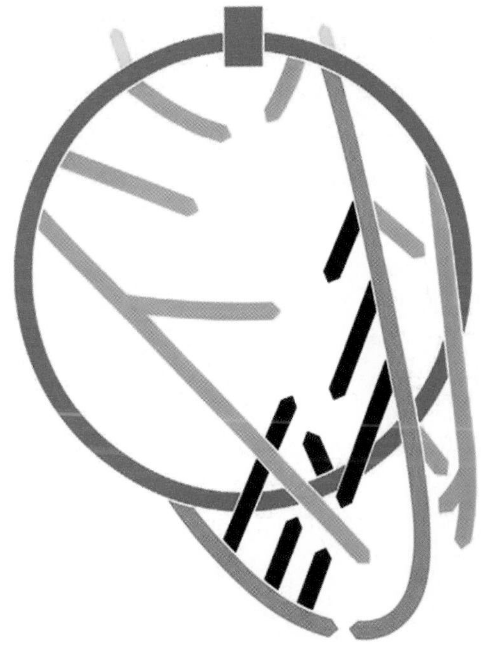

Fig. 7.17. Diagram of coronary arteries

Segmentation of the Right Coranary Artery

- Segment 1 corresponds to the right coronary from the right coronary ostium to the first angle or elbow of the right coronary, beginning at the vertical portion.
- Segment 2 is the vertical portion, from the end of the first angle to the second angle.

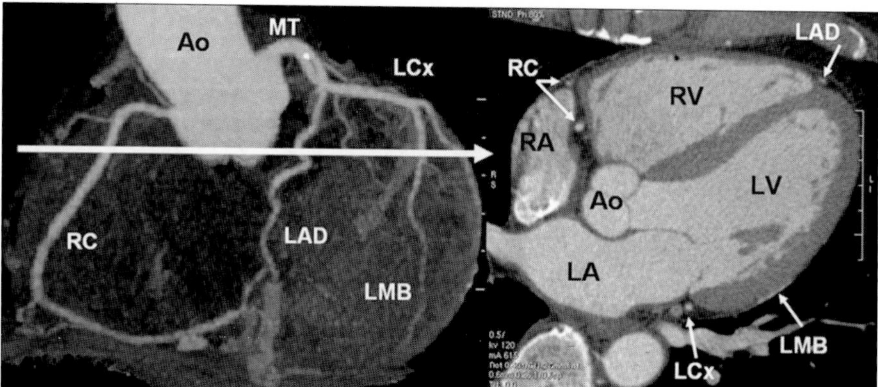

Fig. 7.18. Identification of coronaries in axial view

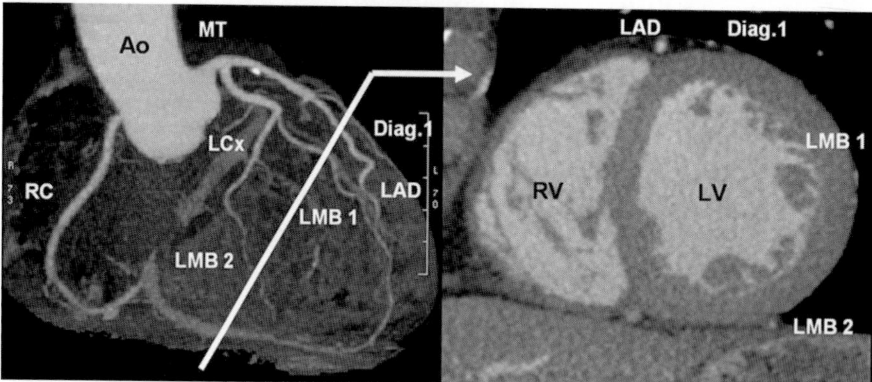

Fig. 7.19. Identification of coronaries in short axis view

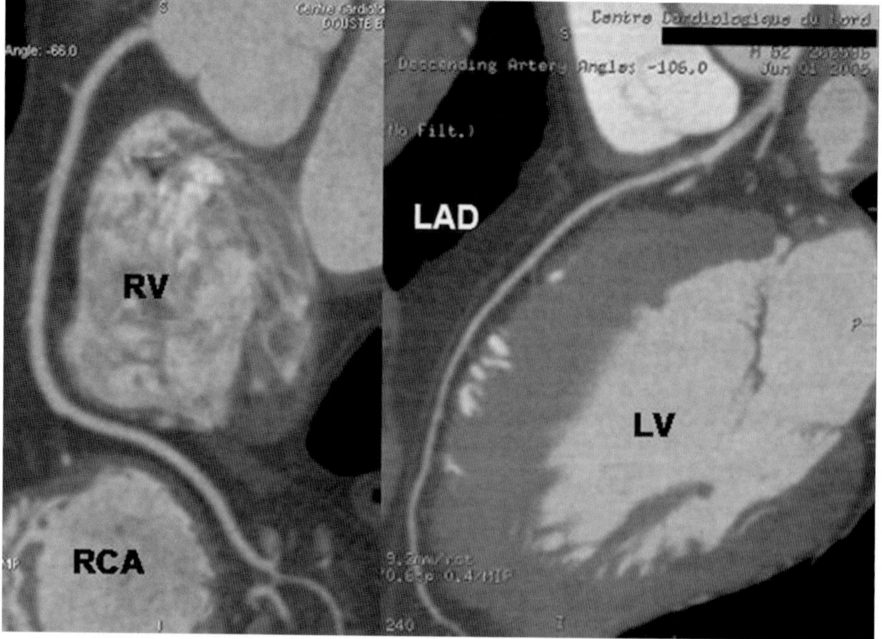

Fig. 7.20. Identification of coronaries in 2D curved view

- Segment 3 is the vertical portion from the end of the second angle up to the cross of the heart, i.e., the PDA/PLA bifurcation.
- Segment 4 is the PDA, and segment 5 is the PLA (Fig. 7.21).

Segmentation of the Left Coranary Artery

- Segment 11 is the left main trunk, from the ostium to the LAD/LCx bifurcation.
- Segment 12 is the LAD, from the proximal part of the LAD to the first septal (but some prefer to say to the first large branch that may be the first diagonal).
- Segment 13 of the LAD corresponds to the middle part of the IVA included between the first septal and the origin of the second diagonal.
- Segment 14 of the LAD is the second diagonal at the tip of the heart.
- The diagonal and septal branches (segments 15, 16, 29) are numbered in ascending order according to their anatomical locations with respect to the proximal LAD.
- Segment 18 of the LCx is the LMT/LAD bifurcation at the first marginal.
- Segment 19 is from the first marginal to the second marginal if it exists. On the other hand, some speak of the medial LCx just after the origin of the first marginal and of a distal LCx as we get farther from it. The marginal branches are numbered in ascending order according to their anatomical locations with respect to the proximal LCx (Fig. 7.22).

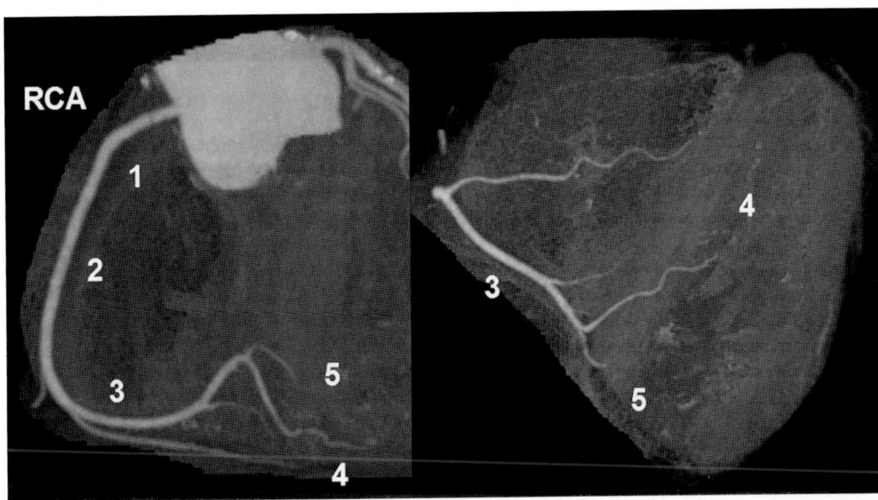

Fig. 7.21. 3D MIP, RCA segmentation

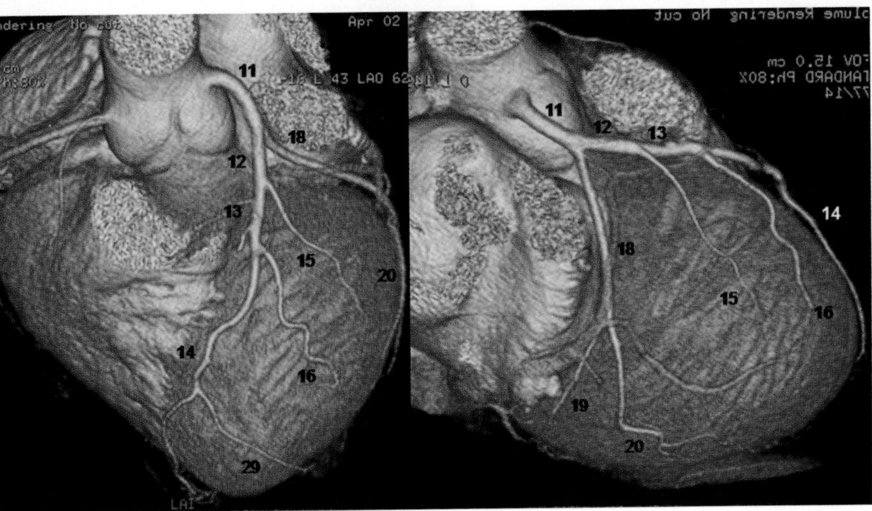

Fig. 7.22. 3D VR views, LCA segmentation

7.1.3.5 Myocardium Segmentation

Each coronary artery irrigates different segments of the myocardium:

The walls of the left ventricle are divided into 16 segments:

There are three main segments: basal, medial and apical.

- the apical segment is divided into four segments: anterior, lateral, posterior, septal.
- the medial segment into six segments: anterior, antero-lateral, postero-lateral, posterior, postero-septal, antero-septal.
- the basal segment is divided in the same way as the medial segment
- The LAD irrigates the apex and the antero-septal wall of the myocardium.
- The left circumflex irrigates the lateral wall of the myocardium.
- The RCA irrigates the inferior wall of the myocardium.
- The apico-lateral segment is vascularized either by the LAD or by the left circumflex.
- Distribution varies according to which network is dominant (Figs. 7.23, 7.24).

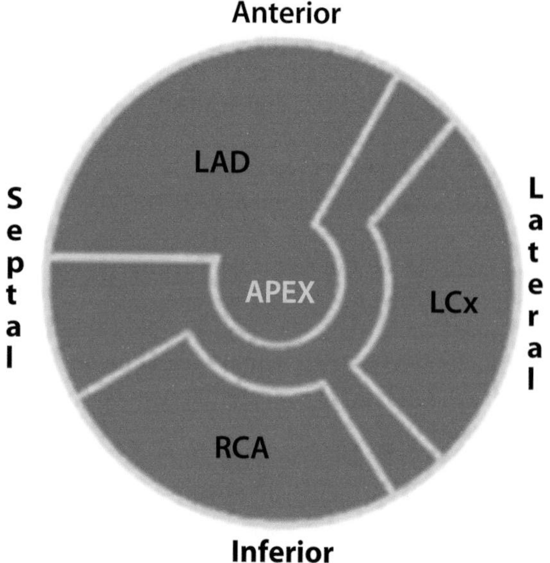

Fig. 7.24. CA and segmentation, bull's eye

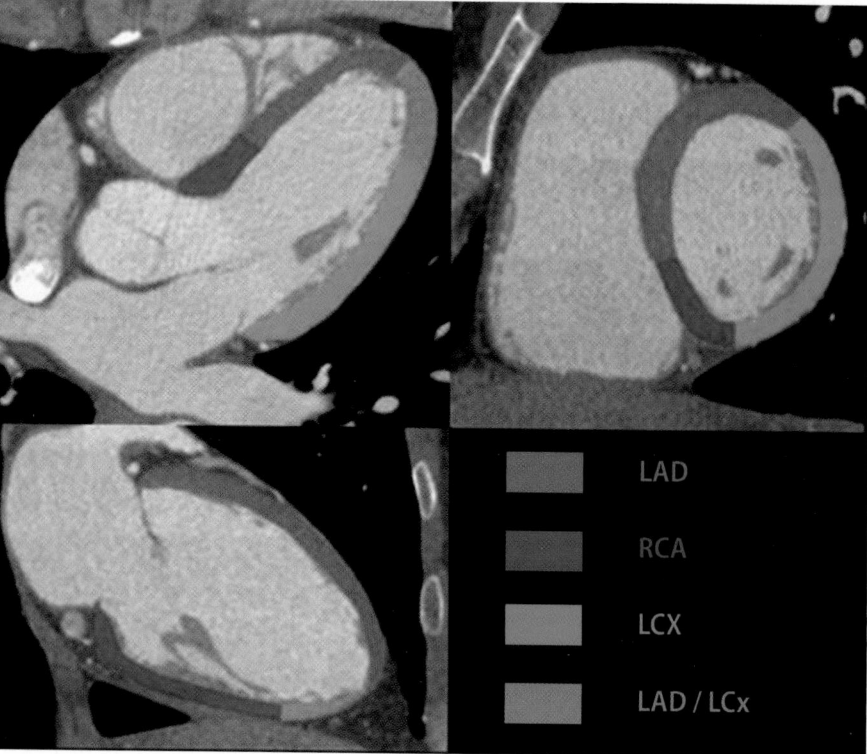

Fig. 7.23. Each coronary artery irrigates different segments of the myocardium

7.1.4
Coronary Vein Anatomy

The veins of the heart are even more variable than the arteries. Approximately 80% of venous blood return is achieved via coronary veins. The great cardiac vein parallel to the left anterior artery) begins at the tip of the heart, follows the anterior interventricular sulcus, then in the auriculo ventricular sulcus or coronary sulcus (parallel to the left circonflex artery). In its course it receives affluents, in particular the left marginal vein and posterior vein of the left ventricle. It then turns into the coronary sinus.

The coronary sinus is a terminal collector measuring 3 cm in length located in the porterior portion of the coronary sulcus. It empties in the right atrium. Immediately before this ostium, the middle cardiac vein (which has a course alongside the posterior descending artery) and the small cardiac vein (parallel to the right coronary artery) also drain into the right atrium. One third of venous blood is drained by the small veins of the heart, primarily the anterior veins of the right ventricle that empty into the right atrium. Some parietal veins empty directly into the cardiac chambers (Fig. 7.25).

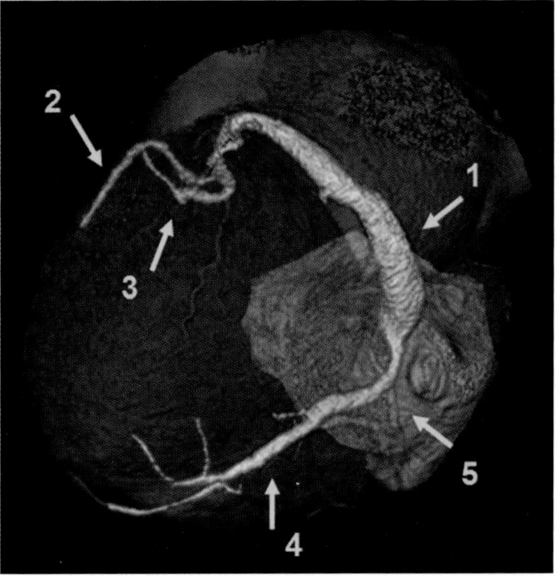

Fig. 7.25. Coronary veins. Diaphragmatic view: (*1*) coronary sinus, (*2*) great cardiac vein, (*3*) LV posterior vein, (*4*) middle cardiac vein, (*5*) small cardiac vein

7.2
Physiological Basis: Reminder of Heart Physiology and Physiopathology Aspects

7.2.1
Cardiac Cycle Chronology

For a given heart rate (HR), the duration of one cycle in milliseconds is 60,000/HR (R-R interval, in reference to the ECG R-wave), e.g., HR = 75/min, R-R = 800 ms. In the case of a cardiac scanner, the starting point for the cardiac cycle is defined as the bottom of the QRS (R-R Phase 0%), and the R-R interval is usually divided into ten phases of 10% of the cycle. The cycles of the right and left heart are not totally synchronous, in particular in pathological situations of conduction disorders or severe cardiopathy, but this asynchronism represents only some tens of milliseconds, which, at the resolution of the cardiac scanner and for current applications, has no practical consequences.

Two successive phases can be identified:

- Ventricular systole, including isovolumic contraction and ventricular ejection.
- Ventricular diastole, including isovolumic relaxation and ventricular filling.

I – Ventricular Systole

The electrical stimulation originates from the sinusal node/auriculoventricular node/bundle of the His/Purkinje network circuit. It results in the depolarization of ventricular cells, the sudden increase in the cellular Ca2+ concentration, the creation of actin-myosin bridges and the contraction of myocardial ventricular cells.

This simultaneous contraction of ventricular cells produces a tensioning of the ventricular walls, responsible for a rapid pressure increase in the ventricle with closure of the auriculoventricular valve (auricular pressure being low, the associated lead time is negligible). Neuro-hormonal factors influence the speed of contraction of the fibers and the pressure generated in the ventricle.

Phase 1: Isovolumic contraction (R-R about 0 to 10%). Pressure rises rapidly, but the arterial and auriculoventricular valves being closed, the ventricular volume remains constant.

Phase 2: Ventricular ejection (R-R about 10 to 40%). When the ventricular pressure becomes greater than the arterial pressure, the arterial valve opens, allowing systolic ventricular ejection. At the end of ejection, given that the shortening of the muscular fibers is at its maximum and the volume is decreasing, the pressure generated in the ventricular cavity falls, resulting in the re-closure of the arterial valve.

II – Ventricular Diastole

Phase 1: Isovolumic relaxation (R-R about 40 to 50%). The active recapture of calcium in the sarcoplasmic reticulum during ventricular repolarization stops the formation of actin-myosin bridges. Ventricular pressure drops rapidly, whereas the ventricular volume remains constant, the valves being closed.

Phase 2: Diastolic filling (R-R about 50 to 0%). When the ventricular pressure drops below the auricular pressure, the auriculoventricular valve opens, and the ventricle starts to fill with the blood accumulated in the atrium during valve closure.

During a Doppler heart exam, during diastolic filling, two flows can be distinguished, called E (early) and A (atrial).

E: The first part of the filling (R-R about 50 to 70%) is passive, given that the blood flow between the atrium and ventricle is simply the result of the pressure difference between these two cavities. At the end of passive filling, this flow can run out.

A: Auricular contraction occurs after the ECG P-wave (R-R about 80 to 0%), responsible for a re-increase in auricular pressure (auricular systole) with a continuation of A-V flow (active filling).

Diastolic filling of the ventricle is equal to the sum of these two passive and active components (E+A).

The E/A ratio between these two components is linked to two principal determinants:

(1) The intrinsic qualities of the ventricular muscle: relaxation (active mechanism of calcium recapture in the sarcoplasmic reticulum, the opposite of myocardial cell contraction, occurring at the beginning of diastole, at the same time as the E-wave) and compliance (elastic properties of the ventricular wall, allowing it to passively distend at low pressure, occurring after relaxation at the end of diastole, at the same time as the A-wave).

(2) Left auricular pressure, which itself changes over the diastole, but is closely correlated to the pulmonary capillary pressure.

The E/A ratio therefore physiologically changes with age, heart rate, volume, and then as a result of the onset of a cardiopathy (deterioration of intrinsic heart muscle properties) and its decompensation (increase in pulmonary capillary pressure).

For healthy and young subjects, the E/A ratio is greater than 1.

7.2.2 Pressure/Volume Curves

The contraction force of the myocardial cell is generated by the interaction between the proteins of the sarcomer: actin, myosin, troponin and tropomyosin. For the heart muscle, as for the skeletal muscle, the force generated varies as a function of the initial length of the sarcomer when contraction starts. There is a range of optimum values in which tension is maximum given that the interaction between the actin and myosin filaments is optimal. Below and above this range, tension drops (due to the fact that confrontation between filaments drops or becomes redundant).

The elastic elements of the muscular wall add to these contractile elements, positioned in series and in parallel with respect to the sarcomers. The tension generated by the elastic elements increases with rest length. In physiology, the functioning of the myocardial cell is below the maximum contraction tension zone, such that the increase of ventricular end-diastolic blood volume (EDV – end-diastolic volume, also called preload) results in an increase in the force generated by the heart muscle (on the rising part of the curve). This additional force allows a larger ejection of end systolic blood (ESV – end-systolic volume) and allows a partial compensation of the increase in the preload (tending to correct ESV).

Similarly, an increase in the ejection resistance (increase in "afterload") is responsible for an initial decrease in the systolic ejection volume (SEV) and therefore an increase in end-systolic volume (ESV). Diastolic filling adds to ESV, and the end-diastolic volume is also increased, triggering the same regulation mechanism by an increase in actin-myosin interactions.

This adaptation of the heart to preload and afterload changes by modulating contraction force is called the Frank-Starling law. Secondarily, the increase in systolic tensioning of sarcomers results in hypertrophy through the increase in the synthesis of contractile proteins, which allow an increase in contractile force with normalization of stress per sarcomer, at the cost of a thickening and therefore rigidification of the wall (reduction of compliance).

The pressure-volume curves are the graphical translation of the Frank-Starling law and allow us to understand the cycle-to-cycle adaptation of cardiopathies and predict their evolutive profile depending on their mechanisms (modification of preload, afterload and change in sarcomer contractile properties – contraction and relaxation, elastic properties of the wall, etc.). This graphic (Fig. 7.26) shows the four stages of the cardiac cycle: isovolumic contraction (1), ejection (2), isovolumic relaxation (3) and filling (4).

7.2.3 Systolic and Diastolic Functions

The heart is a double pump placed in series between the pulmonary and systemic circulations. In the absence of a shunt between the right and left cavities, the pulmonary flow rate is equal to the systemic flow rate and the right cardiac flow rate is equal to the left cardiac flow rate.

Cardiac flow rate (CF) is equal to the product of the blood volume ejected with each cardiac cycle

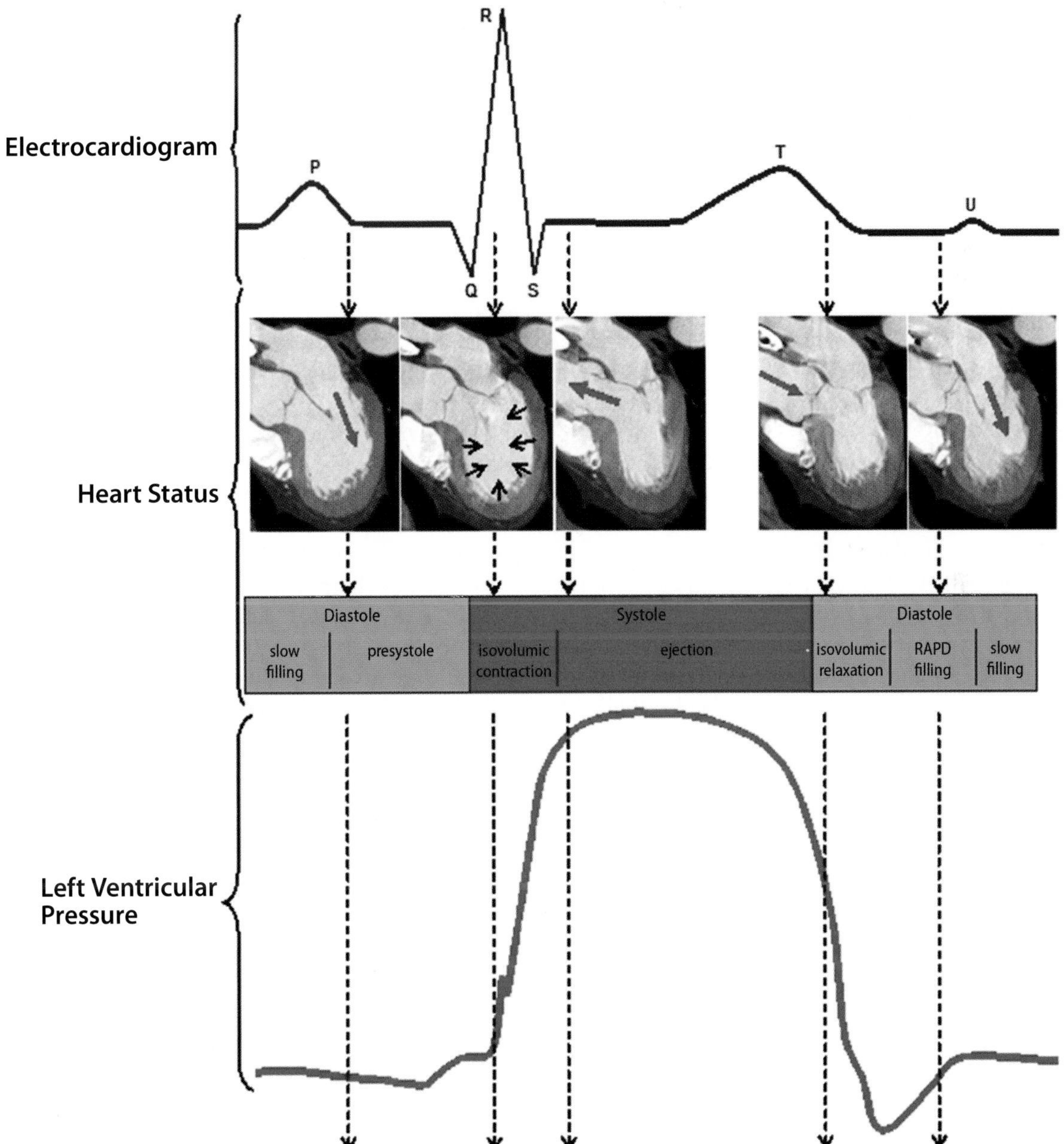

Fig. 7.26. Four stages of the cardiac cycle. RAPD = rapid

(systolic ejection volume–SEV) and the cardiac frequency (CF). The normal value is close to 5 l/min (about 3 l/min/m^2). CF = SEV × CF.

The pulmonary circulation represents a resistance (Rp) that is significantly lower than that of systemic circulation (Rs): the pressure required to ensure pulmonary flow, which is ensured by the right ventricle, is therefore much less than the pressure generated by the left ventricle (dP = R × CF). In a physiological situation, the maximum pressures generated at rest are not greater than 40 mmHg in the right ventricle (RV) and 140 mmHg in the left ventricle (LV) in systole.

The term "systolic function" designates, in general, the capacity of the muscle of a cardiac cavity to eject its content during its contraction (systole). It may be applied to each of the four cavities, but usually designates the contractile function of the left ventricle, the main determining factor for cardiac flow rate.

Left ventricular systolic function is usually expressed in the form of an ejection fraction (left ventricular ejection fraction – LVEF), which is the ratio of the systolic ejection volume (SEV) to the end diastolic volume (EDV). But it can be expressed as a derivative of intra-ventricular pressure, work or power.

In the case of a cardiac scanner, the determination of the end-systolic (40% R-R) and end-diastolic (0% R-R) left ventricular cavity volume is easy and allows the calculation of LVEF. The same principle can be applied to the right ventricular ejection fraction (RVEF).

The term "diastolic function" designates, in general, the capacity of a cardiac cavity to fill at low pressure during diastole. It may also be applied to the four cavities, but is mainly applied to the left ventricle for which the walls are the thickest of the heart and for which the risk of diastolic dysfunction is the highest.

There is no one simple tool for quantifying the left ventricular diastolic function, given that diastole is a complex sequence involving numerous mechanisms. As discussed above, and in schematic terms, the first half of the left ventricular diastole is essentially dependent upon:

- The left ventricle's relaxation capacity (calcium recapture in the reticulum).
- The left intra-auricular static pressure.
- The second half is dependent upon:
- The elastic compliance of the left ventricular walls (passive phenomenon).
- The pressure generated by the auricular contraction.

The only cardiac scanning tool that is currently available for studying diastolic function and the respective contribution of these two filling components is the analysis of ventricular volume variation during diastole (between 40% and 100% of R-R).

The correlation between this fill profile and data obtained by cardiac catheterization or sonogram is being studied. By analogy with the E/A ratio for cardiac Doppler exams, this characteristic profile could contribute to restrictive cardiopathy diagnosis (amylosis, hemochromatosis), decompensated heart failure, tamponade, pericardial constriction, etc.

7.2.4 Rhythmology Aspects

This chapter addresses some of the basic notions of rhythmology that are useful for cardiac scanner applications and, in particular, for the resolution of difficulties that arise as a result of gating. Cardiac rhythm recognition for synchronization is based on the signal acquired by a limited number of electrodes, giving a limited number of electrocardiogram derivations. Given that filtering differs for a system designed for rhythmology analysis, the goal here is not to perform a medical diagnosis, but to optimize the use of the signal through gating.

For a sinus rhythm, cardiac depolarization comprises three principal deflections on the surface ECG, separated by isoelectrical intervals:

- The P-wave, corresponding to the electrical activation of the atrium, and which slightly precedes their effective contraction.
- The QRS complex, which corresponds to the depolarization of the ventricular myocardium, contraction of the muscle with a certain shift (electro-mechanical delay) and atrium re-polarization, is not very high or synchronous with the QRS and is therefore not visible.
- The T-wave, which corresponds to the ventricular re-polarization that precedes ventricular relaxation (Fig. 7.27).

Difficulty of QRS Detection

Gating is based on QRS detection, which is normally the largest deflection. Certain pathological situations in which the T-wave is particularly large (subendocardial ischemia, hyperkalemia, etc.) can confuse the algorithm, resulting in a double detection: the reconstruction produces an incoherent fusion of data making the acquisition unusable. In rare instances, the same phenomenon can be observed with a very large P-wave (auricular hypertrophy). Inversely, a QRS axis that is perpendicular to the coronal plane can result in small amplitudes that are difficult for the software to recognize. This problem can usually be avoided by adjusting the voltage, changing the ECG derivation or repositioning the electrodes.

The Presence of a Non-Sinus Supraventricular Rhythm Can Compromise Exam Quality in Two Ways

- The high heart rate (supraventricular tachycardia): depending on manufacturer, the upper limit of acceptable heart rate for acquisition varies between 65 and 100 cycles/min, but because of the segmentation algorithms used, the quality of the result is not reliable in this range for a given system. In most cases, a medical treatment to reduce atrial tachycardia or auricular fibrillation, prescribed in advance by the treating cardiologist, allows this problem to be managed.
- Rhythm irregularity: This is the principal limitation for gating; the exact chronology of a short cycle is not simply the transposition of a long cycle at another timescale, and the fusion of data from short and long cycles results in 'stacked' artifacts and an image that is difficult to exploit.

Currently, we do not recommend cardiac scans for patients with auricular fibrillation. Relative sinus tachycardia, regular flutter and regular atrial tachycardia can be envisaged if the ventricular rate is below 100 cycles/min.

With regard to preparation by oral or intravenous beta-blocker, it is necessary to take particular care that there are no contraindications:

- Bronchospasm (asthmatic, spastic COPD; bradycardic calcium inhibitors can then be used).
- Conduction disorders or associated antiarrhythmic therapy.
- But above all patent or latent heart failure.

The administration protocols vary depending on the team. In the absence of oral beta-blockers, we recommend an injectable short-duration beta-blocker: esmolol (BreviblocR), with scope monitoring before and after scan (elimination occurs within a few minutes by intraplasmatic metabolization). Auricular and ventricular extrasystoles (AES and VES) result in the same problem as for cardiac arrhythmia. If these are limited in number, certain systems allow the exclusion of the corresponding acquisition data, but with an associated loss of quality (noise).

The Presence of a Pacemaker Is Responsible for Two Types of Problems

- Artifacts due to the metallic probes placed in the right cavities (atrium, ventricle) and sometimes

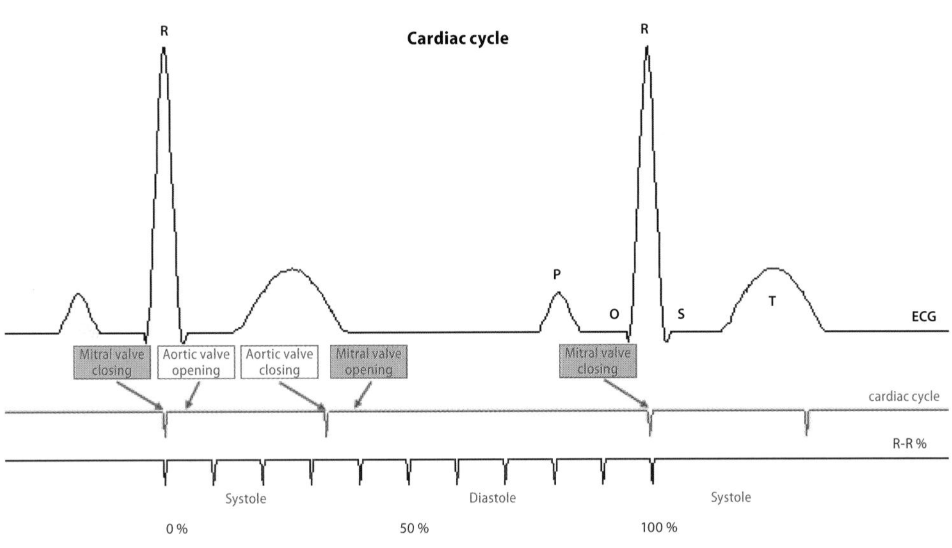

Fig. 7.27. The T-wave, which corresponds to the ventricular re-polarization that precedes ventricular relaxation

in the coronary sinus branches (multi-site stimulation).

- Spikes on the ECG, vertical lines corresponding to the delivery of the electrical impulse preceding the depolarization of heart cells. These spikes may result in gating detection errors. Again in this case, the adjustment of the voltage, a change in derivation or re-positioning of electrodes can resolve certain problems. Occasionally, temporary re-programming of the pacemaker by the cardiologist can resolve the problem.

7.2.5 Opacification of Coronary Arteries

The heart is mobile around its axis, with rotation during systole. Its volume varies between systole and diastole. The heart's volume is affected by displacement of the diaphragm. Coronary filling is easier during diastole. In systole, the opening of the aortic valves and the ventricular ejection creates a "vacuum pump" effect at the aortic coronary sinuses, which makes movement of blood through the ostia of the coronary arteries more difficult.

Cardiac diastole represents the moment of muscular and valvular silence: the heart is immobile, positions are fixed (apart from movements of the diaphragm controlled by the breath-hold), and there is better filling of the coronary arteries. On the ECG, the period of cardiac immobility or diastole begins slightly later than the R-wave and lasts until the Q-wave (on the ECG, the center of diastole is situated at about 70% of an R-R complex).

The time of coronary circulation, from the ostium to the myocardial capillaries, must be taken into account. Coronary venous return is continuous. The transit time of a bolus of blood through the coronary network must be accurately assessed. In coronography, it may take one, two, three or more "systole-diastole" complexes. During these "systole-diastole" cycles, one must take advantage of the moments when the coronary arteries are opacified and the heart is fixed and with maximum aspiration, i.e., during diastole. The number of "systole-diastole" cycles necessary to fill the whole coronary network will require 5–10 s. The faster the heart rate, the slower coronary filling will be (this is one of the factors leading to ischemia in fast-beating hearts) and the longer the required acquisition time. Slowing of the heart rate favors coronary filling. It also lengthens the period of diastolic immobility that can be used for acquisition. The regulation and slowing of heart rate are factors that favor good quality imaging: oxygen therapy, hypotensive agents and beta blockers. The heart rate should be slowed as much as is possible without discomfort for the patient.

Reference

Bernard Y (2002) Echocardiographie normale et pathologique. Encycl Med Chir Radiodiagnostic Coeur-Poumon. 32-006-A-10, p 37

Cluzel P, Brochu B, Izzillo R et al. (2004) Evaluation de la fonction cardiaque en imagerie par résonance magnétique et scanner hélicoïdal multicoupe. J Radiol 85:1766–1782

Delmas A, Rouviere H (2002) Anatomie humaine. Tome 2

Garcier JM, Trogrlic S, Boyer L, Crochet PD (2004) Anatomy of the heart and coronary arteries. J Radiol 85:1758–1763

Manuel D, Cerqueira MD, Weissman NJ, Dilsizian V, Jacobs AK, Kaul S, Laskey WK, Pennell DJ, Rumberger JA, Ryan T, Verani MS (2002) Standardized myocardial segmentation and nomenclature for tomographic imaging of the heart. Circulation 105:539–542

Sablayrolles JL, Bouvier E, Feignoux J, Sénéchal Q (2005) Cardiac CT. GE Healthcare

Part III:

Heart-Lung Interactions

Physiological Interactions

8

Francois Laurent and Michel Montaudon

CONTENTS

F. Laurent, MD
M. Montaudon, MD
Unité d'Imagerie Thoracique et Cardiovasculaire, Hôpital Cardiologique du Haut Lévèque, Avenue de Magellan, 33604 Pessac, France

8.1 Introduction

Improvement in both temporal and spatial resolution of MDCT has brought the ability to explore both the heart and lung within a single examination and opened the field of functional evaluation. However, interactions between heart and lung have long been identified as important physiological phenomena in pathology (Pinsky 2005). For the radiologist, they are involved in difficulties of interpretation in a MDCT thorax examination and in the understanding of observations in physiological normal or near-normal clinical situations. In this chapter, after a brief overview of physiological heart-lung interactions, we will overview the consequences in imaging the heart and lung with the effects of the beating heart on thoracic organs, those of respiratory maneuvers, and of cardiac functional parameters on vascular enhancement. Then, interactions among the pulmonary, systemic circulation, and lymphatic circulations in normal subjects will be considered. Finally, near-normal conditions, such as clinically silent right-left shunts by patent foramen ovale, deformities, or postoperative conditions, will be described in this physiologic perspective.

8.2 Physiological Basis of Heart-Lung Interactions

The basic physiological heart-lung interactions can be understood as the effects of lung volume variations on both the cardiac rhythm and function and are mainly explained by variations of pressure. Lung volume varies in a tidal fashion during spontaneous respiration. During inspiration, intrathoracic pressure decreases owing to the contraction of the respiratory muscles. Inflation induces immediate changes in autonomic output, causing cardiac acceleration (Glick et al. 1969). This is otherwise known as respiratory sinus arythmia, a normal responsiveness that is lost in diabetic peripheral neuropathy. Lung inflation to larger tidal volume (> 15 ml/g) increases heart rate by sympathetic withdrawal and reflex arterial vasodilatation (Pinsky 2005). Thus, the heart has the intrinsic ability to vary its rate in synchrony with ventilation. Changes, or the rate of changes, in myocardial wall stretch might alter intrinsic heart rate independently of autonomic tone (Bernardi et al. 1989).

Interactions between respiration and cardiac function can be understood based on the effects of changes in intrathoracic pressure and lung volume on both venous return and left ejection fraction. During spontaneous ventilation, venous return increases when intrathoracic pressure decreases, that is, during inspiration (Pinsky 1984a). When filling increases on the right side, less filling occurs on the left side. In addition, the pooling of blood in the pulmonary circulation decreases filling pressure on the left side of the heart (Pinsky 1984b). The reverse occurs during expiration, and an increase in intrathoracic pressure augments the left ventricular afterload (Pinsky 1984a). This phenomenon, called interventricular dependence, is anatomically in relation to the presence of the constraining pericardium and the fact that ventricles share the interventricular and interatrial septum. Interventricular dependence works both ways even if the right side of the heart is more vulnerable to compressive forces. Interventricular dependence is increased when ventricular volumes are increased, i.e., in dilated cardiomyopathies or when the pericardium is relatively resistant to stretch, such as the stiffer pericardium of constrictive pericarditis or increased intrapericardial pressure of tamponade. In this setting, increasing right ventricular volume shifts the intraventricular septum into the left ventricle and simultaneously decreases left ventricular diastolic compliance and end-diastolic left volume.

Sustained increase in intrathoracic pressure, as seen with the Valsalva maneuver, will eventually decreases aortic blood pressure and arterial pressure because venous return decreases. Hyperinflation compresses the heart between the expanding lungs (Butler 1983) and increases juxtacardiac intrathoracic pressure more than the lateral chest wall intrathoracic pressure.

Ventilation alters pulmonary vascular resistance by a process known as hypoxemic pulmonary vasoconstriction. If regional alveolar PO^2 decreases below 60 mmHg, local pulmonary vasomotor tone increases, then reducing blood flow. Decrease in end-expiratory volume promotes alveolar collapse, stimulating hypoxemic pulmonary vasoconstriction. However, changes in intrathoracic pressure that occur without changes in lung volume, as may occur with obstructive inspiratory effort or Valsalva maneuver, will not alter pulmonary vascular resistance (Pinsky 2005, 1984b).

8.3 Influence of the Moving Heart on Thoracic Organs

The transmitted motion of the beating heart is the origin of many pitfalls in imaging the aorta, the coronary arteries, and the pulmonary vessels. This knowledge is essential for the radiologist since for obvious reasons of radiation dose, non-ECG-gated scans will continue to be performed. In addition, their occurrence is not entirely suppressed by using ECG gating.

8.3.1 Aorta

Pendular and circular aortic motion that can lead to false-negative or false–positive diagnoses of aortic dissection has long been identified (Batra et al. 2000). These artifacts are viewed as more or less prominent double contours of the vessels (Fig. 8.1) or as a hypodense curvilinear interface or a crescent-like thin flap along the wall of the aortic root or sometimes along the pulmonary artery trunk (Fig. 8.2). They mainly affect the aortic root and ascending aorta and the left anterior and right posterior quadrants and are of variable prominence (Batra et al. 2000; Ko et al. 2005). Intricate interferences among heart rate, aortic motion, and simultaneous rapid helical data volume acquisition by multiple-detector rows are involved in its origin. The occurrence of aortic motion artifacts is diminished in elderly patients by the age-related reduced distensibility of the aorta, after a previous surgery, and in pathologic situations, such as mediastinal masses and aortic aneurysms (Set et al. 1993).

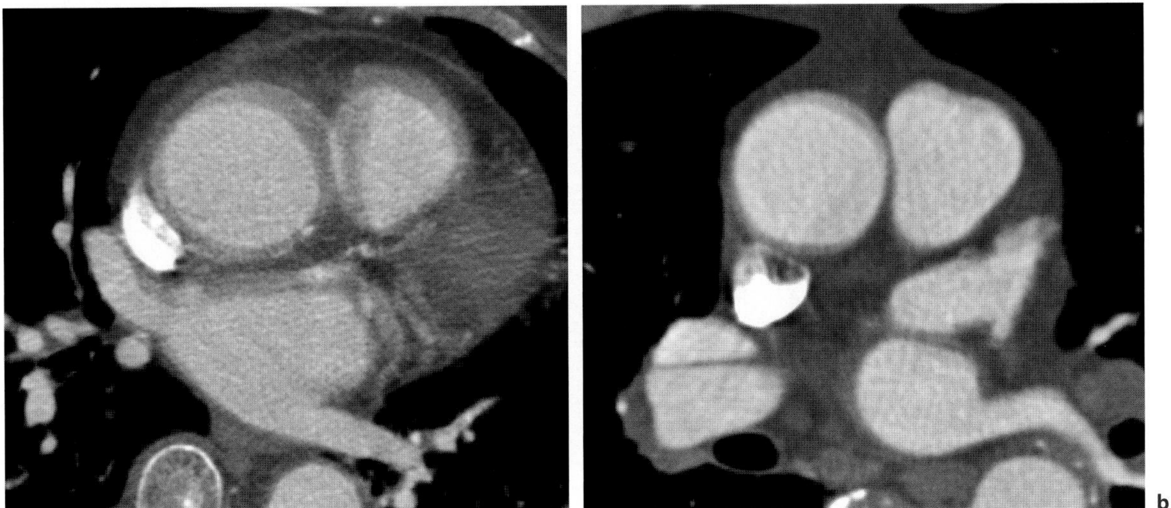

Fig. 8.1.a,b. Aortic motion artifacts of variable prominence in two different patients with non-ECG-gated thoracic MDCT. **a** A pulsation artifact visible in all four quadrants in ascending aorta and in pulmonary artery trunk. **b** Slight crescent-shaped hypodense artifact along the anterior aspect of ascending aorta

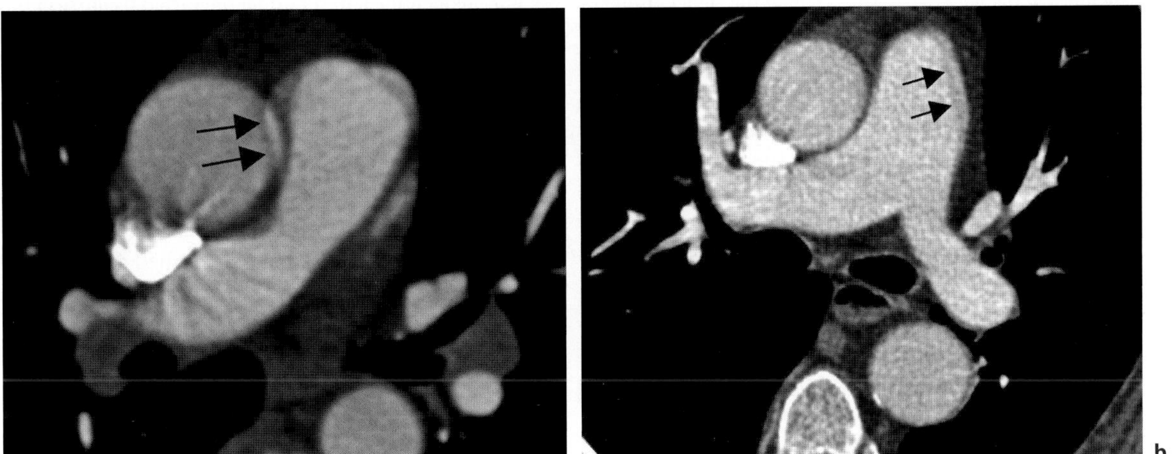

Fig. 8.2a,b. Non-ECG-gated thoracic MDCT. Aortic motion artifact visible as a pseudo-dissection image (*arrows*) in the ascending aorta (**a**) and in another patient in the pulmonary trunk (**b**)

On conventional CT with 1-s scanning time, aortic root artifacts were reported in 37% to 57% of sections, but were usually limited to two or three images, with a mean maximum amplitude of 3–4 mm (Burns et al. 1991; Duvernoy et al. 1995; Qanadli et al. 1999). With the development of MDCT technology, they remained a potential pitfall present in 91.9% of images despite the decrease in scanning time to 0.5 s and simultaneous use of multiple channels (Roos et al. 2002). Ko et al. (2005) have evaluated the influence of the cardiac cycle for different heart rates in generating motion artifacts using non-ECG-assisted MDCT. They found greater amplitude and more sections affected in patients with heart rates ranging from 56 to 65 bpm (beat per minutes). With a 0.5-s scanning time and a heart rate of approximately 60–65 bpm, reconstructed CT images may encompass full diastole and systole for each heart beat, resulting in more obvious motion artifacts during image reconstruction. Transmitted cardiac beats are also responsible for an artifact simulating an aberrant origin of the right coronary artery from the left sinus (Fig. 8.3). This abnormality is considered a malignant variant potentially responsible for sudden cardiac death because of the interarterial course between the aorta and pulmonary trunk.

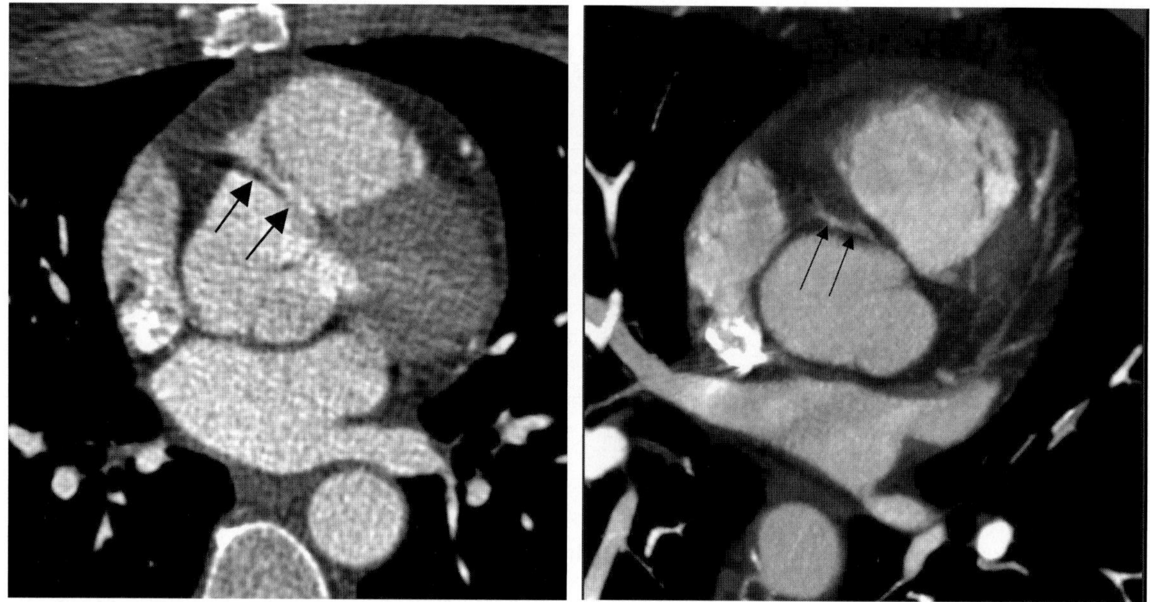

Fig. 8.3. a Artifact in front of aortic root simulating the abnormal interarterial course of the right coronary artery (*arrows*) on a non-ECG-gated MDCT. The origin of the right coronary artery was not identified. **b** Abnormal interarterial course of the right coronary artery (*arrows*) on ECG-gated acquisition and MIP oblique reconstruction in another asymptomatic patient

The lack of depiction of the normal origin of the right coronary artery reinforces the suspicion, but the right coronary artery is frequently unidentified on a non-gated examination. This false abnormal origin has been reported in 5.9% in a population of subjects who underwent non-ECG-gated thoracic MDCT (Katoh et al. 2005).

The use of ECG-gating reduces aortic motion artifacts (Roos et al. 2002), but the patient heart rate has to be slow to maximize its effect (Fig. 8.4) (Morgan-Hughes et al. 2003a). Although no study has been dedicated to the assessment of the aortic motion artifacts within the complete cardiac cycle, all have shown a negative correlation between the heart rate and image quality (Flohr et al. 2002; Morgan-Hughes et al. 2003b).

8.3.2 Lung

Transmitted cardiac pulsations and respiratory motion are the most common causes of motion artifacts in the lung. Whereas shortening of acquisition time has suppressed the latter from most of examinations, the effective suppression of cardiac motion would need an acquisition time of less than 19.1 ms, a temporal resolution not yet achieved even by the newest machines (Ritchie et al. 1992). On non-ECG-gated examinations, cardiac motion results in the appearance of a doubling fissure and in focal areas of low attenuation adjacent to pulmonary vessels (Fig. 8.5). On lung windows, they have been described as the twinkling star artifact and can mimic the appearance of bronchiectasis or thickened bronchial walls (Kuhns and Borlaza 1980; Mayo et al. 1987; Tarver et al. 1988). They are more prominent at the base of the lung in the paracardiac regions close to the heart, where there is direct transmission of the left ventricular movement. Pulmonary arteries experience a decay of the amplitude of displacement that increases with their distance from the heart. ECG-gated scanning, which allows acquisition windows to be set to the quietest period of the cardiac cycle, usually mid-diastole, has been reported as a potential method of reducing cardiac motion artifacts (Fig. 8.6), but at the expense of the radiation dose (Montaudon et al. 2001; Schoepf et al. 1999). The benefit is, however, partially lost when the heart rate is faster than 75–80 bpm (Schoepf et al. 1999), and the advantage using ECG-gating for evaluation the lung parenchyma remains minimal regarding the increased radiation dose (Boehm et al. 2003). A major factor in reduction of motion artifacts is the shorter gantry rotation time (Fig. 8.6) as assessed by some studies (Montaudon et al. 2001; Yanagawa et al. 2007).

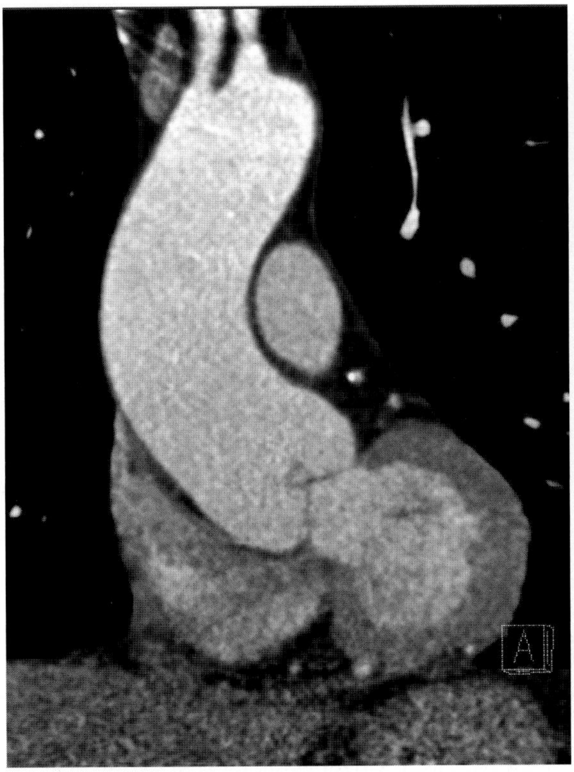

Fig. 8.4a–c. ECG-gated MDCT of the thoracic aorta. Heart rate: 58 bpm. Phase reconstruction at 70% of RR. No artifact is visible, and excellent evaluation of the aortic valve on two in the oblique coronal planes (**a**,**b**), and within the valvular plane (**c**)

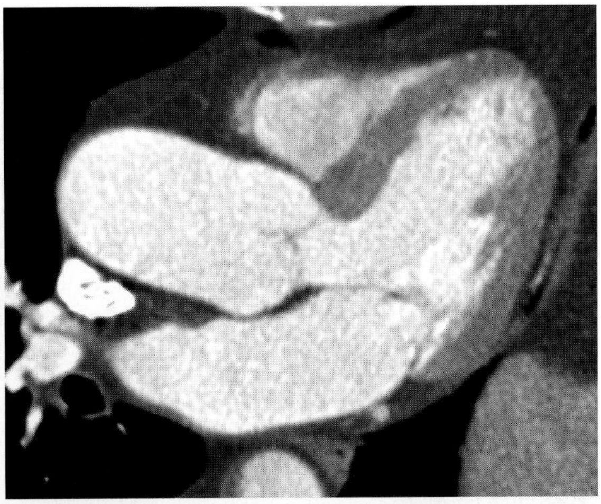

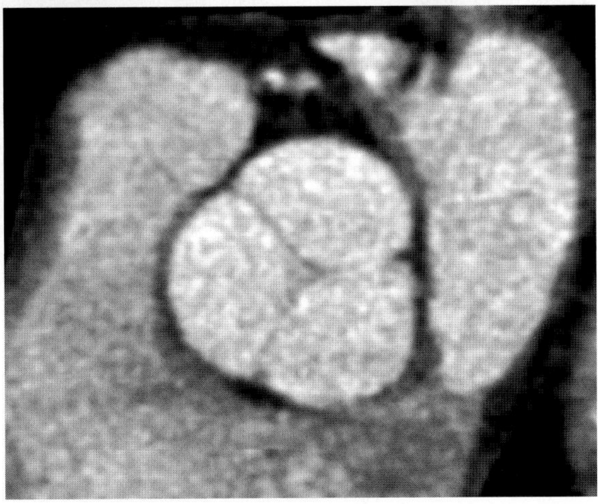

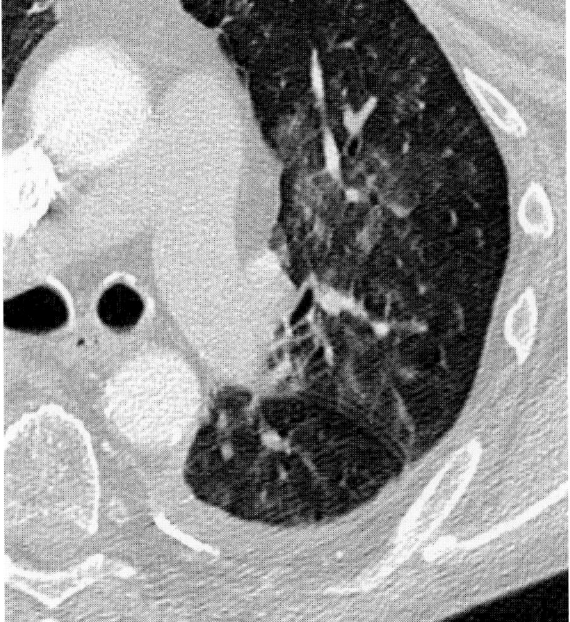

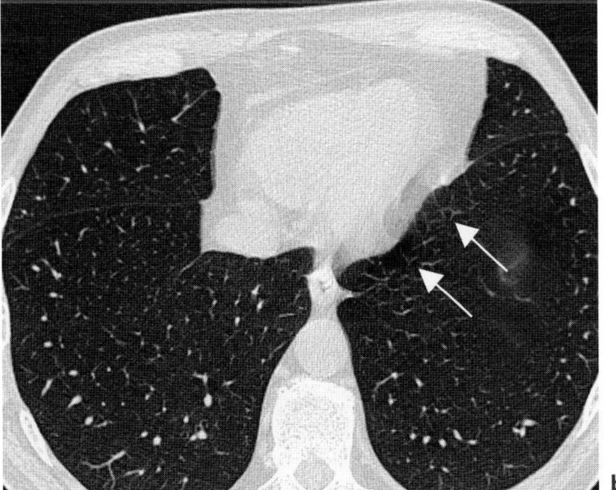

Fig. 8.5a,b. Lung artifacts on non-ECG gated MDCT. Doubling of the left main fissure (**a**) and "twinkling star" artifacts (*arrows*) due to transmitted cardiac pulsations to the pulmonary arteries running close to the heart

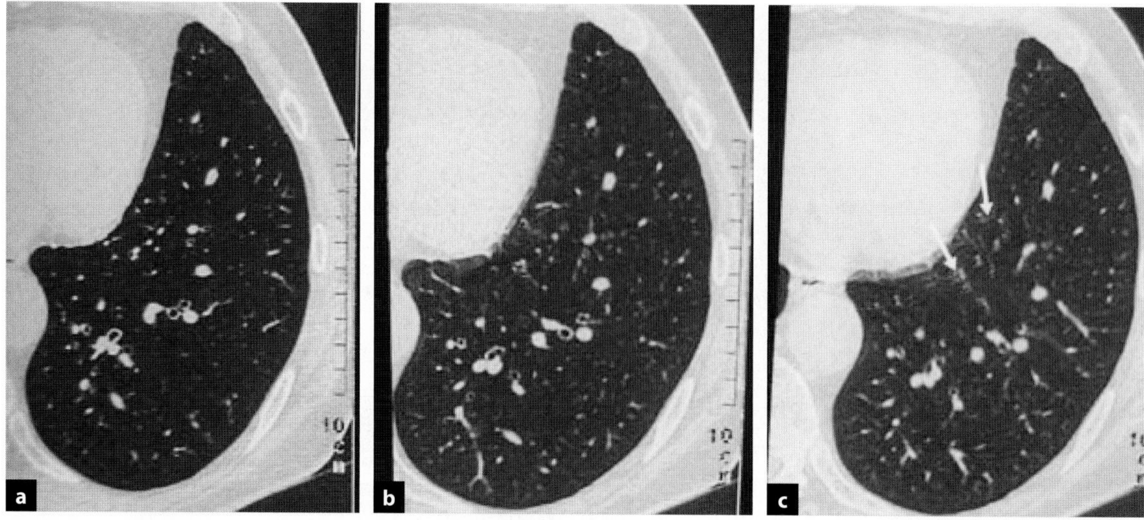

Fig. 8.6a–c. A 35-year-old man with suspicion of pulmonary infection after a bone marrow graft. Thin section of the left lung. **a** ECG-gated 0.5-s scan; **b** 0.5-s scan; **c** 1-s scan. No abnormalities are seen in the lung parenchyma. Note the clear delineation of the cardiac border compared with the blurred images in **b** and **c**. Several artifacts due to distorted vessels are visible in **b** and more prominent (*arrows*) in **c**. Bronchi are better visualized and defined than in **c**. From Montaudon et al. (2001) with permission

The effect of transmitted cardiac pulsation on pulmonary arteries has been recognized as a major cause of pitfalls in angio-computed tomography in the clinical setting of pulmonary embolism, generating pseudo-filling defects on angio-CT of pulmonary arteries (Fig. 8.7). Whereas in-plane displacement results in an overestimation of the size of a structure and loss of edge detail, out-displacement is responsible for size underestimation and reduced contrast resolution (Reinhardt and Hoffman 1998). Therefore, horizontal and obliquely running pulmonary arteries are the most susceptible for reduced contrast resolution and impaired contrast enhancement. Despite its frequent mention in the literature, few studies have reported a systematic observation of this cardiac effect. Bruzzi et al. (2005) have shown that, using a 16-slice scanner, 81% of patients having at least one pulmonary artery affected showed the main pulmonary trunk and right main pulmonary artery being concerned in 41 and 33% in this series, respectively. However, neither blurring nor doubling the arterial wall of these major vessels closely resembled intravascular filling defect. In the same study, most of the artifacts of various severities were, however, found at the segmental or subsegmental level, the lingula and the left lower lobe being affected in 74% and 88% of cases, respectively. In addition, the reduction of rotation gantry rotation time from 0.5 to 0.375 s reduced cardiogenic motion artifacts at all arterial levels and the frequency of pseudofilling defects from 54% to 25%, especially when patients had a heart rate lower than 75 bpm. A virtually complete suppression of cardiac pulsation artifacts can be achieved with ECG-gated 64-section CT (Remy-Jardin et al. 2005).

8.3.3 Coronary Arteries

Coronary arteries undergo heterogeneous movement and deformation throughout the cardiac cycle, which cause motion artifacts on CT images when the velocity exceeds the temporal resolution of the scanner. The major responsibility of heart rate has recently been identified in the generation of motion artifacts in coronary angio-CT (Hong et al. 2001; Schroeder et al. 2002) (Fig. 8.8). Actually, two cardiac factors should be considered, heart rate and heart rate variability. In a study thought to examine heart rate and heart rate variability during CT coronary angiography, breath-holding during cardiac CT scan acquisition was shown to significantly lower the mean heart rate by approximately 4 bpm, but the heart rate variability was observed to be similar or even diminished to that detected during normal breathing (Zhang et al. 2008).

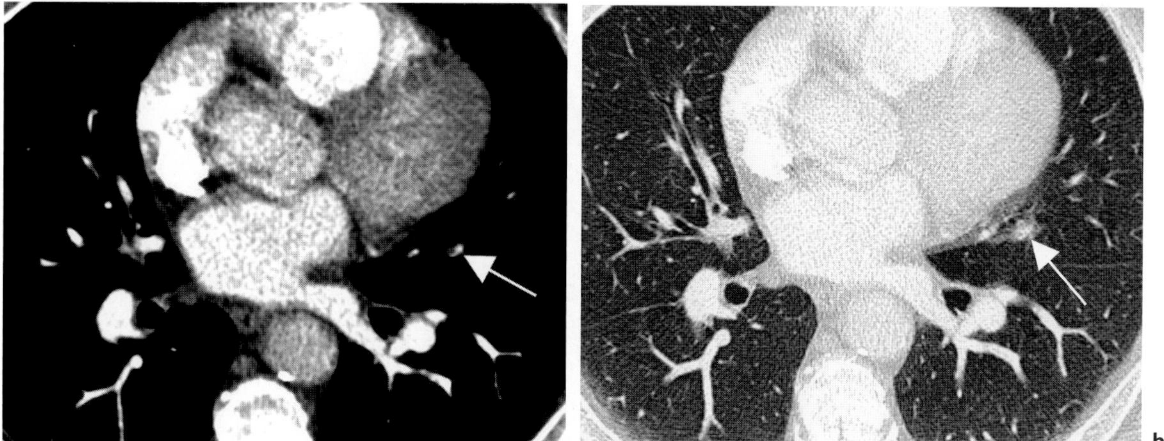

Fig. 8.7a,b. Pseudo filling defect (*arrow*) in a lingular artery on mediastinal window (**a**). Motion artifact transmitted from heart beat is responsible for the blurring of the vessel (*arrow*) on lung window (**b**)

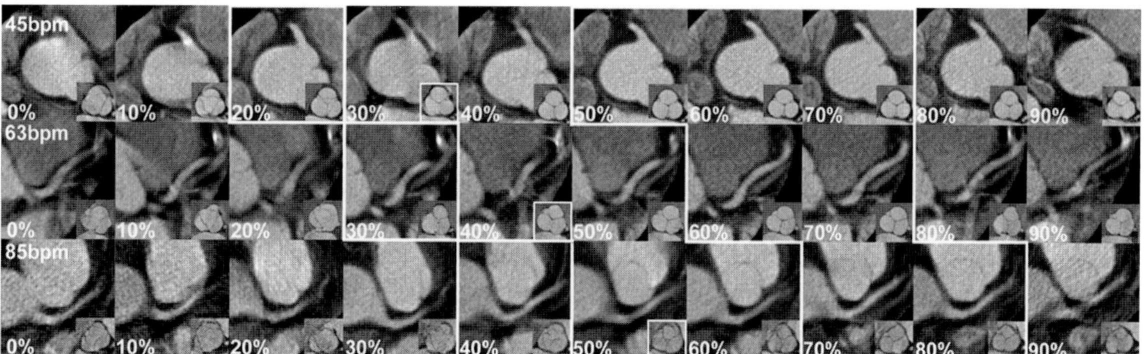

Fig. 8.8. Effects of increasing heart rate on image quality at 64-section CT angiography and duration of systole and diastole regarding reconstruction intervals. Transverse images in three patients with heart rates of 45 bpm (*top row*), 63 bpm (*middle row*), and 85 bpm (*bottom row*). With increasing heart rate, best image quality (*large white squares*) shifts to later percentage phases of the R-R intervals (indicated by *number* in *left corner* of the image). This is accompanied by an increased length in systole and decreased length in diastole. *Boxes* in *lower right corners* show opening and closing of aortic valve throughout R-R interval; *small white squares* show percentage of aortic valve closure. From Husman et al. (2007) with permission

Motion of the coronary arteries in three dimensions during the cardiac cycle is complex and follows that of the whole beating heart. However, there are differences in velocities and course between arteries and segments. Our knowledge about coronary artery motion comes from studies evaluating the locations of coronary artery bifurcation points on biplane coronary cine angiograms and from data that have been obtained using electron beam CT (Mao et al. 2000; Lu et al. 2001) and MRI (Hofman et al. 1998). The latter, however, were restricted to the transverse plane. The recent study of Husman et al. (2007), performed using MDCT, has fully improved our understanding of the motion of coronary arteries during the cardiac cycle. The authors have shown that motion artifacts are minimized when the course of the coronary arteries is minimal. By determining the beginnings of diastole and systole, coronary motion could be related to the physiologic changes caused by different heart rates (Fig. 8.9). The study has shown that the duration of systole lengthens from 30% at low heart rates (45 bpm) to 60% at high heart rates (100 bpm), accompanied by shifts of the mid-diastolic and mid-systolic velocity troughs and shift of the early diastolic peak of velocity. The early systolic peak remained at a constant interval, probably because the preceding isovolumic contraction phase is relatively heart rate independent. The mid-diastolic velocity trough was found to shorten and even disappear at heart rates greater than 80 bpm,

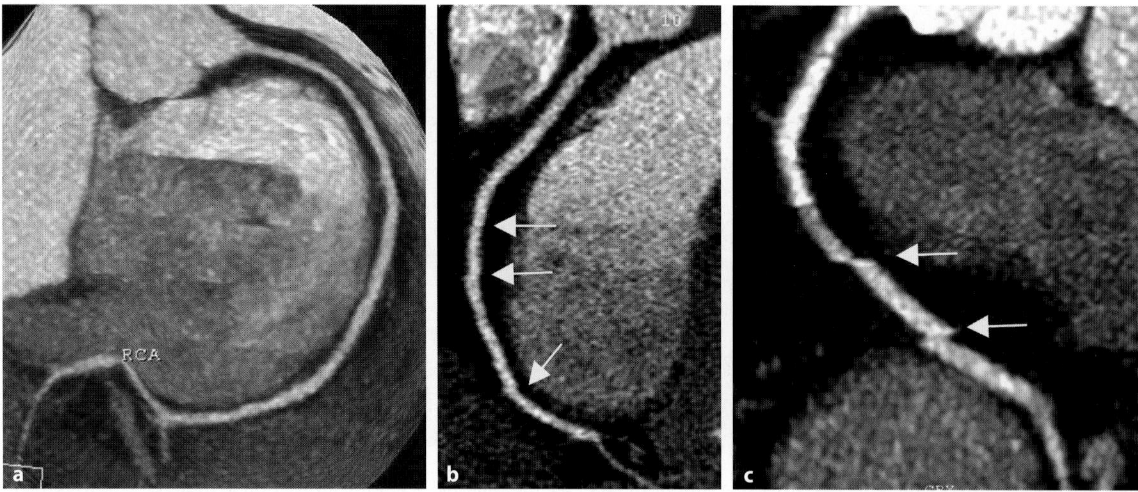

Fig. 8.9a–c. Curved MPR of the right coronary artery performed with a 16-section CT acquisition in three patients with heart rates of 52 bpm (**a**), 64 bpm (**b**), and 75 bpm (**c**). The right coronary artery is visualized along its whole course without artifact at low heart rate (**a**). Slight stair-step artifacts (*arrows*) and minimal vessel blurring are visible at moderate heart rate (**b**). Large stair-step artifacts (*arrows*) at higher heart rate do not permit proper interpretation (**c**)

close to the 82 bpm already known from physiologic studies (Chung et al. 2004).

Velocity troughs were found at end systole (20–30%) in the phase of reduced ejection and in the mid-diastole (60–70%), which represents the diastasis of the diastole. Therefore, the 50% phase of the cardiac cycle can either be a part of systole or a part of diastole, depending on individual patient's heart rate.

A cutoff of 83 bpm has been found for the heart rate at which the minimal velocity in systole becomes smaller than minimal velocities in diastole (Husman et al. 2007). Therefore, coronary CT angiography should be reconstructed at 50–60% of the RR interval in patients with heart rates less than 60 bpm, at 70–80% in patients with heart rates from 71 to 83 bpm, and at 30–40% in patients with heart rates greater than 83 bpm of the RR interval. Also the placement of the center for full-tube output should be done accordingly when ECG pulsing is used for dose saving (Jakobs et al. 2002). Other studies have found that, at 165-ms temporal resolution, systole offers the best overall image quality in patients with heart rates higher than 75 bpm (Wintersperger et al. 2006).

8.3.3.1 Optimal Reconstruction Window for Coronary Angio-Computed Tomography

The coronary artery motion has consequences in the choice of best reconstruction phase, but is also related to the type of scanner used and to the presence of stent or bypass graft. With the limited rotation speed of 370–500 ms/360°, used in 16-slice CT, the heart rate needs to be markedly reduced to less than 60–65 bpm, or multisegment reconstruction methods allowing the merging of data of adjacent cardiac cycles have to be employed (Hong et al. 2001; Dewey et al. 2004; Flohr and Ohnesorge 2001; Hoffmann et al. 2005). Different optimal reconstruction time points in four-section CT have been reported for the RCA, LCX, and LAD, at 40–50, 50–60, and 60–80% of the cardiac cycle, respectively (Hong et al. 2001; Dewey et al. 2004; Flohr and Ohnesorge 2001; Hoffmann et al. 2005). In a study designed to examine the influence of heart rate and a multisector reconstruction algorithm on the image quality of coronary arteries using an anthropomorphic adjustable moving heart phantom on an ECG-gated MDCT unit, image quality of the coronary arteries was not only related to the heart rate, and the influence of the multisector reconstruction technique becomes significant above 70 bpm (Greuter et al. 2005). Wintersperger et al. (2006) found that at 165-ms temporal resolution, there is no significant gain in overall image quality using separate reconstruction time points for each coronary artery and no significant difference in the relative timing of optimized reconstruction for individual coronary artery. The new generation of scanners enable coronary artery imaging with a spatial resolution of $0.4 \times 0.4 \times 0.4$ mm^3 with a temporal resolution of 83–165 ms and high diagnostic image quality over a wide range of heart rates up to 92 bpm with only 3–4% of no diagnostic segments, but motion artifacts of coronary arteries still occur (FLOHR et al. 2005; LEBER et al. 2005; LESCHKA et al. 2005; RAFF et al. 2005).

Temporal windows providing the best image quality of different segments and types of coronary artery bypass grafts with 64-slice computed tomography (CT) were evaluated in an experimental setup. Image quality of proximal segments did not significantly vary with the temporal window, whereas for all other segments image quality was significantly better at 60%, compared with other temporal windows (Fig. 8.10) (DESBIOLLES et al. 2007).

Coronary artery stent lumen visibility was assessed as a function of cardiac movement and temporal resolution with an automated objective method using an anthropomorphic moving heart phantom. According to this study, the cardiac movement during data acquisition is responsible for approximately twice as much blurring compared with the influence of temporal resolution on image quality (GROEN et al. 2007).

8.4 Influence the Bolus of Contrast Media by Heart-Lung Interactions

Several physiological heart and lung parameters can influence the bolus flow of contrast media, i.e., effects of respiration on venous systemic return, cardiac output, circulatory blood flow, and pulmonary arterial resistance.

8.4.1 Effect of the Systemic Venous Return

Variations of the systemic venous return have major impacts on the pulmonary circulation. The superior vena cava and inferior vena cava contributions to systemic venous return to the thorax vary with different respiratory maneuvers. When intrathoracic pressure remains constant, as during breath-holds at end inspiration and expiration, the superior vena cava/inferior vena cava flow ratio is about 2:1, very similar to that observed during free breathing. When intrathoracic pressure be-

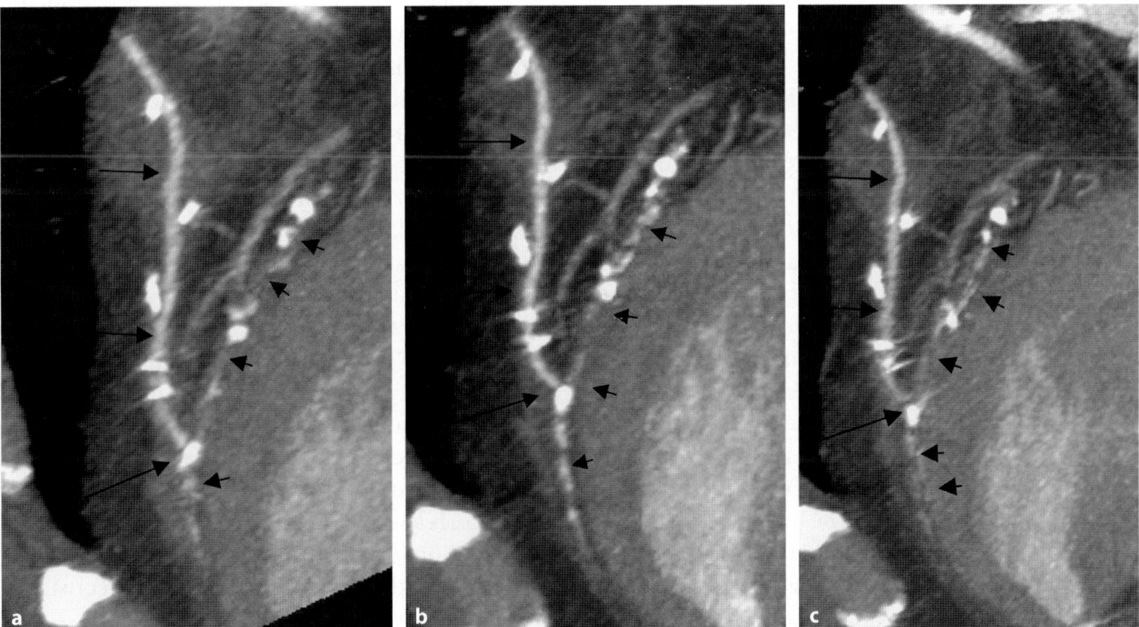

Fig. 8.10a–c. A 67-year-old patient after coronary artery bypass graft surgery with left internal mammary artery grafted to the middle segment of the left anterior descending artery with diffuse infiltration by atheroma and mural calcifications (*short arrows*). MIP projection shows the distal part of the graft (*long arrows*) at 40% (**a**), 60% (**b**), and 70% (**c**) of the R-R interval. Visualization of the distal anastomosis is impaired at 40% and 70 % because of blurring artifacts, but acceptable at 60% of the R-R interval. Note the clip artifacts, which minimally hinder the distal anastomosis

comes negative during continuous inspiration, the venous return to the right atrium increases nearly 50% as shown by measurements performed using flow-encoded cine MR (Kuzo et al. 2007). Since the contribution to this increase is significantly greater from the inferior vena cava, the relative increase of unopacified blood dilutes contrast media generally injected through an arm vein. After a deep inspiration, the blood volume with a lesser concentration of contrast media traveling to the pulmonary arteries by the time scans are acquired at the level of pulmonary arteries. The consequence is a transient interruption of contrast material in a portion of the pulmonary artery compared to the proximal and distal portions of the same vessel. This artifact has been reported with frequency varying from 3% (Wittram 2003) to 37% (Gosselin et al. 2004), the large range being likely related to the type of instruction given to the patient to hold his breath. Both hyperventilation before scanning and deep inspiration are the exacerbating factors of this artifact and should be avoided before scanning (Wittram and Yoo 2007). Otherwise, patient age, body weight, and the amount of contrast medium are the most important factors associated with vessel enhancement in CT pulmonary angiography (Arakawa et al. 2007).

8.4.2 Effect of the Pulmonary Resistance

Pulmonary artery pressure has been reported to increase with patient age (Ghali et al. 1992). The pulmonary blood is consequently more stagnant, and the transit time of a small amount of contrast media through the pulmonary circulation becomes significantly longer with patient age after adjustment for differences in blood pressure, body surface area, and cardiac function (Hartmann et al. 2002). A frequent observation is that opacification of pulmonary arteries is greater in older subjects compared to that observed in the young (Fig. 8.11). Resistance can be increased unilaterally and induces a swirl of contrast media in one arterial branch (Fig. 8.12). Retrograde enhancement of the inferior vena cava or hepatic veins during IV contrast-enhanced studies is a common finding, and elevated pulmonary resistances explain its association with right-sided heart disease, such as tricuspid regurgitation, pulmonary hypertension, and right ventricular systolic dysfunction in small series (Collins et al. 1995). However, this feature has also been observed in normal subjects, and the volume of contrast and rate of injection have both been shown to be involved in this finding (Yeh et al. 2004). With an intravenous contrast injection rate less than 3 ml/s, the contrast reflux into the inferior vena cava or hepatic veins on CT is highly specific, but not sensitive for right-sided heart disease, and unmasks decreased cardiac output reserve (Yeh et al. 2004).

8.4.3 Effect of Cardiac Output

The systemic vascular enhancement response to IV-injected contrast media is characteristic for a given territory and for a given patient. It depends on the anatomic distance between the injection site and the vascular territory of interest and on the encountered physiologic flow rates between these landmarks. Arterial enhancement is lower in patients with high cardiac output and stronger in patients with low cardiac output despite increased contrast media transit time (interval needed for the contrast media to arrive in the arterial territory of interest). In subjects with a high cardiac output, more blood is ejected per unit of time, and consequently the contrast media per unit of time is more diluted.

Clinically, it has been observed that reduced cardiac output results in delayed and increased vascular enhancement (Sivit et al. 1992), but the body of evidence on the role of cardiac output has been shown by experimental investigation. Using a porcine model, Bae et al. (1998a) investigated how reduced cardiac output affects the timing of aortic and hepatic contrast medium enhancement. With reduction in cardiac output, the time from the injection start to the arrival of contrast medium bolus in the aorta and the time from injection completion to peak aortic and the peak hepatic enhancement increased significantly. The time delay to the arrival of the contrast media bolus in the abdominal aorta was highly correlated with and linearly proportional to the reduction in cardiac output. This finding reflects an increase in the circulation time with a decrease in cardiac output.

The time from the start of injection to peak aortic enhancement was related directly to the injection duration (Bae et al. 1998b). The peak hepatic enhancement increased only slightly, but the time delay to peak hepatic enhancement correlated highly

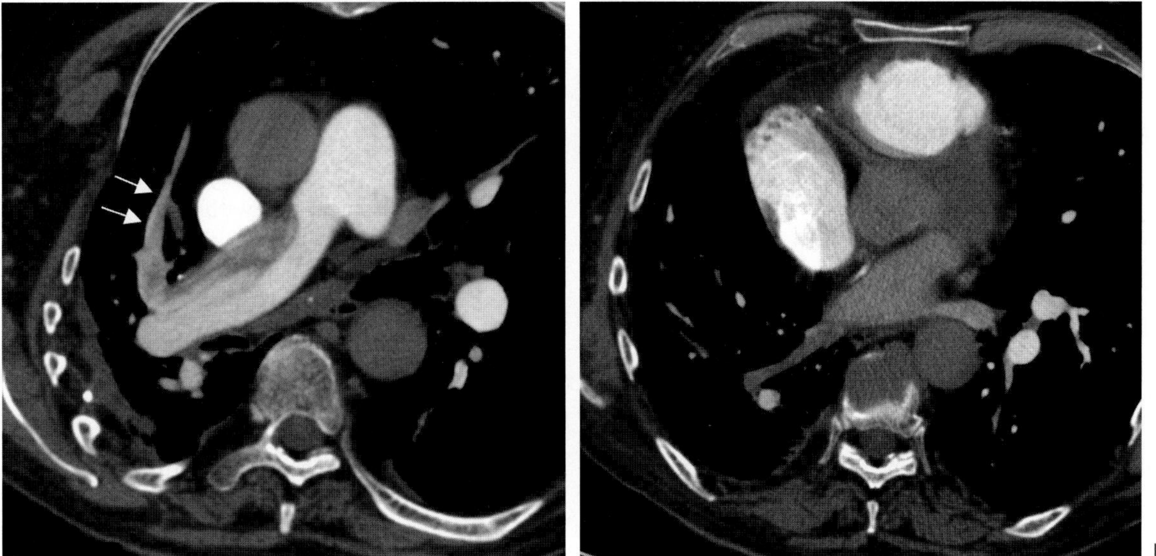

Fig. 8.11a,b. Pulmonary artery angio-CT in a patient with a previous right middle lobe pulmonary resection with thoracoplasty for thoracic wall and pleural tuberculosis. **a** Low attenuation area is visible in the right main pulmonary artery and in the anterior segmental pulmonary artery (*arrows*) and is attributed to the slowed down circulation in the right arterial tree. At a lower level, the right inferior pulmonary vein remains unopacified, conversely to the left one (**b**)

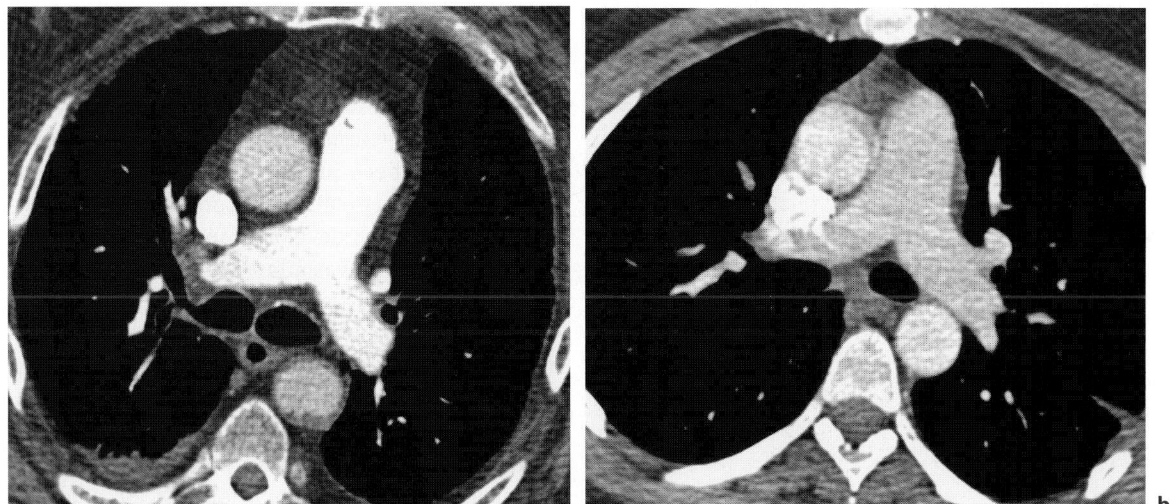

Fig. 8.12a,b. CT angiography performed on a 16-row multidetector CT in two different patients of 75 (**a**) and 23 (**b**) years old. Both examinations were negative for pulmonary embolism. None had a detectable cardiac or pulmonary disease. Technical parameters were similar. The difference in the degree of enhancement was attributed to the increase of pulmonary resistance occurring with age

with a reduction in cardiac output (Bae et al. 1998a). This reflects the longer circulatory distance and greater dispersion of contrast media between the injection and sampling site for the liver as compared with those in the aorta. The magnitude of both aortic and hepatic enhancement increased with reduced cardiac output, but magnitudes were different in the aorta and liver. The latter was not significant, and the former was proportional to the decrease in cardiac output. Reduction of cardiac output results in decreased peripheral perfusion. The overall tissue enhancement represents the amount of contrast media in the capillary and interstitial compartment divided by the total organ volume. With a slower cardiac output, the contrast media stays longer in the capillary space, resulting in increased contrast media in that compartment. However, the capillary space volume is small relative to the organ volume, and contrast media delivery to the interstitial space is slower with decreased cardiac output. Therefore, the overall contrast media concentration in tissue is not substantially increased with decreased cardiac output.

8.4.4 Effect of Circulatory Blood Volume

In parenchymal organs, the peak enhancement occurs when the maximum amount of contrast media in the central blood volume is delivered to the capillary and interstitial compartments of the organ. Contrast media flows from the central blood volume compartment to the parenchymal interstitial compartment until the contrast media concentration gradient between the two compartments equilibrates, that is, at the distribution equilibrium. Central blood volume is inversely related to arterial enhancement, but affects recirculation rather than the first-pass effect (Dawson and Blomley 1996). Central blood volume correlates with body weight, and studies have shown that body weight is the most important for the magnitude of contrast medium enhancement, with an inverse relationship between contrast enhancement and patient weight (Heiken et al. 1995). The clinical effect of reduced circulation on contrast media enhancement can be observed in hypovolemic shock and systemic hypertension, where typical CT findings include dense opacification of arteries, bowel wall, and kidneys (Sivit et al. 1992).

8.4.5 Consequences in Designing Protocols

These results are useful for designing strategies to optimize contrast medium enhancement of aorta and coronary arteries as well as myocardium enhancement in patients with reduced cardiac function. Achieving optimal contrast enhancement is necessary in coronary angiography to insure sufficient contrast between the coronary lumen and plaques or arterial wall and to assess stent potency based on intraluminal enhancement measurements (Hong et al. 2004).

High injection rates increase the attenuation values of the aorta and coronary arteries. However, the attenuation value reaches a plateau at rates over 5 ml/s in the aorta and over 4 ml/s in the coronary arteries (Kim et al. 2008).

The time delay between the start of injection and scanning can be calculated with a bolus test or using semi-automated bolus-tracking software. Semi-automated software typically requires a predetermined enhancement threshold for a given organ of interest, and scanning is initiated when contrast media enhancement reaches this threshold. In case of severely compromised cardiac output, contrast media cannot sometimes reach the threshold because of overestimation, and scanning may be performed too early when peak enhancement has not been reached.

Several methods of designing the injection rate have been proposed. The constant rate, uniphasic method results in a steadily rising vascular contrast enhancement profile with a single peak of enhancement occurring shortly after completion of the injection. However, vascular enhancement is not uniform throughout the entire image acquisition, and uniform enhancement is useful for image processing and display because some 3D post-processing techniques are based on a threshold CT attenuation value (Rubin et al. 1998). Other injection methods have been proposed to generate uniform vascular enhancement. The exponentially decelerated technique was developed mathematically and is based on cardiovascular properties and pharmacokinetics. The basic premise is that uniform vascular enhancement occurs when the constant medium outflow rate is balanced by the contrast media infusion rate. This steady-state contrast media accumulation in vessels is achieved by administering contrast media into the central blood compartment at an exponentially decelerated rate to compensate for the dissipation of contrast media from the central blood compartment to the interstitial compartment (Bae et al. 2000, 2004). The optimal decay coefficient is proportional to the cardiac output per body weight and has been estimated to be 0.01% for humans with normal cardiac output. The biphasic or triphasic injection techniques can be considered as a simplified form of the described multiphasic exponential method. Durations and rate of injections of each phase can be tailored by calculating the transfer function of the system from the Fourier transform of a test bolus (Fleischmann et al. 2000).

However, streak artifacts arising from densely opacified brachiocephalic veins or superior vena cava during contrast media administration may obscure neighboring structures and pathology. Similarly, artifacts arising from the right atrium and ventricle of the heart may obscure the right coronary artery. They can be removed when acquisition is performed after contrast media is already removed from the large veins by flushing the venous system with saline immediately after the contrast media injection, a method also known as the bolus chaser (Haage et al. 2000). The use of a bolus chaser is also expected to allow volume reduction of contrast media at coronary angiography (Han et al. 2000; Yamashita et al. 2000).

8.4.6 Effect of Physiological Parameters on Pulmonary Perfusion

MDCT has the ability and has the resolution to explore the relationships between lung ventilation, regional lung flow, and lung structure at a regional level with a unique spatial resolution. While the physiologist has access to a number of techniques to evaluate lung function, such as multiple inert gas elimination technique or the injection of microspheres, these techniques have significant disadvantages, including lack of spatial information or low spatial resolution and, in the case of microspheres, an inability to make measurements in humans. The functional imaging techniques based on magnetic resonance (MR), computed tomography (CT), or positron emission tomography (PET) hold substantial promise. Early studies were conducted thanks to Ultrafast or Cine CT (Imatron Corporation, San Francisco, CA). Today, MDCT 64 section scanners can acquire volumetric images in a single rotation completed in as little as 0.3 s within a breath hold of 5 s or less and with a z-axis coverage of four centimetres (cm). With the two tubes mounted orthogonally in dual-source CT, both spiral acquisitions can run simultaneously, which largely excludes changes in contrast enhancement or patient movement between the acquisitions. With dual-energy CT, the separate 80 and 140 KVp images are analyzed using specific software to determine the iodine content of every voxel based on the decomposition for soft tissue, air, and iodine (Johnson et al. 2007). Images are displayed on a workstation with the virtual enhancement as greyscale background and iodine content superimposed and color-coded (Chon et al. 2006).

The concept of measurement of pulmonary blood flow has been established using a single-compartment model of indicator transport in which flow is proportional to maximal enhancement, in which the assumption is that tissue accumulation of the indicator is nearly completed before the onset of the wash-out (Wolfkiel and Rich 1992). The signal within a single voxel related to microvascular blood flow can be extracted from CT images. Time-attenuation curves in the feeding artery and in the peripheral region are used to extract the transfer function, which expresses the mathematical function serving to convert the arterial curve into the parenchymal curve. The transfer function is of bimodal type, and this reflects the partial volume microvascular bed. Once eliminated, the first portion of the transfer function, the arterial curve, can be reconvolved using the second portion, and a time-attenuation curve reflecting microvascular perfusion can be derived (Hoffman and Chon 2005).

Although clinical use of the assessment of pulmonary perfusion by MDCT has been so far limited to pulmonary embolism and to the evaluation of tumor vascularity, there are many potential applications in the field of physiology and physiopathology. The main physiological characteristic of pulmonary perfusion is matching between ventilation (V) and perfusion (Q), which is critical for adequate gas exchange. However, regional heterogeneity of V/Q exists, and posture, breath holding, and exercise have substantial effects on regional blood flow (Hopkins 2004). The distribution of blood flow is posture dependent in the right lung, but not in the left one, and the heart weight may play a role in this difference (Chon et al. 2006). Gravity-related gradients in the lung can be demonstrated (Wolfkiel and Rich 1992), but the effects of gravity are modified in the supine and lower decubitus position because perfusion is more uniformly distributed (Amis et al. 1984). Although important, gravity is, however, not the predominant determinant of pulmonary perfusion heterogeneity (Glenny et al. 1999). The relative effect of vascular branching morphometry has been shown to be a dominant factor in flow distribution, whereas that of gravity is only minor (Burrowes et al. 2005). Many of these physiological results have been obtained by using experimental data obtained from MDCT.

8.5 Interaction among Pulmonary, Systemic, and Lymphatic Circulations

The basis of understanding the pathophysiology of pulmonary edema relies on the knowledge of the three circulations of the lung, pulmonary, bronchial, or systemic and lymphatic. Actually, the lymphatic system provides an important drainage mechanism for fluid being filtered from pulmonary blood vessels and from bronchial blood vessels.

The structural architecture of the lung influences the amount and direction of water within the lung. In the normal lung, the surface area of gas exchange is about 70 m^2, and capillaries form a network of about 10 μ in diameter ramifying over the surface of the alveoli and containing a volume per lung of only 90 to 120 ml of blood. The basement membrane of the endothelial wall of a capillary facing the alveolus is fused with the basement membrane of the alveolar epithelium (thin side of the alveolocapillary interface). By contrast, the capillary wall facing away from the alveolar wall is separated from the neighboring alveolus by the interstitial space (the thick side of the alveolocapillary interface) (Fig. 8.13). To support the stress of various physiological respiratory maneuvers, alveolar septa have remarkable strength due to the extracellular matrix, particularly the presence of type IV collagen (Milne and Pistolesi 1993).

The alveolar septa do not contain lymphatics, but the nearby peribronchiolar sheaths do, the end of the lymphatics capillaries having a fenestrated endothelial layer and discontinuous basement membrane. These anatomic features combine to provide in normal circumstances the filtering of efficient drainage liquid from the capillaries and at the same time permits gas exchange between capillaries and alveoli.

Four potential pathways by which this fluid can leave the lung exist: (1) via resorbtion directly back into the vasculature, (2) by moving through the interstitium directly into the peribronchial cuffs, (3) through lymphatics directly adjacent to large pulmonary vessels, or (4) by bulk transport into the airway lumen and subsequent clearance via mucociliary removal.

The physiologic factors determining the rate of liquid and solute exchange across a capillary wall are (1) intravascular hydrostatic pressure (HPiv), (2) extravascular hydrostatic pressure (HPev), (3) intravascular oncotic pressure (OPiv), and (4) extravascular oncotic pressure (OPev). Oncotic pressure acts in an opposite direction to hydrostatic pressure. The theoretical amount of fluid Qf filtered per unit area and per unit of time is given by the Starling equation Qf = Kf (HPiv – Hpev) – t(OPiv – Opev). *Kf* represents the conductance of the capillary wall and *t* the oncotic reflexion coefficient, expressing the permeability of the capillary membranes to macromolecules. The greater the reflection coefficient is, the more the passage of macromolecules will be restricted, thus decreasing overall fluid filtration. The net flow Fnet is defined as Qf-Ql, in which *Ql* represents lymphatic absorption and *Qf* fluid transudation or fluid filtration. Although in normal conditions the endothelial cells are relatively impermeable to protein but remain permeable to water and solutes, the tight intercellular junctions of the alveolar epithelium remain impermeable to water and solutes, thus constituting an effective barrier that is a major factor in preventing the development of pulmonary edema (Milne and Pistolesi 1993) (Fig. 8.14).

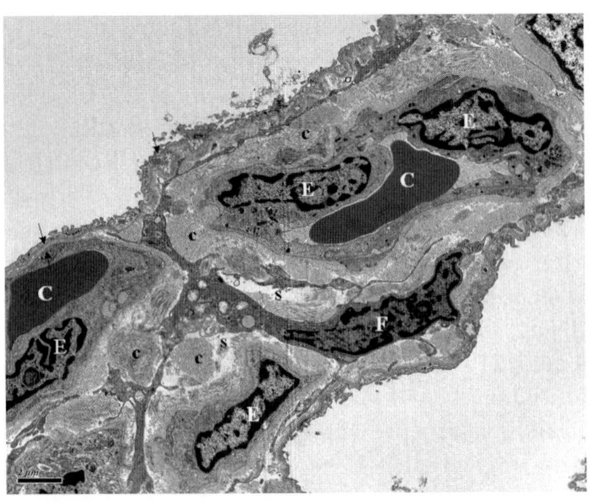

Fig. 8.13. Ultrastructure of a subnormal lung septum between two alveoli. On one side, the alveolus is separated from the capillary (C) by only the fused basement membranes (small arrows) of the alveolar epithelium and of the capillary endothelium. On the other side, the alveolus is separated from the capillary (C) by the alveolar epithelium (E), the interstitial space filled with fibroblasts (F) containing a few collagen fibers (C) and small pools of free liquid (S). Small arrow indicates a pneumocyte type I cytoplasmic expansion. Bar is 2 microns length (Courtesy of H. Begueret, Bordeaux)

There are two ways in which flow of water out of the capillaries can be increased: (1) increased transmural pressure (hydrostatic and/or oncotic), the most common causes being left heart failure and mitral valve

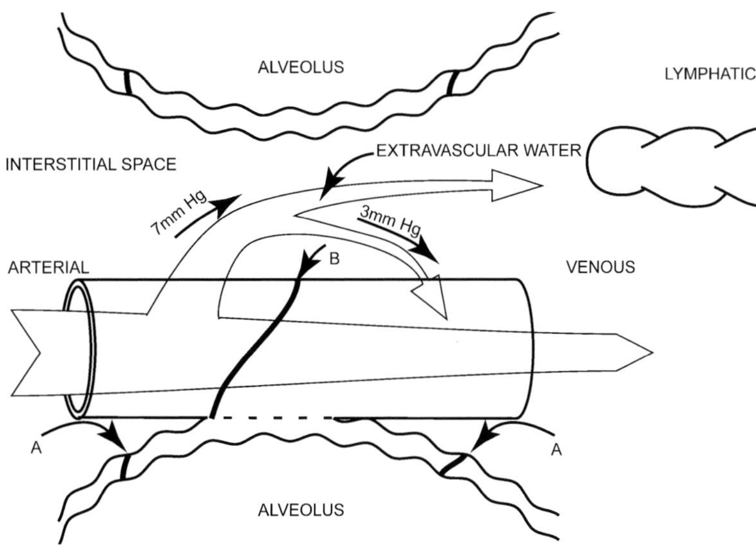

Fig. 8.14. Schematic drawing of the interstitial space between two alveoli. Unfused basement membrane (*thick*) side of the alveolus. Alveolar epithelial junctions are tight (*A*) and endothelial cell loose (*B*). Starling forces operating on the capillaries result in fluid transudate out of the arterial end of the capillary (approximate transmural pressure +7 mmHg) and is partially reabsorbed (transmural pressure −3 mmHg) at the venous end of the capillary. The continual excess water formed flows toward the lymphatics where it is picked up and removed (modified from Milne and Pistolesi 1993)

disease and (2) reversible or irreversible damage of the endothelial cell junctions. Elevated pressure edema is characterized by two pathophysiologic and radiological phases: interstitial edema and alveolar flooding. The intensity and duration of each phase are clearly related to the degree of increased pressure, determined by the hydrostatic-oncotic pressure ratio. Pulmonary edema is traditionally divided into hydrostatic or cardiogenic caused by an increase capillary pressure and high-permeability edema due to an increased permeability of the capillary wall. There is, however, substantial overlap between these two groups (West and Mathieu-Costello 1995). Experimental conditions have shown that there is a spectrum of types of pulmonary edema as the capillary pressure is raised from low to high values. Fluid moves from the capillary lumen into the alveolar wall interstitium and possibly into the alveolar space. The result is the so-called hydrostatic edema. Finally, at even higher pressures, stress failure occurs with disruption of the capillary endothelial and/or alveolar epithelial layers and results in a high-permeability edema type. Thus, as the capillary pressure gradually rises from normal to high levels, the first stage is a hydrostatic edema, but this is followed by a high-permeability edema type. Clinical conditions involving stress failure of pulmonary capillaries include those in which an increased capillary pressure is sufficiently high to cause permeability edema, neurogenic edema, high-altitude pulmonary edema, and ARDS following trauma. Occasionally, it can also be encountered in human athletes after extreme exercise (West and Mathieu-Costello 1995) (Fig. 8.15).

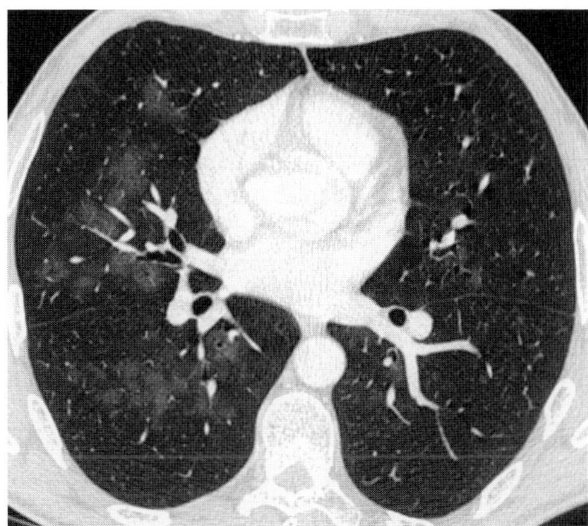

Fig. 8.15. Exercise-induced pulmonary hemorrhage. A 42-year-old marathon runner repeatedly developed a small amount of hemoptysis after extreme physical exertion. Extensive investigations revealed no abnormalities, but ground-glass opacities consistent with alveolar bleeding 24 h after a new hemoptysis. Abnormalities are bilateral, but less visible on the left lung due to motion artifacts. A high-permeability-type edema induced by elevated pulmonary pressure due to the very high cardiac output needed for oxygen consumption was suggested based on these findings

The extent of lymphatic clearance regarding the bronchial circulation is less known. Recent work, however, has reported that a substantial fraction of lymph flow originates from leakage of bronchial blood vessels, that is, from the airway wall, but is unlikely to cause airway obstruction (Wagner et al. 1998).

8.6 Heart-Lung Interactions in Near-Normal Anatomical Conditions

In the previous paragraphs, we have described physiological interactions between heart and lung. There are, however, some particular situations in which heart-lung interactions play a significant role in revealing symptoms that would not occur without the conjoined effect of an anatomical change and physiological interactions. Such a condition is the patent foramen ovale (PFO), which may cause an intermittent right-left shunt when right atrial pressure exceeds the left atrial pressure.

PFO is the most frequent asymptomatic right-left shunt, found to have an autopsy incidence of 27–29% in the general population, and has no hemodynamic significance at rest (Hagen et al. 1984). It has been shown to be associated with several clinical conditions, including cryptogenic stroke, unexplained decompression sickness in divers, and recently migraine headache (Hara et al. 2005). PFOs are often associated with atrial septum aneurysms, defined as a total septal excursion of 15 mm or more. PFO is an oblique slit-like valve, a remnant of the fetal circulation incompletely fused after birth. Before birth, the oxygenated placental blood enters the right atrium via the inferior vena cava and then crosses the valve of the foramen ovale to enter the systemic system. Anatomically, inferior vena cava flow is directed to the interatrial septum and foramen ovale, whereas superior vena cava and coronary sinus flows are directed away. The amount of shunting is below the threshold level for oximetry detection. Today, echocardiography is the principle method of assessment, particularly TTE and TEE. Both are used with saline contrast, and saline contrast appearing in the left heart within three cardiac cycles of its appearance within the right heart during normal breathing is consistent with shunting and a resting PFO. The method can be sensitized by Valsalva maneuver or repeated cough because of an increase in heart pressure (Dubourg et al. 1984). Measurement of anatomical size by direct measurement of slit width or color Doppler is also possible. Both the largest sized PFO and resting PFO are more frequently noted in pathological conditions. Direct detection of large PFOs has been performed thanks to the high spatial and temporal resolution of MDCT (Manghat et al. 2007) (Fig. 8.16). Dynamic study of the fossa ovalis during the relapse of Valsalva maneuver and comparison with MDCT in a population with cryptogenic stroke has shown that MDCT was able to

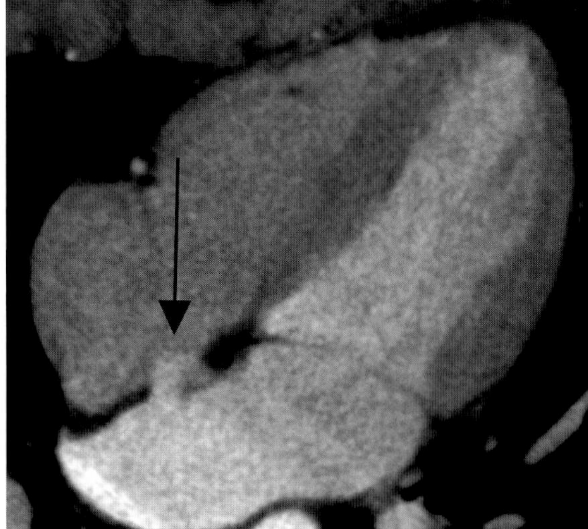

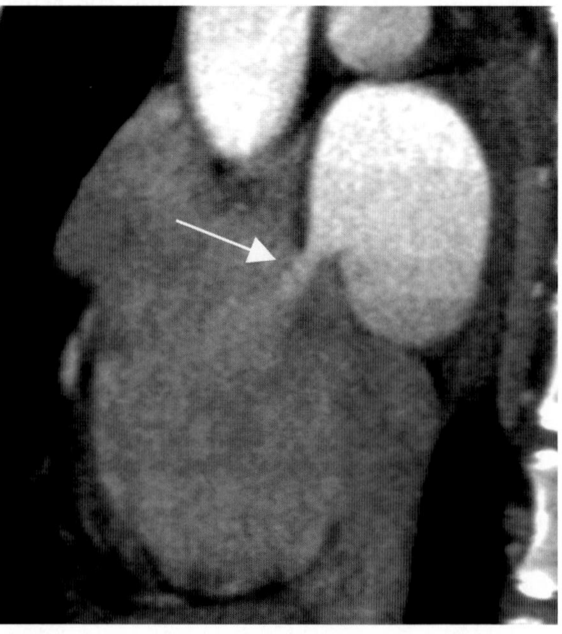

Fig. 8.16a,b. Patent foramen ovale incidentally discovered in a patient prior to atrial radio-frequency ablation procedure and subsequently confirmed by contrast echocardiography. ECG-gated CT with contrast medium enhancement and saline bolus chaser. A subtle flush of contrast in the right atrium and a defect of the interatrial septum (*arrow*) are visible on transverse section (**a**) and sagittal oblique multplanar reformation (**b**)

depict high-grade PFOs thanks to the enhancement of left atrium before pulmonary veins (Revel et al. 2007).

The presence of an anatomical and physiological PFO has been proposed as the main explanation for poor enhancement of pulmonary arteries at CT angiography when seen in combination associated with early and strong enhancement of the thoracic aorta and sufficient contrast media within the superior vena cava (Fig. 8.17). The physiological right-to-left shunt happens during deep inspiration, after the Valsalva maneuver, or coughing when the right atrial pressure exceeds the left atrial pressure. In a result of a study of 244 patients suspected for PE, 16% of the patients were found with this abnormal contrast dynamic on their scans and an intracardiac right-to-left shunt (Henk et al. 2003). These results support the fact that, in patients with a prior detected PFO, subsequent CT examination should be performed during slow respiration or near-end expiration. Most recent scanners allow decreasing imaging times and therefore enabling dyspneic patients to hold their breath in expiration throughout the whole study.

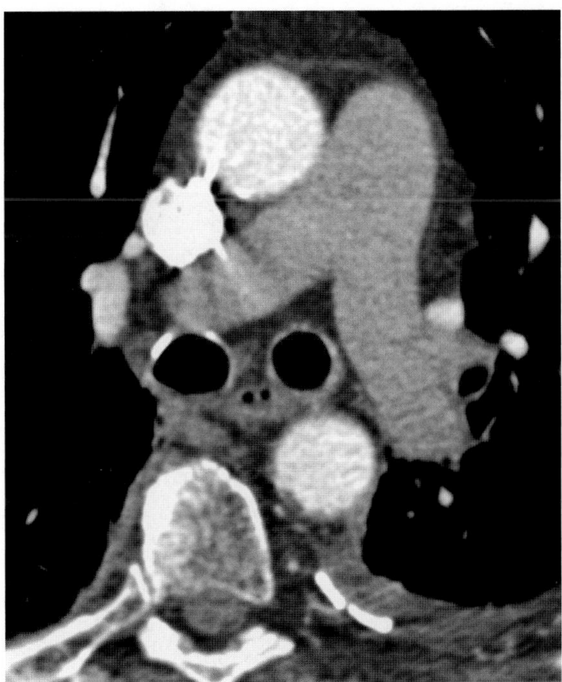

Fig. 8.17. Poor enhancement of pulmonary trunk and main arteries, whereas aorta and superior vena cava are well opacified in a pulmonary artery CT angiography performed for suspected pulmonary embolism. A patent PFO was found at transesophageal echocardiography

PFOs can play an important role in hemodynamic changes after lung surgery and are a potential cause of the clinical deterioration that may be observed after pulmonary resection. Increased gradient across the PFO could be induced by restriction of the pulmonary vascular bed and by compression of the right atrium by the weight of the postoperative hydrothorax, and a symptomatic right-to-left shunt can occur after pulmonary resection. This rare clinical condition is called platypnea-orthodeoxia syndrome, which is almost exclusively observed after right a pneumonectomy (Marini et al. 2006). It typically evolves after an interval of a few months without relevant symptoms after the operation and is posture-dependant with worsening of dyspnea and arterial oxygen desaturation in the upright position and relief by recumbency. Various hemodynamic explanations have been proposed, but the precise mechanism remains unclear today. Proposals are that the vertical position causes a decrease in the venous oxygen saturation and generates a cycle of elevated right atrial pressure, increased pulmonary vascular resistance caused by the reduced vascular bed, which causes elevation of the right ventricular end-diastolic pressure and increases right atrial pressure, and the weight of the heart in the shifted position pulling downward on the interatrial septum and causing the foramen ovale to open or widen. However, anatomic relationships among the right atrium, superior and inferior vena cava after pneumonectomy cause preferential flow through a PFO or ASD, even in the absence of a pressure gradient (Bakris et al. 1997; Mercho et al. 1994). The detection of PFO has been proposed before performing a pneumonectomy in order to prevent hemodynamic impairment (Aigner et al. 2008).

Other causes of hemodynamic impairment can occur after pneumonectomy. The massive relaxation and consecutive elevation of the diaphragm and the compression of the right atrium or inferior vena cava (Fig. 8.18) can be observed after diaphragmatic resection as well as with intact diaphragm and may be responsible for changes with sometimes clinical significance (Huwer et al. 2006; Patane et al. 2007).

Other thoracic deformities can be susceptible to inducing hemodynamic changes involving respiratory consequences. The study of cardiac function in subjects with pectus has shown an impairment in right ventricular diastolic filling, which may be especially evident at exercise and is related to the severity of the chest wall deformity (Sigalet et al. 2003, 2007). This has been demonstrated using a variety of functional and imaging techniques, such as echocardiography, nuclear medicine, and angiography, and improvement after open and closed repair has been shown (Sigalet et al. 2003, 2007; Shamberger 2000; Shamberger and Welch 1988; Xiao-Ping et al. 1999). Since MDCT is nowadays required for evaluating the severity and therefore selecting patients for surgery, it has the ability to identify and even quantify the degree of compression of the right ventricle, the shift of the heart on the left side, and the effects on left lower lobe ventilation and perfusion (Fig. 8.19). Congenital absence of the left pericardium can be responsible for deformity of the right ventricle (Fig. 8.20) and may be symptomatic for similar reasons, and in addition conveys the risk of heart herniation (Montaudon et al. 2007).

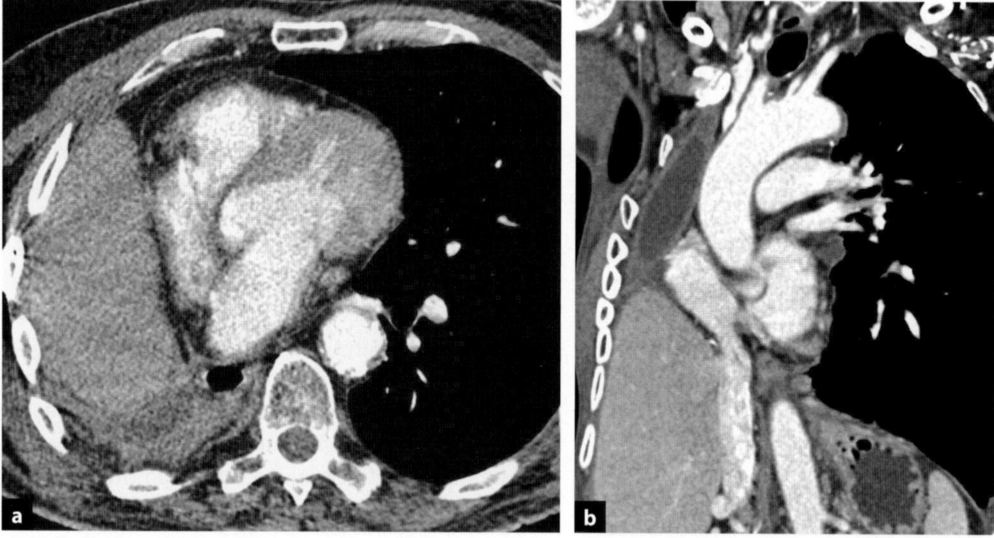

Fig. 8.18a,b. CT scan 6 months after right pneumonectomy for bronchial squamous cell carcinoma cancer in a 64-year-old male patient explored for progressively increasing dyspnea. Massive elevation of the right diaphragm and consecutive obstruction of inferior vena cava were thought to be responsible for the dyspnea. Neither pulmonary nor recurrence causes were found, nor was a patent foramen ovale discovered at contrast echocardiography

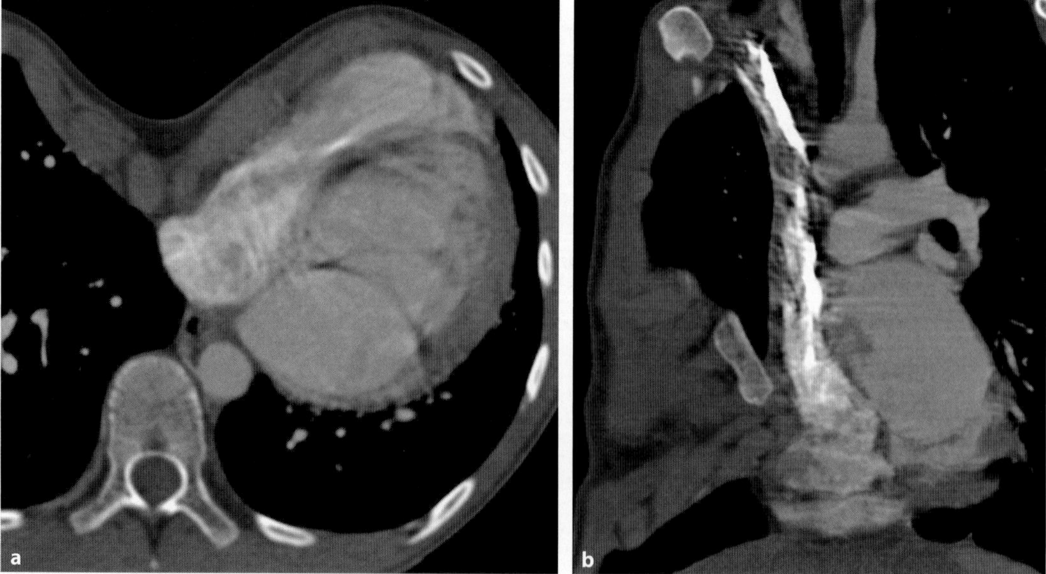

Fig. 8.19a,b. Severe pectus excavatum in an 18-year-old male patient. The patient complained of exercise-induced dyspnea. CT angiography shows the deformed and compressed right atrium

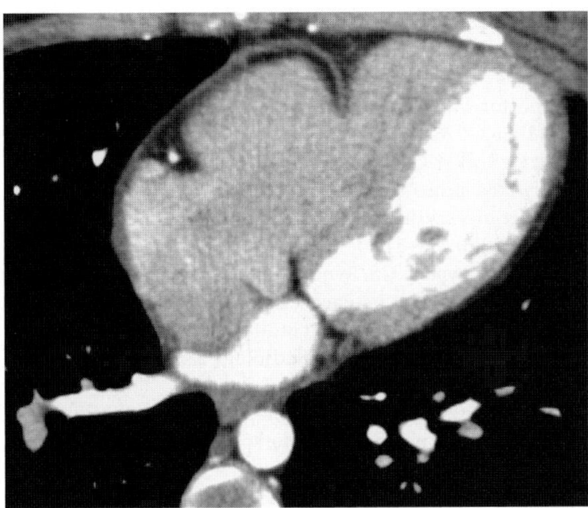

Fig. 8.20. Congenital absence of the left pericardium in a 17-year-old woman referred for a rapidly progressive dyspnea. CT showed a large defect of the pericardium from which a cul-de-sac made a marked impression on the right ventricle wall. After surgical repair, symptoms disappeared

References

Aigner C, Lang G, Taghavi S et al. (2008) Haemodynamic complications after pneumonectomy: atrial inflow obstruction and reopening of the foramen ovale. Eur J Cardiothorac Surg 33(2):268–2671

Amis TC, Jones HA, Hughes JM (1984) Effect of posture on inter-regional distribution of pulmonary perfusion and VA/Q ratios in man. Respir Physiol 56(2):169–182

Arakawa H, Kohno T, Hiki T, Kaji Y (2007) CT pulmonary angiography and CT venography: factors associated with vessel enhancement. AJR Am J Roentgenol 189(1):156–161

Bae KT, Heiken JP, Brink JA (1998a) Aortic and hepatic contrast medium enhancement at CT. Part II. Effect of reduced cardiac output in a porcine model. Radiology 207(3):657–662

Bae KT, Heiken JP, Brink JA (1998b) Aortic and hepatic peak enhancement at CT: effect of contrast medium injection rate–pharmacokinetic analysis and experimental porcine model. Radiology 206(2):455–464

Bae KT, Tran HQ, Heiken JP (2000) Multiphasic injection method for uniform prolonged vascular enhancement at CT angiography: pharmacokinetic analysis and experimental porcine model. Radiology 216(3):872–880

Bae KT, Tran HQ, Heiken JP (2004) Uniform vascular contrast enhancement and reduced contrast medium volume achieved by using exponentially decelerated contrast material injection method. Radiology 231(3):732–736

Bakris NC, Siddiqi AJ, Fraser CD Jr, Mehta AC (1997) Right-to-left interatrial shunt after pneumonectomy. Ann Thorac Surg 63(1):198–201

Batra P, Bigoni B, Manning J et al. (2000) Pitfalls in the diagnosis of thoracic aortic dissection at CT angiography. Radiographics 20(2):309–320

Bernardi L, Keller F, Sanders M et al. (1989) Respiratory sinus arrhythmia in the denervated human heart. J Appl Physiol 67(4):1447–1455

Boehm T, Willmann JK, Hilfiker PR et al. (2003) Thin-section CT of the lung: does electrocardiographic triggering influence diagnosis? Radiology 229(2):483–491

Bruzzi JF, Remy-Jardin M, Kirsch J et al. (2005) Sixteen-slice multidetector computed tomography pulmonary angiography: evaluation of cardiogenic motion artifacts and influence of rotation time on image quality. J Comput Assist Tomogr 29(6):805–814

Burns MA, Molina PL, Gutierrez FR, Sagel SS (1991) Motion artifact simulating aortic dissection on CT. AJR Am J Roentgenol 157(3):465–467

Burrowes KS, Hunter PJ, Tawhai MH (2005) Investigation of the relative effects of vascular branching structure and gravity on pulmonary arterial blood flow heterogeneity via an image-based computational model. Acad Radiol 12(11):1464–1474

Butler J (1983) The heart is in good hands. Circulation 67(6):1163–1168

Chon D, Beck KC, Larsen RL, Shikata H, Hoffman EA (2006) Regional pulmonary blood flow in dogs by 4D X-ray CT. J Appl Physiol 101(5):1451–1465

Chung CS, Karamanoglu M, Kovacs SJ (2004) Duration of diastole and its phases as a function of heart rate during supine bicycle exercise. Am J Physiol Heart Circ Physiol 287(5):H2003–2008

Collins MA, Pidgeon JW, Fitzgerald R (1995) Computed tomography manifestations of tricuspid regurgitation. Br J Radiol 68(814):1058–1060

Dawson P, Blomley MJ (1996) Contrast agent pharmacokinetics revisited: I. Reformulation. Acad Radiol 3 (Suppl 2):S261–263

Desbiolles L, Leschka S, Plass A et al. (2007) Evaluation of temporal windows for coronary artery bypass graft imaging with 64-slice CT. Eur Radiol 17(11):2819–2828

Dewey M, Laule M, Krug L et al. (2004) Multisegment and half-scan reconstruction of 16-slice computed tomography for detection of coronary artery stenoses. Invest Radiol 39(4):223–229

Duvernoy O, Coulden R, Ytterberg C (1995) Aortic motion: a potential pitfall in CT imaging of dissection in the ascending aorta. J Comput Assist Tomogr 19(4):569–572

Dubourg O, Bourdarias JP, Farcot JC et al. (1984) Contrast echocardiographic visualization of cough-induced right to left shunt through a patent foramen ovale. J Am Coll Cardiol 4(3):587–594

Fleischmann D, Rubin GD, Bankier AA, Hittmair K (2000) Improved uniformity of aortic enhancement with customized contrast medium injection protocols at CT angiography. Radiology 214(2):363–371

Flohr T, Ohnesorge B (2001) Heart rate adaptive optimization of spatial and temporal resolution for electrocardiogram-gated multislice spiral CT of the heart. J Comput Assist Tomogr 25(6):907–923

Flohr T, Prokop M, Becker C et al. (2002) A retrospectively ECG-gated multislice spiral CT scan and reconstruction technique with suppression of heart pulsation artifacts for cardio-thoracic imaging with extended volume coverage. Eur Radiol 12(6):1497–1503

Flohr TG, Stierstorfer K, Ulzheimer S, Bruder H, Primak AN, McCollough CH (2005) Image reconstruction and image quality evaluation for a 64-slice CT scanner with z-flying focal spot. Med Phys 32(8):2536–2547

Ghali JK, Liao Y, Cooper RS, Cao G (1992) Changes in pulmonary hemodynamics with aging in a predominantly hypertensive population. Am J Cardiol 70(3):367–370

Glenny RW, Bernard S, Robertson HT, Hlastala MP (1999) Gravity is an important but secondary determinant of regional pulmonary blood flow in upright primates. J Appl Physiol 86(2):623–632

Glick G, Wechsler AS, Epstein SE (1969) Reflex cardiovascular depression produced by stimulation of pulmonary stretch receptors in the dog. J Clin Invest 48(3):467–473

Gosselin MV, Rassner UA, Thieszen SL, Phillips J, Oki A (2004) Contrast dynamics during CT pulmonary angiogram: analysis of an inspiration associated artifact. J Thorac Imaging 19(1):1–7

Greuter MJ, Dorgelo J, Tukker WG, Oudkerk M (2005) Study on motion artifacts in coronary arteries with an anthropomorphic moving heart phantom on an ECG-gated multidetector computed tomography unit. Eur Radiol 15(5):995–1007

Groen JM, Greuter MJ, van Ooijen PM, Oudkerk M (2007) A new approach to the assessment of lumen visibility of coronary artery stent at various heart rates using 64-slice MDCT. Eur Radiol 17(7):1879–1884

Haage P, Schmitz-Rode T, Hubner D, Piroth W, Gunther RW (2000) Reduction of contrast material dose and artifacts by a saline flush using a double power injector in helical CT of the thorax. AJR Am J Roentgenol 174(4):1049–1053

Hagen PT, Scholz DG, Edwards WD (1984) Incidence and size of patent foramen ovale during the first 10 decades of life: an autopsy study of 965 normal hearts. Mayo Clin Proc 59(1):17–20

Han JK, Kim AY, Lee KY et al. (2000) Factors influencing vascular and hepatic enhancement at CT: experimental study on injection protocol using a canine model. J Comput Assist Tomogr 24(3):400–406

Hara H, Virmani R, Ladich E et al. (2005) Patent foramen ovale: current pathology, pathophysiology, and clinical status. J Am Coll Cardiol 46(9):1768–1776

Hartmann IJ, Lo RT, Bakker J, de Monye W, van Waes PF, Pattynama PM (2002) Optimal scan delay in spiral CT for the diagnosis of acute pulmonary embolism. J Comput Assist Tomogr 26(1):21–25

Heiken JP, Brink JA, McClennan BL, Sagel SS, Crowe TM, Gaines MV (1995) Dynamic incremental CT: effect of volume and concentration of contrast material and patient weight on hepatic enhancement. Radiology 195(2):353–357

Henk CB, Grampp S, Linnau KF et al. (2003) Suspected pulmonary embolism: enhancement of pulmonary arteries at deep-inspiration CT angiography–influence of patent foramen ovale and atrial-septal defect. Radiology 226(3):749–755

Hoffman EA, Chon D (2005) Computed tomography studies of lung ventilation and perfusion. Proc Am Thorac Soc 2(6):492–498, 506 Review

Hoffmann MH, Shi H, Manzke R et al. (2005) Noninvasive coronary angiography with 16-detector row CT: effect of heart rate. Radiology 2005;234(1):86–97. Epub 2004 Nov 18. Write to the Help Desk NCBI | NLM | NIH Department of Health & Human Services Privacy Statement | Freedom of Information Act | Disclaimer

Hofman MB, Wickline SA, Lorenz CH (1998) Quantification of in-plane motion of the coronary arteries during the cardiac cycle: implications for acquisition window duration for MR flow quantification. J Magn Reson Imaging 8(3):568–576

Hong C, Becker CR, Huber A et al. (2001) ECG-gated reconstructed multi-detector row CT coronary angiography: effect of varying trigger delay on image quality. Radiology 220(3):712–717

Hong C, Chrysant GS, Woodard PK, Bae KT (2004) Coronary artery stent patency assessed with in-stent contrast enhancement measured at multi-detector row CT angiography: initial experience. Radiology 233(1):286–291. Epub 2004 Aug 10

Hopkins SR (2004) Functional magnetic resonance imaging of the lung: a physiological perspective. J Thorac Imaging 19(4):228–234

Husmann L, Leschka S, Desbiolles L et al. (2007) Coronary artery motion and cardiac phases: dependency on heart rate–implications for CT image reconstruction. Radiology 245(2):567–576

Huwer H, Winning J, Isringhaus H, Kalweit G (2006) Post-pleuropneumonectomy herniation of liver mimicking major pulmonary embolism. Asian Cardiovasc Thorac Ann 14(3):e60–62

Jakobs TF, Becker CR, Ohnesorge B et al. (2002) Multislice helical CT of the heart with retrospective ECG gating: reduction of radiation exposure by ECG-controlled tube current modulation. Eur Radiol 12(5):1081–1086

Johnson TR, Nikolaou K, Wintersperger BJ et al. (2007) Optimization of contrast material administration for electrocardiogram-gated computed tomographic angiography of the chest. J Comput Assist Tomogr 31(2):265–271

Katoh M, Wildberger JE, Gunther RW, Buecker A (2005) Malignant right coronary artery anomaly simulated by motion artifacts on MDCT. AJR Am J Roentgenol 185(4):1007–1010

Kim DJ, Kim TH, Kim SJ et al. (2008) Saline flush effect for enhancement of aorta and coronary arteries at multidetector CT coronary angiography. Radiology 246(1):110–115

Ko SF, Hsieh MJ, Chen MC et al. (2005) Effects of heart rate on motion artifacts of the aorta on non-ECG-assisted 0.5-s thoracic MDCT. AJR Am J Roentgenol 184(4):1225–1230

Kuhns LR, Borlaza G (1980) The "twinkling star" sign: an aid in differentiating pulmonary vessels from pulmonary nodules on computed tomograms. Radiology 135(3):763–764

Kuzo RS, Pooley RA, Crook JE, Heckman MG, Gerber TC (2007) Measurement of caval blood flow with MRI during respiratory maneuvers: implications for vascular contrast opacification on pulmonary CT angiographic studies. AJR Am J Roentgenol 188(3):839–842

Leber AW, Knez A, von Ziegler F et al. (2005) Quantification of obstructive and nonobstructive coronary lesions by 64-slice computed tomography: a comparative study with quantitative coronary angiography and intravascular ultrasound. J Am Coll Cardiol 46(1):147–154

Leschka S, Alkadhi H, Plass A et al. (2005) Accuracy of MSCT coronary angiography with 64-slice technology: first experience. Eur Heart J 26(15):1482–1487

Lu B, Dai RP, Jiang SL et al. (2001) Effects of window and threshold levels on the accuracy of three-dimensional rendering techniques in coronary artery electron-beam CT angiography. Acad Radiol 8(8):754–761

Manghat NE, Kakani N, Morgan-Hughes GJ (2007) Incidental patent foramen ovale detected by 64-detector row CT before radiofrequency ablation therapy. Heart 93(11):1356

Mao S, Lu B, Oudiz RJ, Bakhsheshi H, Liu SC, Budoff MJ (2000) Coronary artery motion in electron beam tomography. J Comput Assist Tomogr 24(2):253–258

Marini C, Miniati M, Ambrosino N et al. (2006) Dyspnoea and hypoxaemia after lung surgery: the role of interatrial right-to-left shunt. Eur Respir J 28(1):174–181

Mayo JR, Muller NL, Henkelman RM (1987) The double-fissure sign: a motion artifact on thin-section CT scans. Radiology 165(2):580–581

Mercho N, Stoller JK, White RD, Mehta AC (1994) Right-to-left interatrial shunt causing platypnea after pneumonectomy. A recent experience and diagnostic value of dynamic magnetic resonance imaging. Chest 105(3):931–933

Milne EN, Pistolesi M (1993) Reading the chest radiograph. A physiologic approach. Mosby, St Louis, pp 9–50

Montaudon M, Berger P, Blachere H, De Boucaud L, Latrabe V, Laurent F (2001) Thin-section CT of the lung: influence of 0.5-s gantry rotation and ECG triggering on image quality. Eur Radiol 11(9):1681–1687

Montaudon M, Roubertie F, Bire F, Laurent F (2007) Congenital pericardial defect: report of two cases and literature review. Surg Radiol Anat 29(3):195–200

Morgan-Hughes GJ, Marshall AJ, Roobottom CA (2003a) Refined computed tomography of the thoracic aorta: the impact of electrocardiographic assistance. Clin Radiol 58(8):581–588

Morgan-Hughes GJ, Owens PE, Marshall AJ, Roobottom CA (2003b) Thoracic aorta at multi-detector row CT: motion artifact with various reconstruction windows. Radiology 228(2):583–588

Patane S, Anfuso C, Marte F, Minutoli F, Bella GD, Coglitore S (2007) An unusual presentation of a right atrial Chiari network. Int J Cardiol 2007 Nov 13 [Epub ahead of print]

Pinsky MR (1984a) Instantaneous venous return curves in an intact canine preparation. J Appl Physiol 56(3):765–771

Pinsky MR (1984b) Determinants of pulmonary arterial flow variation during respiration. J Appl Physiol 56(5):1237–1245

Pinsky MR (2005) Cardiovascular issues in respiratory care. Chest 128 (5 Suppl 2):592S–597S

Qanadli SD, El Hajjam M, Mesurolle B et al. (1999) Motion artifacts of the aorta simulating aortic dissection on spiral CT. J Comput Assist Tomogr 23(1):1–6

Raff GL, Gallagher MJ, O'Neill WW, Goldstein JA (2005) Diagnostic accuracy of noninvasive coronary angiography using 64-slice spiral computed tomography. J Am Coll Cardiol 46(3):552–557

Reinhardt JM, Hoffman EA (1998) Quantitative pulmonary imaging: spatial and temporal considerations in high-resolution CT. Acad Radiol 5(8):539–546

Remy-Jardin M TA, Kirsh J, Bruzzi J, Khalil C, Remy J (2005) Cardiogenic artifacts on multidetector CT angiograms of the pulmonary circulation: comparison wit ECG-gated and non-gated acquisitions. In: Radiological Society of North America Scientific Assembly and Annual Meeting Program. Oak Brook, Ill. Radiological Society of North America 2005:327

Ritchie CJ, Godwin JD, Crawford CR, Stanford W, Anno H, Kim Y (1992) Minimum scan speeds for suppression of motion artifacts in CT. Radiology 185(1):37–42

Roos JE, Willmann JK, Weishaupt D, Lachat M, Marincek B, Hilfiker PR (2002) Thoracic aorta: motion artifact reduction with retrospective and prospective electrocardiography-assisted multi-detector row CT. Radiology 222(1):271–277

Rubin GD, Leung AN, Robertson VJ, Stark P (1998) Thoracic spiral CT: influence of subsecond gantry rotation on image quality. Radiology 208(3):771–776

Set PA, Lomas DJ, Maskell GF, Flower CD, Dixon AK (1993) Artifacts in the ascending aorta on computed tomography: another measure of aortic distensibility? Eur J Radiol 16(2):107–111

Revel MP, Remy-Jardin M, Hennon H, Deklunder G, Remy J (2007) Diagnosis of patent foramen ovale using 64-multidetector row CT. Study in 105 patients. In: Radiological Society of North America Scientific Assembly and Annual Meeting Program. Oak Brook, Ill. Radiological Society of North America, 2007: 606

Schoepf UJ, Becker CR, Bruening RD et al. (1999) Electrocardiographically gated thin-section CT of the lung. Radiology 212(3):649–654

Schroeder S, Kopp AF, Kuettner A et al. (2002) Influence of heart rate on vessel visibility in noninvasive coronary angiography using new multislice computed tomography: experience in 94 patients. Clin Imaging 26(2):106–111

Shamberger RC, Welch KJ (1988) Cardiopulmonary function in pectus excavatum. Surg Gynecol Obstet 166(4):383–391

Shamberger RC (2000) Cardiopulmonary effects of anterior chest wall deformities. Chest Surg Clin N Am 10(2):245–252, v–vi

Sigalet DL, Montgomery M, Harder J (2003) Cardiopulmonary effects of closed repair of pectus excavatum. J Pediatr Surg 38(3):380–385; discussion 380–385

Sigalet DL, Montgomery M, Harder J, Wong V, Kravarusic D, Alassiri A (2007) Long term cardiopulmonary effects of closed repair of pectus excavatum. Pediatr Surg Int 23(5):493–497

Sivit CJ, Taylor GA, Bulas DI, Kushner DC, Potter BM, Eichelberger MR (1992) Posttraumatic shock in children: CT findings associated with hemodynamic instability. Radiology 182(3):723–726

Tarver RD, Conces DJ Jr, Godwin JD (1988) Motion artifacts on CT simulate bronchiectasis. AJR Am J Roentgenol 151(6):1117–1119

Wagner EM, Blosser S, Mitzner W (1998) Bronchial vascular contribution to lung lymph flow. J Appl Physiol 85(6):2190–2195

West JB, Mathieu-Costello O (1995) Vulnerability of pulmonary capillaries in heart disease. Circulation 92(3):622–631

Wintersperger BJ, Nikolaou K, von Ziegler F et al. (2006) Image quality, motion artifacts, and reconstruction timing of 64-slice coronary computed tomography angiography with 0.33-s rotation speed. Invest Radiol 41(5):436–442

Wittram C (2003) Pulmonary artery enhancement at CT pulmonary angiography. Radiology 229(3):932; author reply 932–933

Wittram C, Yoo AJ (2007) Transient interruption of contrast on CT pulmonary angiography: proof of mechanism. J Thorac Imaging 22(2):125–129

Wolfkiel CJ, Rich S (1992) Analysis of regional pulmonary enhancement in dogs by ultrafast computed tomography. Invest Radiol 27(3):211–216

Xiao-Ping J, Ting-Ze H, Wen-Ying L, Fu-Kang W, Yu-Ru Y, Jie-Xiong F, Qi-Cheng L, Ming L, Yun-Man T (1999) Pulmonary function for pectus excavatum at long-term follow-up. J Pediatr Surg 34(12):1787–1790

Yamashita Y, Komohara Y, Takahashi M, Uchida M, Hayabuchi N, Shimizu T, Narabayashi I (2000) Abdominal helical CT: evaluation of optimal doses of intravenous contrast material–a prospective randomized study. Radiology 216(3):718–723

Yanagawa M, Tomiyama N, Sumikawa H et al. (2007) Thin-section CT of lung without ECG gating: 64-detector row CT can markedly reduce cardiac motion artifacts which can simulate lung lesions. Eur J Radiol [Epub ahead of print]

Yeh BM, Kurzman P, Foster E, Qayyum A, Joe B, Coakley F (2004) Clinical relevance of retrograde inferior vena cava or hepatic vein opacification during contrast-enhanced CT. AJR Am J Roentgenol 183(5):1227–1232

Zhang J, Fletcher JG, Scott Harmsen W et al. (2008) Analysis of heart rate and heart rate variation during cardiac CT examinations. Acad Radiol 15(1):40–48

Drug-Induced Respiratory Disease in Cardiac Patients

9

Philippe Camus, Clio Camus, and Pascal Foucher

CONTENTS

P. Camus, MD
C. Camus, MD
P. Foucher, MD
Department of Pulmonary and Critical Care Medicine, Hôpital Universitaire du Bocage, 21000 Dijon, France, and Pneumotox®

9.1 Introduction

By definition, adverse reactions to drugs develop unpredictably in patients exposed to therapeutic doses of 'drugs,' which include such respiratory gases as dioxygen (O_2) and nitric oxide (NO). Accordingly, misuse, disuse, drug interactions, deliberate or accidental overdoses, illicit drugs, and radiation therapy are outside the province of this chapter. Notwithstanding that, it is difficult to cover this topic without mentioning the features of respiratory reactions occasioned by abused substances, herbals, radiation therapy, overdoses of drugs, and procedures when these overlap with the features or are in the differentials list for drug-induced respiratory disease (Hagan and Burney 2007).

Drug-induced respiratory injury has become an important area of pulmonary medicine, with 406 drugs overall capable of causing a constellation of distinct patterns of respiratory involvement, among which interstitial lung disease, pulmonary edema, alveolar hemorrhage, and pleural involvement are the most common (Pneumotox® 1997). The level of evidence for drugs as the cause of respiratory disease is wide ranging and depends on the incidence rate and distinctiveness of the adverse reaction, and on the possibility that other causes may cause it, or that it may occur idiopathically. Several methodologies exist (Rothman 2000; Etminan et al. 2006), even for isolated case reports (Srihari and Lee 2008). The full list of causal drugs along with an estimate of incidence is available at www.pneumotox.com (Pneumotox®) (Pneumotox® 1997). The list of cardiac drugs is shown in Table 9.1.

Drug-induced respiratory disease in cardiac patients has changed with time. Reports in the 1950s and 1960s focused on organizing pneumonia as a complication of treatments with the early ganglionic blockers (hexamethonium, mecamylamine),

Table 9.1. Cardiac drugs and the corresponding patterns of respiratory involvement

Drug	Pattern of respiratory involvement
Adenosine	Bronchospasm Cardiac arrest ECG changes
Amiodarone	Interstitial pneumonia with dyslipidosis Organizing pneumonia/BOOP Pulmonary fibrosis ARDS Lone pleural effusion SLE
Analgesics	Pulmonary edema Propofol infusion syndrome or PRIS
Anesthetic agents (systemic)	Anaphylaxis Violent coughing
Anesthetic agents (topical)	Anaphylaxis Methemoglobinemia
Angiotensin-converting enzyme inhibitors	Angioedema ≥ upper airway obstruction Cough Eosinophilic pneumonia SLE
Anorectic agents	Pulmonary hypertension
Antibiotics	Anaphylaxis Eosinophilic pneumonia
Anticoagulants (oral)	Alveolar hemorrhage Hematoma compressing the major airway
Aprotinin	Anaphylaxis
Aspirin/NSAIDs	Anaphylaxis Bronchospasm, sudden asthma attack Eosinophilic pneumonia Pulmonary edema
Beta-blocking agents	Bronchospasm, sudden asthma attack Interstitial pneumonia Pleural effusion SLE
Blood, blood products	Pulmonary edema TRALI/ARDS
Dextran	Anaphylaxis
Doxorubucin	Acute myocardial failure, pulmonary edema
Epinephrine (adrenaline)	Pulmonary edema
Ergolines	Pleural effusion/thickening
Factor VIIa	Thromboembolism
Fibrinolytic agents (systemic, intracoronary)	Alveolar hemorrhage Hematoma compressing the major airway
Flecainide	Interstitial pneumonia
Glitazones	Pulmonary congestion/edema Pleural effusion
Glycoprotein IIB/IIIA receptor inhibitors	Alveolar hemorrhage
Heparin	Alveolar hemorrhage Anaphylaxis
Hydrochlorothiazide	Pulmonary edema (relapsing with rechallenge)
Latex*	Asthma* Bronchospasm* Anaphylaxis
Lupus-inducing drugs (Rubin 2005)	Pleural, pericardial effusion Interstitial pneumonia
Nafazoline (topical)	Pulmonary edema
Neuromuscular blocking drugs	Anaphylaxis Respiratory failure Upper airway obstruction
Opiates	Pulmonary edema Respiratory failure
Radiation therapy	Mediastinal fibrosis Pulmonary vein stenosis Pericardial/pleural effusion Pulmonary fibrosis
Radiographic contrast agents	Anaphylaxis Bronchospasm Pulmonary edema
Statins	Interstitial pneumonia BOOP SLE
Vasopressin	Pulmonary edema

* Can affect health-care workers as well. ARDS: adult respiratory distress syndrome; BOOP, bronchiolitis obliterans organizing pneumonia; SLE: systemic lupus erythematosus; TRALI, transfusion-related acute lung injury

drug-induced lupus, hydrochlorothiazide-induced pulmonary edema, and anticoagulant-induced complications (Foucher et al. 1997). In the 1980s, amiodarone emerged as a significant cause for pulmonary toxicity, and the disease is still prevalent today (Ernawati et al. 2008). Recent additions include angiotensin-converting enzyme inhibitor (ACEI)-induced cough (Dicpinigaitis 2006) and upper airway obstruction (Sondhi et al. 2004), statin-induced interstitial lung disease (Fernandez et al. 2008), glycoprotein IIB/IIIA receptor inhibitor-induced alveolar hemorrhage (Iskandar et al. 2006), transfusion-related lung injury (TRALI) (Popovsky 2008), and sirolimus-, temsirolimus-, and everolimus-induced pneumonitis (Pneumotox® 1997).

The clinical expression of drug-induced respiratory disease and the way it impacts lung functions depend upon its suddenness, nature, and location, with laryngeal edema, acute pulmonary edema, alveolar hemorrhage, and progressive parenchymal fibrosis ranking highest in terms of severity. The untoward consequences of adverse respiratory reactions can be further compounded by drug-induced hemorrhage, hemodynamic instability, or shock, and also depend upon the underlying disease for which the drug was exactly prescribed.

Notable features of drug-induced respiratory disease in cardiac patients include the following:

- The diagnosis of drug-induced lung disease is against the pulmonary manifestations of left ventricular failure, which at times are difficult to differentiate from the drug-induced disease on imaging (Gluecker et al. 1999). Cardiac ultrasound examination, judicious use of drug therapy withdrawal, corticosteroid therapy, and diuresis help segregate these conditions.
- Subclinical left ventricular failure and the confounding influence of smoking may impact lung volumes, diffusing capacity for carbon monoxide, and inspiratory muscle force (Johnson et al. 2001; Stelfox et al. 2004), causing deviations in baseline lung function from predicted values that are difficult to predict. Therefore, measurement of pulmonary physiology is a useful step before commencing treatments with drugs that commonly cause pulmonary toxicity (e.g., amiodarone) (Stelfox et al. 2004), as any data during treatment can then be compared to pre-therapy evaluation to separate adverse drug effects from previous abnormalities.
- Drug-induced effects in lung can be nonspecific. Thus, histopathology may not be an adequate means to prove or disprove drug-induced disease (Flieder and Travis 2004). Accordingly, due to the risks inherent to the procedure, a lung biopsy is rarely justified, and in the majority of pulmonary drug reactions, the diagnosis is suggested using clinical, laboratory, and radiologic features, and confirmed by the dechallenge test.
- A number of adverse respiratory reactions to drugs develop acutely and unexpectedly shortly after drug administration, causing life-threatening respiratory emergencies (Bonniaud et al. 2006). Instant recognition is an essential guide to proper management and avoidance of re-exposure. Thus, physicians and nurses in cardiology, anesthesia, intensive care, and surgery should be cognizant of the multiple possibilities of drug-induced respiratory involvement.
- Several drug classes as a whole (e.g., angiotensin convertase inhibitors, beta-blocking drugs, statins, anticoagulants, and glycoprotein IIB/IIIA receptor inhibitors) occasion similar adverse respiratory reactions. Thus, patients who present with adverse reactions to one drug should probably not be challenged with drugs of the same family, since chances are that they may adversely cross-react.
- The risk associated with drug therapy withdrawal (an essential diagnostic tool in drug-induced disease) should be balanced against its benefits. For instance, amiodarone withdrawal may require coverage with another antiarrhythmic drug to prevent recurrence of ventricular arrhythmia.
- A number of drugs and physical agents cause cardiac injury (Hagan and Burney 2007; Prosnitz et al. 2005; Yahalom and Portlock 2008), which may manifest with the classic features of left ventricular failure, valvular involvement, pericardial effusion, or tamponade. Although the present chapter does not address this area specifically, cardiac and pulmonary toxicity of drugs share several features.
- Due to their age range, patients with cardiac conditions may suffer from or develop other medical conditions requiring treatment with other drugs. Typical examples include drugs used to treat high blood pressure, type II diabetes mellitus, rheumatoid arthritis, or depression. It is incumbent upon clinicians to review all drugs capable of causing respiratory injury using appropriate sources of information (Pneumotox® 1997).
- Medical, imaging, or surgical procedures (e.g., placement of venous catheter, Swan-Ganz line,

pacemaker, coronary stents, coronary angiography, cardiac catheterization, coronary artery bypass graft, and gastric banding) may cause pleural, cardiac, or vascular injury (PLATAKI and BOUROS 2004), which may manifest with pneumothorax, serous or sanguineous pleural effusion, hemopericardium, air embolism, or pulmonary artery aneurysm, not to mention acupuncture, injections of street drugs, and self-inflicted damage (HAGAN and BURNEY 2007; PLATAKI and BOUROS 2004; NEWCOMB and CLARKE 2005).

9.2 Causal Drugs

Table 9.1 lists the main cardiac drugs that may cause adverse respiratory reactions, along with corresponding patterns of involvement (PNEUMOTOX® 1997). Not mentioned in this list are herbals, illicit, laced, or abused substances, solvents, chemicals, and radiation therapy to the breast or chest, which may also cause lung or heart injury. History taking should include exposure to the latter agents, the list of which is expanding (HU et al. 2005; NANDA and KONNUR 2006; ALAPAT and ZIMMERMAN 2008).

9.3 Diagnostic Criteria

Causality assessment is the crux of the diagnosis of alleged adverse reaction to drugs.

9.3.1 Hill Criteria

In 1965, HILL delineated the following criteria to separate causation from association between environment (to which drugs are related) and signal (disease) that still stand today:

Strength of signal, which is reflected by the number of published reports or, if available, by incidence rates in patients exposed to the drug as opposed to unexposed controls.

Consistency, i.e., the signal is repeatedly observed by different persons, in different places, settings, ethnic groups, circumstances, and times.

Specificity, reflected by the distinctive clinical, biological, imaging, or histopathological features of the signal, or alternatively, reflected by the magnitude of the association of the signal with exposure to the specific drug or agent.

Temporality, when a definite timing of therapy (latency period, time to onset of pulmonary symptoms, effect of therapy withdrawal, and recurrence with rechallenge).

Drug-induced diseases having a gradual and insidious onset, those that develop following a free interval after termination of treatment, or those that occasion an irreversible and progressive pattern of involvement that is uninfluenced by drug withdrawal may fail to meet this criterion.

Biological gradient, when a dose-versus-signal relationship can be evidenced.

Plausibility, which depends on knowledge of the day.

Coherence, when the adverse reaction results from a foreseeable pharmacologic effect of the drug (e.g., anticoagulation and alveolar hemorrhage).

Supportive experimental evidence when the disease can be reproduced in animal models.

Analogy, if chemically or pharmacologically related drugs produce analogous adverse effects.

Tests of significance when controlled studies are available.

9.3.2 Naranjo Criteria

The Naranjo scale (NARANJO et al. 1981) articulates approximately ten questions:

1. Are there previous conclusive reports on this reaction?
2. Did the adverse event appear after the suspected drug was administered?
3. Did the adverse reaction improve when the drug was discontinued or a specific antagonist was administered?
4. Did the adverse reaction reappear when the drug was re-administered?
5. Are there alternative causes (other than the drug) that could on their own have caused the reaction?
6. Did the reaction reappear when a placebo was given?
7. Was the drug detected in the blood or other fluids in concentrations known to be toxic?

8. Was the reaction more severe when the dose was increased or less severe when the dose was decreased?
9. Did the patient have a similar reaction to the same or similar drugs in any previous exposure?
10. Was the adverse event confirmed by any objective evidence?

Scoring (−1 to +2) is assigned to each question depending on whether the answer is 'yes,' 'no,' or 'do not know.' The reaction is judged definite, probable, possible, or doubtful if the total score is >9, 5–8, 1–4, and ≤0, respectively. Numbers are less subject to variability and are generally preferred to words to gauge plausibility.

9.3.3 Irey Scoring

The scoring system by Irey (1976) consists of the following:

1. Correct identification of the drug, with evidence for exposure to the agent, and estimates of dose and duration of exposure.
2. Exclusion of other primary or secondary lung diseases.
3. Temporal eligibility and appropriate latent period.
4. Remission of symptoms with removal of drug. Recurrence with rechallenge.
5. Singularity of drug: can other drugs the patient is taking compete to explain the clinical-imaging picture?
6. Characteristic pattern of reaction to a specific agent from previous documentation.
7. Quantification of drug levels that confirms abnormal levels.

The degree of certainty is then deduced: causative, probable, or possible.

9.3.4 Proposal

A scoring system specific to adverse respiratory reactions has yet to be tested. A tentative list could include the following:

- Correct identification of the drug(s) the patient is exposed to, including batch number and route of administration (almost no route renders patients immune to the development of drug-induced respiratory disease).
- Drug singularity. If the patient was concomitantly exposed to several drugs, it is necessary to evaluate the possible contribution of each drug taken in isolation or in combination to the reaction under scrutiny.
- Risk evaluation. Were there any risk factors, such as advanced age, atopy, ethnicity, a history of abnormal pulmonary function, or infiltrative lung disease? Was the daily or cumulative dosage of the drug within the above-recommended range?
- Availability of pretherapy pulmonary evaluation to which imaging or pulmonary function can be compared during treatment. This will confirm that the observed changes did occur concomitantly with treatment and do not reflect previous abnormalities independent from treatment with the drug under evaluation.
- Evidence-based evaluation of the signal in the literature in terms of magnitude and distinctiveness. For example, the signal of amiodarone pulmonary toxicity with several hundred reported cases, distinctive histopathology, and significantly increased risk of pneumonitis in patients exposed to the drug is strong. Although not many cases of eosinophilic pneumonia are associated with ACEI, the distinctiveness of this pattern of reaction and positive dechallenge test make drug causality plausible (Etminan et al. 2006; Srihari and Lee 2008; Rothman et al. 2004).
- Symptom-exposure relationship or temporality. A prerequisite for entertaining the diagnosis of drug-induced disease is the occurrence of symptoms after commencement of treatment with the suspected drug. Hence, pretherapy evaluation is useful to make sure the changes are not spurious. A very short time to onset of a few minutes or hours suggests the drug etiology. Drug-induced bronchospasm, anaphylaxis, or pulmonary edema typically demonstrate a short to very short exposure-symptom relationship, while it takes a few days, weeks, or months for alveolar hemorrhage, interstitial lung disease, or pleural involvement to develop, and up to several years for amiodarone pulmonary toxicity to do so. Ideally, abatement of all signs and symptoms [including abnormal blood tests such as antinuclear antibodies (ANA)] should follow drug discontinuation. Drug conditions that are rapidly progressive (e.g., acute pulmonary edema, alveolar hemorrhage, interstitial lung disease) or irreversible (e.g., fatal reactions, pulmonary fibrosis) may fail to meet this criterion. Likewise, amiodarone withdrawal may not

translate into improvement, owing to the persistence of the drug in lung tissue. Corticosteroids interfere with assessment of the effect of drug discontinuance and for that reason are reserved for patients with symptomatic or extensive disease. Relapse upon rechallenge with the suspected drug is considered irrefutable evidence for a drug condition. However, deliberate rechallenge rarely is performed for diagnostic purposes because the risks of the procedure are unknown. However, history-taking should inquire about previous relapse(s) following iterative exposure to the drug, as has been described with ACEI-induced angioedema and hydrochlorothiazide-induced pulmonary edema. When present, this finding has a diagnostic contribution nearly identical to a positive rechallenge.

- Quantification of the drug [and metabolite(s) if applicable] levels in blood, other fluids, or tissues. Although this step is easily missed at the time of admission, it is useful to the diagnosis of aspirin-induced pulmonary edema, where blood levels are classically above the therapeutic range, and in the evaluation of patients suspected of drug abuse.
- Appropriate differentiation and labeling the respiratory reaction (Tables 9.1, 9.2, and 9.3). Since a pathological specimen rarely is available for review, attempts at characterizing adverse reactions are made using the combination of minimally invasive tests [imaging, bronchoalveolar lavage (BAL)]. Drug-induced reactions express themselves with many patterns. However, predicting the histopathological pattern (Tables 9.2, 9.3) from imaging and BAL is not entirely reliable (Cleverley et al. 2002).
- Consistency of the clinical, biological, imaging, and pathological pattern of involvement with the specific drug. Pneumotox® is an attempt at summarizing the literature, and the repository includes >11,500 references at this time (Pneumotox® 1997).
- Exclusion of causes other than drug(s) that may explain the clinical scenario. Main competing diagnoses in cardiac patients include cardiac pulmonary edema, a coincidental infection, an opportunistic infection in heart transplant recipients on immunosuppressives or in patients on even small doses of corticosteroids, reactions to other drugs, and, less often, a neoplastic condition.
- Make room for a follow-up period of a few weeks for acute reactions (e.g., bronchospasm) to a few months for interstitial lung disease to confront the diagnosis of drug-induced lung disease to the test of time.
- In vitro tests. These rarely can support the diagnosis of the drug-induced condition.
  - The predominance of lymphocytes, neutrophils, or eosinophils may help relate a pattern of interstitial lung disease with a specific drug. The finding of lipid-laden foam cells in the BAL is suggestive of amiodarone pulmonary toxicity (APT) (Costabel et al. 2004).
  - Circulating ANAs characterize those patients with drug-induced lupus, especially if ANA levels diminish following drug withdrawal (Rubin 2005).
  - Lymphocyte stimulation with the drug is now considered unreliable, if not misleading (Matsuno et al. 2007).
  - Acetylator phenotyping, measurement of circulating KL-6 or TGF-ß1 have not demonstrated sufficient diagnostic utility yet.
- Criteria more specific to certain situations or drugs are described in the appropriate sections below.

Any scoring system tacitly capitalizes on the accuracy of each criterion, particularly the differential. At any rate, review of data by an external observer is worthwhile. In many western countries, reporting the adverse effect to drug agencies is mandatory.

9.4 Patterns of Drug-Induced Injury

Any classification has limitations. We rely on a mixed classification resting on severity, pattern of reaction, and drugs. The severity of adverse drug reactions ranges from mild (e.g., ACEI cough) to moderate (e.g., amiodarone-induced pulmonary toxicity), life threatening (acute amiodarone pulmonary toxicity, severe alveolar hemorrhage), or fatal (e.g., anaphylaxis, acute upper airway obstruction, and catastrophic bronchospasm). Outcomes depend on the type of adverse reaction, its association with adverse systemic effects (bleeding, shock), the effect of drug withdrawal, response to treatment, and setting where the reaction occurs, for instance when a cataclysmic reaction occurs intraoperatively or at a distance from point of care.

Table 9.2. Main patterns of drug-induced respiratory involvement in cardiac patients

Site of involvement	Clinical-pathological pattern	Incidence	TTO	ARF	Clinical presentation	Endoscopy - BAL	C.A.	Imaging
Lung								
	Classic interstitial pneumonia	Uncommon	V	+	Dyspnea	Increase in BAL lymphocytes	Easy	Diffuse pulmonary infiltrates
	APT	Common	V	++	Dyspnea, constitutional symptoms	Foam cells ± lymphocytes or neutrophils in BAL	Easy	Asymmetrical infiltrates, scattered opacities, masses
	Eosinophilic pneumonia	Uncommon	V	+	Dyspnea	Eosinophils in BAL	Easy	Peripheral or diffuse pulmonary infiltrates
	Pulmonary edema	Uncommon	VS/S	++	Dyspnea	BAL mainly used to rule out an infection	Easy	Transient pulmonary infiltrates <-> whiteout, ARDS
	Alveolar hemorrhage	Not uncommon	S/V	++	Dyspnea, pallor	Hemorrhage confirmed by BAL	Difficult	pulmonary infiltrates and hemoglobin loss
	Diffuse alveolar damage	Not uncommon	V	+++	Acute respiratory failure	BAL mainly used to rule out an infection		Dissuse whiteout
Upper airway								
	Angioedema	Common	V/L	+++	Stridor	Loss of patency	Easy	ND
	Anaphylaxis	Not uncommon	VS	+++	Stridor, shock, bronchospasm	NUD	Easy	ND
	Hematoma	Rare	V	++	Stridor	Bulging, narrowing, discoloration	Easy	Airway narrowing on CT
Lower airway								
	Acute asthma attack	Common	VS/S	+++	Wheezing	NR	Easy	Hyperinflation
	Lone cough	Very common	V	-	Cough	Normal	Easy	Normal
Pleura								
	Pleural effusion	Uncommon	L	+	Dyspnea, chest pain	NR	Easy	Pleural effusion
	Pleural thickening	Uncommon	L	-	Dyspnea, chest pain, friction rubs	NR	Easy	Pleural thickening
Pulmonary circulation								
	Pulmonary thrombo-embolism	Not uncommon	V	++	Dyspnea, RVF	NR	Difficult	Abnormal V/Q scan and contrast CT
	Chronic obliterative vasculopathy	Rare	L	++	Signs of PHTn	NR	Difficult	Normal V/Q scan
Hemoglobin								
	Methemoglobinemia£	Not uncommon	VS	++	Cyanosis, low SaO2, normal PaO2	NR	Easy	NR

APT: amiodarone pulmonary toxicity; ARF: propensity to produce acute respiratory failure; BAL (– to ++ scale): bronchoalveolar lavage; C.A.: causality assessment; ND: no data; NR not relevant; NUD: not usually done because symptoms tend to predominate elsewhere; RVF: right ventricular failure; PHTn: pulmonary arterial hypertension; TTO: time to onset; VS: very short; S: short; V variable; L: long; V/Q scan: ventilation-perfusion scan; CT : computer tomography; £: arterial blood has a brownish discoloration instead of the normal bright red color

Table 9.3. Imaging-oriented table of drug-induced parenchymal lung disease in cardiac patients with the corresponding drugs and histopathological patterns of involvement

Pattern on imaging	Histopathological correlates	Prototypical drugs (see Pneumotox® for cardiac and noncardiac drugs)
1-Chest radiograph		
Bilateral haze/ground glass	Alveolitis (alveolar/interstitial inflammatory cell infiltrate) Pulmonary edema (early stage) DAD (early stage)	E.g., beta-blocking agents, amiodarone
Micronodular/miliary pattern	Granuloma	Sirolimus
Bilateral alveolar opacities with or without the batwing pattern and air bronchograms	Pulmonary edema Alveolar hemorrhage with or without capillaritis Diffuse alveolar damage	Adrenaline/epinephrine Anticoagulants, abciximab, and related drugs Amiodarone
Peripheral subpleural opacities	Eosinophilic pneumonia Organizing pneumonia	ACEI Amiodarone
Alveolar opacities with a recognizable lobar or segmental distribution with or without volume loss	Amiodarone pulmonary BOOP toxicity	Amiodarone
Lone consolidation or mass	Organizing or eosinophilic pneumonia Amiodarone pulmonary toxicity Amiodaronoma	ACEI, amiodarone Amiodarone Amiodarone
Migratory opacities	Organizing or eosinophilic pneumonia	ACEI, amiodarone
Multiple nodules	Amiodarone pulmonary toxicity	Amiodarone
2-HRCT		
Diffuse ground glass	Cellular interstitial pneumonia, alveolitis Pulmonary edema, DAD early stage	Hydrochlorothiazide, amiodarone
Smooth mosaic lung attenuation	Cellular nonspecific interstial pneumonia Pulmonary edema Alveolar hemorrhage	Beta-blockers Hydrochlorothiazide Anticoagulants, fibrinolytic agents, abciximab, and related drugs
Patchy or diffuse pulmonary shadows showing increased attenuation	Amiodarone pulmonary toxicity, foamy macrophages	Amiodarone
Prominent intralobular thickening	?	Amiodarone
Prominent interlobular thickening		Drugs that produce pulmonary edema (e.g., adrenaline) Amiodarone
Lone consolidation or mass	Organizing- or eosinophilic pneumonia Amiodarone pulmonary toxicity « Amiodaronoma »	ACEI, amiodarone Amiodarone Amiodarone
Migratory opacities	Organizing or eosinophilic pneumonia	ACEI, amiodarone
Multiple (shaggy) nodules	Amiodarone pulmonary toxicity	Amiodarone
Honeycombing and traction bronchiectasis	Pulmonary fibrosis (UIP pattern)	Amiodarone, late

ACEI: angiotensin-converting enzyme inhibitors; DAD: diffuse alveolar damage; OP: organizing pneumonia; PIE: pulmonary infiltrates and eosinophila; UIP: usual interstitial pneumonitis

Several drugs cause a stereotypical, hence recognizable, clinical, imaging, and pathological pattern of involvement. Amiodarone produces pneumonitis with an insidious onset, ACEI occasions chronic cough or acute upper airway obstruction, hydrochlorothiazide produces short-lived "allergic" pulmonary infiltrates or pulmonary edema, and anticoagulants, fibrinolytic agents, and platelet glycoprotein IIB/IIIA receptor inhibitors cause alveolar hemorrhage. Some drugs can cause more than one pattern of involvement (Table 9.1).

9.4.1 Drug-Induced Respiratory Emergencies

Drug-induced respiratory emergencies may result from involvement of the upper or lower airways, lung parenchyma, pulmonary circulation, pleura, pericardium, heart, or neuromuscular system. Involvement is in the form of inflammation, edema, a cellular infiltrate, thromboembolism, effusion, hemorrhage, fat embolism, or hematoma. Radiographic appearances depend on the location of pathological process, and there is little correlation between imaging features and severity: parenchymal (e.g., infiltrative lung disease, pulmonary edema, alveolar hemorrhage) and pleural involvement is visible on imaging, while upper airway involvement or bronchospasm, albeit severe, may produce only subtle changes on imaging.

9.4.1.1 Upper Airway Involvement

9.4.1.1.1 Drug-Induced Angioedema

Typically, angioedema cases with significant upper airway obstruction (UAO) are admitted to the Emergency Department for stridor and/or asphyxia (Sondhi et al. 2004). The majority of angioedema cases occur in patients who are being exposed to ACEI. Annunciating symptoms include a sore throat, progressive lip or tongue edema, and a change in voice. These symptoms may progress at an unpredictable rate to laborious breathing and asphyxia. Education of patients receiving ACEI, discussing with them an appropriate action plan, regular monitoring for even mild adverse effects during follow-up visits, and early recognition are warranted. If left unrecognized, the drug is not discontinued promptly, and appropriate therapy is not undertaken, airway compromise may progress to a point where endotracheal intubation cannot be achieved because airway landmarks cannot be identified; tracheostomy may be required. There is no known association with ACEI-induced cough. ACEI may account for 30–60% of all cases of angioedema. Enalapril appears to be the most common ACEI associated with this complication, but virtually every marketed ACEI has been reported. The incidence has been reported to be from 0.1% to 0.2% of the treated population. In the United States, nine out of ten patients are dark skinned, and most are women. Although most series emanate from the USA, series of affected patients have been reported in Caucasians as well. Otherwise, no clinical profile reliably identifies which patients are at risk for this adverse effect. Having a recent history of upper airway trauma, perhaps a lupus diathesis, and being an atopic may be additional risk factors. The incidence of ACEI-induced angioedema seems higher in recipients of heart and kidney transplants, with odds 24 and 5 times those in controls, respectively. Having demonstrated an earlier, even milder, reaction with these agents is a strong predictor of subsequent episodes, dictating drug discontinuance. No triggering factor is identified in about a third of the cases. In about a third of the cases, angioedema develops within 12 h following the first administration of the drug, and the majority of cases develop within 4 weeks of initiation of therapy. Angioedema may occur intra- or perioperatively, with potentially serious consequences. Less commonly, ACEI-induced angioedema develops without much notice after months or years of treatment. In patients who develop the condition late into treatment, it is not unusual to elicit a history of prior episodes of spontaneously resolving tongue swelling known as 'episodic macroglossia' or hoarseness, which probably represents *formes frustes* of angioedema and deserves consideration in the perspective of drug discontinuance. For unknown reasons, angioedema may resolve despite the patient continuing treatment with the ACEI, erroneously prompting an alternative cause. A commonly made error is to ascribe angioedema to other causes. This may be why in half the patients, the ACEI is continued despite one (and up to seven in one case) previous documented episode(s) of UAO.

Clinical presentation: The pathology has a special predilection for the tongue. Initially, patients complain of pruritus and/or edema of the lips or mouth floor, and of dysphagia. In mild cases, the condition manifests itself with sore throat, slight facial or mouth edema, macroglossia, or drooling of saliva. The edema may resolve, wax and wane, or proceed to more pronounced or extensive adverse angioedematous reactions and breathing difficulties in hours, days, or months. Edema in distant organs and episodes of abdominal pain can occur, erroneously focusing attention on other sites. In severe cases, which represent about 10% of all cases of ACEI-induced angioedema, there is rapidly evolving edema of the upper air passages. The severity of tongue edema may make orotracheal intubation impossible as anatomic landmarks are distorted. No study has addressed the imaging characteristics of ACEI-induced angioedema. In the suspect patient, it is crucial that a careful ear, nose, and throat (ENT) endoscopy be performed to quantify the degree of obstruction and determine if the patient requires a monitored unit, particularly when laryngeal or combined laryngeal and pharyngeal swelling is present. On ENT endoscopy, involvement is of the mouth floor, tongue, supraglottic area, and, less often, laryngeal or tracheal walls. Angioedema can be classified as: type 1, limited to the face; type 2, to the floor of the mouth, base of tongue, and uvula; type 3, oropharayngeal, glottic and supraglottic edema. In one study, these occurred in 57%, 26%, and 17% of patients, respectively. Rarely, bronchospasm or anaphylaxis develops in association with angioedema. Angioedema can be a life-threatening adverse reaction, with 40 percent of patients requiring admission to the ICU, and the pathology has a 5 percent mortality rate. In an autopsy study of seven cases of ACEI-induced angioedema in African-American men and women aged 50–65 years, massive edema of the tongue was present in all. Only a fraction displayed laryngeal or pharyngeal swelling (Dean et al. 2001). Improvement of symptoms follows drug withdrawal and treatment with i.v. corticosteroids, antihistamines, and, in severe cases, adrenaline. However, symptoms sometimes progress despite optimized medical therapy, necessitating endotracheal intubation or tracheostomy. It is advisable not to discharge patients before 24 or 48 h, since in a few a rebound following successful medical therapy may occur unexpectedly. Rechallenge with the drug exposes patients to recurrence with increased severity after variable periods of time and is contraindicated. Once even minor angioedema is attributed to an ACEI, an alternative class of medication should be chosen. The angioedema that occurs in association with ACEI being mechanism based (enhanced sensitivity to bradykinin) rather than drug based, it is likely to occur upon rechallenge with different ACEIs, and treatment with any other ACEI is contraindicated. Contrary to expectations based on a bradykinin-based mechanism of involvement, treatments with an angiotensin II receptor antagonist may sometimes be complicated by severe angioedema (Chiu et al. 2001). Thus, therapy with an angiotensin II receptor antagonist in the patient with a history of ACEI-induced angioedema should be started with caution, only if no alternative drugs can be used.

Less common inducers of angioedema include amiodarone, betalactam antibiotics, corticosteroids, NSAIDs, cycloxygenase 2 inhibitors (COX-2 or coxibs), omeprazole, and radiographic contrast media (Pneumotox® 1997).

9.4.1.1.2 Anaphylaxis

Drug-induced anaphylaxis is an unexpected and explosive reaction, which results from IgE-, IgG-, or non-Ig-mediated release of preformed mediators on the mast cell surface in response to various stimuli, including drugs [analgesics, anesthetic agents, antibiotics (amoxicillin, chlorhexidine, ciprofloxacin, penicillin, sulfamides, sulfamethoxazole-trimethoprim, vancomycin), aprotinin, aspirin, blood products, calcium and phosphate replacement therapy, colloid plasma expanders, cortisone, coxibs, fluorescein, heparin, immunoglobulins, infliximab, latex, lepirudin, neuromuscular blocking drugs, NSAIDs, opiates, patent blue, protamine, psyllium, and radiographic contrast media] and foreign proteins in addition to the above (Pumphrey 2000; Gruchalla and Pirmohamed 2006; Webb and Lieberman 2006; Levy and Adkinson 2008). A particularly difficult situation is intraoperative anaphylaxis (Levy and Adkinson 2008). In a study of 20 yearly deaths from anaphylaxis, half were caused by drugs (Pumphrey 2000). In another series of 25 fatal anaphylaxis cases, 13 were due to medications (drugs: 7; radiocontrast material: 6) (Greenberger et al. 2007). Most accidents occur following exposure to analgesics, NSAIDs, radiographic contrast agents, and antibiotics, with an increased risk of occurrence in females and in atopics, and an increased vital risk in the elderly with comorbidities. Clinical manifestations include the rapid onset of any of the following: malaise, dizziness, urticaria, itching of the nose or palate, abdominal cramping, vomiting, diarrhea, ocular symptoms, bronchospasm, angioedema, pulmonary vasoconstriction, and hypotension.

The full-blown reaction is characterized by laryngeal and/or tracheal edema compromising airway patency, pulmonary edema, bronchospasm, frothy sputum, hemoptysis, internal organ edema, circulatory collapse, shock, and seizures, followed by cardiac arrest (Levy and Adkinson 2008). Severity may not increase in patients who present with repeated episodes of anaphylaxis. Short of being managed properly and aggressively, anaphylaxis can lead to death within minutes of exposure to the causal agent. Autopsy studies of fatal anaphylaxis cases indicate edema of the epiglottis, larynx, and trachea, pulmonary hyperinflation, and/or edema and hemorrhage (Pumphrey and Roberts 2000; Low and Stables 2006). In a study in the UK, time to respiratory or cardiac arrest averaged 5 min, and even though about a third of the patients were resuscitated, most suffered hypoxic brain damage and died within 30 days of the accident, mostly from hypoxic brain damage (Pumphrey 2000). In another study, the anaphylactic reaction began within 30 min of exposure in the vast majority of the cases, and death occurred within 60 min in half the cases. Adrenaline/epinephrine was self-administered in only one out of five cases (Greenberger et al. 2007). Clinically, anaphylaxis can be mistaken for Münchausen syndrome, panic attack, hysteria, or vocal cord dysfunction. This may unnecessarily delay appropriate treatment (Pumphrey 2000). Management of anaphylaxis requires preparedness, immediate recognition, alertness, volume therapy through a central line, and drugs. Parenteral adrenaline is to be repeated every 15 min until blood pressure is restored and stabilizes. High-dose parenteral corticosteroids and correction of cardiac arrhythmias are indicated. Ensuring early access to the airway is crucial, as when significant laryngeal edema has developed, attempts at orotracheal intubation may fail, as it does in angioedema. Adrenaline/epinephrine often is not administered in time or properly, being injected subcutaneously, or is outdated. Adrenaline/epinephrine can induce adverse effects on its own, including pulmonary edema, vomiting with consequent aspiration of gastric content, and myocardial infarction (Pumphrey 2000; Levy and Adkinson 2008).

9.4.1.1.3
Hematoma

Life-threatening hematoma compromising airway patency can involve the tongue, sublingual area, mouth floor, tonsils, valleculae, arytenoids, laryngeal wall, vocal cords, thyroid, or the retropharyngeal and mediastinal space (Di Pasquale et al. 1990; al-Fallouji et al. 1993; Kaynar et al. 1999; Shojania 2000; Ahmed et al. 2005). Anticoagulant-induced hematomas have the reputation for producing misleading symptoms. Although the onset of hematomas may be elicited by sneezing, violent coughing, or insertion of a central venous line, most seem to occur spontaneously. At an early stage, patients complain of such vague symptoms as sore throat and/or changes in voice, which can be mistaken as upper respiratory tract infection. Early symptoms are followed in a few days by expansion of the hematoma into the sublingual, oral, cervical, retropharyngeal, or mediastinal space, causing further airway compromise. Examination of the oral cavity and/or ENT endoscopy may reveal a reddish submucosal swelling involving the mouth floor and the ventral aspect of the tongue, or the whole muscle. Examination of the pharyngeal area or tracheal endoscopy may show compression and/or submucosal hematoma of the laryngeal or tracheal walls. Subcutaneous bruising may be present on the neck, progressively spreading down to the chest. Digital examination may reveal anterior displacement of the posterior pharyngeal wall in patients with retropharyngeal hematoma. On the lateral chest radiograph, anterior displacement of the posterior aspect of the pharynx or tracheal wall is sometimes visualized. CT studies may show the hematoma, with consequent compression of the airway lumen. Coagulation studies may indicate values well above the accepted therapeutic range, with INR up to 60 or more, but in some cases, coagulation studies are in the therapeutic range. Management includes control of the airway, reversal of the coagulopathy when it is present, needle aspiration, or surgical debridement of the hematoma if required.

9.4.1.2
Lower Airway Involvement

9.4.1.2.1
Acute Bronchospasm

Aetylsalicylate (aspirin), NSAIDs, beta-blockers, and other cardiovascular drugs account for most cases of drug-induced bronchospasm, a potentially life-threatening adverse effect (Vaszar and Stevenson 2001; Babu and Salvi 2000).

- Aspirin and NSAIDs
  Patients who are intolerant to these drugs may adversely react to the first or subsequent admin-

istration of these compounds in the form of moderate or catastrophic bronchospasm with consequent respiratory failure. The gravity of this condition resides in its unpredictability, explosive nature, its possible association with anaphylaxis, and the acute respiratory failure with consequent irreversible hypoxic brain damage and death. Although most accidents occur after oral intake or parenteral injection, cases are described following dermal applications or intra-articular injections. Aspirin-induced asthma (in fact, aspirin/NSAIDs exacerbated bronchospasm would better label this pathology) usually develops in the 3rd or 4th decade of life and is more common in women at a ratio of about two to one. Rhinitis usually precedes the clinical onset of the asthma, with aspirin/NSAID sensitivity becoming apparent only later. The asthma often is difficult to control, with about 50% of those afflicted requiring regular treatment with oral corticosteroids. In a few patients, drug-induced bronchospasms occur *de novo* with no prodromal symptoms, producing sudden catastrophic bronchospasm as the response to the first intake of a tablet of aspirin or other NSAIDs with COX-1 inhibitory properties. Occasionally, the response is anaphylactic. Severe bronchoconstriction may lead to 'locked lung,' hypoxia, and death within minutes of exposure to the drug. Estimates based on history and challenge tests suggest sensitivity to aspirin and NSAIds in 1–3% or 5–10% of asthmatics, respectively. Prevalence is higher among subjects who suffer from chronic rhino-sinusitis or nasal polyps. Prevalence of aspirin/NSAID sensitivity is also greater in patients with a history of severe asthma attacks. It is estimated that 8% of patients admitted to the ICU for an acute asthma attack requiring mechanical ventilation have been exposed to asthma-triggering drugs immediately prior to admission (Picado et al. 1989). The weak COX-1 inhibitors acetaminophen and salsalate would require higher concentrations to trigger bronchospasm. The preferential COX-2 inhibitors nimesulide and meloxicam cross-react poorly with aspirin or classic NSAIDs. In controlled challenge tests, the selective COX-2 inhibitors [celecoxib, rofecoxib (now recalled), etoricoxib] cross-react with aspirin in 1.5 to 2% of NSAID-sensitive individuals and are generally considered safe. Treatment of acute bronchospasm induced by the above drugs requires antihistamines, H2 blockers, corticosteroids, and ß2-receptor agonists, and sometimes adrenaline and mechanical ventilation are required. Following the bronchospastic episode, the history often is straightforward enough for further investigation to be unnecessary, since a challenge test may be risky. When the association is less clear, or when treatment with aspirin or an NSAID is desirable, a controlled challenge test is discussed and should be conducted close to an ICU. The patient should have a venous access placed, and therapy drugs for bronchospasm, anaphylaxis, and resuscitation equipment should be available. Desensitization to aspirin/NSAIDs can be practiced in patients who are intolerant and need these drugs for the treatment of their underlying cardiac condition, and several protocols are available. Since tolerance to aspirin and cross-tolerance to other NSAIDs depend on the continued presence of the drug, uninterrupted treatment is needed to maintain the desensitized state as, otherwise, sensitivity may return in a few days (Pleskow et al. 1982). Since aspirin-exacerbated airways disease seldom resolves spontaneously (Rosado et al. 2003), patients with a clear history of intolerance to aspirin/NSAIDs should be formally advised to avoid all aspirin-containing products and other COX-1 inhibitors. They should also be given a comprehensive list of prohibited drugs to wear at all times. Paracetamol (acetaminophen) and COX-2 inhibitors pose a substantially lower risk, although crossed reactions have been described in a few patients. Pretreatment with a leukotriene receptor antagonist antagonizes aspirin-induced bronchospasm, and some advocate the use of leukotriene receptor antagonists to lower the bronchoconstriction elicited by aspirin provocation challenge.

- ß-blockers (Spitz 2003)
  The early nonselective beta-blockers, particularly propranolol, produce greater bronchospasm than the drugs available now. In addition, propranolol blunts the bronchodilatory response to ß2-agonists to a greater degree than do mordern cardioselective drugs. Oral cardioselective ß1-blockers are considered safe (Salpeter 2003), if not beneficial (Salpeter et al. 2003; Dransfield et al. 2008) in patients with mild to moderate asthma or COPD (safety extends to ophtalmic instillations), provided these patients can take bronchodilator drugs, and as long as appropriate follow-up is possible. However, this view is disputed as far as asthmatics are concerned, because the likelihood and magnitude of bronchospasm during treatments with ß-blockers are difficult to predict

in these patients and may vary with time. Even though patients may not exhibit a significant drop in FEV1 when challenged in the clinic, they may suffer a more severe episode later during chronic treatment with the beta-blockers due to the unstable nature of the asthma after an encounter with a potent asthma trigger or if they fail to take their asthma medications. Treatments with ß-blockers also increase the risk of anaphylactoid reactions to radiographic contrast material or anesthetic agents, and attenuate or blunt the response to ß2-receptor agonists should these drugs be needed if an asthma attack or anaphylaxis develops. Due to these uncertainties, many will err on the safe side and consider that ß-blockers are not indicated in most asthmatics. A risk-benefit evaluation is necessary on a case-by-case basis. Rare cases of fatal bronchospasm still occur, mainly following accidental exposure of asthmatics to propranolol.

- Other drugs (Pneumotox® 1997)
  Orally or parenterally administered ACEI, antibiotics, narcotics, and radiographic contrast material sometimes occasion severe bronchospasm. Less often, inhaled corticosteroids or bronchodilators cause an asthma attack (Leuppi et al. 2001; Babu and Marshall 2004).

9.4.1.3 Infiltrative Lung Disease

Diffuse pulmonary opacities in the context of acute respiratory failure is relatively common an illness. Many non-cardiac and a few cardiac drugs can produce the syndrome. Patients may fall within several distinct clinical-pathological categories (Pneumotox® 1997).

9.4.1.3.1 Severe Interstitial Pneumonitis

Drug-induced severe pneumonitis with a lymphocytic BAL pattern and a dense infiltrate of mononuclear cells on histology is an uncommon occurrence in cardiac patients, as opposed to rheumatology, where it is frequent with the use of methotrexate (Pneumotox® 1997).

Interstitial pneumonitis has occasionally been reported during treatments with beta-blocking agents (Pneumotox® 1997).

The patterns may be more common in heart transplant patients who are being treated with sirolimus or congeners (Champion et al. 2006). The incidence rate of sirolimus-induced pneumonitis is as high as 10%, and time to onset ranges from 1 to 51 months into treatment, with half the cases occurring within the first 6 months of treatment. Risk factors for the condition include a daily dose >5 mg, trough levels >15 ng/ml, a recent increase in dosage, starting treatment with a loading dose of sirolimus, renal failure, and in kidney transplant recipients allograft dysfunction, advanced age, and male gender. Signs and symptoms include cough in 95% of the patients, fever in two thirds, dyspnea in a third 33%, and hemoptysis in 8%. On imaging, ground-glass opacities, a fine reticulation, disseminated mottling, a nodular appearance, or consolidation may be visualized. BAL studies indicate lymphocytosis in an overwhelming majority of patients [80%; range of lymphocyte percentages 0–075%, while an eosinophilic pattern is seen in 12% (range of eosinophil percentages 0–14%)]. Interestingly, features consistent with diffuse alveolar hemorrhage are seen in approximately 10% of the patients. On pathology, cellular nonspecific interstitial pneumonia, a lymphocytic interstitial or organizing pneumonia are the most frequent pattern, followed by intraalveolar granulomas, alveolar hemorrhage, a desquamative interstitial pneumonia, or, rarely, a pulmonary alveolar proteinosis pattern or vasculitis. Management includes drug therapy withdrawal, diminution of drug dosage, switching to everolimus and/or corticosteroid therapy. Everolimus and temsirolimus can also occasion interstitial lung disease, although the number of cases is still less.

9.4.1.3.2 Acute Eosinophilic Pneumonia

The clinical presentation of acute eosinophilic pneumonia is similar to the above pattern, except that eosinophils are present either in the peripheral blood or in the BAL and/or lung tissue (Pneumotox® 1997). No cardiac drug produces the syndrome of acute eosinophilic pneumonia, but several drugs that may be used incidentally in cardiac patients (mostly antibiotics, particularly minocycline) can produce this syndrome. Acute eosinophilic pneumonia can also occur in smokers, particularly those who recently started the habit, or those who resume after cessation. Clinical presentation is that of respiratory failure with high fevers, diffuse pulmonary opacities, and BAL eosinophilia, while eosinophilia in blood is not a constant finding. On imaging, there is dense bilateral shadowing that sometimes assumes a peripheral subpleural distribution, and moderate bilateral pleural effusion is common. The BAL may exhibit a percentage of eosinophils as high as 80%. The main differential of acute eosinophilic pneumonia is parasitic infestation, which needs to be ruled out before corticosteroid therapy is contemplated. An open lung biopsy is rarely needed for diagnosing this condition and would show the characteristic features of dense interstitial inflammation. Tissue eosinophilia with sometimes overlapping features of organizing pneumonia or vasculitis. A few drugs, mostly leukotriene receptor antagonists, can produce a perfect mimic of naturally occurring Churg-Strauss syndrome, with pulmonary infiltrates and internal organ involvement (including cardiac involvement in about a third of patients) (Pneumotox® 1997; Hauser et al. 2008). Drug discontinuance and corticosteroid therapy are indicated.

Severe cases of acute eosinophilic pneumonia in conjunction with cutaneous and deep organ involvement raise the question of "Drug Rash and Eosinophilia with Systemic Symptoms" or DRESS, a generalized, life-threatening drug-induced eosinophilic condition mainly caused by minocycline and anticonvulsants (Pneumotox® 1997).

9.4.1.3.3
Acute Amiodarone Pulmonary Toxicity

There are two distinct patterns of amiodarone pulmonary toxicity with an acute onset (Pneumotox® 1997; Camus et al. 2004):

- Early acute APT can occur after a few days or weeks of the intravenous loading dose of amiodarone particularly, but not exclusively so, if there is a history of recent thoracic surgery (Skroubis et al. 2005). Investigators showed that the incidence of ARDS thought to represent acute APT (fatal in two out of three patients and unrelated to amiodarone or desethylamiodarone blood levels) increased six-fold in patients who were receiving amiodarone compared to unexposed controls (van Mieghem et al. 1994). Thus, the use of amiodarone for arrhythmia prophylaxis in the postoperative period should be considered with caution. Acute APT manifests with dyspnea, diffuse alveolar shadowing, and ground-glass, volume loss, hypoxemia, with or without respiratory failure or an ARDS picture. Pulmonary edema, a coincidental infection, postoperative atelectasis, and thromboembolic disease must be ruled out carefully by means of cardiac ultrasound, diuresis, and, if needed, measurement of pulmonary capillary wedge pressure. Interestingly, the BAL in acute APT may exhibit lipid-laden macrophages, a hallmark of subacute APT, even though patients have been exposed to the drug for only a few days. Once the diagnosis is secured, corticosteroid therapy is indicated. A few patients will not respond to this form of therapy, and for those who do, this is a diagnostic test. The clinical and imaging features of acute APT will reverse quickly in a few days, in some with discernible improvement as early as within a few hours. In selected cases, an open lung biopsy is indicated, and histological findings include resolving diffuse alveolar damage, fibrinous organizing pneumonia, interstitial edema, and interstitial fibrosis, superimposed on the background of dyslipidotic changes typical of APT. Mortality in early series of acute APT was 40–50 percent, despite amiodarone therapy withdrawal and high-dose corticosteroid therapy. Careful daily monitoring of imaging in patients on amiodarone in the postoperative period and early recognition are essential.
- Classic APT during chronic treatments with amiodarone can present rather acutely, after months or years into treatment. Symptoms include dyspnea, fever, diffuse fluffy opacities, and hypoxemia. Amiodarone pneumonitis with an acute presentation is characterized by lymphocytosis in the BAL and a consistent response to corticosteroid therapy.

9.4.1.3.4
Acute Organizing Pneumonia

Acute organizing pneumonia is a rare pattern of involvement with an ominous prognosis (Pneumotox® 1997). The condition is characterized by dyspnea, acute respiratory failure, volume loss, dense pulmonary infiltrates, and air bronchograms on imaging and alveolar-ductal fibrosis on histopathogy. Circumstantial evidence relates exposure to amiodarone and HMG-CoA-reductase inhibitors or statins to acute organizing pneumonia. Since a confirmatory lung biopsy is needed, acute organizing pneumonia is rarely diagnosed. Causality assessment is difficult, since acute organizing pneumonia can occur sporadically with or without an identifiable cause. Response to drug therapy withdrawal and corticosteroid therapy is unpredictable.

Acute fibrinous organizing pneumonia (AFOP) is a recently recognized entity that shares several features with classic OP, including exposure to drugs, including amiodarone (Beasley et al. 2002). On histology in AFOP, there is intra-alveolar fibrin and OP associated with varying amounts of type II cell hyperplasia, interstitial edema, and acute or chronic interstitial inflammation.

9.4.1.3.5
Acute Pulmonary Edema

Pulmonary edema with or without the features of acute lung injury or ARDS can complicate treatments with adrenaline/epinephrine, ASA or aspirin, buprenorphine, dextran, hydrochlorothiazide, iodinated contrast agents, nafazoline, nicardipine, phenyephrine, propofol, propranolol, protamine, vasopressin, and verapamil, or it may follow transfusion of blood or blood products (Pneumotox® 1997). Pulmonary edema has also been reported in patients with pulmonary hypertension who were receiving nifedipine, prostacyclin, or nitric oxide (NO). Traditionally, drug-induced pulmonary edema closely follows drug administration (typically given by the i.v. route) except with aspirin, which produces a delayed form of pulmonary edema that is somehow related to high aspirin levels in the blood. Pulmonary edema also may follow overenthusiastic administration of fluids (overload edema). Drug-induced pulmonary edema manifests with sudden dyspnea, cough, and, sometimes, an abundant pink, frothy, blood-tinged, or bloody sputum. On imaging, early cases exhibit a combination of linear interstitial infiltrates, Kerley A, B, and/or C lines, diffuse blurring or haze with, at times, thickened fissures. In more advanced cases, there is widespread shadowing or whiteout, which sometimes assumes a batwing distribution, and, as the disease advances, alveolar flooding and air bronchograms may occur. When a foamy exudate is present at the mouth or in ventilator tubing, the fluid may exhibit a high fluid:plasma protein ratio. Drug-induced pulmonary edema is generally of the noncardiogenic type and results from a drug-induced loss of endothelial integrity, with a consequent increase in pulmonary capillary permeability. The noncardiac nature is confirmed by the normal size of the heart and pedicle on imaging, ultrasound evaluation, and pulmonary capillary wedge pressure. Histopathological appearances at autopsy or, rarely, via the lung biopsy include interstitial edema or resolving edema or organizing pneumonia in early cases, and bland edema with proteinaceous fluid filling the alveolar spaces and inconspicuous inflammation in more advanced cases.

A peculiar form of pulmonary edema follows transfusion of whole blood or blood products, including packed red blood cells, platelets, fresh frozen plasma, plasma-derived coagulation factors, and immunogobulins (Popovsky 2008). Transfusion-related acute lung injury or TRALI develops within a few hours of transfusion, in the form of chills, fever, low blood pressure, dyspnea, bilateral alveolar opacities, hypoxemia, leucopenia, and mild eosinophilia. Based on the severity of pulmonary involvement, which may culminate in an ARDS picture, oxygen therapy and mechanical ventilation are required. Transfusion-related pulmonary edema can be linked to circulatory overload, in which case it is coined 'TACO' for transfusion-associated circulatory overload. The more distinctive transfusion-related lung injury (TRALI) can be subdivided into immune and nonimmune TRALI (Silliman et al. 2005). In immune TRALI, granulocyte-binding alloantibodies (complement-activating HLA class I or II granulocyte-specific, or lymphocytotoxic antibodies) are transferred from one donor in the pool of donors to the recipient, whose leukocytes express the cognate antigens. This results in antibody:antigen interaction, complement-mediated activation of neutrophils, loss of integrity of the endothelial barrier, and capillary leak. Nonimmune TRALI results from the transfer of biologically active lipids or CD40 ligand present in stored blood. These substances also have neutrophil-priming activity and also produce endothelial cell damage and capillary leakage. Immune TRALI occurs mainly after the transfusion of fresh-frozen plasma and platelet concentrates, is less common (incidence about 1 per 5,000 transfusions), and is more severe (mechanical ventilation required in about 70% of cases; fatality rate 6–10%) than nonimmune TRALI. In contrast, nonimmune TRALI occurs mainly after the transfusion of stored platelet and erythrocyte concentrates. Management of post-transfusional pulmonary edema rests on oxygen therapy, ventilatory support, and supportive care. In TACO, fluid restriction and diuresis are indicated. In TRALI, the exaggerated capillary permeability may have caused fluid loss. Diuretics are not indicated without hemodynamic evaluation, as they may cause further hemodynamic compromise. Diagnosing immune TRALI has far-reaching consequences. Since the condition results from the transfer of antibodies, the specific donor should be identified, and blood products from that donor should be quarantined until the diagnosis of TACO vs. nonimmune or immune TRALI is clarified. When identified, the donor (generally a woman with a history of two or more pregnancies) is permanently deferred from blood donation. In surgical patients, a policy that banned blood products from female donors was associated with a significant decrease in the frequency of postoperative acute lung injury from 36% before to 21% after the implementation (Wright et al. 2008).

- The antidiabetic rosiglitazone and other members of this family of drugs can cause weight gain, cardiomegaly, pulmonary congestion, pulmonary edema, and pleural effusion. Experimentally, these drugs augment pulmonary endothelial permeability. The above manifestations resolve upon drug withdrawal (Pneumotox® 1997). The beneficial effect of diuretics is debated.
- A few cases of pulmonary edema due to drug-induced acute heart failure have been described following administration of cyclophosphamide, doxorubicin, fluorouracil, interleukin-2, propranolol, and thyroid hormone abuse (Hayek et al. 2005).

9.4.1.3.6 Alveolar Hemorrhage

Diffuse alveolar hemorrhage (DAH) is an elective complication of treatments with oral anticoagulants (coumadin, warfarin), fibrinolytic agents including rTPA and intracoronary urokinase, heparin, and the novel inhibitors of glycoprotein IIB/IIIA surface receptors on platelets (abciximab, a human-mouse chimeric biologic, and the ligand-mimetic drugs clopidogrel, petifibatide, tirofiban, clopidrogrel, and ticlopidine) (Pneumotox® 1997). Accidental or deliberate poisoning with superwarfarins such as brodifacoum (a pest-eliminating oral anticoagulant with duration of action of weeks) also causes DAH. The condition consists of synchronous bleeding from the pulmonary microcirculation into the alveoli. Clinical presentation includes dyspnea, cough, moderate-to-severe blood loss, and bilateral shadowing, which may assume a batwing pattern on imaging. Hemoptysis is not a constant finding, even though significant alveolar bleeding has occurred. An increase in the diffusing capacity suggesting free hemoglobin in airspaces may be present in patients with active alveolar bleeding; however, this is not a consistent or reliable finding. Alveolar hemorrhage is diagnosed by BAL, which shows increased staining in serial aliquots. Microscopically, the BAL shows red cells with hemosiderin-laden macrophages characterizing those cases with sub-acute bleeding prior to full-blown DAH. A lung biopsy is not indicated to diagnose alveolar hemorrhage. Diffuse alveolar hemorrhage requires expeditious management, as the disease can be rapidly progressive, producing clotting in the airspaces and the "stone lung," or in the major airways, causing a difficult to remove "foreign body." Management includes holding the anticoagulation, supportive care including mechanical ventilation, and, depending on the causal agent, infusion of vitamin K, platelets, packed red blood cells, fresh frozen plasma, cryoprecipitate, activated factor VII, and whole lung lavage with ice-cold saline.

The incidence rate with abciximab is 0.3%, with a risk ratio of 5.5 to 12 vs. unexposed controls. Diffuse alveolar hemorrhage related to glycoprotein IIB/IIIA receptor inhibitors generally, but not always, occurs independently from the thrombocytopenia that may complicate treatments with this class of agents. Incidence of alveolar hemorrhage is greater with abciximab than it is with tirofiban or eptifibatide. Risk factors include concomitant treatment with heparin, an activated clotting time >250 s, and a background of left ventricular failure, smoking, or COPD. The mortality rate is 0 to 28%.

Alveolar hemorrhage occurs in approximately 10% of patients who develop sirolimus-induced pneumonitis. Alveolar hemorrhage as a form of amiodarone pulmonary toxicity is seldom reported.

9.4.1.3.7 Pulmonary Circulation

Aprotinin, clozapine, factor VIIa, and oral contraceptives have been associated with an increased risk of thrombo-embolic disease (Pneumotox® 1997). Treatments with mitomycin, protamine, calcium replacement therapy, and protamine have been associated with acute, sometimes fatal episodes of pulmonary hypertension, as has the abrupt termination of NO inhalation, which may cause rebound of pulmonary hypertension.

9.4.1.3.8 Methemoglobinemia

Methemoglobin or ferrihemoglobin is a ferric (Fe+++) instead of ferrous (Fe++) form of hemoglobin (Pneumotox® 1997; Wright et al. 1999; Moore et al. 2004; Stalnikowicz et al. 2004). Methemoglobin is a poor oxygen carrier, hence the cyanosis in afflicted patients. The purple or dark brown appearance of methemoglobin and of the blood drawn is distinctive, and should raise the suspicion. Several oxidizing agents can produce methemoglobinemia, including amyl nitrite, NO, nitroglycerin, and several local anesthetics. Patients with methemoglobinemia develop cyanosis shortly after drug administration. The condition can be fatal if >40–50% methemoglobin is present. Paradoxically but logically, partial pressure of oxygen in blood (PaO_2) remains near normal. Transcutaneous oxygen saturation may remain in the normal range, and only actual measurement of methemoglobin will diagnose the condition. Mild cases respond to drug withdrawal and oxygen. More advanced cases may require infusion of methylene blue, mechanical ventilation, hyperbaric oxygen, or blood replacement. Patients should be tested for glucose-6-phosphate dehydrogenase deficiency, a predisposing factor for methemoglobinemia in which methylene blue is contraindicated.

9.4.1.3.9 Acute Chest Pain

Of interest to the cardiologist, treatments with 5-fluorouracile, sumatriptan, or statins can occasion acute isolated chest pain with or without ST-segment elevation or myocardial infarction (Pneumotox® 1997).

9.4.2 Subacute Drug-Induced Respiratory Involvement

All of the above patterns of drug-induced involvement of the airways or lung can occur in a diminutive form. Early recognition is warranted to avoid progression toward more severe involvement.

9.4.2.1 Cellular Interstitial Pneumonia

Clinical presentation also is with cough, dyspnea, fever, disseminated or diffuse pulmonary infiltrates, and hypoxemia (Pneumotox® 1997). Cardiac drugs causing this condition include ß-blockers, flecainide, procainamide, statins as a group, sirolimus, everolimus, and temsirolimus. It generally takes weeks or months for drug-induced pneumonitis to be revealed. Imaging studies indicate bilateral, roughly symmetrical linear or, less often, micronodular interstitial opacities or alveolar infiltrates. On CT, radiographic attenuation can be discrete haze or ground-glass or dense patchy areas of consolidation. The opacities may localize in the caudal, mid- or upper zones of the lung, or they can be diffuse. Depending on the patient, HRCT studies may also indicate intra- or interlobular septal thickening, a crazy-paving appearance, or zonal increases in attenuation with a ground-glass or mosaic pattern. Restricted lung volumes, low carbon monoxide diffusion, and hypoxemia generally parallel changes on imaging. The BAL is indicated to exclude an infection and supports the drug etiology when it shows lymphocyte predominance and an increase in either CD4+ or CD8+ lymphocyte subsets, although an increase in neutrophils, or an increase in lymphocytes, neutrophils, and/or eosinophils can sometimes be found. Cases of drug-induced pneumonia with a benign course do not require tissue confirmation of the diagnosis and respond well to drug withdrawal and, when needed, adjunctive corticosteroid therapy. Outcomes are good, provided the causal drug is discontinued early. Corticosteroid therapy is discussed if extensive opacities or hypoxemia is present, and for patients for whom drug discontinuance does not translate into betterment in a few days. It is reasonable to contraindicate rechallenge with the drug, which would lead to relapse of unpredictable severity.

Recently, attention has been directed to the adverse pulmonary effects of sirolimus, mainly in recipients of heart and kidney transplant. Details on sirolimus-, everolimus-, and temsirolimus-induced pneumonitis are given above in Sect. 4.1.3.1.

9.4.2.2 Pulmonary Infiltrates and Eosinophilia

Benign pulmonary infiltrates and eosinophilia (PIE) or eosinophilic pneumonia can be caused by ACEI, aspirin, NSAIDs, iodinated radiographic contrast material, and minocycline in addition to several dozen other drugs (Pneumotox® 1997). Evidence is now unfolding that leukotriene receptor antagonists produce a Churg-Strauss-like vasculitis with pulmonary infiltrates, eosinophilia, and deep organ involvement. Patients who develop drug-induced PIE generally do so after weeks to months into treatment. Clinical presentation is with malaise, dyspnea, dry cough, low-grade fever, chest discomfort, pulmonary infiltrates, and sometimes a skin rash is present. Involvement of organs other than the lung (e.g., heart or nervous system) can be present, particularly in patients with marked blood eosinophilia or in those with Churg-Strauss vasculitis or the DRES syndrome. Opacities may localize in the apices, mid-lung zones, bases, or they can be diffuse or wander from one area of the lung to another, or appear as discreet shadowing with a ground-glass appearance or as bibasilar Kerley 'B' lines. The classic pattern of biapical subpleural opacities known as the photographic negative of pulmonary edema is a distinctive (Souza et al. 2006), but inconstant feature of PIE. On HRCT, the opacities in PIE have a predilection for the external subpleural zones of the lung and range from a discreet haze to patchy subpleural crescentic shadowing, or multifocal areas of consolidation with air bronchograms. The imaging features of PIE may be at times difficult to separate from those of organizing pneumonia, cellular interstitial pneumonia, or interstitial pulmonary edema (Cleverley et al. 2002). PIE is diagnosed by peripheral and BAL eosinophilia, and/or eosinophilia in lung tissue. Relating PIE to drug exposure is straightforward in patients exposed to one eligible drug and/or if drug therapy withdrawal is demonstrably followed by improvement of symptoms, imaging, and eosinophilia. Corticosteroids accelerate the resolution of PIE, albeit at the expense of drug causality assessment, since PIE of other causes may also respond to corticosteroid therapy. Rechallenge with the drug leads to malaise, fever, and blood eosinophilia, and relapse of pulmonary infiltrates follows within hours or a few days. Although rechallenge in PIE has the reputation for being benign, the diagnostic merit of the test is unclear, particularly if an alternate drug is available to treat the underlying condition.

9.4.2.3 Amiodarone Pneumonitis – Amiodarone Pulmonary Toxicity (APT)

Amiodarone pulmonary toxicity was first reported in 1980 and is the most common form of drug-induced pulmonary toxicity (Pneumotox® 1997; Camus et al. 2004). Amiodarone toxicity is thought to result from sequestration of the parent compound, and its main metabolite desthylamiodarone in several tissues, with the lung and liver ranking ahead of other organs. The two iodines on each molecule of both amiodarone and desethylamiodarone account for the high attenuation numbers that may be found in the liver and in areas of amiodarone pneumonitis on CT, a suggestive feature of amiodarone exposure and toxicity, respectively. The amiodarone and metabolite impair the physiologic processing of endogenous phospholipids. Consequently, phospholipids accumulate in the lung, causing a form of lipid storage disease superimposed on features of interstitial pneumonitis. Upon drug withdrawal, amiodarone and metabolite efflux slowly from pulmonary and other tissues. The above features account for the characteristics of APT, with its gradual and insidious onset, target organs corresponding to tissues where amiodarone accumulates most, high attenuation numbers on CT, evidence for dyslipidosis in BAL cells and in lung tissue, slow improvement following drug discontinuance, relapse when steroids are tapered (even though the drug has been withdrawn months earlier), and delayed onset after termination of treatment with the drug. The beneficial effect of corticosteroid therapy in many patients indicates that APT is also likely an inflammatory condition.

The incidence rate of APT increases with the degree of exposure from 0.1% in patients on low dose (100–200 mg per day) to almost 50% in patients exposed to high dosages (>1,200 mg/day). The average is three to five percent (Stewart et al. 2008). Abnormal pulmonary physiology or abnormal chest radiograph do not constitute a contraindication to treatments with the drug. Onset of APT can be after a few weeks and up to several years into treatment, but most cases are diagnosed in the 6–12-month time frame and within the 101–150-g dose range. APT is generally diagnosed after an average of 2 months of clinical symptoms on average. Clinically, APT manifests insidiously, with gradual weight loss, malaise, dyspnea, dry cough, and slight fever, and sometimes pleuritic chest pain is present. Crackles or moist rales are common findings at auscultation, and a friction rub may be present. Adverse effects of amiodarone in the liver or thyroid are occasionally present in association with the pulmonary toxicity, and appropriate tests are required to detect these complications. Leukocytosis, an increased blood LDH level, and a raised erythrocyte sedimentation rate are common, and the two latter findings can predate the clinical onset of APT. The role of serum brain natriuretic peptide levels in distinguishing APT from pulmonary edema is imprecise, inasmuch as (1) patients may present with an association of both conditions and (2) drugs including amiodarone may interfere with BNP levels (Troughton et al. 2007). A concomitant hyperthyroid state may increase the perception of dyspnea in APT and may also deteriorate left ventricular function, complicating the diagnosis of APT. APT may develop post-lung transplantation, raising complex diagnostic issues. Imaging studies indicate interstitial, alveolar, or mixed opacities. Typical amiodarone pulmonary toxicity manifests with recognizable changes on imaging, including dense uni- or bilateral, often asymmetrical interstitial, patchy areas of condensation or fluffy alveolar infiltrates, which may involve any area of one or both lungs, including the apices, and often abut the pleura, which can be thickened *en face* the involved area. Volume loss is generally present in the areas of greatest involvement. Opacities in APT may assume a recognizable lobar or segmental distribution, with partial atelectasis of one segment or lobe, simulating an infection, organizing pneumonia, primary lung cancer, bronchoalveolar carcinoma, or pulmonary lymphoma. There is an impression that the right lung (mainly the right upper lobe) is more frequently involved than the left lung. While some patients present with unilateral involvement on the chest radiograph, involvement of the opposite lung often is detectable on HRCT. Less common patterns of APT include subtle or unilateral involvement, a coin lesion, a lone mass simulating primary lung cancer (which has been coined "amiodaronoma" by analogy with paraffinoma), multiple masses with a central area of decreased attenuation on CT, and multiple shaggy nodules with the halo sign corresponding to tissue necrosis. The halo corresponds to attenuated amiodarone pneumonitis peripherally. On HRCT, the involvement in APT often is scattered, patchy, and asymmetrical, with areas of haze, ground glass, alveolar shadowing, inter- or intralobular linear opacities with crazy paving, or dense consolidation or mass(es), sometimes with high attenuation numbers. These changes can coexist in different areas of the lung, or one of the above can be the dominant feature throughout the lung fields. In a study of 20 symptomatic patients with moderate APT (Vernhet et al. 2001), ground-glass opacities were present in all 20 patients, areas of consolidation were found in 4, and intralobular reticulations in 5. A subpleural distribution of the opacities was more common than a central distribution (in 18 vs. 2 patients). High density in the area of APT was present in 8 of the 20 patients. In more advanced disease, increased attenuation seems a more consistent finding (Mason 2001). The disease may overlap, resemble, or simulate pulmonary edema, cellular or fibrotic nonspecific interstitial pneumonia, organizing pneumonia, eosinophilic pneumonia, pulmonary alveolar proteinosis, or lipid storage disease. A paucicellular pleural exudate occurs in up to a third of patients with amiodarone lung involvement, but rarely occurs in isolation. The expression of APT on imaging may be attenuated and the clinical presentation more severe in amiodarone toxic patients with a background of emphysema.

Interpretation of pulmonary function tests in APT is against a background of airway obstruction from prior smoking or restrictive dysfunction from heart failure, two common conditions in patients on amiodarone. Pre-therapy evaluation will considerably ease the interpretation of these tests. Restrictive lung dysfunction, decreased diffusing capacity for carbon monoxide (CO), and hypoxemia are present in virtually any patient with clinically significant APT, and these changes are more in patients with extensive disease. The earliest functional abnormality in APT is a precipitous and consistent decrease in the diffusing capacity for carbon monoxide that takes place over a few weeks. Left ventricular failure, pulmonary edema, and simple exposure to amiodarone do alter this measurement, but to a far lesser extent than APT. Conversely, an isolated documented decrease of the diffusing capacity does not necessarily indicate disease, as overt toxicity will develop in about a third of such patients.

A range of abnormalities can be found in the BAL in APT (Costabel et al. 2004; Coudert et al. 1992). The most consistent finding is the presence of numerous foam cells that contain osmiophilic lamellar inclusions if examined on electron microscopy, a cumbersome technique that is now rarely used to diagnose APT. Foam cells are a routine finding during treatments with amiodarone and indicate exposure to the drug, not necessarily toxicity (Bedrossian et al. 1997). To a certain degree, the absence of foam cells in the BAL is against the diagnosis of APT, but the specificity of this finding depends on technical factors and is not absolute. Therefore, one should not overly rely on the presence or absence of these cells to establish or refute the diagnosis of APT. In addition, amiodarone-toxic patients may exhibit an increase in neutrophils, lymphocytes, or both cell types in the BAL. Lymphocytosis suggests inflammation, denotes a shorter time to onset, correlates with diffuse fluffy opacities on imaging, and is associated with response to corticosteroid therapy. Lone eosinophilia and alveolar hemorrhage are rare findings in APT. A normal distribution of lymphocytes, neutrophils, and eosinophils can also be found.

Like any drug-induced lung disease, APT is a diagnosis of exclusion. An open lung biopsy is rarely deemed necessary, and a risk benefit is not available. A lung biopsy is indicated in patients with severe ventricular arrhythmias in whom pulmonary opacities develop, and there is no substitute for amiodarone, or in patients considered for valvular replacement or heart transplantation, in whom the diagnosis of pulmonary infiltrates (amiodarone pulmonary toxicity vs. neoplasia) must be secured before surgery or transplantation is contemplated. The histopathological appearances of amiodarone toxicity include septal thickening by interstitial edema, nonspecific inflammation, interstitial fibrosis, lipids in interstitial, endothelial and alveolar cells and lying free in alveolar spaces (Myers et al. 1987; Donaldson et al. 1998), and significant numbers of free-floating foamy macrophages in alveolar spaces. Foam cells may be so numerous as to mimic a pattern of desquamative interstitial pneumonia. Other reported findings include organizing, or fibrinous organizing pneumonia, a reactive epithelium, and mutilating interstitial fibrosis. Active or resolving diffuse alveolar damage and hyaline membranes characterize those cases with acute presentation.

In most patients in whom APT is suspected, it is reasonable to trim down the diagnostic possibilities by BAL, diuresis, and cardiac ultrasound. If the diagnosis of APT is high enough on the list, one may proceed with drug therapy withdrawal, underlying arrhythmia permitting, using corticosteroid therapy as a diagnostic test if drug withdrawal does not suffice. The main competing diagnoses of APT are not supposed to resolve under the influence of corticosteroid therapy. Since amiodarone withdrawal alone often is not followed by improvement, owing to the pharmacokinetics of the drug in lung, and because persistent APT may lead to a picture of irreversible pulmonary fibrosis, corticosteroid therapy is advised in the majority of cases with 'significant' APT. Although a consensus about 'significant amiodarone pulmonary toxicity' does not exist, a starting proposal might include the combination of sluggish response to drug withdrawal and involvement of >40% of the lung fields on frontal chest radiograph. Hypoxemia would indicate those cases in which waiting for the effect of drug withdrawal can be bypassed. Corticosteroid therapy should be given for extended periods of time although, again, no consensus and no controlled study exist. Six-month duration seems the lower end in terms of duration. Twelve months may suffice. Eighteen months may be required. A slow taper is essential in all cases to avoid relapse of the condition. In most cases, relapse of APT following steroid tapering can be controlled by reinstatement or augmentation of corticosteroid therapy. Rarely, relapse is resistant to corticosteroid therapy, and this is the reason why a relapse-avoiding strategy should be planned for each amiodarone-toxic patient. Amiodarone-toxic patients on corticosteroids must be monitored clinically and by appropriate imaging and physiologic studies. They should also be monitored for the development of adverse effects, including myopathy and infections. Care should also be taken to prevent the risk of arrhythmic death following amiodarone withdrawal. Mortality in APT is in the range of 10% in ambulatory patients. The attrition rate is higher (20-to-33%) in patients who require hospital admission for the treatment of their condition and nears 50% in cases with an ARDS picture.

Asymptomatic patients on amiodarone may present with subclinical disease in the form of pulmonary opacities on imaging, mainly HRCT. Such infiltrates may correspond to actual areas of APT or are incidental findings. Their significance often is unclear, because they cannot be accessed easily. Amiodarone therapy withdrawal is not an absolute requisite. A positive 67-Ga scan or dyslipidotic changes in the BAL may help suspect early APT. Serial follow-up with continued exposure to the drug is advisable to monitor whether the infiltrates progress or disappear with time.

Should regular chest radiographs be taken and pulmonary physiology measured in patients receiving amiodarone long term (Sunderji et al. 2000). No guidelines have been validated, and practices vary widely (Stelfox et al. 2004). A chest radiograph is indicated prior to the commencement of treatment with amiodarone to detect prior abnormalities to which any change occurring later can be compared. Ideally, two to three sets of lung volumes and diffusing capacity at the time amiodarone is instituted will serve as reference baseline. The chest radiograph can be monitored during treatment at regular intervals, e.g., every 4 to 12 months, and the frequency is adjusted depending on amiodarone dosage and/or if otherwise unexplained symptoms develop. Routine monitoring of pulmonary function is not cost effective, since APT is likely to develop swiftly between two sets of measurements. Furthermore, if modest decrements in lung function and diffusing capacity are detected, and these are common during chronic treatments with amiodarone, they may not equate clinical toxicity and may raise unnecessary investigation. An isolated reduction of the diffusing capacity should not prompt discontinuation of amiodarone unless there is clinical or imaging evidence for APT, particularly because an "amiodarone holiday" carries a risk of recurrence of arrhythmia. Instead, an isolated reduction of the diffusing capacity commands repeated measurement of this parameter and serial imaging over a shorter period of time. A stable diffusing capacity and imaging with time will indicate a lack of clinically meaningful APT. In summary, it is wise to monitor pulmonary function and diffusing capacity solely if unexplained symptoms or pulmonary infiltrates develop. Self-reporting of symptoms, serial clinical evaluation, and periodical chest radiographs are an easy and meaningful way to detect early APT, particularly during the first year of exposure, in patients over 60 years of age, and in those who receive >200 mg amiodarone daily.

9.4.2.4 Organizing Pneumonia

Organizing pneumonia [OP, or bronchiolitis obliterans organizing pneumonia, (BOOP)] is diagnosed on ductal and/or alveolar fibrosis in conjunction with interstitial inflammation as the dominant histopathological feature (Pneumotox® 1997). The main problem with OP is that the disease has many recognized causes and contexts other than drugs, making evaluation of causality difficult. Drug-induced OP was described during treatments with hexamethonium and mecamylamine in the 1950s. These drugs have been recalled. Later, organizing pneumonia was temporally associated with exposure to amiodarone, ß-blockers, and statins. Clinically, OP manifests with malaise, weight loss, dyspnea, low-grade fever, and sometimes pleuritic chest pain, which may simulate coronary artery disease. Typically, the disease is suspected when migratory opacities are seen on serial films. There may be intervening periods with a normal chest radiograph despite continued exposure to the causal drug. In some cases, the opacities are in the form of a fixed lone mass or masses, which may assume a recognizable segmental or lobar distribution. Other imaging patterns include multiple shaggy nodules and dense diffuse infiltrates. Although lymphocytes and sometimes neutrophils and/or eosinophils can dominate in be BAL differential, no distinctive BAL pattern reliably identifies OP of the drug-induced variant of it. Relying on a small sample of lung tissue obtained via the transbronchial route is problematic, since OP can be an incidental finding in many other conditions, including nonspecific interstitial pneumonia, eosinophilic pneumonia, infectious pneumonia, aspiration, and atelectasis upstream from an obstructed airway. Dyslipidosis suggestive of APT can be present in conjunction with the classic features of OP in amiodarone-induced OP. Otherwise, no histopathological feature will reliably differentiate OP due to drugs vs. OP of other causes. Some tissue eosinophilia is at times present, making the recognition of organizing from eosinophilic pneumonia difficult.

Most patients who present with migratory opacities and a background of compatible exposure to drugs in whom drug-induced OP is considered will not undergo a confirmatory lung biopsy. Careful follow-up after drug discontinuance will indicate whether signs and symptoms of OP abate, supporting the drug etiology. If drug discontinuance is not followed by improvement within a few weeks, then a trial of corticosteroids therapy or a lung biopsy is indicated. Traditionally, OP responds to corticosteroid therapy, regardless of its cause. However, this form of therapy may be ineffective in drug-induced OP, unless or until the culprit drug is eventually withdrawn. It is wise to look for the drug etiology in any patient presenting with OP, particularly if the conditions respond suboptimally to corticosteroid therapy.

9.4.2.5 Pulmonary Fibrosis

Pulmonary fibrosis is a complication of treatments with amiodarone, chemotherapy agents, and radiation therapy to the chest (Pneumotox® 1997). Ascribing pulmonary fibrosis to drugs is difficult, due to the confounding influence of idiopathic pulmonary fibrosis. This is the reason why pretherapy evaluation is so important in patients who are going to be exposed to amiodarone. Drug-induced pulmonary fibrosis manifests with cough, dyspnea, noisy Velcro® basilar crackles, and weight loss. On the chest radiograph, there are basilar or more diffuse linear or streaky shadows and volume loss. On HRCT, coarse reticular perilobular and/or subpleural thickening and traction bronchiectasis dominate in the lung bases, with honeycombing as a late and inconstant feature. Amiodarone-induced pulmonary fibrosis can develop after an episode of nonresolving APT, especially if corticosteroids are not given, or it occurs as a *de novo* phenomenon. Criteria for diagnosis of amiodarone-induced fibrosis include a normal chest radiograph prior to institution of treatment with the drug, timing with exposure, compatible imaging, and, if lung tissue is available, evidence for pulmonary fibrosis. The presence of dyslipidotic changes depends on time from the discontinuation of amiodarone to the lung biopsy. Drug therapy withdrawal is indicated. This is rarely followed by improvement. Response to corticosteroids is limited and/or transient.

9.4.2.6
Pleural Involvement

- The pleura and lung can be involved in the drug-induced lupus (Rubin 2005), a complication of treatments with about 60 chemically unrelated drugs, including the cardiac drugs amiodarone, ACEI, ß-blockers, dihydralazine, methyldopa, statins, and ticlopidine (Pneumotox® 1997; Morelock and Sahn 1999; Camus 2004). Drugs may cause 5 to 30% of all cases of lupus. The prevalence of pleuropulmonary involvement in drug-induced SLE is between 15 and 60%, depending on the causative drug (Rubin 1999). Clinical manifestations of the drug-induced lupus include chest pain, cough, dyspnea, arthralgias, skin changes, fever, malaise, pleuritis, pericarditis, and pleural or pericardial effusion. Pulmonary infiltrates without the pleural manifestations of the disease occur in a small minority of patients. The lupus anticoagulant and antiphospholipid antibodies may produce thromboembolic phenomena or the hypercoagulable state. The scarcity of drug-induced lupus cases with renal impairment, neurological involvement, and alveolar hemorrhage separate the drug condition from naturally occurring lupus. Diagnostic criteria for drug-induced lupus include (1) treatment with an SLE-inducing drug, (2) a suggestive clinical picture, and (3) a positive antinuclear antibody or antihistone test without, generally, the presence of anti-double-strand DNA antibodies. Management of drug-induced SLE consists of drug therapy withdrawal, with corticosteroid therapy, immunosuppressives, and plasma exchange reserved for severe cases. Clinical manifestations reverse more rapidly than do ANA levels, which decrease slowly over months after drug therapy withdrawal.
- Drugs can occasion exudative pleural effusion with elevated pleural lymphocytes, neutrophils or eosinophils, or pleural thickening without the above features of the drug lupus. These include amiodarone, beta-blockers, ergolines (e.g., bromocriptine, pergolide), hydralazine, imidapril, minoxidil, procainamide, simvastatin, and troglitazone. The pleural fluid in amiodarone-induced pleural effusion is typically unilateral and moderate in volume. It is either lymphocyte or lymphocyte and neutrophil predominant. Foam cells have been evidenced in pleural fluid and in pleural tissue. The effusion usually resolves upon discontinuation of the drug.

9.4.2.7
Pulmonary Hypertension

Old-fashioned anorectics of the 1980s have produced a similar pattern of pulmonary hypertension, and abused cocaine and amphetamines may produce the same syndrome (Pneumotox® 1997).

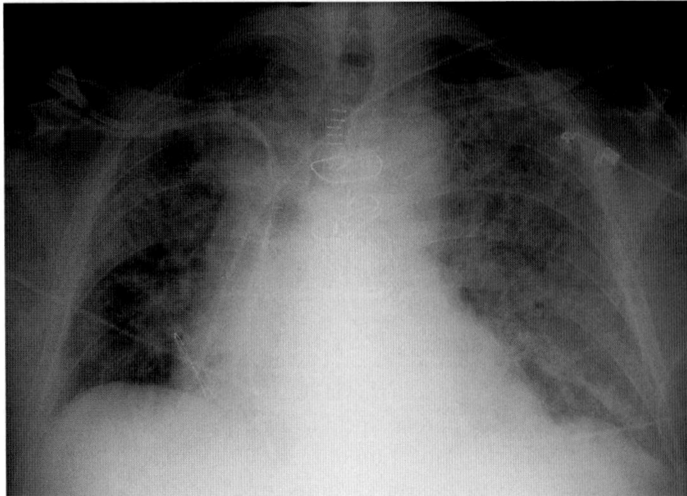

Fig. 9.1. Amiodarone pulmonary toxicity may occur acutely after a few days or weeks into treatment with elevated dosages of the drug, typically in the postoperative period of thoracic surgery. Diagnosis is by exclusion of other causes and is aided by the finding of foam cells in the bronchoalveolar lavage (see Fig. 9.5). Corticosteroid therapy is indicated

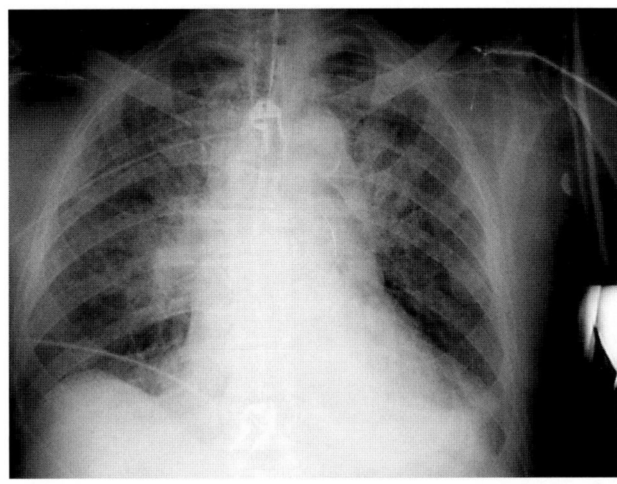

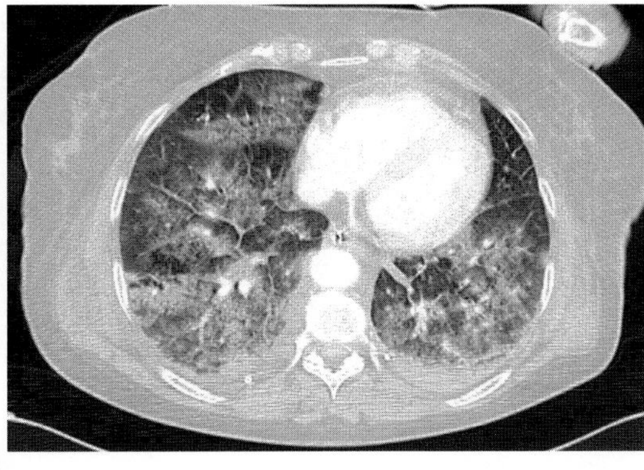

Fig. 9.2a,b. Acute pulmonary edema (**a**,**b**) can complicate treatments with several cardiac drugs including aspirin, epinephrine/adrenaline, hydrochlorothiazide and transfusion of blood and blood products (see Pneumotox®. On imaging (**a**,**b**), the opacities of pulmonary edema typically display a batwing pattern and, on CT, there is thickening of inter- and/or intralobular septa, alveolar shadowing and pleural effusion. Drug-induced pulmonary edema typically closely follows drug administration, and resolves in a few hours or days after drug discontinuation, except in cases which evolve to an ARDS picture. With aspirin, pulmonary edema may occur during longterm exposure to the drug. Drug withdrawal is the mainstay of treatment

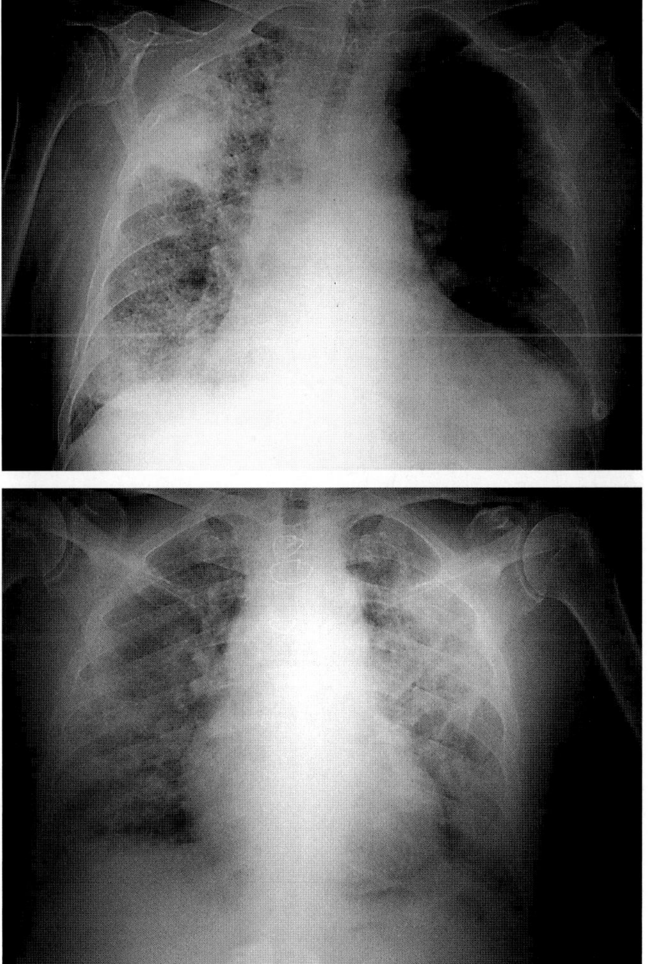

Fig. 9.3a,b. The expression of subacute (classic) amiodarone pulmonary toxicity may be assymmetrical (**a**), symmetrical (**b**), basilar or apical, localized or diffuse

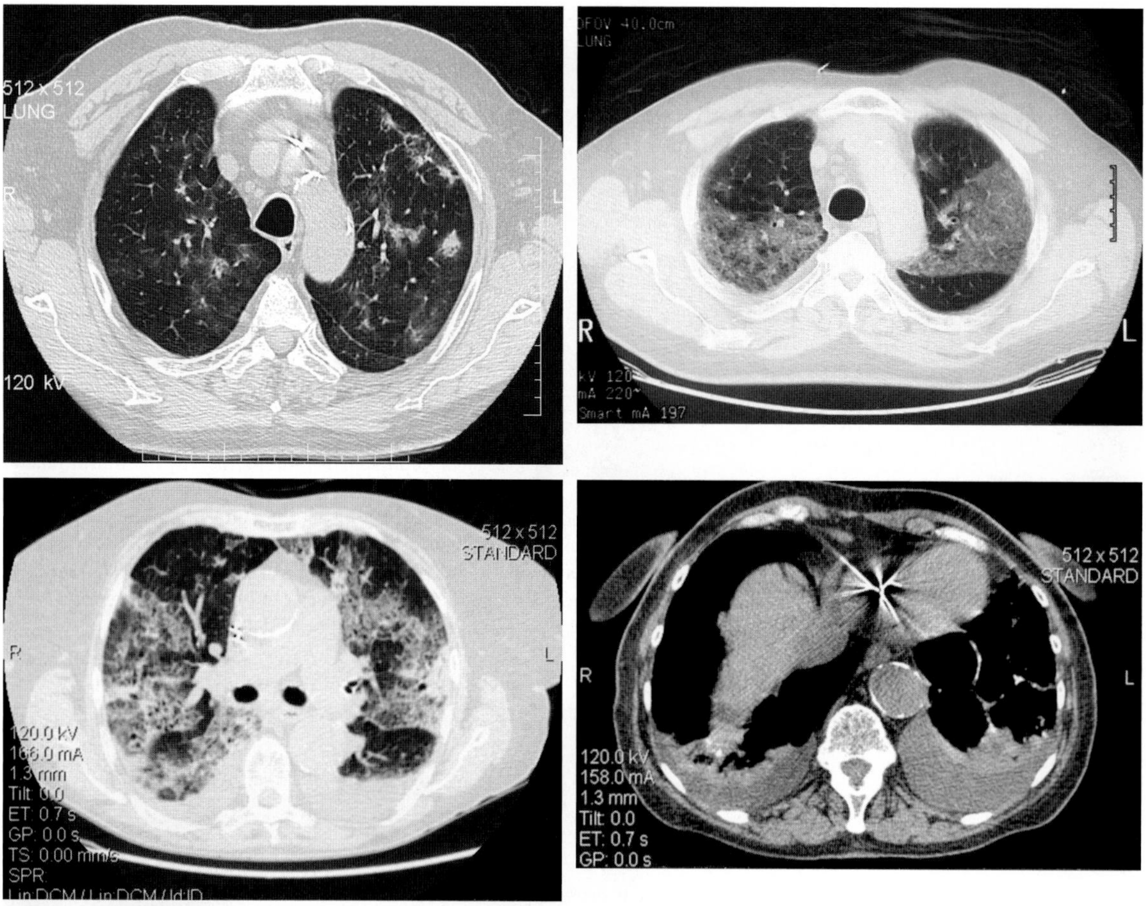

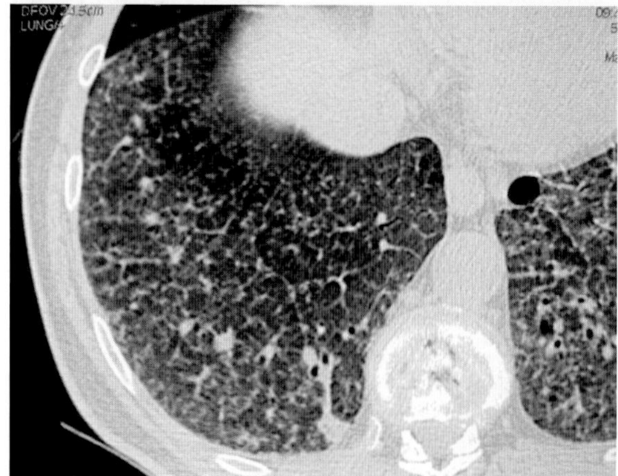

Fig. 9.4a–e. On HRCT, early cases are in the form of patchy, stellate opacities with intervening ground-glass or normal lung (**a**). In more advanced cases, the disease may manifest with segmental or lobar shadowing (**b**), inter- and intralobular thickening resembling the opacities of pulmonary congestion or interstitial pulmonary fibrosis (**c**,**e**). Pleural thickening (**b**) or effusion (**d**) is relatively common a finding. Prolonged corticosteroid therapy is indicated if drug therapy withdrawal is not associated with reversal of the manifestations of the disease in a few weeks

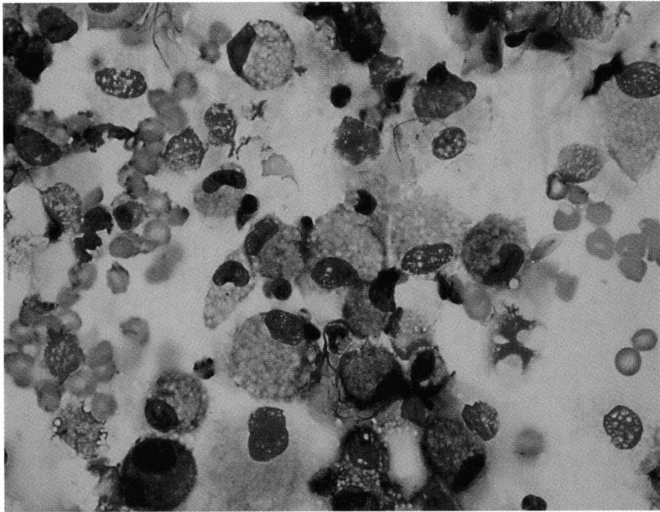

Fig. 9.5. The presence of characteristic foam cells in the BAL is a dinctinctly useful finding, that helps separate amiodarone pulmonary toxicity from other conditions such as pulmonary edema, alveolar hemorrhage or incidental disease processes

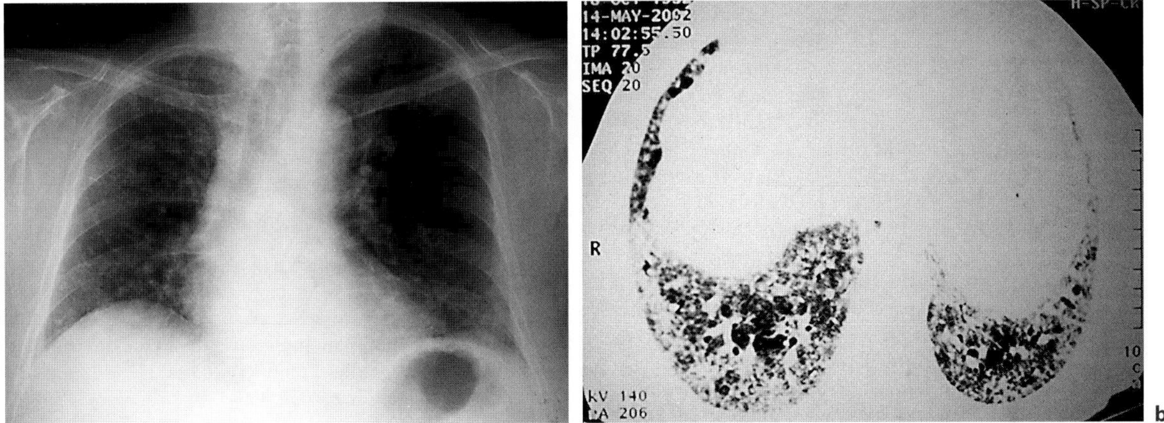

Fig. 9.6a,b. Amiodarone induced pulmonary fibosis (**a**,**b**) often is an irreversible process, that resembles pulmonary fibrosis that occurs spontaneously or in the context of connective tissue diseases. Bilateral streaky opacities, volume loss and hypoxemia are present. Relatedness with amiodarone is best established when the pretherapy pulmonary evaluation (chest radiograph and physiology) showed a normal chest radiograph

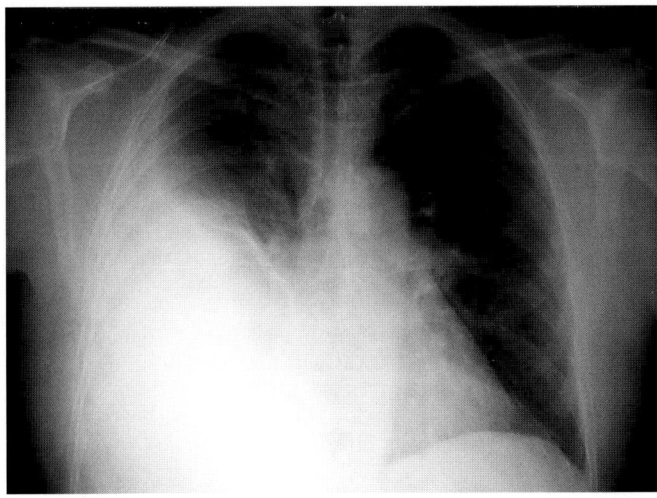

Fig. 9.7. Pleural effusion and pericardial effusion may occur with or without the features of lupus erythematosus and antinuclear antibodies. The effusion resolves after drug withdrawal in a few weeks or months. It may take several months for antinuclear antibodies to come back to normal values

References

Ahmed J, Philpott J, Lew GS, Blunt D (2005) Airway obstruction: a rare complication of thrombolytic therapy. J Laryngol Otol 119:819–821

Alapat PM, Zimmerman JL (2008) Toxicology in the critical care unit. Chest 133:1006–1013

al-Fallouji HK, Snow DG, Kuo MJ, Johnson PJ (1993) Spontaneous retropharyngeal haematoma: two cases and a review of the literature. J Laryngol Otol 107:649–650

Babu KS, Salvi SS (2000) Aspirin and asthma. Chest 118:1470–1476

Babu KS, Marshall BG (2004) Drug-induced airways diseases. Clin Chest Med 25:113–122

Beasley MB, Franks TJ, Galvin JR, Gochuico B, Travis WD (2002) Acute fibrinous and organizing pneumonia. A histologic pattern of lung injury and possible variant of diffuse alveolar damage. Arch Pathol Lab Med 126:1064–1070

Bedrossian CW, Warren CJ, Ohar J, Bhan R (1997) Amiodarone pulmonary toxicity: cytopathology, ultrastructure, and immunocytochemistry. Ann Diagn Pathol 1:47–56

Bonniaud P, Camus C, Jibbaoui A, Kazambu K, Baudouin N, Foucher P, Camus P (2006) Drug-induced respiratory emergencies. In: Fein A, Kamholz S, Ost D (eds)Respiratory emergencies. Edward Arnold, London, pp 269–290

Camus P, Martin WJ II, Rosenow EC III (2004) Amiodarone pulmonary toxicity. Clin Chest Med 25:65–76

Camus P (2004) Drug-induced pleural disease. In: Bouros D (ed) Pleural disorders. M Dekker, New York, pp 317–352

Champion L, Stern M, Israel-Biet D, Mamzer-Bruneel MF, Peraldi MN, Kreis H, Porcher R, Morelon E (2006) Sirolimus-associated pneumonitis: 24 cases in renal transplant recipients. Ann Intern Med 144:505–509

Chiu AG, Krowiak EJ, Deeb ZE (2001) Angioedema associated with angiotensin II receptor antagonists: challenging our knowledge of angioedema and its etiology. Laryngoscope 111:1729–1731

Cleverley JR, Screaton NJ, Hiorns MP, Flint JD, Müller NL (2002) Drug-induced lung disease: high-resolution CT and histological findings. Clin Radiol 57:292–299

Costabel U, Uzaslan E, Guzman J (2004) Bronchoalveolar lavage in drug-induced lung disease. Clin Chest Med 25:25–36

Coudert B, Bailly F, André F, Lombard JN, Camus P (1992) Amiodarone pneumonitis: bronchoalveolar lavage findings in 15 patients and review of the literature. Chest 102:1005–1012

Dean DE, Schultz DL, Powers RH (2001) Asphyxia due to angiotensin-converting enzyme (ACE) inhibitor mediated angioedema of the tongue during the treatment of hypertensive heart disease. J Forensic Sci 46:1239–1243

Di Pasquale G, Salpietro V, Boaron M (1990) Spontaneous mediastinal hematoma during therapy with oral anticoagulants. G Ital Cardiol 20:972–975

Dicpinigaitis PV (2006) Angiotensin-converting enzyme inhibitor-induced cough: ACCP evidence-based clinical practice guidelines. Chest 129:169S–173S

Donaldson L, Grant IS, Naysmith MR, Thomas JS (1998) Acute amiodarone-induced lung toxicity. Intensive Care Med 24:626–630

Dransfield MT, Rowe SM, Johnson JE, Bailey WC, Gerald LB (2008) Use of beta blockers and the risk of death in hospitalised patients with acute exacerbations of COPD. Thorax 63:301–305

Ernawati DK, Stafford L, Hughes JD (2008) Amiodarone-induced pulmonary toxicity. Br J Clin Pharmacol 66:82–87

Etminan M, Gill S, Fitzgerald M, Samii A (2006) Challenges and opportunities for pharmacoepidemiology in drug-therapy decision making. J Clin Pharmacol 46:6–9

Fernandez AB, Karas RH, Alsheikh-Ali AA, Thompson PD (2008) Statins and interstitial lung disease: A systematic review of the literature and of FDA adverse event reports. Chest 08-0943 (Epub ahead of print)

Flieder DB, Travis WD (2004) Pathologic characteristics of drug-induced lung disease. Clin Chest Med 25:37–46

Foucher P, Biour M, Blayac JP, Godard P, Sgro C, Kuhn M, Vergnon JM, Vervloet D, Pfitzenmeyer P, Ollagnier M, Mayaud C, Camus P (1997) Drugs that may injure the respiratory system. Eur Respir J 10:265–279

Gluecker T, Capasso P, Schnyder P, Gudinchet F, Schaller MD, Revelly JP, Chiolero R, Vock P, Wicky S (1999) Clinical and radiologic features of pulmonary edema. RadioGraphics 19: 1507–1531; discussion 1532–1503

Greenberger PA, Rotskoff BD, Lifschultz B (2007) Fatal anaphylaxis: postmortem findings and associated comorbid diseases. Ann Allergy Asthma Immunol 98:252–257

Gruchalla RS, Pirmohamed M (2006) Clinical practice. Antibiotic allergy. N Engl J Med 354:601–609

Hagan IG, Burney K (2007) Radiology of recreational drug abuse. RadioGraphics 27:919–940

Hauser T, Mahr A, Metzler C, Coste J, Sommerstein R, Gross WL, Guillevin L, Hellmich B (2008) The leucotriene receptor antagonist montelukast and the risk of Churg-Strauss syndrome: a case-crossover study. Thorax 63:677–682

Hayek ER, Speakman E, Rehmus E (2005) Acute doxorubicin cardiotoxicity. N Engl J Med 352:2456–2457

Hill AB (1965) The environment and disease: association or causation? Proc Roy Soc Med 58:295–300

Hu Z, Yang X, Ho PC, Chan SY, Heng PW, Chan E, Duan W, Koh HL, Zhou S (2005) Herb-drug interactions: a literature review. Drugs 65:1239–1282

Irey NS (1976) Tissue reactions to drugs. Am J Pathol 82:613–647

Iskandar SB, Kasasbeh ES, Mechleb BK, Garcia I, Jackson A, Fahrig S, Albalbissi K, Henry PD (2006) Alveolar hemorrhage: an underdiagnosed complication of treatment with glycoprotein IIb/IIIa inhibitors. J Interv Cardiol 19:356–363

Johnson BD, Beck KC, Olson LJ, O'Malley KA, Allison TG, Squires RW, Gau GT (2001) Pulmonary function in patients with reduced left ventricular function. Chest 120:1869–1876

Kaynar AM, Bhavani-Shankar K, Mushlin PS (1999) Lingual hematoma as a potential cause of upper airway obstruction. Anesth Analg 89:1573–1575

Leuppi JD, Schnyder P, Hartmann K, Reinhart WH, Kuhn M (2001) Drug-induced bronchospasm: analysis of 187 spontaneously reported cases. Respiration 68:341–351

Levy JH, Adkinson NF Jr (2008) Anaphylaxis during cardiac surgery: implications for clinicians. Anesth Analg 106:392–403

Low I, Stables S (2006) Anaphylactic deaths in Auckland, New Zealand: a review of coronial autopsies from 1985 to 2005. Pathology 38:328–332

Mason JW (2001) Amiodarone pulmonary toxicity and Professor Hounsfield. J Cardiovasc Electrophysiol 12:437–438

Matsuno O, Okubo T, Hiroshige S, Takenaka R, Ono E, Ueno T, Nureki S, Ando M, Miyazaki E, Kumamoto T (2007) Drug-induced lymphocyte stimulation test is not useful for the diagnosis of drug-induced pneumonia. Tohoku J Exp Med 212:49–53

Moore TJ, Walsh CS, Cohen MR (2004) Reported adverse event cases of methemoglobinemia associated with benzocaine products. Arch Intern Med 164:1192–1196

Morelock SY, Sahn SA (1999) Drugs and the pleura. Chest 116:212–221

Myers JL, Kennedy JI, Plumb VJ (1987) Amiodarone lung: pathologic findings in clinically toxic patients. Hum Pathol 18:349–354

Nanda S, Konnur N (2006) Adolescent drug and alcohol use in the 21st century. Pediatr Ann 35:193–199

Naranjo CA, Busto U, Sellers EM, Sandor P, Ruiz I, Roberts EA (1981) A method for estimating the probability of adverse drug reactions. Clin Pharmacol Ther 30:239–245

Newcomb AE, Clarke CP (2005) Spontaneous pneumomediastinum: a benign curiosity or a significant problem? Chest 128:3298–3302

Picado C, Castillo JA, Montserrat JM, Agusti-Vidal A (1989) Aspirin-intolerance as a precipitating factor of life-threatening attacks of asthma requiring mechanical ventilation. Eur Respir J 2:127–129

Plataki M, Bouros D (2004) Iatrogenic and rare pleural effusion. In: Bouros D (ed) Pleural disorders. M Dekker, New York, pp 897–913

Pleskow WW, Stevenson DD, Mathison DA, Simon RA, Schatz M, Zeiger RS (1982) Aspirin desensitization in aspirin-sensitive asthmatic patients: clinical manifestations and characterization of the refractory period. J Allergy Clin Immunol 69:11–19

Pneumotox® (1997, 2008) http://www.pneumotox.com: (Website). Producers: P Foucher, P Camus. Last update: August 2008

Popovsky MA (2008) Transfusion-related acute lung injury: Incidence, pathogenesis and the role of multicomponent apheresis in its prevention. Transfusion Med Hemother 35:76–79

Prosnitz RG, Chen YH, Marks LB (2005) Cardiac toxicity following thoracic radiation. Semin Oncol 32:S71–S80

Pumphrey RSH (2000) Lessons from management of anaphylaxis from a study of fatal reactions. Clin Exp Allergy 30:1144–1150

Pumphrey RS, Roberts IS (2000) Postmortem findings after fatal anaphylactic reactions. J Clin Pathol 53:273–276

Rosado A, Vives R, Gonzalez R, Rodriguez J (2003) Can NSAIDs intolerance disappear? A study of three cases. Allergy 58:689–690

Rothman RB (2000) The age-adjusted mortality rate from primary pulmonary hypertension, in age range 20 to 54 years, did not increase during the years of peak "Phen/Fen" use. Chest 118:1516–1517

Rothman KJ, Lanes S, Sacks ST (2004) The reporting odds ratio and its advantages over the proportional reporting ratio. Pharmacoepidemiol Drug Safety 13:519–523

Rubin RL (2005) Drug-induced lupus. Toxicology 209:135–147

Rubin RL (1999) Etiology and mechanisms of drug-induced lupus. Curr Opin Rheumatol 11:357–363

Salpeter SR, Ormiston TM, Salpeter EE, Poole PJ, Cates CJ (2003) Cardioselective beta-blockers for chronic obstructive pulmonary disease: a meta-analysis. Respir Med 97:1094–1101

Shojania KG (2000) Coumadin-induced lingual hemorrhage mimicking angioedema. Am J Med 109:77–78

Silliman CC, Ambruso DR, Boshkov LK (2005) Transfusion-related acute lung injury. Blood 105:2266–2273

Skroubis G, Galiatsou E, Metafratzi Z, Karahaliou A, Kitsakos A, Nakos G (2005) Amiodarone-induced acute lung toxicity in an ICU setting. Acta Anaesthesiol Scand 49:569–571

Sondhi D, Lippmann M, Murali G (2004) Airway compromise due to angiotensin-converting enzyme inhibitor-induced angioedema: clinical experience at a large community teaching hospital. Chest 126:400–404

Souza CA, Muller NL, Johkoh T, Akira M (2006) Drug-induced eosinophilic pneumonia: high-resolution CT findings in 14 patients. AJR Am J Roentgenol 186:368–373

Spitz DJ (2003) An unusual death in an asthmatic patient. Am J Forensic Med Pathol 24:271–272

Srihari VH, Lee TW (2008) Evidence based case report – Pulmonary embolism in a patient taking clozapine. Br Med J 336:1499–1501

Stalnikowicz R, Amitai Y, Bentur Y (2004) Aphrodisiac drug-induced hemolysis. J Toxicol Clin Toxicol 42:313–316

Stelfox HT, Ahmed SB, Fiskio J, Bates DW (2004) Monitoring amiodarone's toxicities: Recommendations, evidence, and clinical practice. Clin Pharmacol Ther 75:110–122

Stewart JI, Chawla R, Lloyd JM, Kane GC (2008) Amiodarone pneumonitis. Respir Care 53:370–375

Sunderji R, Kanji Z, Gin K (2000) Pulmonary effects of low dose amiodarone: a review of the risks and recommendations for surveillance. Can J Cardiol 16:1435–1440

Troughton RW, Richards AM, Yandle TG, Frampton CM, Nicholls MG (2007) The effects of medications on circulating levels of cardiac natriuretic peptides. Ann Med 39:242–260

van Mieghem W, Coolen L, Malysse I, Lacquet LM, Deneffe GJD, Demedts MGP (1994) Amiodarone and the development of ARDS after lung surgery. Chest 105:1642–1645

Vaszar LT, Stevenson DD (2001) Aspirin-induced asthma. Clin Rev Allergy Immunol 21:71–87

Vernhet H, Bousquet C, Durand G, Giron J, Senac JP (2001) Reversible amiodarone-induced lung disease: HRCT findings. Eur Radiol 11:1697–1703

Webb LM, Lieberman P (2006) Anaphylaxis: a review of 601 cases. Ann Allergy Asthma Immunol 97:39–43

Wright SE, Snowden CP, Athey SC, Leaver AA, Clarkson JM, Chapman CE, Roberts DRD, Wallis JP (2008) Acute lung injury after ruptured abdominal aortic aneurysm repair: The effect of excluding donations from females from the production of fresh frozen plasma. Crit Care Med 36:1796–1802

Wright RO, Lewander WJ, Woolf AD (1999) Methemoglobinemia: etiology, pharmacology, and clinical management. Ann Emerg Med 34:646–656

Yahalom J, Portlock CS (2008) Long-term cardiac and pulmonary complications of cancer therapy. Hematol Oncol Clin North Am 22:305–318,VII

Part IV:

Medical Applications of Integrated Cardiothoracic Imaging

Cardiac Complications of Thoracic Disorders

Diseases of the Pulmonary Circulation

10

Martine Rémy-Jardin, Andrei-Bogdan Gorgos, Vittorio Pansini, Jean-Baptiste Faivre, and Jacques Rémy

CONTENTS

M. Rémy-Jardin, MD, PhD, Professor
A.-B. Gorgos, MD
V. Pansini, MD
J-B. Faivre, MD
J. Remy, MD, Professor
Department of Thoracic Imaging, C.H.R.U. de Lille, Hôspital Calmette, Boulevard du Prof. Leclercq, 59037 Lille Cédex, France

Introduction

Over the last decades, CT angiography has become the first-line noninvasive imaging modality of the pulmonary circulation, particularly well exemplified in the management of acute pulmonary embolism (Remy-Jardin et al. 2007). Multidetector-row CT systems with fast scanning capabilities can acquire images of the thorax with reduced cardiac motion artifact, enabling improved evaluation of the heart and surrounding structures in the course of routine thoracic CT imaging (Bruzzi et al. 2006a, 2006b). Moreover, the introduction of fast rotation speed and dedicated cardiac reconstruction algorithms exploiting the multislice acquisition scheme of the data has opened the possibility of integrating cardiac functional information into a diagnostic CT scan of the chest, providing prognostic information in the management of patients with a wide variety of acute or chronic respiratory disorders. This chapter describes the additional information that can be obtained at the level of the heart in the course of chest CT examinations indicated for the management of pulmonary vascular diseases.

10.1 Obstructive Diseases of the Pulmonary Circulation

10.1.1 Acute Pulmonary Embolism

10.1.1.1 Cruoric Emboli

Once the diagnosis of acute PE is made, prognostic assessment is required for risk stratification and therapeutic decision making. Risk stratification consists of clinical evaluation of the patient's hemodynamic status followed by the search for markers of right ventricular (RV) dysfunction and injury (ESC Task Force 2008). In the clinical context of massive acute PE, it is well established that acute pulmonary embolism increases the pressure of the pulmonary arterial tree and right ventricle, which, in turn, may cause acute right heart dysfunction and failure. Such severe hemodynamic situations may lead to the patient's death caused by circulatory collapse secondary to acute right heart failure, defining the category of high-risk patients. Whereas CT does not play any role in the diagnostic approach of right ventricular dysfunction secondary to massive acute PE, it may provide important prognostic information in cases of nonmassive acute PE, a category characterized by patients hemodynamically stable at presentation. In this latter category, patients with right heart dysfunction and/or myocardial injury define the intermediate-risk category owing to the well-established link between the presence of RV dysfunction and the higher risk of PE-related early mortality. Recognition of this category of patients usually relies on the measurement of biological markers of RV dysfunction or injury, but also on the search for echocardiographic and/or CT features of RV dysfunction. With echocardiography suffering from several limitations (Burgess et al. 2002), great interest has been directed toward depiction of RV dysfunction on the same CT examination as that used for diagnosing acute PE.

Following the initial descriptions by Oliver et al. (1998) and Reid and Murchison (1998), CT can give information regarding the status of the heart by showing the size of the right ventricle and the position of the interventricular septum (Fig. 10.1). The normal right ventricle has a limited ability to handle an acute increase in afterload. In the event of a sudden increase in afterload, right ventricular wall tension becomes elevated, followed by dilatation and hypokinesis of the right ventricle and secondary tricuspid regurgitation. The interventricular septum, which normally bows toward the right ventricle, may shift toward the left ventricle because of the restraints of the pericardium. This shift causes decreased left ventricular filling and cardiac output, which may lead to a vicious circle of falling systemic pressure, ventricular ischemia, and further dilatation of the right ventricle. The CT features suggestive of right ventricular dysfunction on cross-sectional imaging are summarized in Table 10.1. Several studies have shown that right ventricular enlargement on CT, based on the assessment of the right-ventricular-to-left-ventricular dimension ratio, predicted subsequent admission to the intensive care unit, adverse clinical events, and early death (Contractor et al. 2002; Collomb et al. 2003; Araoz et al. 2003; Schoepf et al. 2004; Quiroz et al. 2004; van der Meer et al. 2005; Ghuysen et al. 2005; Ghaye et al. 2006; He et al. 2006). However, data recently reported by Araoz et al. (2007) failed to confirm the prognostic value of a CT-based RV/LV ration for risk stratification. In this study, these authors observed that RV/LV diameter ratio and embolic burden were not associated with short-term death due to PE. Explanations for such discrepancies can be found in the variety of planes of reformation on which these measurements can be made, which include transverse CT scans, four-cavity chamber views, or short-axis images of the ventricular cavities. Moreover, one should underline the variety of cut-off values above for which an adverse patient outcome has been reported. In addition, whereas an increased RV/LV diameter ratio may result from acutely elevated RV pressures secondary to PE, it may also result from a preexisting process that is independent of acute PE. In a recent study, Lu et al. (2008) have shown that the interval increase of the right ventricular-left ventricular (RV-LV) diameter ratio was more accurate than the diameter ratio of the CT examination with positive findings for PE alone for mortality prediction after acute PE. Consequently, in the absence of universally accepted criteria, the current consensus on the contribution of CT in risk stratification of patients with confirmed PE focuses on the recognition of low-risk patients based on the lack of RV dilatation (ESC Task Force 2008). Other CT-derived indices, such as interventricular septum shape or pulmonary artery dimensions, have not been found to be of prognostic relevance.

The introduction of high-speed ECG gated acquisitions of the entire thorax has enlarged the concept of cardiothoracic imaging with the subsequent possibility of providing quantitative information on right ventricular function. The ideal scanning protocol should allow the radiologist to evaluate both morphology and function from a single image data set, an objective currently achievable with 16-slice, but more easily with 64-slice MDCT technology. Using segmentation methods to calculate right ventricular ejection fraction (RVEF) with CT, several studies have investigated the accuracy of CTA compared to MRI (Lembcke et al. 2005), radionu-

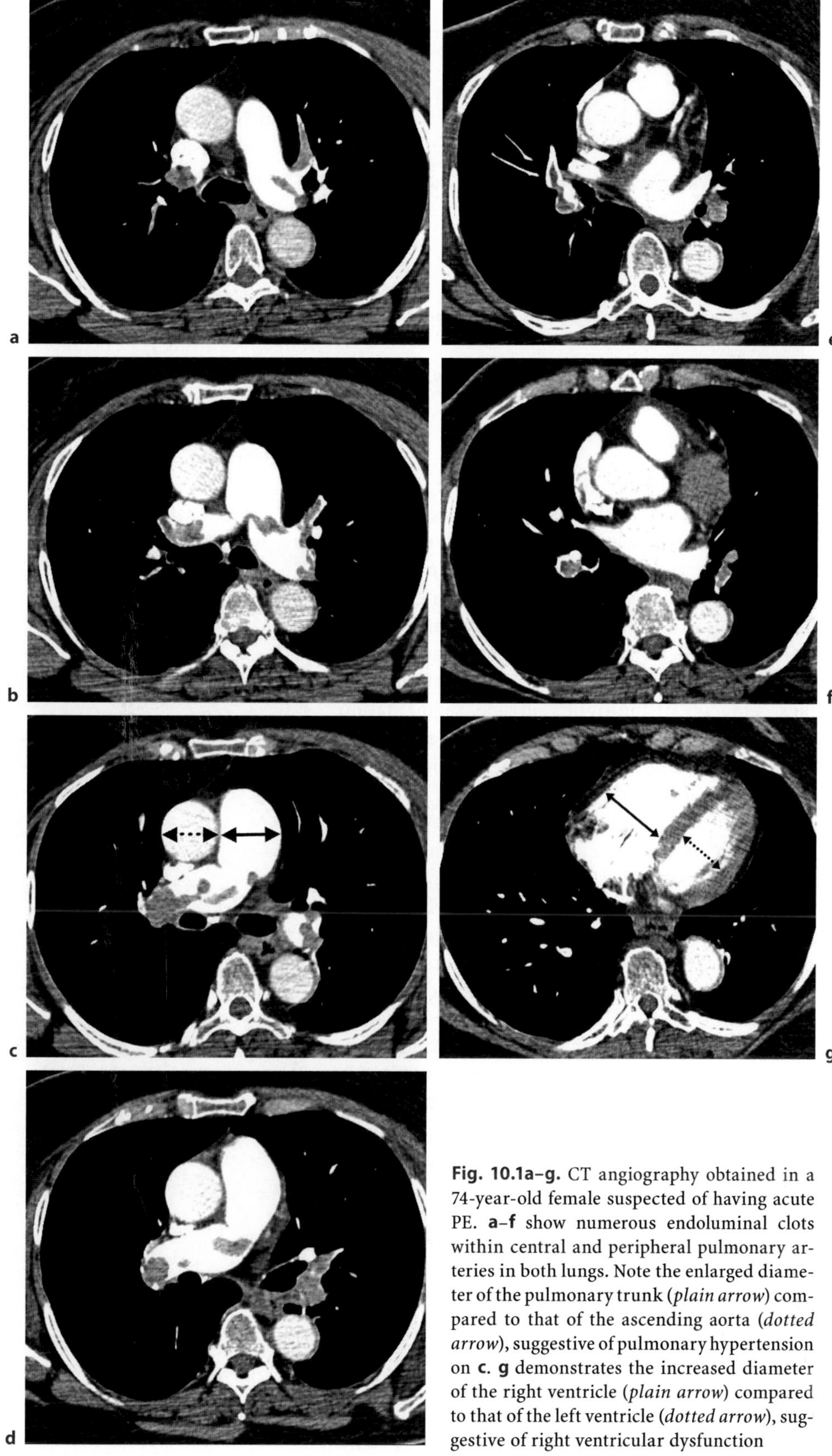

Fig. 10.1a–g. CT angiography obtained in a 74-year-old female suspected of having acute PE. **a–f** show numerous endoluminal clots within central and peripheral pulmonary arteries in both lungs. Note the enlarged diameter of the pulmonary trunk (*plain arrow*) compared to that of the ascending aorta (*dotted arrow*), suggestive of pulmonary hypertension on **c**. **g** demonstrates the increased diameter of the right ventricle (*plain arrow*) compared to that of the left ventricle (*dotted arrow*), suggestive of right ventricular dysfunction

Table 10.1. CT features of right ventricular dysfunction

- Morphological changes at the level of the cardiac cavities
  - Right ventricle enlargement
  - Right ventricular–left ventricular diameter ratio >1
  - Leftward displacement of the interventricular septum
- Additional morphological changes
  - Right atrium enlargement
  - Dilatation of the systemic veins (inferior and/or superior vena cava; coronary sinus)
  - Reflux of contrast medium into the systemic veins

clide ventriculography (Kim et al. 2005; Coche et al. 2005; Delhaye et al. 2006), and echocardiography (Dogan et al. 2006). In the clinical context of chronic respiratory impairment, these studies have demonstrated that MDCT was an accurate and reliable noninvasive technique for evaluating right ventricular function and offered certain advantages over other imaging modalities. Because of the complex geometry of the right ventricle, segmentation of the right ventricular cavity cannot be automated and requires manual drawing of the ventricular contours in systole and diastole (Fig. 10.2). The overall duration of postprocessing to calculate RVEF using this method is approximately 15 min. A more rapid means of estimating RVEF with CT has recently been investigated based on the measurement of tricuspid annulus displacement between systole and diastole. Because of the orientation of muscle fibers, RV contraction occurs mainly along its longitudinal axis, between the tricuspid annulus and the RV apex. Consequently, measurement of the tricuspid annulus excursion, known under the acronym of TAPSE, reflects the strength of RV contraction. On the basis of transthoracic echocardiography, this parameter has been found to provide a reliable estimation of RV systolic function (Forfia et al. 2006; Lamia et al. 2007). Using ECG-gated 64-slice MDCT, Delhaye et al. (2008) have recently demonstrated that TAPSE measurements on four-chamber views of the cardiac cavities provide an accurate and rapid estimation of RV function (Fig. 10.3). It should be emphasized that ECG-gated examinations of the chest do not require administration of beta-blockers (Salem et al. 2006; Delhaye et al. 2007) and can be obtained without excessive radiation exposure to the patient (D'Agostino et al. 2006).To date, a single study has evaluated ECG-gated and non-gated MDCT examinations in the assessment of RV dysfunction in patients suspected of having acute PE at initial presentation (Dogan et al. 2007). Measuring dimension ratios for the RV and LV on non-synchronized transverse and angulated four-chamber views and calculating RV end-systolic volumes and RV/LV volume ratios on ECG-gated scans, the authors concluded that ECG-synchronized MDCT facilitates detection of RV dysfunction in patients with PE. Two current limiting factors for ECG-gated acquisitions–namely longer scanning times compared to non-ECG-gated acquisitions and image quality degradation due to irregular and/or high cardiac rhythms – are expected to be overcome with the newly introduced dual-source CT technology, which should allow the

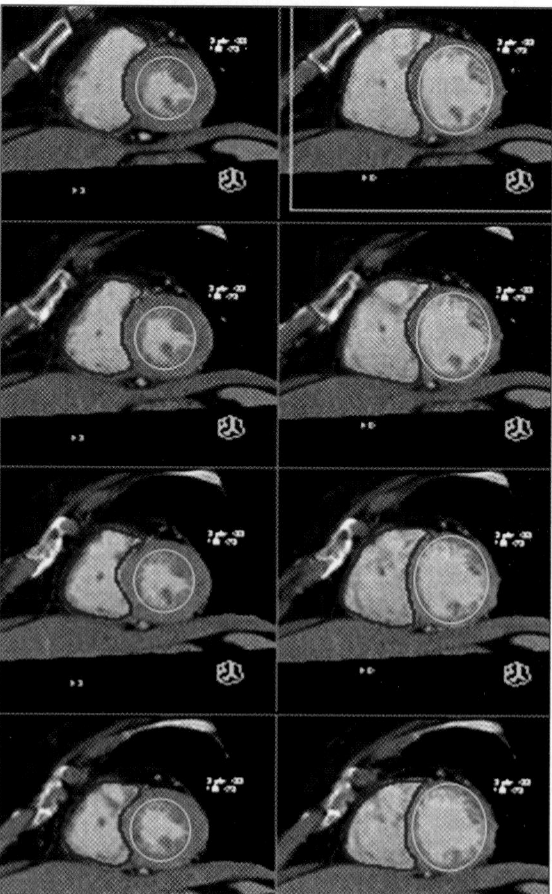

Fig. 10.2. Short-axis images of the ventricular cavities in systole (*left column*) and diastole (*right column*). On both series of images, the *red lines* illustrate the manual segmentation of the right ventricle and the *yellow lines* to the semi-automatic segmentation of the left ventricular cavity

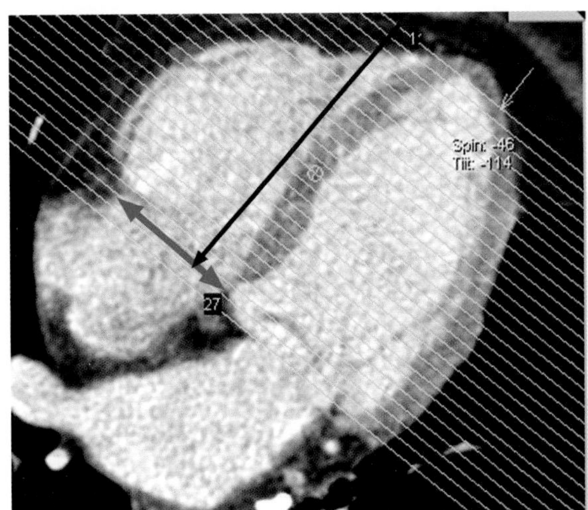

Fig. 10.3. Long-axis image of the ventricular cavities. The *red line* illustrates the anatomical position of the tricuspid valve and the *black arrow* the orientation of the displacement of the tricuspid valve during right ventricular contraction

radiologists to provide clinicians with cardiac functional information in routine clinical practice.

Special mention should be added to the possibility for ECG-gated MDCT to depict mobile clots in the right heart. Their presence is synonymous with a particularly severe form of acute PE, with a mortality rate of up to 27% in a 2002 metaanalysis (Rose et al. 2002). It has been hypothesized that the migration of these clots to the lungs is temporarily slowed down by high pulmonary pressure, low cardiac output, and considerable tricuspid regurgitation, which may result in the clot remaining in the right atrium (Ferrari et al. 2005).

10.1.1.2 Noncruoric Emboli

Although less frequently encountered than cruoric emboli, septic and tumoral emboli are worth considering as they may involve both right cardiac cavities and pulmonary arteries. Septic emboli are rare but important complications in patients with septicemia. Predisposing conditions include bacterial endocarditis, infected venous catheters or pace-maker wires, septic thrombophlebitis, and ondotogenic infections. The CT appearance of septic emboli has been well described, including nodules and wedge-shaped subpleural opacities with or without cavitation and the feeding vessel sign (Dodd et al. 2006). In the context of infective endocarditis, ECG-gated MDCT examinations of the entire chest may be useful for identifying in one CT acquisition the various components of the disease. Fellah et al. (2007) have recently reported a case of tricuspid valve endocarditis complicated by septic pulmonary embolism documented on ECG-gated 40-MDCT of the entire chest. Similarly to that already reported for the aortic valve (Willmann et al. 2002; Bootsveld et al. 2004), it is likely that ECG-gated acquisitions of the chest will lead to incidental depiction of valvular lesions (Fig. 10.4).

Although metastatic spread of tumor to the lung is common, pulmonary tumor emboli are unusual.

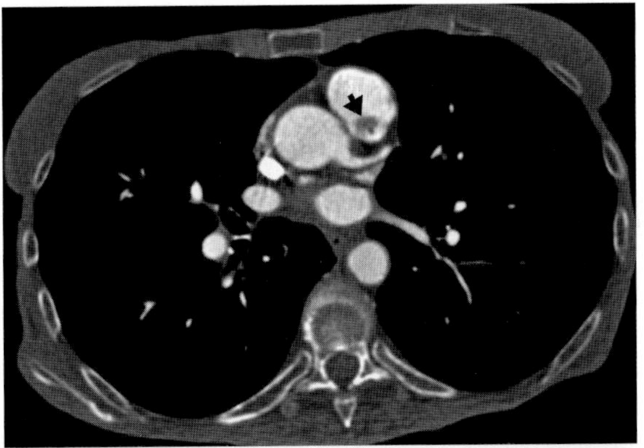

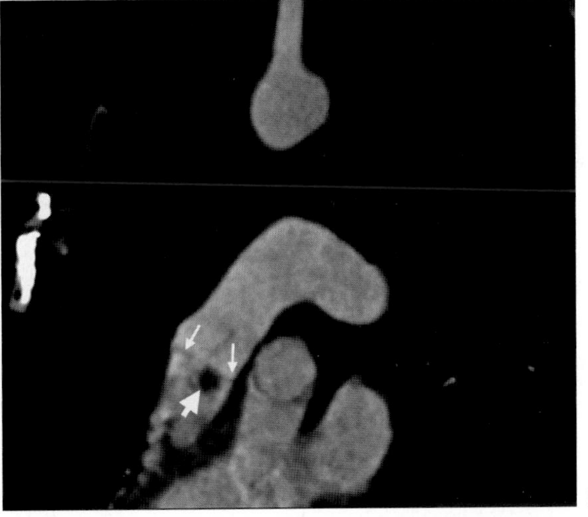

Fig. 10.4a,b. Transverse CT scan obtained below the level of the pulmonary valve (**a**) and sagittal oblique reformation obtained along the main axis of the pulmonary trunk (**b**), both in diastolic phase. Note the presence of a rounded, hypoattenuated mass (*large arrow* **a**,**b**), adjacent to the inferior wall of the pulmonary valve (*small arrows* **b**). Transthoracic echocardiography confirmed the presence of a mass adjacent to the pulmonary valve, suggestive of papillary fibroelastoma (no histologic confirmation owing to the presence of severe underlying respiratory disease; stable over a 3-year follow-up)

Their CT features are often undistinguishable from those of cruoric emboli, except when delayed acquisitions over the embolic material are obtained, showing increased attenuation values within tumoral emboli (Hauret et al. 2000; Wanatabe et al. 2002; Wong et al. 2004). Another origin for tumoral pulmonary emboli can be found at the level of the cardiac cavities. Secondary cardiac neoplasias are 20 to 40 times more common than primary tumors, and almost every type of malignant tumor has been shown to metastasize to the heart. Leukemia is the most frequent cause of cardiac tumors, with cardiac lesions developing in 50% of patients with leukemia. Other neoplasias that produce cardiac metastases include breast, lung melanoma, and lymphoma. Abdominal and pelvic tumors can also grow in a cephalad direction via the inferior vena cava to reach the right cardiac cavities. Embolization of cardiac metastases into the pulmonary circulation may then occur. Less frequently observed, such material may also migrate through a patent atrial septal defect, leading to paradoxic tumoral embolism (Dumont et al. 2002). Primary tumors of the right cardiac cavities can also lead to pulmonary embolism, and several cases of pulmonary migration of right atrial myxoma fragments have been reported (McCoskey et al. 2000; Parsons and Detterbeck 2003).

10.1.2 Chronic Thromboembolic Disease

10.1.2.1 Evaluation of Cardiac Consequences at the Time of Initial Diagnosis

Chronic thromboembolic pulmonary hypertension (CTEPH) is an infrequent outcome of acute pulmonary embolism. Several mechanisms have been postulated to be responsible for the development of chronic pulmonary hypertension after an acute event, including a recurrence of embolism, an incomplete resolution of endoluminal clots, as well as an in situ thrombus growth. CTEPH causes right ventricular pressure overload, which leads to functional and morphologic alterations of both right and left ventricles. These changes result in a decreased cardiac index. Table 10.2 summarizes the pathophysiology of right and left heart failure in patients with CTEPH (Menzel et al. 2000).

Table 10.2. Pathophysiology of left heart failure and right heart failure in patients with CTEPH undergoing pulmonary thromboendarterectomy (from Menzel et al. 2000)

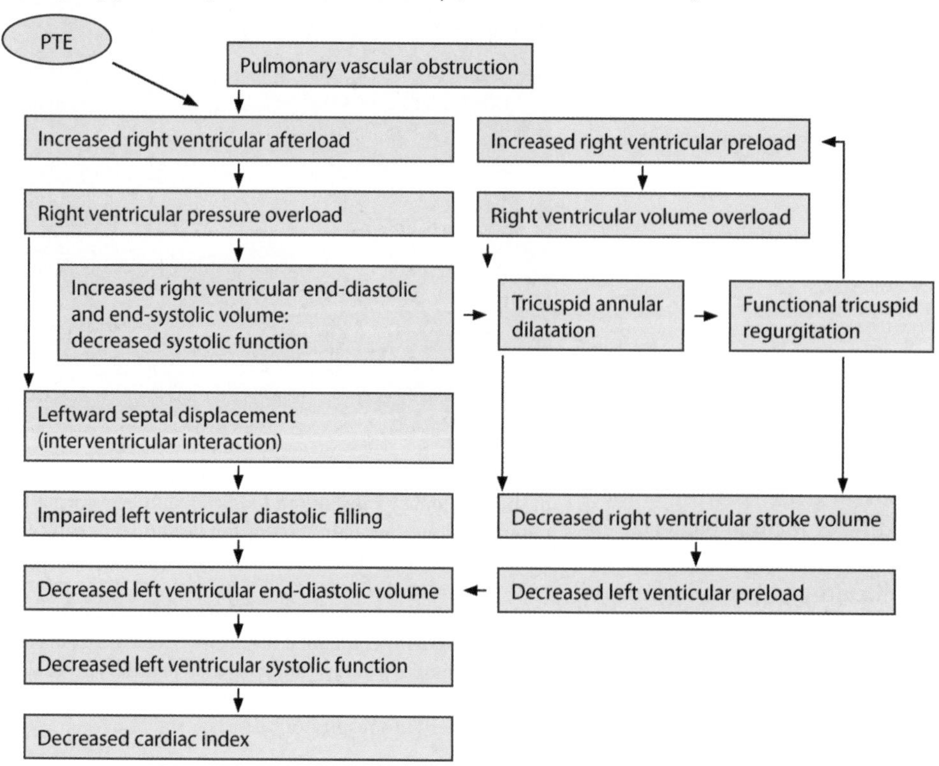

10.1.2.2 Changes Observed after Thromboendarterectomy

The hemodynamic and cardiac changes remain partially reversible, even after years of illness (Chow et al. 1988; Dittrich et al. 1988; Jamieson et al. 1993; Menzel et al. 2000). In a study investigating 39 patients before and after pulmonary thromboendarterectomy (PTE), improved lung perfusion and the reduction of right ventricular pressure overload have been shown to be direct results of PTE, which in turn bring a profound reduction of right ventricular size and a recovery of systolic function (Menzel et al. 2000). Normalization of interventricular septal motion as well as improved venous return to the left atrium lead to a normalization of left ventricular diastolic and systolic function, and the cardiac index improves. To date, cardiac morphology as well as alterations of right and left ventricular function RV have been investigated noninvasively mainly by echocardiography and, more recently, by magnetic resonance imaging (Menzel et al. 2000; Reesink et al. 2007). As the morphologic features of RV remodeling, namely RV dilatation, hypertrophy, and leftward ventricular septal bowing, are also accessible to MDCT, it is likely that this noninvasive imaging tool will be more extensively used in the follow-up of patients who undergo thrombendarterectomy (Fig. 10.5).

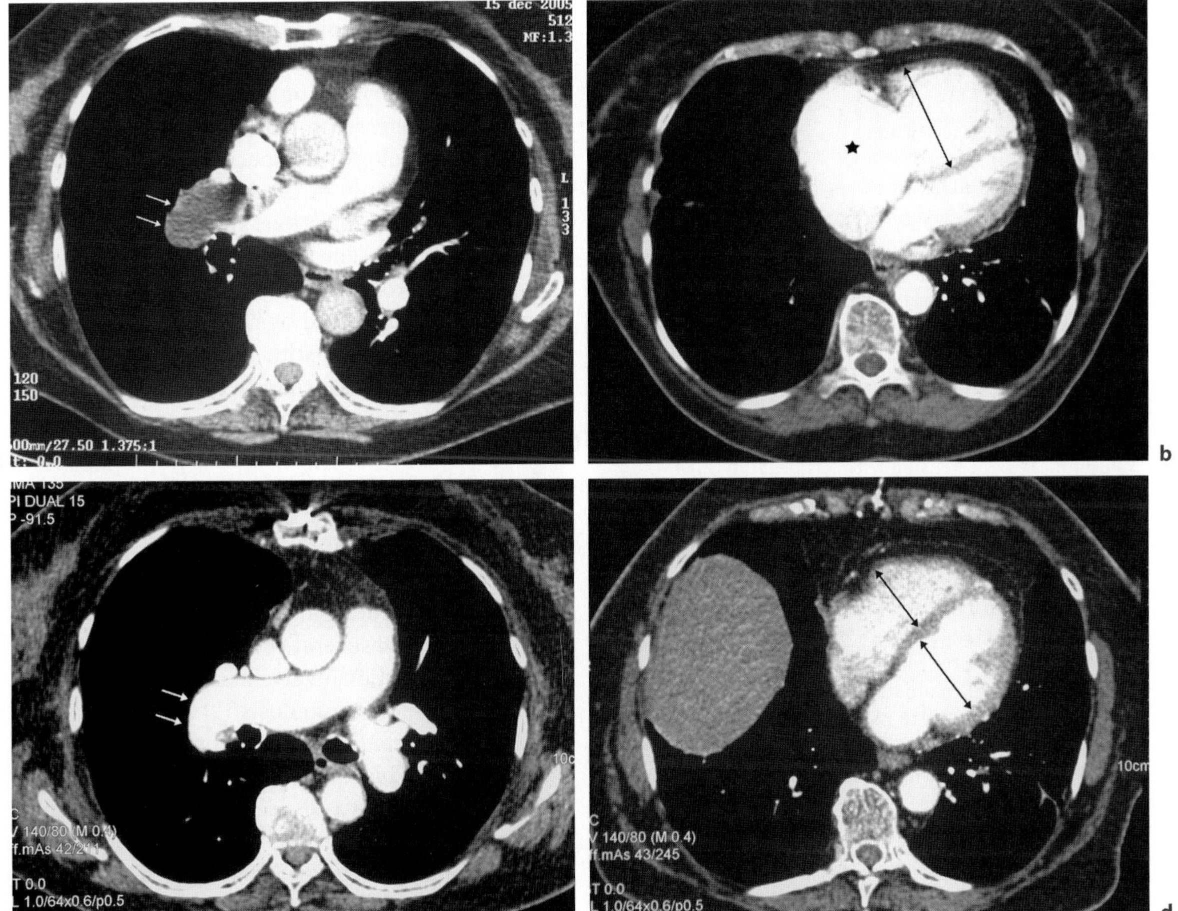

Fig. 10.5a–d. Chronic thromboembolic disease in a 78-year-old female treated by thromboendarterectomy. Preoperative transverse CT scans (**a**,**b**) showing a large endoluminal filling defect at the level of the right interlobar pulmonary artery (*arrows* **a**), right ventricular enlargement with septal bowing toward the left ventricle (*arrow* **b**). Note the additional presence of an enlarged right atrium (*star*) on **b**. Postoperative CT scans obtained at the same anatomical levels as those of **a** and **b** (**c**,**d**) illustrating the successful removal of endoluminal clots (*arrows* c) and the resolution of the CT features of right ventricular dysfunction, suggested by a right ventricle-left ventricle ratio <1 (*arrows* **d**)

10.1.3 Cardiac Changes in Other Causes of Pulmonary Hypertension

The classification of pulmonary hypertension was modified during the Third World Symposium on pulmonary hypertension (SIMONNEAU et al. 2004) (Table 10.3). The various causes of pulmonary hypertension can also be considered according to their relationships and/or impact on cardiac function. There are a few situations in which pulmonary hypertension has no impact on cardiac function, as observed with pulmonary veno-occlusive disease and pulmonary capillary hemangiomatosis at the beginning of their development. In some other circumstances, pulmonary hypertension can be observed with left heart disease, including left-sided atrial or ventricular heart disease as well as left-sided valvular heart disease. Whereas left heart disease is usually diagnosed before its impact on the level of pulmonary artery pressure, it may be unknown at the time of the initial patient's management. In such circumstances, the link between pulmonary hypertension and left heart disease can be suspected on the basis of left heart abnormalities on CT scans. Specific mention should be made for the late diagnosis of some congenital cardiac diseases, such as atrial septal defects, patent ductus arteriosus and partial anomalous pulmonary venous return, which may become clinically symptomatic in adulthood secondary to the development of pulmonary hypertension. Consequently, it is worth analyzing the cardiac cavities when performing a chest CT examination for a patient referred for pulmonary hypertension of unknown etiology with specific attention directed toward the anatomy of the interatrial septum and pulmonary vein connections and a search for patent ductus arteriosus. The largest subgroup to consider comprises disorders for which pulmonary hypertension can be complicated by right heart dysfunction as observed with idiopathic and familial hypertension, hypertension associated with collagen vascular disease, most chronic lung diseases and hypoxemia, and specific etiologies such as sarcoidosis. In this subgroup, the functional capacity of the right ventricle is a major prognostic determinant in pulmonary hypertension. Estimation of right ventricular function follows the same technical principles as those developed for acute pulmonary embolism. Lastly, one should quote several specific situations: (1) the specific myocardial involvement observed in systemic sclerosis and sarcoidosis; (2) the cardiac origin of COPD exacerbations; (3) the presence of cardiovascular comorbidities, such as those reported in patients with COPD and sleep apnea syndromes.

Table 10.3. Revised clinical classification of pulmonary hypertension (VENICE 2003) (from SIMONNEAU et al. 2004)

1. Pulmonary arterial hypertension (PAH)
- 1.1. Idiopathic (IPAH)
- 1.2. Familial (FPAH)
- 1.3. Associated with (APAH)
  - 1.3.1. Collagen vascular disease
  - 1.3.2. Congenital systemico-to-pulmonary shunts
  - 1.3.3. Portal hypertension
  - 1.3.4. HIV infection
  - 1.3.5. Drugs and toxins
  - 1.3.6. Other (thyroid disorders, glycogen storage disease, Gaucher disease, hereditary hemorrhagic telangiectasis, hemoglobinopathies, myeloproliferative disorders, splenectomy)
- 1.4. Associated with significant venous or capillary involvement
  - 1.4.1. Pulmonary veno-occlusive disease (PVOD)
  - 1.4.2. Pulmonary capillary hemangiomatosis (PCH)
- 1.5. Persistent pulmonary hypertension of the newborn

2. Pulmonary hypertension with left heart disease
- 2.1. Left-sided atrial or ventricular heart disease
- 2.2. Left-sided valvular heart disease

3. Pulmonary hypertension associated with lung diseases and/or hypoxemia
- 3.1. Chronic obstructive pulmonary disease
- 3.2. Interstitial lung disease
- 3.3. Sleep-disordered breathing
- 3.4. Alveolar hypoventilation disorders
- 3.5. Chronic exposure to high altitude
- 3.6. Development abnormalities

4. Pulmonary hypertension due to chronic thrombotic and/or embolic disease
- 4.1. Thromboembolic obstruction of proximal pulmonary arteries
- 4.2. Thromboembolic obstruction of distal pulmonary arteries
- 4.3. Non-thrombotic pulmonary embolism (tumor, parasites, foreign material)

5. Miscellaneous

Sarcoïdosis, histiocytosis X, lymphangiomatosis, compression of pulmonary vessels (adenopathy, tumor, fibrosing mediastinitis)

In addition to the recognition of the etiology of pulmonary hypertension, there is a need for improvement in the noninvasive depiction of pulmonary hypertension. Recently, it has been shown that criteria derived from right ventricle morphology can be used to estimate noninvasively the level of pulmonary artery pressure. Using MRI, SABA et al. (2002) have reported that a calculated ventricular mass index could provide an accurate and practical means of estimating pulmonary artery pressure in pulmonary hypertension. These authors suggested that MRI could provide a reliable assessment of long-term disease progression and response to treatment because ventricular mass will not respond to transient changes in pulmonary artery pressure. Using MDCT, a similar approach for subsequent depiction of pulmonary artery hypertension can be followed by studying pulmonary artery wall distensibility. Investigating a cohort of 45 patients, Revel et al. (2008a) have shown that right pulmonary artery distensibility was an accurate predictor for PHT on ECG-gated 64-slice MDCT scans of the chest. Its diagnostic value was found to be superior to that of the single measurement of pulmonary trunk diameter.

10.1.4 Pericardial Abnormalities Associated with Pulmonary Arterial Hypertension

Several studies have already shown that asymptomatic pericardial effusion is associated with both idiopathic and secondary forms of pulmonary hypertension (Park et al. 1989; Bacque-Juston et al. 1999; Raymond et al. 2002; Fischer et al. 2007). However, little is known about the pathophysiologic mechanism of pericardial effusion in the presence of pulmonary hypertension. One hypothesis is that increased right atrial pressure could contribute to the production of pericardial fluid via the direct drainage of some cardiac veins into the right atrium (Bacque-Juston et al. 1999). Alternatively, pericardial fluid accumulation could be a passive transudative process resulting from increased pulmonary artery pressure (Gibson and Segal 1978).

10.1.5 Foramen Ovale Patency (FOP)

Foramen ovale patency is due to the incomplete closure of the interatrial septum at birth. Based on autopsy studies, frequency is around 27% in the general population and decreases with age, from 34% in patients less than 30 years to 20% at 90 years (Hagen et al. 1984). Patients with chronic obstructive pulmonary disease have an increased frequency of FOP because they have increased right atrial pressure, compared to controls (Soliman et al. 1999). FOP is a factor of impairment in these patients because it contributes to chronic hypoxemia (Hacievliyagil et al. 2006).The gold standard technique for diagnosing FOP is transesophageal echocardiography (TEE) (Schneider et al. 1996), which is superior to transthoracic echocardiography, although it is less well tolerated. The reported proportion of unsuccessful TEE is 1.9% in a large multicentric study including 10,419 examinations (Daniel et al. 1991). Moreover, TEE has certain contraindications, especially history of dysphagia, current pathologic conditions of the esophagus, esophageal varices, and recent esophageal operations. Because TEE is not possible in all patients, there is the need for alternative, less invasive diagnostic modalities. Magnetic resonance imaging (MRI) has been evaluated in comparison with TEE, with a large range in the reported sensitivities varying from 19 to 100% (Mohrs et al. 2005; Nusser et al. 2006). In a recent study, Revel et al. (2008b) have investigated non-gated MSCT for the detection of patent foramen ovale (PFO) and atrial septum aneurysm (ASA) in comparison to transesophageal echocardiography (TEE) in patients with recent stroke (Fig. 10.6). These authors have found that MSCT allowed visual assessment of PFO with 96% specificity and an overall sensitivity of 55%, ranging from 28% in grade 1 shunts to 91% in grade 4 shunts. Sensitivity for detection of ASA is only 11%, making MSCT inappropriate for evaluating the risk of stroke recurrence. Because of its better tolerance compared to TEE, MSCT could be used for the detection of high-grade shunts, especially in the investigation

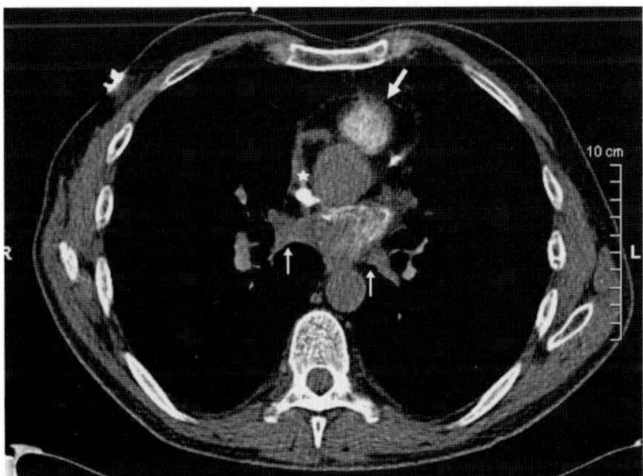

Fig. 10.6. Diagnosis of patent foramen ovale using 64-multidetector-row CT. Early left atrium enhancement (*double arrow*) is present on visual assessment. Contrast enhancement is also observed in the pulmonary trunk (*large single arrow*), but not in the pulmonary veins (*small single arrow*). The *star* indicates the presence of contrast medium in the lower part of the superior vena cava. Transesophageal echocardiography demonstrated a grade 4 patent foramen ovale

of unexplained hypoxemia as CT evaluation of lung parenchyma is part of the usual diagnostic workup in patients with such symptoms.

10.2 Hereditary Hemorrhagic Telangiectasia (HHT)

HHT is characterized clinically by recurrent epistaxis, mucocutaneous telangiectases, and visceral arteriovenous malformations. More than 20% of patients with HHT develop pulmonary arteriovenous malformations (PAVMs), ranging from diffuse PAVMs to large complex structures (Shovlin and Letarte 1999). Whereas PAVMs per se are not directly responsible for cardiac impairment, the concurrent presence of diffuse hepatic arteriovenous malformations may result in high-output congestive heart failure (Bernard et al. 1993; Stocks et al. 1999; Chavan et al. 2004). In the liver, the arteriovenous shunts are often numerous and may exist between the hepatic arterial branches and branches of the hepatic and portal veins. The superior and inferior mesenteric arteries and the left gastric artery, as well as direct collaterals of the aorta, are other potential arterial feeders. Possible therapeutic options of symptomatic patients include surgical ligation or transcatheter embolization of the feeding arteries with subsequent decrease in cardiac output. When pulmonary arteriovenous malformations are seen with the concurrent presence of symptomatic hepatic malformations, liver treatment is recommended prior to PAVM occlusion. The technical procedure and therapeutic results are facilitated by cardiac output normalization and subsequent reduction in the pulmonary arterial blood flow. Cardiac dysfunction in the clinical context of HHT can also be observed as a consequence of longstanding pulmonary arterial hypertension. This rare association between HHT and pulmonary arterial hypertension occurs predominantly in hereditary hemorrhagic telangiectasia type 2 (HHT2) in which mutations in ALK1, i.e., activin receptor-like kinase 1, are seen (Harrison et al. 2003). A few cases of HHT and pulmonary hypertension have also been reported in hereditary hemorrhagic telangiectasia type 1 (HHT1), the latter being linked to mutations in ENG, i.e., endoglin (Chaouat et al. 2004; Mache et al. 2008).

10.3 Diseases of Pulmonary Veins

Partial anomalous pulmonary venous connections are congenital anomalies in which one or more of the pulmonary veins drain into the right atrium or one of its tributaries instead of the left atrium, thus creating a left-to-right shunt. Most cases involve the right lung; most cases of right partial anomalous pulmonary venous return connect the superior vena cava or right atrium (Hijii et al. 1998). These malformations are often associated with other congenital heart defects, especially atrial septal defect. Depending on the magnitude of the left-to-right shunt, cardiomegaly can be depicted on CT scans as a consequence of right heart overload (Haramati et al. 2003). As previously emphasized, it is possible that the partial anomalous pulmonary venous return may not be clinically important. However, in patients with this anomaly in combination with lung cancer, this may present some serious problems. Black et al. (1992) reported a patient with fatal right heart failure after right pneumonectomy for lung cancer with a missed controlateral partial anomalous pulmonary venous return. When the anomaly is present in the other lobe, major lung resection (especially pneumonectomy) for lung cancer can result in acute right heart failure due to increased shunting through the anomalous venous return. Consequently, it has been recently advocated that the partial anomalous venous return should be corrected before lung resection, especially if major lung resection is considered, to prevent fatal postoperative heart failure (Sakurai et al. 2005).

From a practical standpoint, one can exemplify a few situations illustrating the clinical impact of an anomalous pulmonary venous return depending on its functional importance. A partial anomalous pulmonary venous return involving one pulmonary vein corresponds to a left-to-right shunt representing approximately 25% of the cardiac output. In a subject devoid of any respiratory disease, this shunt will have no cardiac consequences. In a patient presenting with controlateral extensive lung parenchymal disease, such as atelectasis, or pneumonia, there will be a redistribution of pulmonary blood flow towards the anomalous venous return, which will subsequently increase the importance of the left-to-right shunt. A partial anomalous pulmonary venous return involving two pulmonary veins corresponds to a left-to-right shunt representing approximately

50% of the cardiac output. This shunt is not only responsible for cardiac dysfunction, but it represents a high-risk situation in case of contralateral lung resection.

10.4 Diseases of the Systemic Circulation

Cardiac complications can be observed in the context of pulmonary sequestrations, rare congenital malformations of the lung characterized by a pulmonary lobe or segment that receives its blood supply directly from the aorta. The venous drainage of an intralobar sequestration invariably occurs via the pulmonary veins, thus producing a left-to-left shunt. The venous drainage of an extralobar pulmonary sequestration usually runs via the systemic venous system (inferior vana cava, azygos, hemiazygos or portal vein), creating a left-to-right shunt. Cardiac complications of pulmonary sequestrations may be caused by the high cardiac output, the diastolic volume overload to the left ventricle caused by the left-to-right shunt through the pulmonary sequestration, or both (Marti et al. 2001). The magnitude of the shunt influences the moment of appearance of cardiac symptoms and thus the time of diagnosis, most often made during childhood rather than in adults. The clinical benefit of MDCT in the diagnosis of bronchopulmonary sequestrations has recently been emphasized, enabling a noninvasive depiction of all the anatomical components of the malformation (Ahmed et al. 2004).

Cardiac symptoms may also reveal a rare form of pulmonary sequestration in which a pulmonary segment is supplied by a coronary artery. In such circumstances, myocardial ischemia caused by vasospasm and stealing from the coronary circulation may lead to the diagnosis of this entity. Until now, cross-sectional imaging has been mostly used to recognize lung parenchymal abnormalities, while depiction of the abnormal coronary supply has relied on coronary angiography (Silverman et al. 1994; Bertsch et al. 1999; Nakayama et al. 2000; Tsitouridis et al. 2005). It is likely that the most recent generations of MDCT scanners will allow the simultaneous depiction of the sequestrated lung and its systemic supply from the coronary circulation on the basis of ECG-gated acquisitions.

The shunting of blood flow from the coronary to the bronchial or pulmonary arterial circulation can deprive the myocardium of a considerable amount of its blood supply, and thus is responsible for a "coronary steal syndrome." The occurrence of an angina-like chest pain can be observed in patients with normal coronary arteries in whom coronary-to-bronchial artery anastomoses or shunts between coronary, bronchial, and pulmonary arteries have developed. Table 10.4 summarizes the diseases in which stealing from the coronary circulation can be observed.

Table 10.4. Diseases potentially associated with a coronary steal syndrome (from Matsunaga et al. 1993; Kochiadakis et al. 2002)

- Chronic pulmonary inflammatory diseases
- Bronchiectasis
- Chronic pulmonary thromboembolism
- Takayasu arteritis
- Behcet's disease
- Pulmonary sequestrations
- Unilateral absence of a pulmonary artery
- Congenital heart diseases with decreased pulmonary flow
- Primary tumors of a pulmonary artery

References

d'Agostino AG, Remy-Jardin M, Khalil C, Delannoy-Deken V, Flohr T, Duhamel A, Remy J (2006) Low-dose ECG-gated 64-slice helical CT angiography of the chest: evaluation of image quality in 105 patients. Eur Radiol 16:2137–2146

Ahmed M, Jacobi V, Vogl TJ (2004) Multislice CT and CT angiography for noninvasive evaluation of bronchopulmonary sequestration. Eur Radiol 14:2141–2143

Araoz PA, Gotway MB, Harrington JR, Harmsen WS, Mandrekar JN (2007) Pulmonary embolism: prognostic CT findings. Radiology 242:889–897

Araoz PA, Gotway MB, Trowbridge RL et al. (2003) Helical CT pulmonary angiography predictors of in-hospital morbidity and mortality in patients with acute pulmonary embolism. J Thorac Imaging 18:207–215

Bacque-Juston MC, Wells AU, Hansell DM (1999) Pericardial thickening or effusion in patients with pulmonary artery hypertension: a CT study. AJR 172:361–364

Bernard G, Mion F, Henry L, Plauchu H, Paliard P (1993) Hepatic involvement in hereditary hemorrhagic telangiectasia: clinical, radiological and hemodynamic studies in 11 cases. Gastroenterology 105:482–487

Bertsch G, Market T, Hahn D, Silber RE, Schanzenbächer P (1999) Intralobar lung sequestration with systemic coronary arterial supply. Eur Radiol 9:1324–1326

Black MD, Shamji FM, Golstein W, Sachs HJ (1992) Pulmonary resection and controlateral anomalous drainage: a lethal combination. Ann Thorac Surg 53:689–691

Bootsveld A, Puetz J, Grube E (2004) Incidental finding of a papillary elastoma on the aortic valve in 16-slice multidetector row computed tomography. Heart 90:e35

Bruzzi JF, Remy-Jardin M, Delhaye D, Teisseire A, Khalil C, Remy J (2006a) When, why and how to examine the heart during thoracic CT: Part 1, basic principles. AJR 186:324–332

Bruzzi JF, Remy-Jardin M, Delhaye D, Teisseire A, Khalil C, Remy J (2006b) When, why and how to examine the heart during thoracic CT: Part 2, clinical applications. AJR 186:333–341

Burgess MI, Bright-Thomas RJ (2002) Echocardiographic evaluation of right ventricular function. Eur J Echocardiography 3:252–262

Chaouat A, Coulet F, Simonneau G, Weitzenblum E, Soubrier F, Humbert M (2004) Endoglin germline mutation in a patient with hereditary haemorrhagic telangiectasia and dexfenfluramine associated pulmonary arterial hypertension. Thorax 59:446–448

Chavan A, Caselitz M, Gratz KF, Lotz J, Kirchhoff T, Piso P, Wagner S, Manns M, Galanski M (2004) Hepatic artery embolization for treatment of patients with hereditary hemorrhagic telangiectasis and symptomatic hepatic vascular malformations. Eur Radiol 14:2079–2085

Chow LC, Dittrich HC, Hoit BD et al. (1988) Doppler assessment in right-sided cardiac hemodynamics after pulmonary thromboendarterectomy. Am J Cardiol 61:1092–1097

Coche E, Vlassenbroeck A, Roelants V, D'Hoore W, Verschuren F, Goncette L, Maldague B (2005) Evaluation of biventricular ejection fraction with ECG-gated 16-slice CT: preliminary findings in acute pulmonary embolism in comparison with radionuclide ventriculography. Eur Radiol 15:1432–1440

Collomb D, Paramelle PJ, Calaque O, Bosson JL, Vanzetto G, Barnoud D, Pison C, Coulomb M, Ferretti G (2003) Severity assessment of acute pulmonary embolism. Eur Radiol 13:1508–1514

Contractor S, Maldjian PD, Sharma VK, Gor DM (2002) Role of helical CT in detecting right ventricular dysfunction secondary to acute pulmonary embolism. J Comput Assist Tomogr 26:587–591

Daniel WG, Erbel R, Kasper W et al. (1991) Safety of transesophageal echocardiography. A multicenter survey of 10,419 examinations. Circulation 83:817–821

Delhaye D, Remy-Jardin M, Faivre JB, Deken V, Duhamel A, Remy J (2008) Tricuspid annular displacement: a new indicator of right ventricular function on MDCT scans? Eur Radiol (P):212 (abstract B-321)

Delhaye D, Remy-Jardin M, Teisseire A, Hossein-Foucher C, Leroy S, Duhamel A, Remy J (2006) MDCT of right ventricular function: comparison of right ventricular ejection fraction estimation and equilibrium radionuclide ventriculography. AJR 187:1597–1604

Delhaye D, Remy-Jardin M, Salem R, Teisseire A, Khalil C, Delannoy-Deken V, Duhamel A, Remy J (2007) Coronary imaging quality in routine ECG-gated multidetector CT examinations of the entire thorax: preliminary experience with a 64-slice CT system in 133 patients. Eur Radiol 17:902–910

Dittrich HC, Nicod PH, Chow LC et al. (1988) Early changes in right heart geometry after pulmonary thromboendarterectomy. J Am Coll Cardiol 11:937–943

Dodd JD, Souza CA, Muller NL (2006) High-resolution MDCT of pulmonary septic embolism: evaluation of the feeding vessel sign. AJR 187:623–629

Dogan H, Kroft LJM, Bax JJ, Schuijf JD, van der Geest RJ, Doornbos J, de Roos A (2006) MDCT assessment of right ventricular systolic function. AJR 186:S366–S370

Dogan H, Kroft LJM, Huisman MV, van der Geest RJ, de Roos A (2007) Right ventricular function in patients with acute pulmonary embolism: analysis with electrocardiography-synchronized multidetector row CT. Radiology 242:78–84

Dumont E, Racine N, Ugolini P, Carrier M, Pellerin M, Perrault LP (2002) Paradoxical cerebral emboli of hypernephroma to the right ventricle five years after primary tumor resection. J Thorac Cardiovasc Surg 123:572–573

Fellah L, Waignein F, Wittebole X, Coche E (2007) Combined assessment of tricuspid valve endocarditis and pulmonary septic embolism with ECG-gated 40-MDCT of the whole chest. AJR 189:W228–W230

Ferrari E, Benhamou M, Berthier F, Baudouy M (2005) Mobile thrombi of the right heart in pulmonary embolism. Delayed disappearance after thrombolytic treatment. Chest 127:1051–1053

Fischer A, Misumi S, Curran-Everett D, Meehan RT et al. (2007) Pericardial abnormalities predict the presence of echocardiographically defined pulmonary arterial hypertension in systemic sclerosis-related interstitial lung disease. Chest 131:988–992

Forfia PR, Fisher MR, Mathai SC et al. (2006) Tricuspid annular displacement predicts survival in pulmonary hypertension. Am J Respir Crit Care Med 174:1034–1041

Ghaye B, Ghuysen A, Willems V, Lambermont B, Gerard P, D'Orio V, Gevenois PA, Dondelinger RF (2006) Severe pulmonary embolism: pulmonary artery clot load scores and cardiovascular parameters as predictors of mortality. Radiology 239:884–891

Ghuysen A, Ghaye B, Willems V, Lambermont B, Gerard P, Dondelinger RF, d'Orio V (2005) Computed tomographic pulmonary angiography and prognostic significance in patients with acute pulmonary embolism. Thorax 60:956–961

Gibson AT, Segal MB (1978) A study of the composition of pericardial fluid with special reference to the probable mechanism of fluid accumulation. J Physiol 277:367–377

Hacievliyagil SS, Gunen H, Kosar FM, Sahin I, Kilic T (2006) Prevalence and clinical significance of a patent foramen ovale in patients with chronic obstructive pulmonary disease. Respir Med 100:903–910

Hagen PT, Scholz DG, Edwards WD (1984) Incidence and size of patent foramen ovale during the first 10 decades of life: an autopsy study of 965 normal hearts. Mayo Clin Proc 59:17–20

Haramati LB, Moche IE, Rivera VT, Patel PV, Heyneman L, McAdams P, Issenberg HJ, White CS (2003) Computed tomography of partial anomalous pulmonary venous connection in adults. J Comput Assist Tomogr 27:743–749

Harrison RE, Flanagan JA, Sankelo M, Abdalla SA, Rowell J, Machado RD, Elliot CG, Robbins IM, Olschewski H, McLaughlin V, Gruenig E, Kermeen F, Laitinen T, Morell NW, Trembath RC (2003) Molecular and functional analysis identifies ALK-1 as the predominant cause of pulmonary hypertension related to hereditary haemorrhagic telangiectasia. J Med Genet 40:865–871

Hauret L, Minvielle F, Lévêque C, Jeanbourquin D, Cordoliani YS (2000) Métastases néoplasiques intrartérielles pulmonaires. J Radiol 81:807–809

He H, Stein MW, Zalta B, Haramati LB (2006) Computed tomography evaluation of right heart dysfunction in patients with acute pulmonary embolism. J Comput Assist Tomogr 30:262–266

Hijii T, Fukushige J, Hara T (1998) Diagnosis and management of partial anomalous pulmonary venous connections. Cardiology 89:148–151

Jamieson SW, Auger WR, Fedullo PF et al. (1993) Experience and results in 150 pulmonary thromboendarterectomy operations over 29-month period. J Thorac Cardiovasc Surg 106:116–127

Kim TH, Ryu YH, Hur J, Kim SJ, Kim HS, Choi BW, Kim Y, Kim HJ (2005) Evaluation of right ventricular volume and mass using retrospective ECG-gated cardiac multidetector computed tomography: comparison with first-pass radionuclide angiography. Eur Radiol 15:1987–1993

Kochiadakis GE, Chrysostomakis SI, Igoumenidis NE, Skalidis EI, Vardas PE (2002) Anomalous collateral from the coronary artery to the affected lung in a case of congenital absence of the left pulmonary. Effect on coronary circulation. Chest 121:2063–2066

Lamia B, Teboul JL, Monnet X, Richard C, Chemla D (2007) Relationship between the tricuspid annular plane excursion and right and left ventricular function in critically-ill patients. Intensive Care Med 33:2143–2149

Lembcke A, Dohmen PM, Dewey M, Klessen C, Elgeti T, Hermann KGA, Konertz WF, Hamm B, Kivelitz DE (2005) Multislice computed tomography for preoperative evaluation of right ventricular volumes and function: comparison with magnetic resonance imaging. Ann Thorac Surg 79:1344–1351

Lu MT, Cai T, Ersoy H, Whitmore AG, Quiroz R, Goldhaber SZ, Rybicki FJ (2008) Interval increase in right-left ventricular diameter ratios at CT as a predictor of 30-day mortality after acute pulmonary embolism: Initial experience. Radiology 246:281–287

Mache CJ, Gamillscheg A, Popper HH, Haworth SG (2008) Early-life pulmonary arterial hypertension with subsequent development of diffuse pulmonary arteriovenous malformations in hereditary haemorrhagic telangiectasia. Thorax 63:85–86

Marti V, Pujadas S, Casan P, Garcia J, Guiteras P, Auge JM (2001) Reversible dilated cardiomyopathy after lobectomy for pulmonary sequestration. J Thorac Cardiovasc Surg 121:1001–1002

Matsunaga N, Hayashi K, Sakamoto I, Ogawa Y, Matsuoka Y, Imamura T, Kuriya T (1993) Coronary-to-pulmonary artery shunts via the bronchial artery: analysis of cineangiographic studies. Radiology 186:877–882

McCoskey EH, Mehta JB, Krishnan K, Roy TM (2000) Right atrial myxoma with extracardiac manifestations. Chest 118:547–549

Menzel T, Wagner S, Kramm T, Mohr-Kahaly S, Mayer E, Braeuninger S, Meyer J (2000) Pathophysiology of impaired right and left ventricular function in chronic pulmonary hypertension. Changes after pulmonary thromboendarterectomy. Chest 118:897–903

Mohrs OK, Petersen SE, Erkapic D et al. (2005) Diagnosis of patent foramen ovale using contrast-enhanced dynamic MRI: a pilot study. AJR 184:234–240

Nakayama Y, Kido M, Minami K, Ikeda M, Kato Y (2000) Pulmonary sequestration with myocardial ischemia caused by vasospasm and steal. Ann Thorac Surg 70:304–305

Nusser T, Hoher M, Merkle N, Grebe OC, Spiess J, Kestler HA, Rasche V, Kochs M, Hombach V, Wohrle J (2006) Cardiac magnetic resonance imaging and transesophageal echocardiography in patients with transcatheter closure of patent foramen ovale. J Am Coll Cardiol 48:322–329

Oliver TB, Reid JH, Murchison JT (1998) Interventricular septal shift due to massive pulmonary embolism shown by CT pulmonary angiography: an old sign revisited. Thorax 53:1092–1094

Park B, Dittrich HC, Polikar R et al. (1989) Echocardiographic evidence of pericardial effusion in severe chronic pulmonary hypertension. Am J Cardiol 63:143–145

Parsons AM, Detterbeck FC (2003) Multifocal right atrial myxoma and pulmonary embolism. Ann Thorac Surg 75:1323–1324

Quiroz R, Kucher N, Schoepf UJ et al. (2004) Right ventricular enlargement on chest computed tomography: prognostic role in acute pulmonary embolism. Circulation 109:2401–2404

Raymond RJ, Hinderliter AL, Willis PW et al. (2002) Echocardiographic predictors of adverse outcomes in primary pulmonary hypertension. J Am Coll Cardiol 39:1214–1219

Reesink HJ, Marcus JT, Tulevski II, Jamieson S, Kloek JJ, Noordegraaf AV, Bresser P (2007) Reverse right ventricular remodelling after pulmonary endarterectmy in patients with chronic thromboembolic pulmonary hypertension: Utility of magnetic resonance imaging to demonstrate restoration of the right ventricle. J Thorac Cardiovasc Surg 133:58–64

Reid JH, Murchison JT (1998) Acute right ventricular dilatation: a new helical CT sign of massive pulmonary embolism. Clin Radiol 53:694–698

Remy-Jardin M, Pistolesi M, Goodman LR, Gefter WB, Gottschalk A, Mayo J, Sostman HD (2007) Management of suspected acute pulmonary embolism in the era of CT angiography: A statement of the Fleischner Society. Radiology 245:315–329

Revel MP, Faivre JB, Letourneau T, Henon H, Leys D, Delannoy-Deken V, Duhamel A, Remy-Jardin M, Remy J (2008b) Detection of patent foramen ovale by 64-slice multidetector-row CT. Radiology (in press)

Revel MP, Faivre JB, Remy-Jardin M, Delannoy-Deken V, Duhamel A, Remy J (2008a) ECG-gated 64-slice Multi-Detector CT Angiography of the Chest: Evaluation of new functional parameters as diagnostic criteria of Pulmonary Hypertension? Radiology (in press)

Rose PS, Punjabi NM, Pearse DB (2002) Treatment of right heart thromboemboli. Chest 121:806–814

Saba TS, Foster J, Cockburn M, Cowan M, Peacock AJ (2002) Ventricular mass index using magnetic resonance imaging accurately estimates pulmonary artery pressure. Eur Respir J 20:1519–1524

Sakurai H, Kondo H, Sekiguchi A, Naruse Y, Makuuchi H, Suzuki K, Asamura H, Tsuchiya R (2005) Left pneumonectomy for lung cancer after correction of contralateral partial anomalous pulmonary venous return. Ann Thorac Surg 79:1778–1780

Salem R, Remy-Jardin M, Delhaye D, Khalil C, Teisseire A, Delannoy-Deken V, Duhamel A, Remy J (2006) Integrated cardiothoracic imaging with ECG-gated 64-slice multidetector-row CT: initial findings in 133 patients. Eur Radiol 16:1973–1981

Schneider B, Zienkiewicz T, Jansen V, Hofmann T, Noltenius H, Meinertz T (1996) Diagnosis of patent foramen ovale by transesophageal echocardiography and correlation with autopsy findings. Am J Cardiol 77:1202–1209

Schoepf UJ, Kucher N, Kipfmueller F et al. (2004) Right ventricular enlargement on chest computed tomography: a predictor of early death in acute pulmonary embolism. Circulation 110:3276–3280

Shovlin CL, Letarte M (1999) Hereditary haemorrhagic telangiectasia and pulmonary arteriovenous malformations: issues in clinical management and review of pathogenic mechanisms. Thorax 54:714–729

Silverman ME, White CS, Ziskind AA (1994) Pulmonary sequestration receiving arterial supply from the left circumflex coronary artery. Chest 106:948–949

Simonneau G, Galie N, Rubin LJ, Langleben D, Seeger W, Domenighetti G, Gibbs S, Lebrec D, Speich R, Beghetti M, Rich S, Fishman A (2004) Clinical classification of pulmonary hypertension. J Am Coll Cardiol 43:5S–12S

Soliman A, Shanoudy H, Liu J, Russell DC, Jarmukli NF (1999) Increased prevalence of patent foramen ovale in patients with severe chronic obstructive pulmonary disease. J Am Soc Echocardiogr 12:99–105

Stockx L, Raat H, Caerts B, van Cutsem E, Wilms G, Marchal G (1999) Transcatheter embolization of hepatic arteriovenous fistulas in Rendu-Osler-Weber disease: a case report and review of the literature. Eur Radiol 9:1434–1437

Task Force for the Diagnosis and Management of Acute Pulmonary Embolism of the European Society of Cardiology (ESC) (2008) Guidelines on diagnosis and management of acute pulmonary embolism. Eur Heart J (in press)

Tsitouridis I, Tsinoglou K, Cheva A, Papapostolou P, Efthimiou D, Moschialos L (2005) Intralobar pulmonary sequestration with arterial supply from the coronary circulation. J Thorac Imaging 20:313–315

Van der Meer RW, Pattynama PMT, van Strijen MJL, van den Berg-Huijsmans AA, Hartmann IJC, Putter H, de Roos A, Huisman MV (2005) Right ventricular dysfunction and pulmonary obstruction index at helical CT: prediction of clinical outcome during 3-month follow-up in patients with acute pulmonary embolism. Radiology 235:789–803

Wanatabe SI, Shimokawa S, Sakasegawa KI, Masuda H, Sakata R, Higashi M (2002) Choriocarcinoma in the pulmonary artery treated by emergency pulmonary embolectomy. Chest 121:654–656

Willmann J, Weishaupt D, Lacaht M et al. (2002) Electrographically gated multidetector row CT for assessment of valvular morphology and calcification in aortic stenosis. Radiology 225:120–128

Wong PS, Aye WMM, Lee CN (2004) Pulmonary tumor embolism secondary to osteosarcoma. Ann Thorac Surg 77:341

COPD and Cardiac Comorbidities

11

Jacques Rémy, Anne-Lise Hachulla, and Jean-Baptiste Faivre

CONTENTS

J. Rémy, MD
Professor, Department of Thoracic Imaging, C.H.R.U. de Lille, Hôpital Calmette, Boulevard du Prof. J. Leclercq, 59037 Lille Cédex, France
A.-L. Hachulla, MD
J.-B. Faivre, MD
Department of Thoracic Imaging, University Center of Lille, Boulevard du Prof. J. Leclercq, 59037 Lille Cédex, France

In the last few years, chronic obstructive pulmonary disease (COPD) has been considered as a simultaneous disorder of both the cardio-vascular and the respiratory systems in which cardio-vascular co-morbidities and non-fatal coronary events increase when respiratory function decreases. The main purposes of the following chapter will be to summarize the new concepts of COPD, its cardiac comorbidities and the new technological breakthrough allowing a common approach to CT and to analyze its related cardio-vascular disorders related to pulmonary hypertension, right cardiac cavities, left heart, coronary arteries and coincidental cardio-vascular diseases, having a potential impact on the COPD diagnosis or treatment.

11.1 COPD, Heart and Systemic Vessels: A Disease Prototype for Integrated Cardiothoracic Imaging

11.1.1 Definitions New Concepts of COPD and Cardio-Vascular Comorbidities

According to the Global Initiative for Chronic Obstructive Lung Disease (GOLD), chronic obstructive pulmonary disease (COPD) is now defined as "a preventable and treatable disease ... with significant extrapulmonary effects ... and comorbidities characterized by airflow limitation that is not fully reversible ... usually progressive and associated with an abnormal inflammatory response ..." (Rabe et al. 2007). The clinical indicators for considering a diagnosis of COPD in individuals over age 40 are dyspnea, chronic cough, chronic sputum production and a history of exposure to risk factors, especially tobacco smoke, occupational dusts and chemicals, smoke from home cooking and heating fuels (Rabe et al.2007). Its spirometric classification into four stages is based on forced expiratory volume in 1 s (FEV1) and forced vital capacity (FEV1/FVC). Stage I (mild COPD) corresponds to mild airflow limitation (FEV1/FVC < 0.70; FEV1 ≥ 80% predicted) with chronic cough and sputum production. Stage II (moderate COPD), with FEV1/FVC < 0.70; 50% < FEV1 < 80% predicted, is characterized by cough and sputum production with shortness of breath on exertion. It is the stage at which patients consult. Stage III is severe COPD with FEV1/FVC < 0.70 and 30% ≤ FEV1 < 50% predicted. Stage IV is very severe COPD with the same spirometry as stage III plus chronic respiratory failure with gazometric impact or right heart failure.

Before the 2007 spirometric classification, the first one published in 2001 (Pauwels et al. 2001) included a stage 0 of patients at risk with chronic symptoms (cough, sputum production) and normal spirometry. This category of patients corresponds to healthy smokers in whom an incidental CT scan of the thorax can find COPD lesions. Unfortunately, stage 0 has been removed from the 2007 classification. There was also an intermediary classification for which the stages of severity were renamed in 2003. The global burden of COPD will increase, and the Word Health Organization predicts that COPD will become the third cause of death and the fifth cause of disability. Its socio- and medico-economic impacts are of the utmost importance (Fabbri et al. 2003).

Acute exacerbation of COPD is defined as "an event in the natural course of the disease characterized by a change in the patient's baseline symptoms that is beyond normal day-to-day variations, is acute in onset and may warrant a change in regular medication in a patient with underlying COPD" (Rabe et al. 2007). In 2004, a book entirely dedicated to this topic was published (Siafakas et al. 2004) in which the diseases that provoke, precipitate or mimic an acute exacerbation were summarized (Table 11.1). This table emphasizes the fact that in acute exacerbation a large number of diseases causes increased dyspnea in COPD patients, but are not the causes of it (Hurst and Wedzicha 2007).

Table 11.1. Summary of diseases that provoke, precipitate or mimic an acute exacerbation (Siafakas et al. 2004)

Parenchymal diseases	Pneumoniae and their complications Complicated bullae
Airway diseases	Bronchial carcinoma. Infection of the tracheo-bronchial tree Common pollutants
Cardiac diseases	Congestive cardiac failure. Right heart failure
Lung vessels	Pulmonary hypertension Acute pulmonary embolism Hemoptysis
Pleura	Pleural effusion Pneumothorax
Muscles	Muscular wasting
Mediastinum	Pneumomediastinum

11.1.2 Cardio-Vascular Comorbidities

Over 40% of patients with COPD present comorbid conditions, among which cardio-vascular disorders are frequent. The prevalence of pulmonary embolism in patients hospitalized for acute exacerbation of unknown origin varies from 5 to 25% according to the literature. The worsening of expiratory flow limitation and dynamic hyperinflation has cardio-vascular effects: increased pulmonary arterial pressure, decreased right ventricle preload and increased left ventricle afterload (O'Donnel and Parker 2006).

The GOLD strategy, like multiple other disease-specific guidelines, does not address, in proportion to its frequency, the issue of cardio-vascular comorbidity and does not take into account the concept of cardiothoracic imaging applied to COPD. It has been recently emphasized in an editorial entitled "One heart, two lungs together for ever" (Ceconi et al. 2006), which underlines the high frequency of left ventricular dysfunction in acute exacerbation (Fig. 11.1) and the figure of 20% of unrecognized heart failure in elderly patients with stable COPD. For every 10% decrease in FEV1, cardiovascular mortality increases by 28%, and non-fatal coronary events increase by almost 20% in mild to moderate COPD. In patients with FEV1 <50%, the leading causes of death are predicted to be cardiovascular (Sin and Man 2005). The abnormally functioning lung of COPD has multiple cardiac consequences as demonstrated in Table 11.2 (modified from Rennard 2005).

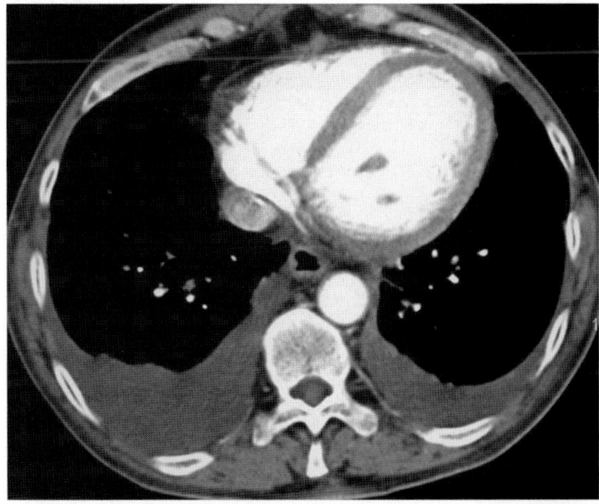

Fig. 11.1. Elderly patient with acute exacerbation of COPD. Pulmonary embolism is suspected because a pleuro-pneumopathy does not correctly respond to antibiotics. The ventricular diameters perpendicular to the interventricular septum are consistent with dilatation of the left ventricle. Associated to bilateral pleural effusions, this left ventricular failure was initially suspected and subsequently confirmed

These four pulmonary pathophysiologic events and their cardio-vascular consequences are increased with exercise.

According to a meta-analysis from a Medline search, the relationship between reduced FEV1 and mortality from ischemic heart disease is striking (Sin et al. 2005). The lung and airway inflammation incite systemic inflammation, which, independent of smoking, can contribute to the progression of atherosclerosis. Low-grade systemic inflammation is a major risk for atherothrombotic plaque genesis, progression and rupture. It is well known that COPD is associated with systemic inflammation (Agusti 2006), but its variation over time and its contribution to the phenotypic characteristic of the disease has not yet been taken into account. Tobacco smoking self-induces systemic inflammation in the absence of COPD, which can contribute to atherosclerosis. Chronic intermittent hypoxia is an expected manifestation of COPD. Pulmonary artery hypertension, absent at rest, may appear during exercise and trigger an intermittent right-to-left shunting through a patent foramen ovale. Experimentally, nine of ten mice exposed to chronic intermittent hypoxia and a high-cholesterol diet developed atherosclerotic lesions (Savransky et al. 2007). The conjunction of stimuli, systemic inflammation and hypoxia-induced atherosclerosis may increase cardio-vascular co-morbidities. Cardiovascular disease in COPD patients may represent a burden greater than that of lung disease itself (Huiart et al. 2005), and it is

Table 11.2. Multiple cardiac consequences of abnormally functioning lung of COPD (modified from Rennard 2005)

Lung dysfunction	Cardiac consequences
Lung hyperinflation	Pulmonary hypertension Decreased RV preload Increased LV afterload
Increased work of breathing	Increased cardiac output
Increased intra-thoracic pressure	Decreased pulmonary venous return LV diastolic dysfunction
Pulmonary hypertension	RV dysfunction

the reason why non-invasive diagnostic strategies should be considered in priority. Left ventricular dysfunction in COPD patients can be attributable to coronary artery disease. Considering a pre-selected group of patients with severe obstructive pattern and after exclusion of known coronary disease, myocardial infarction, cardiomyopathy or vascular disease, the prevalence of significant coronary artery disease is 10.5% (Vizza et al. 1998) in this group. However, in patients with symptomatic deterioration a study found left ventricular dysfunction in 32% of COPD patients (Render et al. 1995). The gap between 10.5% and 32% can be partially explained by two other causes of LV dysfunction: a pre-existent cardio-vascular disease and ventricular independence, which will be reviewed in the following chapters. Increased arterial stiffness increases myocardial oxygen demand and left ventricular afterload. Coronary perfusion is reduced, leading to subendocardial ischemia (Sabit et al. 2007). If there is an evident relationship among the patient's age, stage of COPD and cardiovascular events, this comorbidity should be particularly taken into account prior to surgical treatments (lung transplantation or lung volume reduction surgery). In this high-risk group, the incidence of cardiovascular morbidity after lung volume reduction surgery was recently estimated at 20% (Nauheim et al. 2006).

11.1.3 Technological Impacts of Cardiothoracic Imaging

Cardio-pulmonary interactions are very numerous: embryologic, physiologic, physiopathologic and mechanical. The very fast rotation times of modern CT technologies greatly improve the temporal resolution of cross-sectional and multiplanar imaging. For example, acquisition of the entire thorax with 0.33-s rotation time and a pitch of 1.5 is equivalent to about 165 ms temporal resolution of the reconstructed images. With cardiac gating and single-source CT, the temporal window is also 165 ms (Fig. 11.2). With dual-source CT, it is lowered to 83 ms with cardiac gating, allowing coronary, cardiac and pulmonary imaging with very high cardiac rhythms. The use of both tubes without cardiac gating and with a pitch of 2 has the same temporal resolution (83 ms) and a 3 s acquisition time of the entire thorax (Fig. 11.3). With this technique, the cardiac cavities can be correctly visualized because half the cardiac height is acquired in 0.5 s. In addition, the very short acquisition time of the entire thorax and the monitoring of the contrast bolus in the descending aorta allow for an optimal opacification of all the thoracic vessels and cardiac cavities with only 80 ml contrast medium.

a
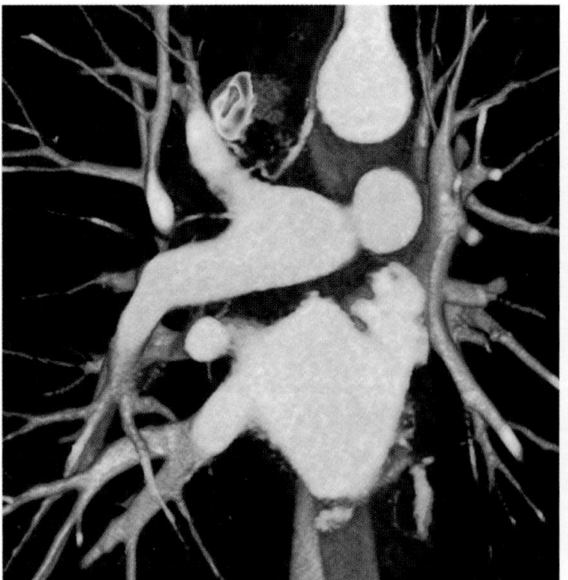
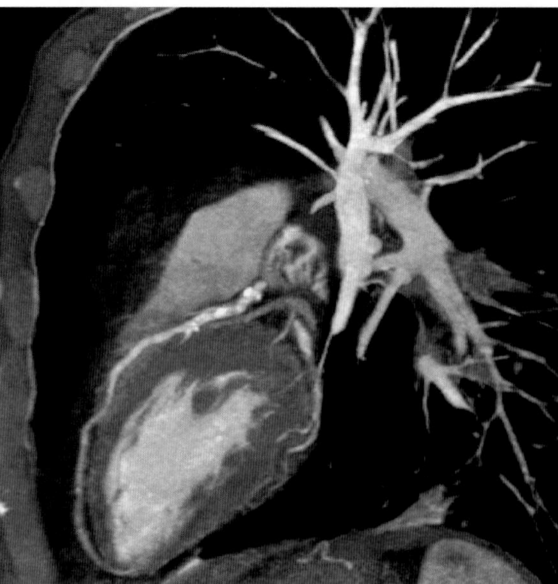
b

Fig. 11.2a,b. Spiral CT angiography performed with cardiac gating in a COPD patient with hemoptysis (temporal resolution: 165 ms). Gating is aimed at precise analysis of the bronchial artery origins. The left subclavian artery origin of the right bronchial artery is precisely demonstrated (**a**). No motion artifact can be identified at the level of the pulmonary artery or aortic arch. The left anterior descending artery is depicted in its entire course on a sagittal planar reformation (**b**)

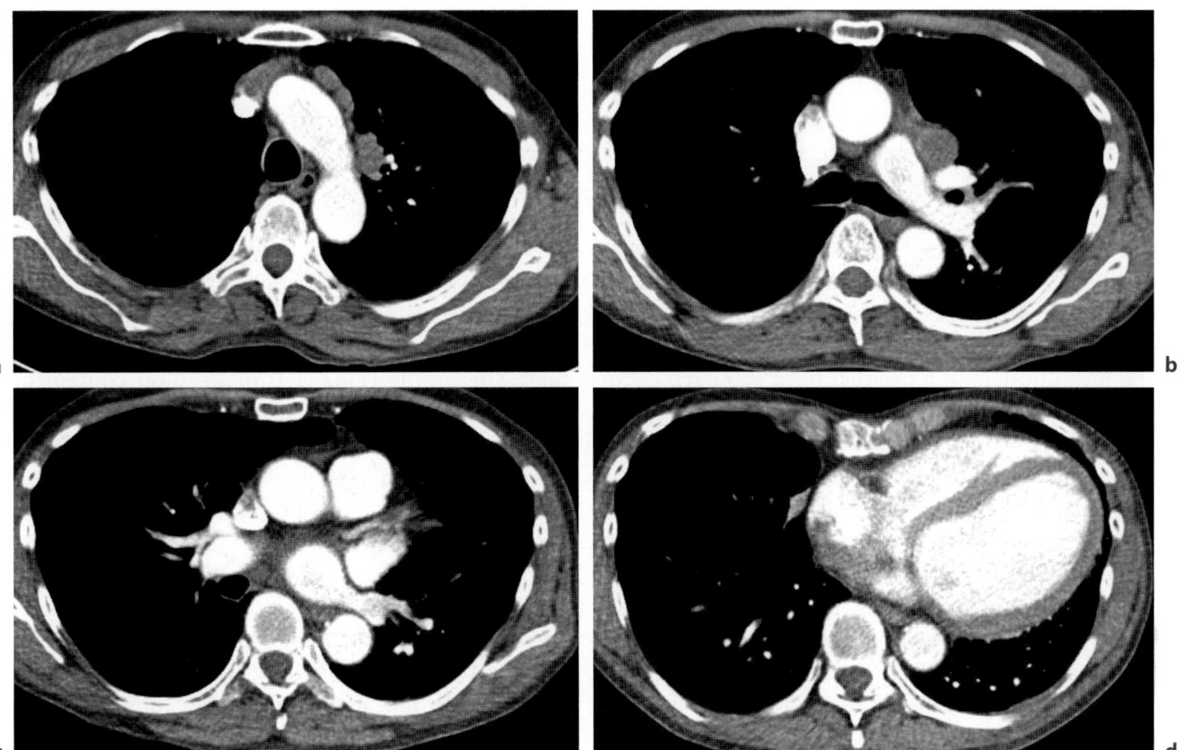

Fig. 11.3a–d. Double source acquisition without cardiac gating or apnea with 100 kV, 90 mAs per tube, care dose 4D, pitch of 2, 80 ml of a 250 mg/ml contrast medium injected at 4 cc/s. The acquisition is triggered at 150 HU in the descending aorta; 75 bpm. DLP: 127 mGycm. The 83-ms temporal resolution allows for an acquisition without motion artifact at the level of the aorta (**a**), pulmonary arteries (**b**,**c**) and right and left ventricles (**d**). No streak artifact from the superior vena cava. Slice thickness: 5 mm

The above-mentioned technical capabilities must be compared to the negative effects of ß blockers on airway responsiveness in COPD patients. In their study, van der Woude et al. (2005) found evidence of the negative effects of ß-blocker treatment on lung function (FEV1) and airway hyper-responsiveness in patients with mild-to-moderate irreversible COPD. Alternatives are some cardio-selective ß blockers, such as celiprolol or metoprolol, which have the least negative consequences on pulmonary function. But with the double-source CT, this drug does not have to be used in the majority of patients.

The breakthrough of new CT technologies counterbalances the limitations of the usual non-invasive cardiac tests in these patients. The stress tests with echocardiography, ECG and nuclear medicine are limited due to the patient inability to perform the necessary efforts. The hypoxic myocardium can keep silent at rest. Marked increase in intrathoracic gas, hyperinflation and alterations in the cardiac position makes Doppler echocardiography frequently inaccurate and leads to overestimation of pulmonary hypertension (Arcasoy et al. 2003). Cardiac catheterization is too invasive to be ethically acceptable. The role of cardiac biomarkers is taken strongly into consideration due to the high prevalence of LV dysfunction in COPD. However, this dysfunction can be present without being the cause of symptoms (Abroug et al. 2006). Finally, the conjunction of these multiple limitations and of the new technological developments of cardiac CT opens new possibilities for cardiothoracic imaging.

If the new CT technologies, in conjunction with the limitations of the non-invasive tests previously mentioned, are the basis for development of cardiothoracic imaging, some considerations about radiation dose must be envisaged. The doses required for morphologic and functional studies of the cardiac cavities are less important than for coronary artery visualization. Nevertheless, this chapter is not dedicated to cardiac CT, which merges as a rapidly developing method of non-invasive cardiac imaging. Its developments can be found elsewhere in this book or in the recent literature (Mahnken et al. 2007). Considering single-source 64-slice helical CT and, apart from patients with bradycardia, the use of cardiac gating of the entire thorax with a pitch of 0.3, adjustment of the mAs setting to the patient size, ECG-controlled dose modulation, no administration of ß blockers, 0.33-s rotation time, 120 KV and 200 mAs, the dose-length product was 260.57±83.67 mGy cm with an estimated average effective dose of 4.95±1.59 mSv (D'Agostino et al. 2006). At the same time and with the same machine, the mean dose length product for a standard CT of the thorax was 200 mGy cm. This low-dose integrated cardiothoracic imaging is able to evaluate right and left ventricular ejection fractions, imaging of the proximal coronary arteries and lung, mediastinum, pleura and chest wall without artifacts in more than 90% of the patients (Salem et al. 2006). With the use of 90 to 120 ml contrast medium, this acquisition obtains sufficient functional and morphologic information in COPD patients for the detection of an unknown cardiac comorbidity. The majority of the previous studies emphasized good correlations with values obtained with MRI (Orakzai et al. 2006), which is not used at a first intention in the management of a COPD patient. Dose performance in double-source CT of the entire thorax with cardiac gating must be evaluated in clinical routine. The technologic factors for dose savings were recently reviewed (Mc Collough et al. 2007). Our first results favor a moderately higher dose for low cardiac rhythms and a lower dose at high rhythms.

With 83 and 165 ms temporal resolution without cardiac gating, using a pitch of 1.5 with single source 64-slice CT and a pitch of 2 with dual-source, coronary calcifications are frequently found in COPD patients. Without the accuracy of well-established calcium scoring techniques, these fast acquisition modes allow for an approximate quantification of the calcifications.

11.1.4 The Opportunity of Developing Biomarkers in Cardiothoracic Imaging

Surrogate markers (parameters that predict the effect of treatment in clinical studies) and imaging biomarkers, providing predictive information on clinical outcome, have gained increasing importance (Rudin 2007). The definition of a biomarker, according to the National Institutes of Health/US Food and Drug Administration, is: "A characteristic that is objectively measured and evaluated as an indicator of normal biological processes, pathogenic processes, or pharmacologic responses to a therapeutic intervention" (Downing 2001). Multiple imaging biomarkers of pulmonary function, such as dynamic imaging, are on the verge of being developed or in clinical evaluation. They can analyze dynamic physiologic processes: ventilation, perfusion, vessels distensibility, ventricular ejection fractions, bronchial reactivity and interventricular septal motion. The iodine (Fig. 11.4) or krypton content of the lung can be depicted with dual-energy CT. The iodine content, similar to perfusion imaging, can be correlated to morphological alterations obtained from the same acquisition (Fig. 11.5). In the very near future, lung microvascular blood flow, myocardial perfusion and cardiac function will be simultaneously analyzed. These new imaging biomarkers are very challenging. They need to be developed in collaboration with industry if the chest radiologists want to take full advantage of their opportunities (Schuster 2007).

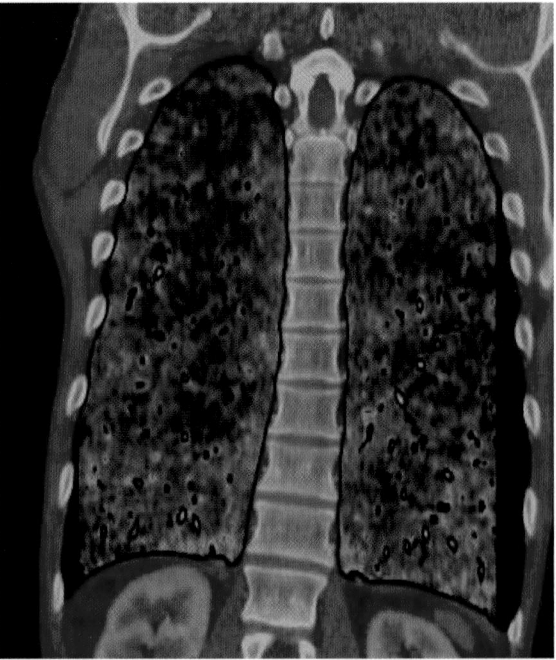

Fig. 11.4. Coronal perfusion image obtained in a COPD patient. Bilateral heterogeneity of the lungs. The *dark areas* correspond to multiple defects of iodine content. The *peripheral black areas* correspond to the parts of non-acquired parenchyma due to the tube B small field of view (26 cm)

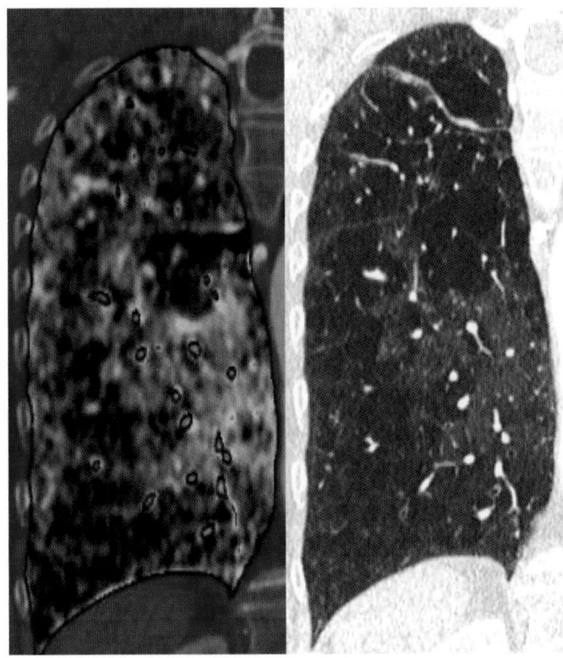

Fig. 11.5. Perfusion-morphology correlation on the same planar reformation of the right lung showing multiple areas of lung destruction with no iodine enhancement. The apical segment of the right lower lobe is relatively spared from emphysema. Nevertheless, multiple small perfusion defects can be identified in this morphologically normal lung

11.2 COPD and Pulmonary Hypertension (PHT)

11.2.1 Pulmonary Hypertension in COPD

The figures of PHT in COPD patients are highly variable, from 20% to 90% according to the publications and disease staging. Its severity depends on the degree of airflow obstruction and pulmonary gas exchange impairment (Barbera et al. 2003). Its evolution is slowly progressive. Pathologic changes in the pulmonary circulation may appear several years before PHT is recognized, even in smokers with normal lung function. Small pulmonary arteries show thickened intima, smooth muscle cell proliferation and elastin and collagen deposition (Peinado et al. 1998; Santos et al. 2002). The arteriolar muscularization of the peribronchiolar centrolobular arteries has no morphologic effect analyzable on HRCT, but the luminal narrowing may have an impact on lung perfusion imaging preceding the development of emphysema (Yamato et al. 1997). There could also be a relationship between systemic inflammation and PHT (Joppa et al. 2006).

PHT in COPD is usually moderate, limited to 25–35 mmHg mean pulmonary artery pressure (mPAP) at rest. It increases at exercise in proportion to resting PAP. The performance of echocardiography in its identification is qualified as "less than optimal" (Naeije 2005). The pathogenesis is complex, bringing together hypoxia, remodeling, amputation of the pulmonary vascular bed, hyperinflation, polycythemia, increased cardiac output and hypercapnic acidosis (Wright et al. 2005). Severe PHT is quite uncommon and is called "disproportionate" PHT, meaning that there is a gap between the benignity of COPD and the severity of PHT. It is estimated in fewer than 5% of COPD patients, many of them having an additional cause of PHT such as obstructive sleep apnea, obesity-hypoventilation syndrome (Chaouat et al. 2005), left heart disease, collagen vascular disease (Weitzenblum and Chaouat. 2005), acute and chronic PE, portal hypertension, HIV infection, appetite-suppressant drugs and recent exacerbation (Thabut et al. 2005). This rare subset of COPD with severe PHT is important to know since it can be treated by pulmonary vasodilators. We will see that left ventricular dysfunction in this group has to be separated into diastolic and systolic dysfunction, the first one being the consequence of right ventricular dysfunction (Scharf et al. 2002). Disproportionate hypoxemia must also be compared to PHT and the importance of lung destruction because it can be due to a patent foramen ovale.

11.2.2 CT Functional Imaging of PHT

11.2.2.1 Pulmonary Artery Distensibility (PAD)

As previously shown, the extensibility of the main pulmonary artery is reduced in PHT. When the pulmonary vascular resistance increases, the vessels become more distended and less distensible (Bogren et al. 1989). Compliance refers to change in cross-sectional area for a given change in pressure. Distensibility refers to fractional change in area for a given change in intra-vascular pressure (McVeigh et al. 2007).

Non-invasive evaluation of the PAD can be performed with US, NMR and CT. When CT angiography is acquired with cardiac gating, the cross-sectional area of the right PA can be visualized, and the distensibility index is calculated as follows (see Fig. 11.6).

Systolic Cross Section Minus Diastolic Cross Section

Systolic Cross Section

Distensibility corresponds to changes in volume between systole and diastole and depends both on the pulmonary vascular resistance and functional value of the right ventricle. It is determined by the elastic properties of the arterial wall. It can also be calculated on the main pulmonary artery and the left one with more difficulties due to its arcuature. In the normally compliant artery, the range in NMR is between 20 and 25% of the minimal diameter whatever the patient's age (Paz et al. 1993). These figures are identical with ultrasonography with the exception that an age-related decline was observed (Visontai et al. 2000). In our experience, PAD calculated on CT is usually well correlated to PA pressure.

11.2.2.2 Measurement of Pulmonary Vascular Resistances

The mean pulmonary transit time (PTTm) can be easily calculated with the monitoring of a minimal bolus of contrast medium flowing from the right ventricular outflow tract to the left atrium obtained on cross-sectional images every 2 s. The cardiac output is determined from the stroke volume and the heart rate. Müller et al. (2000) developed a mathematical model for calculating pulmonary vascular resistances from non-invasive measurements of cardiac output and PTTm.

11.2.2.3 Measurement of the Transverse Diameter of the Main Pulmonary Artery (MPA) on Cross-Sectional Images

Everyone knows this first step evaluation of pulmonary artery pressure, which will not be described in this chapter. The exact value of measurements (MPA transverse diameter or comparison of this diameter with ascending aorta diameter on the same level) depends on the temporal resolution of the machine

a

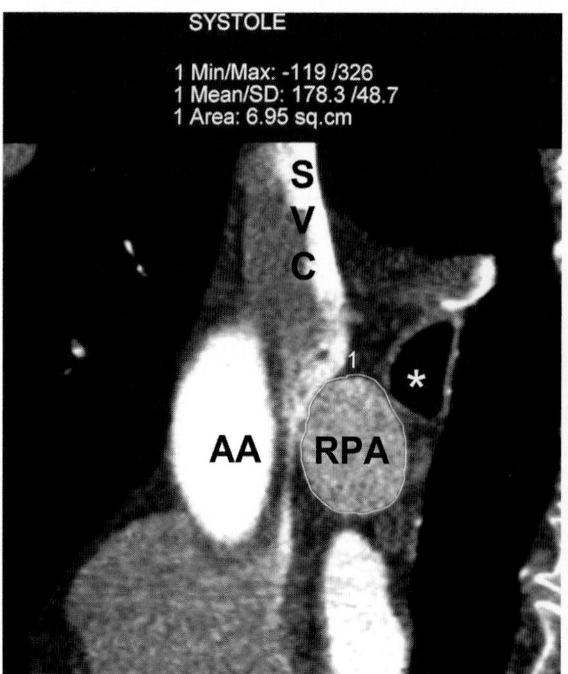

b

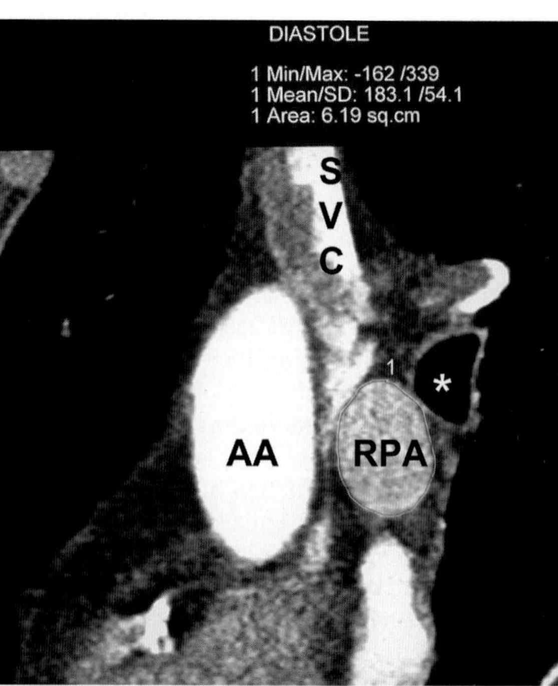

Fig. 11.6a,b. Systolo-diastolic distensibility of the right PA on sagittal reformations. In this patient with PHT, the systolo-diastolic difference in area is limited to 10%. *AA*: Ascending aorta. *RPA*: Right pulmonary artery. *Right main bronchus. *SVC*: superior vena cava

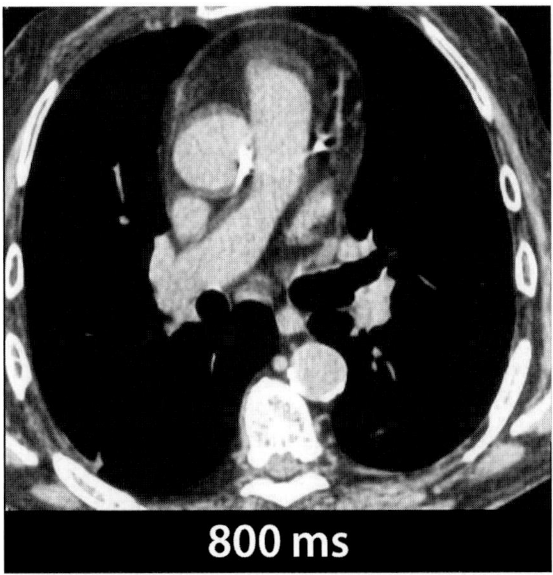

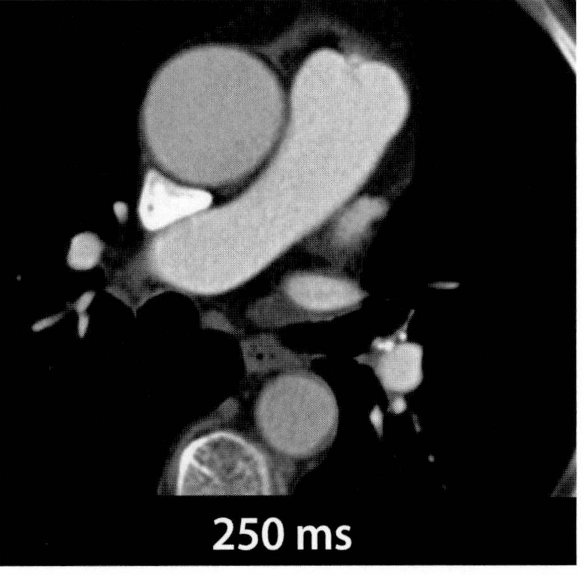

Fig. 11.7a,b. Two different patients with 70 bpm. The acquisition with 800-ms temporal resolution (**a**) shows double contours at the level of all the mediastinal organs: right pulmonary artery, ascending aorta, superior vena cava, left atrial appendage, pericardial recesses and subcarinal lymph node. With 250 ms temporal resolution (**b**) obtained with cardiac gating, all the aforementioned contours are very sharp. Motion artifacts are integrated in the measurements of PA trunk, ascending aorta and lymph nodes

(systolo-diastolic motion artifacts) and on the distensibility of each vessel. Considering that the motion amplitude of the main pulmonary artery wall is about 4 mm between systole and diastole, one can realize the importance of measurement approximation (Fig. 11.7).

11.3 COPD and Right Cardiac Cavities

11.3.1 Patent Foramen Ovale (PFO)

As previously quoted, patients with COPD have an increased patency of their foramen ovale (Soliman et al. 1999). This can be due to increased right atrial pressure. Reduction of pulmonary venous return and thoracic distension can also play a role, the last one being responsible for a malalignment of the interatrial septum. The right-to-left atrial shunt contributes to chronic hypoxemia. The reference for detection of PFO is contrast-enhanced transesophageal echocardiography, which may have some contraindications and is partially invasive. In addition, cough efforts during the procedure may artificially increase the right atrial pressure.

Arrival of bubbles in the left atrium during a Valsalva maneuver or immediately at its end after one to two cardiac cycles is the key point. The same principle can be used in NMR angiography with 10 ml of gadopentetate dimeglumine during a Valsalva maneuver (Mohrs et al. 2005, 2007; Nusser et al. 2006).

PFO can also be visualized during CT angiography with dynamic CT centered on the fossa ovalis after injection of 10 ml of iodinated contrast medium with a low kV technique. The mean dose length product is 140 mGy cm. Images are acquired during the relapse of the Valsalva maneuver showing the left atrial enhancement prior to the pulmonary venous return of iodine (Fig. 11.8). An atrial septal aneurysm bulging in the juxta-atrial part of the left atrium or in the right one can also be identified. Sensitivity of MSCT ranges from 28% in grade 1 to 90% in grade 4 PFO. The specificity is 96% (Revel et al. 2008). CTA of PFO must not be used as a first intention procedure, but has to be kept in mind when TEE is contraindicated or as a first step of a CTA performed in the management of an extra cardiac vascular or parenchymal right-to-left shunting or unexplained hypoxemia.

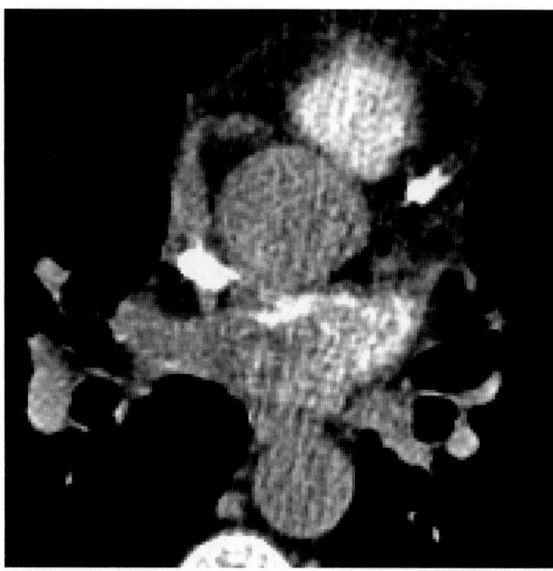

Fig. 11.8. Low-dose dynamic-mode acquisition to detect a patent foramen ovale immediately after a Valsalva maneuver. The small amount of contrast medium found in the left atrium comes from the superior vena cava via the right atrium. The right upper and left lower pulmonary veins are not opacified

11.3.2 Right Ventricular Dysfunction

Adequate assessment of RV performance and morphology is more difficult than that of the left one, and publications about LV largely outnumber those of the right one, by about a factor of 10 (Redington 2002).

Pulmonary hypertension in COPD is the leading cause of right ventricular dysfunction. The old definition of chronic cor pulmonale is now replaced by "alteration in the structure and function of the right ventricle" (MacNee 1994). This imprecise definition implies right ventricular hypertrophy (RVH), which has no clinical precise definition. The incidence and prevalence of RVH are lacking. According to autopsic studies, it may be encountered in 40% of COPD patients (MacNee 1994). It parallels the degree of air-flow limitation and pulmonary hypertension. From a physiologic viewpoint, the blood volume content of the ventricle at the end of the diastole, called end-diastolic volume, is called preload. It is also defined as the force acting on the ventricular muscle before it contracts. Changes in preload impact the end diastolic volume. At the time of the opening of the pulmonary valves, the preload decreases due to blood ejection; this new load is called afterload. It is protosystole dependent. It is related to the intra-ventricular pressure, the ventricular size and inversely related to its wall thickness. The right ventricle ejection fraction is mainly afterload-dependent, but it also depends on the contractility and preload.

The concept of RV dysfunction rests on a right ventricular ejection fraction (RVEF) smaller than 45% on isotopic ventriculography (Weitzenblum and Chaouat 1998). According to these authors, a decreased RVEF probably reflects the consequences of PHT, i.e., an increased afterload. It is a poor indicator of RV function. The anterior wall is not always taken into account in the calculation of RVH because it is often invested with abundant epicardial fat.

The so-called cor pulmonale not only implies RVH, but also dilatation. From a pathologic viewpoint, RVH is defined as a posterior RV wall thickness of 5 mm or greater at the level of the inferior border of the posterior leaflet of the tricuspid valve (Farb et al. 1992). According to Vonk-Noordegraaf (2005) in normoxemic or mildy hypoxemic COPD patients the stroke volume is low, the RV wall mass is higher, and the end-diastolic and the end-systolic volumes are lower than in control group. The RV systolic dysfunction defined as RVEF <45% is present in 20% of the patients.

11.3.3 MSCT and the Right Ventricle

The right ventricle has a complex morphology due to its crescent shape (Fig. 11.9) with a tubular configuration of the right ventricle outflow tract (RVOT). It has a pronounced trabeculation, which is sometimes taken into account, or not, in its volume measurements. In COPD it can be situated at an increased distance from the anterior chest wall due to hyperinflation of the retro-sternal lungs. This can explain why it is not the preferred ventricle for echocardiography. In opposition to echo, MSCT is not restricted by geometrical assumptions. Multiple functional and morphological parameters of the RV can be measured on CT. They cannot be reviewed in extenso in this chapter.

11.3.3.1 RVEF

In a group of 49 patients and for two subgroups of patients with normal and reduced RVEF, comparison of CT with equilibrium radionuclide ventriculography shows similar results. Despite the lack of ß-blockers and the use of ECG pulsing deteriorating the systolic images, MSCT can be used in routine clinical activity (DELHAYE et al. 2006) in unselected patients. The triple rule out or chest pain protocole is able to integrate functional information of the heart into a diagnostic scan. In comparison with scintigraphy, MSCT enables precise identification of the RV tricuspid valves and of the pulmonary valve plane (REMY-JARDIN et al. 2006).

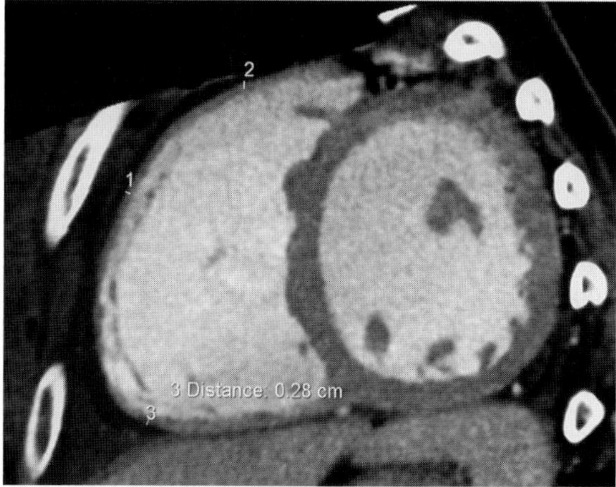

Fig. 11.9. Short axis diastolic reconstruction of normal ventricular cavities. The rightward convexity of the interventricular septum can be visualized and, if necessary, calculated. The difference in thickness between the right and left ventricular myocardium is normal

11.3.3.2
Tricuspid Annular Plane Systolic Excursion (TAPSE)

Complex RV geometry partly limits the application of non-invasive assessment of RV function; however, as contraction occurs mainly along its longitudinal axis between the tricuspid annulus and the RV apex, TAPSE is an excellent measure of RV systolic function (FORFIA et al. 2006). In normal subjects, the displacement of the tricuspid annulus from end-diastole to end-systole is ≥2.5 cm on transthoracic echocardiography. The same author found a linear inverse relationship between TAPSE, and pulmonary vascular resistances, and according to this publication, TAPSE correlates with RVEF, which is the proportion of stroke volume to end-diastolic volume.

Using MCST with cardiac gating, TAPSE can be measured as the annulus displacement on four-chamber views of the cardiac cavities (Fig. 11.10) reconstructed at 20 cardiac phases in step of 5% of the R-R interval, while RVEF is calculated on the short-axis views of the ventricles. TAPSE measurements provide an accurate and rapid estimation of RV function (DELHAYE et al. 2007).

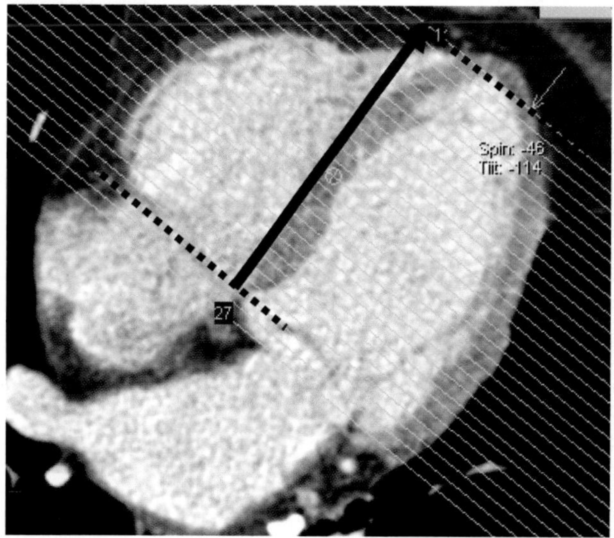

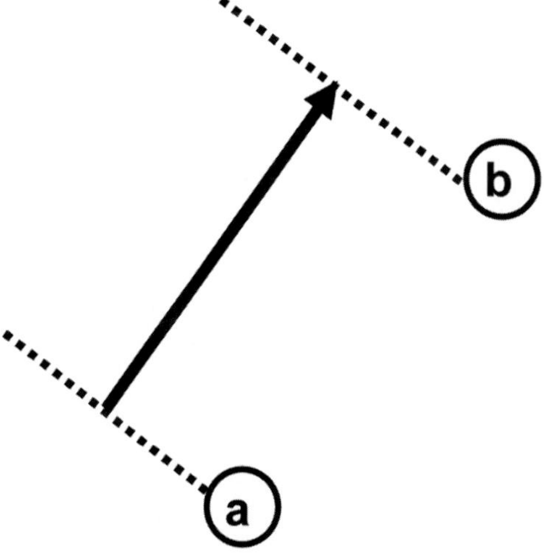

Fig. 11.10a,b. Long axis diastolic reformation of the cardiac cavities. The tricuspid annulus (**a**) is identified at the level of the tricuspid valve and the right atrio-ventricular sulcus. The *sharp triangular shape* of the anterior right ventricular part is depicted (**b**). Line *a* to *b* corresponds to the long axis of the ventricular cavity. The same operation can be performed during diastole. An extracardiac non-mobile reference point can also be chosen, and the axis from *a* to this point is calculated

11.3.3.3 Systolic and Diastolic Evaluation of the Right Ventricular Outflow Tract (RVOT)

On a gated MSCT, one can obtain the systolic and diastolic RVOT wall thickness below the pulmonary valves, the RVOT antero-posterior systolic and diastolic diameters and the cross-sectional area perpendicular to the RVOT long axis. In PHT there is a diastolic increased RVOT myocardial thickness. A thickness of 5.8 mm or above has 100% specificity for PHT. Systolic RVOT diameter and cross-sectional area are significantly larger in patients with PHT (Revel et al. 2008).

11.3.3.4 Interventricular Septal Configuration

Interventricular septal shape is a strong determinant of the RV function. Chronic or acute dilatation of the RV impedes the diastolic function of the left ventricle. Conversely, the LV may contribute from one-fifth to two-thirds of RV function (Klima et al. 2002). Flattening and sometimes bowing of the interventricular septum toward the LV can be seen when the RV systolic pressure is increased (Fig. 11.11). This is in agreement with experimental studies showing that diastolic LV septal bowing occurs with an abnormal transseptal pressure gradient (Beyar et al. 1993).

Setpal bowing can be quantified by its curvature, defined as one divided by the radius of curvature in centimeters (Roeleveld et al. 2005), determined on short-axis views. The curvature calculation is given in the appendix of the above publication. A rightward convexity of the curvature is normal. A systolic pulmonary artery pressure higher than 64 mmHg may be expected when leftward convexity of the curvature is observed (Roeleveld et al. 2005). The interventricular septal curvature (C_{IVS}) can also be compared, on short axis views, to the LV free wall curvature corresponding to the LV poste-

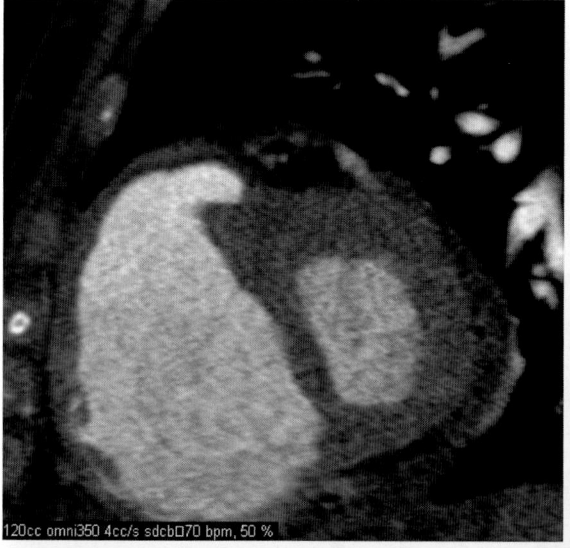

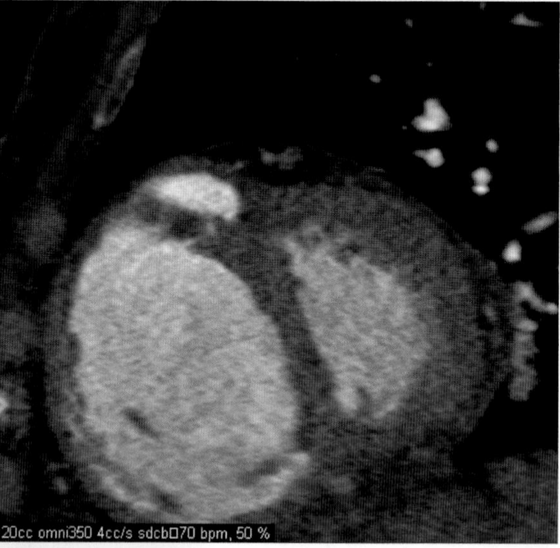

Right Ventricle – Absolute

Cardiac Function			Normal Range (F) (CT)	Units
Ejection Fraction	EF	10.6	47.00 ... 80.00	%
End Diastolic Volume	EDV	231.1	58.00 ... 154.00	ml
End Systolic Volume	ESV	206.6	12.00 ... 68.00	ml
Stroke Volume	SV	24.5	35.00 ... 98.00	ml
Cardiac Output	CO	1.72	2.65 ... 5.98	l/min
Myocardinal Mass (at ED)		----	----	g
Myocardinal Mass (Avg)		----	----	g

Fig. 11.11. Same diastolic reformation axis as in Figure 11.10. Massive dilatation of the right ventricle with leftward diastolic convexity of the interventricular septum. The RV ejection fraction is reduced to 10.6%. The reversed interventricular curvature fully justifies the study of the left ventricular morphology and function

rior wall (C_{FW}). The curvature ratio (R_C) is C_{IVS}/C_{FW}. With cardiac MR, Dellegrottaglie et al. (2007) applied the following formula: RV systolic pressure = systolic blood pressure [1-R_C/1.03] and found an accurate and reproducible index for estimation of RV systolic pressure in patients known to have or suspected of having PHT.

All these aforementioned studies can be performed on CT with some limitations:

- The temporal resolution is not as optimal as MR. However, this limitation is counterbalanced by 83 ms temporal resolution with dual-source CT with single-segment reconstruction. With dual-source single-energy CT, it is possible to perform an acquisition of the heart without cardiac gating in less than 1 s, compared to the diastolic length, which is 0.50 s at 75 bpm.
- Another limitation is radiation exposure. However, MR also has multiple drawbacks in thoracic imaging, and the pre-therapeutic evaluation of COPD, including the heart, needs a CT scan.
- Injection of contrast medium is mandatory in cardiac MR as well as in cardiac CT. The pre-therapeutic evaluation of a COPD patient with CT does not require iodine injection except in three main circumstances: unexplained acute exacerbation, suspected cardio-vascular co-morbidities and perfusion imaging.

With the partial scan algorithms and single segment reconstruction, the heart rate-dependent temporal resolution was 210 ms for a 420-ms gantry rotation with a single-source CT technology (Kim et al. 2005). So, at that time, CT analysis of ventricular volume, function and mass was considered as "not reasonable." Nevertheless, in the same year a maximum gantry speed of 400 ms and a multisegmental reconstruction algorithm, using raw data form up to four cardiac cycles, demonstrated a good agreement among MSCT and MRI for RV end-diastolic volume, end-systolic volume, stroke volume, ejection fraction and myocardial mass (Lembcke et al. 2005). If motion-free cardiac imaging can be obtained with 250-ms temporal resolution at 70 bpm, 150 ms is required at 100 bpm and 50 ms is ideally required for all cardiac phases (Mahesh and Cody 2007). Multisegmental – also called multicycle, multisector or multiphase – reconstruction is usually not recommended for coronary arteries, because it is not precisely at the same site from one cardiac cycle to another. The non-reproducibility of the same volume on successive diastolic volume measurements is not precisely known. In general, MSCT is responsible for an overestimation of the RV end-systolic volumes and for underestimation of the RVEF. As it has been reported that a temporal resolution better than 100 ms is needed for accurate cardiac volumetry (Dogan et al. 2006), we can deduce that 83 ms obtained with DSCT is the last breakthrough toward optimal cardiac volume measurements.

11.4 Left Heart, Coronary Artery Disease and COPD

11.4.1 Pathophysiology

Smoking is responsible for multiple cardio-vascular effects: rise in systemic vascular resistance and blood pressure, increase in coronary resistance, coronary atherosclerosis and reduction in coronary blood flow. The decrease of coronary blood flow impairs LV diastolic function (Lichodziejewska et al. 2007). Doppler echocardiography shows the impairment of LV diastolic relaxation, the early phase of ventricular diastole. Several mechanisms can affect the LV function in COPD: RV disease with septal bowing toward the LV compromises the LV diastolic filling. Reduction of venous pulmonary blood flow also impairs the LV diastolic function. Left ventricular hypertrophy is described in up to 30% of COPD patients at autopsy (Macnee 1994). Coronary artery disease secondary to cigarette smoking or to systemic inflammation can trigger ischemic cardiomyopathy. An alcoholic cardiomyopathy can be superimposed to the previous diseases. Apart from the myocardial contractibility, two mechanisms can explain the LV diastolic dysfunction: impaired relaxation and decreased distensibility.

11.4.2 Left Ventricular Dysfunction (LVD)

The reverse "Bernheim phenomenon" corresponds to a leftward shifting of the interventricular septum (IVS) caused by right ventricular dilatation and hypertrophy. The muscular hypertrophy of the right ventricle can also affect the IVS (Alpert 2001). The IVS bowing toward the left ventricle can be diastolic, while it has its normal rightward convexity during systole (Marcus et al. 2001). The reduced left ventricular volume and diastolic function can be responsible for passive pulmonary hypertension (Fig. 11.12). It is called diastolic heart failure, heart failure with preserved LV function or heart failure with normal ejection fraction, which is the preferred term (Sanderson 2007). Another definition is: (1) presence of signs or symptoms of congestive heart failure, (2) presence of normal or only mildly abnormal left ventricular systolic function and (3) evidence of abnormal left ventricular relaxation, filling, diastolic distensibility or diastolic stiffness (Working Group Report 1998). Patients having precapillary pulmonary hypertension due to COPD may have consequences of their ventricular interdependence. Normally, the LV end-diastolic pressure/volume relationship depends on the LV itself, but also on the RV morphology and function and on the pericardium. A dilated RV may impact on the LV diastolic function and, from it, on the pulmonary venous return. Consequently, the pulmonary capillary wedge pressure can be elevated (Shapiro et al. 2007). Finally, in COPD patients, there may be numerous means of interstitial pulmonary edema: increased vascular and LV diastolic stiffness due to systemic vascular consequences of inflammation and hypoxia in elderly patients, LV diastolic failure related to RV dysfunction, stasis in the lymphatic circulation of the lung draining in the congestive systemic venous return due to RV dysfunction and ischemic cardiomyopathy. Several of them can coexist.

Distinction of dyspnea of cardiac origin from dyspnea due to COPD is not always easy. So an acute or subacute disease exacerbation of unknown cause, occurring in the follow-up of a previously stable disease, must draw attention to the heart. COPD patients who present with increasing dyspnea may have LVD, and only objective measures of ventricular function are able to identify individuals with COPD and COPD plus LVD. LVD was found in 32% of patients with COPD exacerbation (Render et al. 1998). This figure is reduced to 6.4% in end-stage pulmonary disease, including patients with α1-antitrypsine deficiency, COPD, cystic fibrosis, UIP and PHT (Vizza et al. 1998). These authors split the LVD into two parts: the first one, as a consequence of RV dysfunction, is more frequent than isolated LVD. More recently, a MRI study in severe emphysema (FEV1 from 15 to 30% of predicted value) found a significantly decreased LVEF explained by intrathoracic hypovolemia and low LV preload decreasing the LV end-diastolic volume (Jorgensen et al. 2007).

11.4.3 Ischemic Cardiomyopathy

Silent ischemic heart disease is an important manifestation of coronary artery disease. The GRACE registry (Global Registry of Acute Coronary Events) in a group of 20,881 patients with acute coronary syndromes identified 8.4% of patients without chest pain and atypical symptoms (Brieger et al. 2004).

a 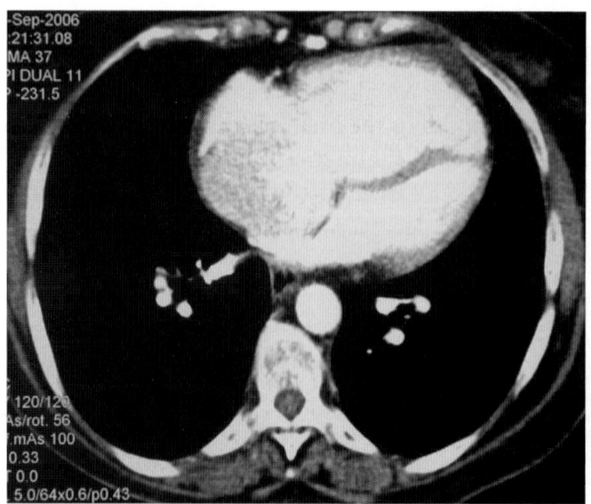

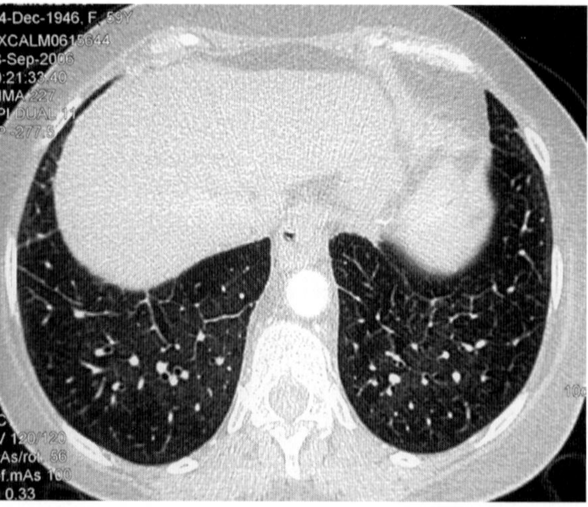 b

Fig. 11.12a,b. A COPD patient with huge dilatation of the right atrium and right ventricle (**a**). Interventricular septal bowing toward the left ventricle. The septal lines of the lung bases (**b**) can be the consequence of the right ventricular dysfunction via left diastolic ventricular impairment

Another proportion of patients may have minimal or no symptoms at all, leading to an incidental discovery of a myocardial infarct. Diabetic patients, with their propensity to autonomic neuropathy, are frequent. The main CT signs of silent ischemic heart disease are here briefly summarized because they are extensively reviewed in another chapter (Chap. 17).

11.4.3.1 Myocardial Fat

Myocardial fat mainly occurs as a result of aging and after myocardial infarct (MI) or chronic ischemia (Fig. 11.13). Lipomatous metaplasia is frequently identified after MI or chronic ischemic heart disease, identified at autopsy in 68 to 84% of left ventricular scars (Jacobi et al. 2007).

This focal fatty infiltration of the LV myocardium has three main sites: the apico-anterior wall, latero-posterior wall and interventricular septum according to the major coronary artery territories. It can also be identified after RV infarct. Those areas can predispose to aneurysm. The fatty area can be transmural or sub-endocardial.

11.4.3.2 Aneurysms and Pseudo-Aneurysms

Post-infarct pseudo-aneurysm (Csapo et al. 1997) has a wall composed of pericardium and epicardial tissue without myocardial muscle. It can be asymptomatic, but is prone to chest pain, rupture, congestive heart failure and embolic events. Its junction with the LV is narrow. This narrow neck, in conjunction with stagnation of contrast medium in the cavity and rapid increase in size, supports the diagnosis of pseudo-aneurysm (Brown et al. 1997). Its inferior or posterior location is usual. When inferior, it can be hidden on cross-sectional images and requires coronal imaging. It can be thrombosed. The wall of a ventricular aneurysm (Fig. 11.14) is composed of myocardial muscle, scarred myocardium and fibrous and calcified tissues. Its insertion on the ventricle is large. It can also include a thrombus. Congestive heart failure, embolic events and ventricular arrhythmia are also possible. It is more often apical or anterolateral. In both lesions, the aneurymal or pseudo-aneurysmal cavity is dyskinetic or akinetic. It does not take part in the ejection. The intra-aneurysmal thrombi, when fused with the myocardial wall, can be difficult to identify, except when calcified.

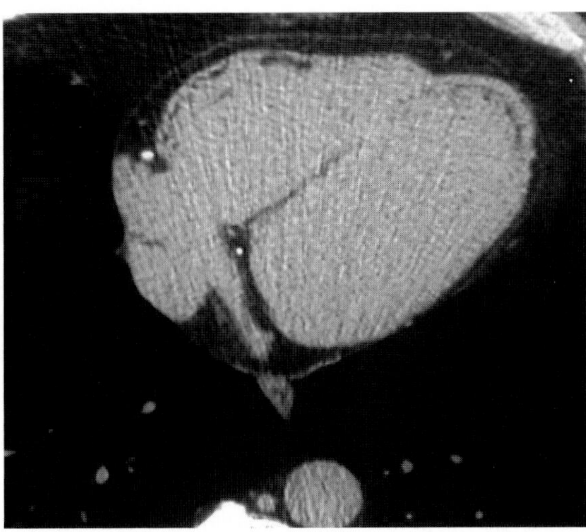

Fig. 11.13. Elderly COPD patient with a previous history of myocardial infarction. The minor fatty infiltration of the right ventricular myocardium is a normal appearance in the elderly. Lipomatous metaplasia of the left ventricular apex consistent with the previous myocardial infarction

11.4.3.3 Coronary Artery Disease

According to the SHAPE (Screening for Heart Attack Prevention and Education) task force, "screening to identify subclinical or asymptomatic atherosclerosis could confer great public health benefit. It may seem surprising that it has not yet been incorporated into national and international clinical guidelines" (Naghavi et al. 2006). COPD patients with smoking history, systemic inflammation, artery stiffness and other comorbidities such as osteoporosis or diabetes are at high risk for heart attack or stroke. Detection and quantification of coronary artery calcifications by CT should consequently be undertaken. There is abundant literature on the detection and quantification of coronary calcifications on prospective or retrospective cardiac CT. Recently, the ability of non-contrast and prospective ECG gated acquisition to detect lipid-rich plaques was emphasized (Dey et al. 2006). The ultrafast acquisition times obtained with dual-source CT (83-ms temporal resolution without cardiac gating) allows for acquisition of half the cardiac height in 0.50 s, the diastolic period in a patient with 75 bpm. Lipids in the plaques increase their biomechanical stresses and their risk of rupture.

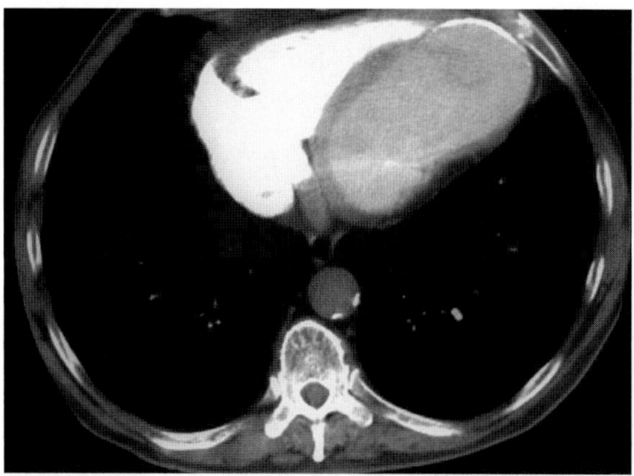

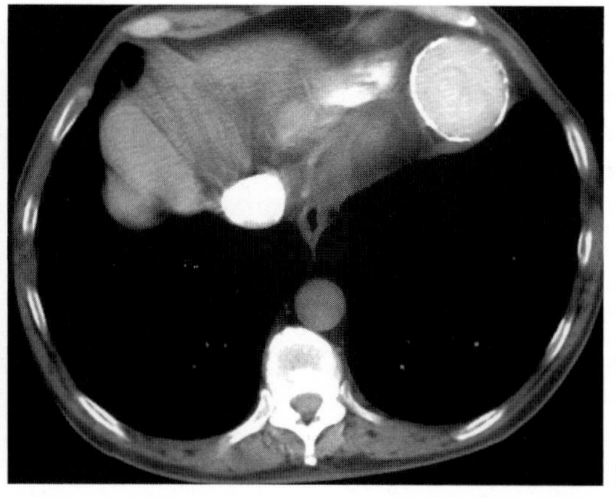

Fig. 11.14a,b. Considering the cranio-caudal acquisition mode, the short acquisition time, the amount and flow rate of contrast medium injection, all the acquisition and injection parameters being kept constant, the stagnation of contrast medium in the right cardiac cavities associated with the poor opacification of the left ventricle and descending aorta (**a**) can cause suspicion of traducing increased pulmonary vascular resistances or cardiac failure. Ballooning of the left ventricular apical lumen and curvilinear superficial myocardial calcification are consistent with left ventricular aneurysm. On a lower level (**b**) the ventricular aneurysm is confirmed

11.4.3.4 Left Ventricle Ejection Fraction (LVEF)

In COPD patients in whom the CT acquisition is obtained with contrast medium injection, low-dose chest pain or triple rule out protocols including cardiac gating should be performed with measurement of LVEF. If this measurement has previously been calculated, it is possible to monitor the LV function follow-up. If not, it could stratify the risks and guide the use of treatment after MI (Lopez-Jimenez et al. 2004).

11.4.3.5 Miscellaneous

Other signs of chronic infarction, such as wall thinning and delayed contrast enhancement occurring 10 min to several hours after contrast injection, can be identified (Nikolaou et al. 2004) as well as signs of acute MI (Moore et al. 2006; Gosalia et al. 2004).

11.4.4 Technical Considerations

Coronary CTA has a high diagnostic accuracy on per patient and per segment analysis (Nikolaou et al. 2006) using the 64 MSCT technology. In patients with a heart rate below 80 bpm, it can be performed without ß blockers contraindicated in COPD (Delhaye et al. 2007, 2007). The performances of cardiac CT with 4-, 8- and 16-channel MDCT on the determination of global and regional LV function is beyond the scope of this review. It is nicely analyzed in the literature (Juergens and Fischbach, 2006). The old poor temporal resolution is no longer a limitation with 83 ms, but a further large evaluation is needed.

11.4.5 Cardio-Vascular Imaging and Invasive Treatments of COPD

In severe emphysema, the diastolic LV function is affected. This can be due to dynamic hyperinflation, which causes reduction of intra-thoracic blood volume. Lung volume reduction surgery increases LV diastolic dimensions and filling and improves LV function (Jorgensen et al. 2003).

Emphysema is the leading cause of lung transplantation. In an evaluation of a group of 210 pretransplant patients with 80% emphysema, noncritical coronary artery disease (CAD) was found in 16% (Choong et al. 2006). Non-critical CAD means single or multivessel mild (<30%) stenosis or moderate 30 to 50% stenosis. In this group of patients, there was no increased perioperative mortality or morbidity. Eighteen percent developed late ischemic events. Pulmonary hypertension is not a significant complication of lung volume reduction surgery (Criner et al. 2007).

11.5 Related or Coincidental Cardiovascular Findings in COPD

Some incidental cardiovascular diseases must be taken into account in the management of COPD because they can simulate or exaggerate its consequences or influence its treatment.

11.5.1 Aortic Calcifications

There is a strong connection between atherosclerosis of the ascending aorta and stroke. It has recently been emphasized in patients undergoing coronary surgery (Van Der Linden et al. 2007). The disease location is often the distal left segment of the ascending aorta. Lee et al. (2007) recommend an aggressive screening of ascending aorta calcifications with non-contrast chest CT to avoid intraoperative manipulation of an atheromatous aorta. Non-rheumatic calcified aortic stenosis is the most frequent valvular disease in the population older than 65 years, occurring in 2 to 7% (Stewart et al. 1997).

In a study by Koos et al. (2006) with routine non-gated chest CT for non-cardiac thoracic indications, aortic valve calcifications were found in 18% of patients with a mean age of 62.5 years. The valve calcifications were scored as follows: grade 0: no calcification; grade 1: small spots: minor; grade 2: mild; grade 3: moderate; grade 4: severe, involving the three cusps. MSCT revealed valves calcifications in 20 of 21 patients with aortic stenosis at echo. They conclude that patients with grade 3 or 4 valve calcifications may require further evaluation. Liu et al. (2006) demonstrated that the severity of commissural calcifications in the central part of the right-left commissure and in the peripheral part of the left-posterior one were at higher risk.

11.5.2 Proximal Anomalies of the Coronary Arteries (PACA)

Among the PACA, the most important one consists of a coronary running between the right ventricular outflow tract (RVOT) and the ascending aorta (Kim et al. 2006) (Fig. 11.15). It can correspond to the RCA, the LCA, the LCx or the LAD. When ectopic, these arteries often orginate at an acute angle from their sinus with a slit-like hypoplastic ostium (Dodd et al. 2007). Those abnormal pathways and diameters have to be imperatively described in COPD patients for the following reasons:

- They have a high frequency of coronary comorbidities.
- The coronary branch running interarterially can be compressed by ascending aorta dilatation or RVOT dilatation, or congenitally stenosed. COPD patients are at high risk of atherosclerosis and PHT. Consequences of PHT on the RVOT can compress the aberrant artery.
- The risk of having a bronchial carcinoma is related to smoking, COPD and systemic inflammation. A treatment or a disease reducing the volume of one lung, such as lobectomy, endoscopic or surgical volume reduction, atelectasis or radiation therapy, can provoke a mediastinal rotation and modify the length and orientation of the straight contact of the ascending aorta and PA trunk. There can be conjunction of:
  (1) Compression or congenital stenosis of the ectopic coronary artery.
  (2) COPD-induced coronary atherosclerosis, arterial stiffness or PHT.
  (3) Mediastinal rotation secondary to pulmonary volume loss.
  (4) Dilatation of the RVOT.
  (5) Reduction of the coronary blood flow may a have an impact on acute coronary events in COPD.

11.5.3 Partial Anomalous Pulmonary Venous Return (PAPVR)

The prevalence of a PAPVR on CT in adults is 0.2% to 0.7%. The abnormal drainage is more often right-sided than left-sided. Its association to COPD is quite possible. The artificial left predominance can be explained by an underestimation of right PAPVR due to the high number of pulmonary vessels normally in close contact to the lower part of the superior vena cava (SVC) (Haramati et al. 2003) and to the streak artifacts coming from the highly concentrated contrast medium in the SVC on CT angiography.

Isolated PAPVR of a single pulmonary vein is responsible for a minor degree of left-to-right shunt,

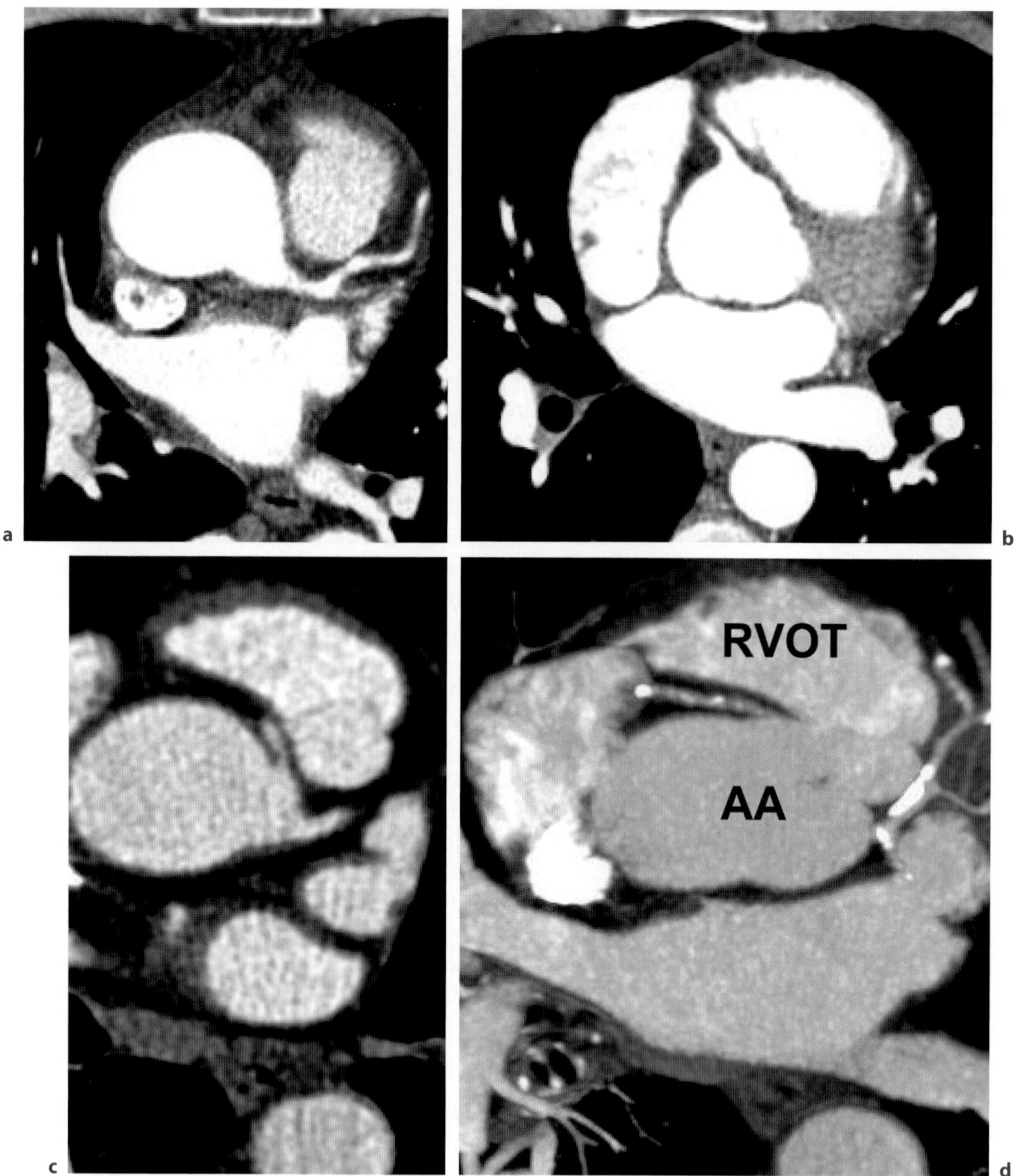

Fig. 11.15a–d. On a thoracic CT angiography with optimal temporal resolution, with or without cardiac gating, the normal origin and proximal course of the coronary arteries must be identified and analyzed (**a**,**b**). A preoperative management of a COPD patient candidate for thoracic surgery for a bronchial carcinoma must be able to detect (with cardiac gating in this patient) an abnormal origin of the right coronary artery from the same sinus as the left one (**c**) and its "malignant" interarterial course (**d**) between the right ventricle outflow tract (*RVOT*) and the ascending aorta (*AA*)

equal to or less than 25% of the total pulmonary venous return. The right atrial pressure being normally lower than the left one, the pulmonary vascular resistance (PVR) is lower in the abnormally drained lung, explaining the usual dilatation of the PAPVR.

An increased pulmonary vascular resistance in COPD can provoke a redistribution of blood flow toward the PAPVR or, conversely, can minimize the left-to-right-shunt, depending on the distribution of COPD lesions. In case of lung volume reduction of the normally drained lung due to a disease complication or treatment, the shunt through the PAPVR can be increased. If responsible for right ventricular overload, the L-R shunt can interact with the RV consequences of the COPD. From a 25% left-to-right shunt, a lobectomy, lobar ateclectasis and multisegmental endoscopic lung volume reduction of a normally drained lobe can major the shunt. The L-R shunt can be minimized when emphysema develops in the ectopically drained lobe. Right heart failure can be responsible for pulmonary edema in that lobe. As previously emphasized, the surgical importance of a PAPVR "should be appreciated by the radiologists" (Black et al. 1992).

11.5.4 Alcoholic Cardiomyopathy (ACM)

ACM can be also found in COPD patients. According to Piano (2002) ACM is the most frequent cause of non-ischemic dilated cardiomyopathy. The average duration of drinking is 15 years. It is characterized by dilatation of the LV, wall thinning, increased LV mass and ventricular dysfunction. A large percentage of patients with ACM is smokers and who may also have a coronary artery disease. Diastolic dysfunction is probably the earliest finding.

References

Abroug F, Ouanes-Besbes L, Nciri N et al. (2006) Association of left-heart dysfunction with severe exacerbation of chronic obstructive pulmonary disease. Diagnostic performance of cardiac biomarkers. Am J Respir Crit Care Med 174:990–996

Agusti A (2006) Chronic obstructive pulmonary disease. A systemic disease. Proc Am Thorac Soc 3:478–483

Alpert JS (2001) The effect of right ventricular dysfunction on left ventricular form and function. Chest 119:1632–1633

Arcasoy SM, Christie JD, Ferrari VA et al. (2003) Echocardiographic assessment of pulmonary hypertension in patients with advanced lung disease. Am J Respir Crit Care Med 167:735–740

Barberà JA, Peinado VI, Santos S (2003) Pulmonary hypertension in chronic obstructive pulmonary disease. Eur Respir J 21:892–905

Beyar R, Dong SJ, Smith ER et al. (1993) Ventricular interaction and septal deformation: a model compared with experimental data. Am J Physiol 256:H2044–H2056

Black MD, Shamji FM, Goldstein W, Sachs HJ (1992) Pulmonary resection and contralateral anomalous venous drainage: a lethal combination. Ann Thorac Surg 52:689691

Bogren HG, Klipstein RH, Mohiaddin RH et al. (1989) Pulmonary artery distensibility and blood flow patterns: a magnetic resonance study of normal subjects and of patients with pulmonary arterial hypertension. Am Heart J 118:990–999

Brieger D, Eagle KA, Goodman SG et al. (2004) Acute coronary syndromes without chest pain. An underdiagnosed and undertreated high-risk group. Chest 126:461–469

Brown SL, Gropler RJ, Harris KM (1997) Distinguishing left ventricular aneurysm from pseudoaneurysm. A review of the literature. Chest 111:1403–1409

Ceconi C, Ferrari R, Mauderi FS (2006) One heart, two lungs together forever. Am J Crit Care Med 174:962–963

Chaouat A, Bugnet AS, Kadaoui N et al. (2005) Severe pulmonary hypertension and chronic obstructive pulmonary disease. Am J Respir Crit Care Med 172:189–194

Choong CK, Meyers BF, Guthrie TJ et al. (2006) Does the presence of preoperative mild or moderate coronary artery disease affect the outcomes of lung transplantation? Ann Thorac Surg 82:1038–1042

Criner GJ, Scharf SM, Falk JA et al. (2007) Effect of lung volume reduction surgery on resting pulmonary hemodynamics in severe emphysema. Am J Respir Crit Care Med 176:253–260

Csapo K, Voith L, Szuk T et al. (1997) Postinfarction left ventricular pseudoaneurysm. Clin Cardiol 20:898–903

D'Agostino AG, Remy-Jardin M, Khalil C et al. (2006) Low-dose ECG gates 64-slice helical CT angiography of the chest: evaluation of image quality in 105 patients. Eur Radiol 16:2137–2146

Delhaye D, Remy-Jardin M, Faivre JB et al. (2007) Excursion systolo-diastolique de l'anneau tricuspidien: un nouvel indicateur TDM de la fonction ventriculaire droite? Annual Meeting of the French Society of Radiology

Delhaye D, Remy-Jardin M, Rozel C et al. (2007) Coronary artery imaging during preoperative CT staging: preliminary experience with 64-slice multidetector CT in 99 consecutive patients. Eur Radiol 17:591–602

Delhaye D, Remy-Jardin M, Salem R et al. (2007) Coronary imaging quality in routine ECG-gated multidetector CT examinations of the entire thorax: preliminary experience with a 64-slice CT system in 133 patients. Eur Radiol 17:902–910

Delhaye D, Remy-Jardin M, Teisseire A et al. (2006) MDCT of right ventricular function: comparison of right ventricular ejection fraction estimation and equilibrium radionuclide ventriculography, part I. AJR 187:1597–1604

Dellegrottaglie S, Sanz J, Poon M et al. (2007) Pulmonary hypertension: accuracy of detection with left ventricular septal-to-free wall curvature ratio measured at cardiac MR. Radiology 243:63–69

Dey D, Callister T, Slomka P et al. (2006) Computer-aided detection and evaluation of lipid-rich plaque on noncontrast cardiac CT. AJR 186:S407–S413

Dodd JD, Ferencik M, Liberthson RR et al. (2007) Congenital anomalies of coronary artery origin in adults: 64-MDCT appearance. AJR 188:W138–W146

Dogan H, Kroft LJM, Bas JJ et al. (2006) MDCT assessment of right ventricular systolic function. AJR 186:S366–S370

Downing G (2001) Biomarkers Definition Working Group. Biomarkers and surrogate endpoints. Clin Pharmacol Ther 69:89–95

Fabbri LM, Hurd SS, for the GOLD Scientific Committee (2003) Global strategy for the diagnosis, management and prevention of COPD: 2003 update. Eur Respir J 22:1–2

Farb A, Burke AP, Virmani R (1992) Anatomy and pathology of the right ventricle (including acquired tricuspid and pulmonic valve disease). Cardiol Clinics 10:1–21

Forfia PR, Fisher MR, Mathai SC et al. (2006) Tricuspid annular displacement predicts survival in pulmonary hypertension. Am J Respir Crit Care Med 174:1034–1041

Gosalia A, Haramati LB, Sheth M et al. (2004) CT detection of acute myocardial infarction. AJR 182:1563–1566

Haramati LB, Moche IE, Rivera VT et al. (2003) Computed tomography of partial anomalous pulmonary venous connection in adults. J Comput Assist Tomogr 27:743–749

Huiart L, Ernst P, Suissa S (2005) Cardiovascular morbidity and mortality in COPD. Chest 128:2640–2646

Hurst JR, Wedzicha JA (2007) What is (and what is not) a COPD exacerbation: thoughts from the new GOLD guidelines. Thorax 62:198–199

Jacobi AH, Gohari A, Zalta B et al. (2007) Ventricular myocardial fat. CT findings and clinical correlates. J Thorac Imaging 22:130–135

Joppa P, Petrasova D, Stancak B, Tkocova R (2006) Systemic inflammation in patients with COPD and pulmonary hypertension. Chest 130:326–333

Jörgensen K, Houltz E, Westfelt U et al. (2003) Effects of lung volume reduction surgery on left ventricular diastolic filling and dimensions in patients with severe emphysema. Chest 124:1863–1870

Jörgensen K, Müller MF, Nel J et al. (2007) Reduced intrathoracic blood volume and left and right ventricular dimensions in patients with severe emphysema. Chest 131:1050–1057

Juergens KU, Fischbach R (2006) Left ventricular function studied with MDCT. Eur Radiol 16:342–357

Kim EY, Seo JB, Do KH et al. (2006) Coronary artery anomalies: Classification and ECG-gated multi-detector row CT findings with angiographic correlation. RadioGraphics 26:317–334

Kim TH, Ryu YH, Hur J et al. (2005) Evaluation of right ventricular volume and mass using retrospective ECG-gated cardiac multidetector computed tomography: comparison with first-pass radionuclide angiography. Eur Radiol 15:1987–1993

Klima UP, Lee MY, Guerrero J et al. (2002) Determinants of maximal right ventricular function: role of septal shift. J Thorac Cardiovasc Surg 123:72–80

Koos R, Kühl HP, Mühlenbruch G et al. (2006) Prevalence and clinical importance of aortic valve calcification detected incidentally on CT scans: Comparison with echocardiography. Radiology 24:76–82

Lee R, Matsutani N, Polimenakos AC et al. (2007) Preoperative noncontrast chest computed tomography identifies potential aortic emboli. Ann Thorac Surg 84:38–42

Lembcke A, Dohmen PM, Dewey M et al. (2005) Multislice computed tomography for preoperative evaluation of right ventricular volumes and function: Comparison with magnetic resonance imaging. Ann Thorac Surg 79: 1344–1351

Lichodziejewska B, Kurnicka K, Grudzka K et al. (2007) Chronic and acute effects of smoking on left and right ventricular relaxation in young healthy smokers. Chest131:1142–1148

Liu F, Coursey CA, Grahame-Clarke C et al. (2006) Aortic valve calcification as an incidental finding at CT of the elderly: Severity and location as predictors of aortic stenosis. AJR 186:342–349

Lopez-Jimenez F, Goraya TY, Hellermann JP et al. (2004) Measurement of ejection fraction after myocardial infarction in the population. Chest 125:397–403

Macnee W (1994) Pathopohysiology of cor pulmonale in chronic obstructive pulmonary disease. Part 1. Am J Respir Crit Care Med 150:833–852

Macnee W (1994) Pathophysiology of cor pulmonale in chronic obstructive pulmonary disease. Am J Respir Crit Care Med 150:1158–1168

Mahesh M, Cody DD (2007) Physics of cardiac imaging with multiple-row detector CT. RadioGraphics 27:1495–1509

Mahnken AH, Mühlenbruch G, Günther RW, Wildberger JE (2007) Cardiac CT: coronary arteries and beyond. Eur Radiol 17:994–1008

Marcus JT, Vonk Noordegraaf A, Roeleveld RJ et al. (2001) Impaired left ventricular filling due to right ventricular pressure overload in primary pulmonary hypertension. Chest 119:1761–1765

McCollough CH, Primak AN, Saba O et al. (2007) Dose performance of a 64-channel dual-source CT scanner. Radiology 243:775–784

McVeigh GE, Bank AJ, Cohn JN (2007) Arterial compliance. In: Willerson JT, Cohn JN, Wellens HJJ, Holmes Jr DR (eds) Cardiovascular medicine, 3rd edn. Springer, Heidelberg Berlin New York, pp 1811–1831

Mohrs OK, Petersen SE, Erkapic D et al. (2005) Diagnosis of patent foramen ovale using contrast-enhanced dynamic MRI: a pilot study. AJR 184:234–240

Mohrs OK, Petersen SD, Erkapic D et al. (2007) Dynamic contrast-enhanced MRI before and after transcatheter occlusion of patent foramen ovale. AJR 188:844–849

Moore W, Fields J, Mieczkowski B (2006) Multidetector computed tomography pulmonary angiogram in the assessment of myocardial infarction. J Comput Assist Tomogr 30:800–803

Müller HM, Tripolt MB, Rehak PH et al. (2000) Noninvasive measurement of pulmonary vascular resistances by assessment of cardiac output and pulmonary transit time. Invest Radiol 35:727–731

Naeije R (2005) Pulmonary hypertension and right heart failure in chronic obstructive pulmonary disease. Proc Am Thorac Soc 2:20–22

Naghavi M, Falk E, Hecht HS et al. (2006) From vulnerable plaque to vulnerable patient–Part III: Executive summary of the Screening for Heart Attack Prevention and Education (SHAPE) Task Force Report. Am J Cardiol (Suppl) 98:2H–15H

Naunheim KS, Wood DE, Krasna MJ et al. (2006) Predictors of operative mortality and cardiopulmonary morbidity in the National Emphysema Treatment Trial. J Thorac Cardiovasc Surg 131:43–53

Nikolaou K, Knez A, Sagmeister S et al. (2004) Assessment of myocardial infarctions using multidetector-row computed tomography. J Comput Assist Tomogr 28:286–292

Nikolaou K, Knez A, Rist C et al. (2006) Accuracy of 64-MDCT in the diagnosis of ischemic heart disease. AJR 187:111–117

Nusser T, Hoher M, Merkle N et al. (2006) Cardiac magnetic resonance imaging and transesophageal echocardiography in patients with transcatheter closure of paten foramen ovale. J Am Coll Cardiol 48:322–329

O'Donnel DE, Parker CM (2006) COPD exacerbation. 3: Pathophysiology. Thorax 61:354–361

Orakzai SH, Orakzai RH, Nasir K, Budoff MJ (2006) Assessment of cardiac function using multidetector row computed tomography. J Comput Assist Tomogr 30:555–563

Pauwels RA, Buist AS, Calverley PMA et al. (2001) Global strategy for the diagnosis, management, and prevention of chronic obstructive pulmonary disease. Am J Respir Crit Care Med 163:1256–1276

Paz R, Mohiaddin RH, Longmore DB (1993) Magnetic resonance assessment of the pulmonary arterial trunk anatomy, flow, pulsatility and distensibility. Eur Heart J 14:1524–1530

Peinado VI, Barberà JA, Ramirez J et al. (1998) Endothelial dysfunction in pulmonary arteries of patients with mild COPD. Am J Physiol 274:L908–l9013

Piano MR (2002) Alcoholic cardiomyopathy. Incidence, clinical characteristics, and pathophysiology. Chest 121:1638–1650

Rabe KF, Hurd S, Anzueto A et al. (2007) Global strategy for the diagnosis, management, and prevention of chronic obstructive pulmonary disease. Am J Respir Crit Care Med 176:532–555

Redington AN (2002) Right ventricular function. Cardiol Clinics 20:341–349

Remy-Jardin M, Delhaye D, Teisseire A et al. (2006) MDCT of right ventricular function: Impact of methodological approach in estimation of right ventricular ejection fraction, part 2. AJR 187:1605–1609

Render ML, Weinstein AS, Blaustein AS (1995) Left ventricular dysfunction in deteriorating patients with chronic obstructive pulmonary disease. Chest 107:162–168

Rennard SI (2005) Clinical approach to patients with chronic obstructive pulmonary disease and cardiovascular disease. Proc Am Thorac Soc 2:94–100

Revel MP, Faivre JB, Remy-Jardin M et al. (2008) Diagnosis of patent foramen ovale using 64-multidetector row CT. Radiology, accepted

Revel MP, Faivre JB, Remy-Jardin M et al. (2008) ECG-gated 64-slice multi-detector row CT angiography of the chest: Evaluation of new functional parameters as diagnostic criteria of pulmonary hypertension. Radiology, admitted

Roeleveld RJ, Marcus JT, Faes TJC et al. (2005) Interventricular septal configuration at MR imaging and pulmonary arterial pressure in pulmonary hypertension. Radiology 234:710–717

Rudin M (2007) Imaging readouts as biomarkers or surrogate parameters for the assessment of therapeutic interventions. Eur Radiol 17:2441–2457

Sabit R, Bolton CE, Edward PH et al. (2007) Arterial stiffness and osteoporosis in chronic obstructive pulmonary disease. Am J Respir Crit Care Med 175:1259–1265

Salem R, Remy-Jardin M, Delhaye D et al. (2006) Integrated cardio-thoracic imaging with ECG-gated 64-slice multidetector-row CT: initial findings in 133 patients. Eur Radiol 16:1973–1981

Sanderson JE (2007) Heart failure with a normal ejection fraction. Heart 93:155–158

Santos S, Peinado VI, Ramirez J et al. (2002) Charactezisation of pulmonary vascular remodelling in smokers and patients with mild COPD. Eur Respir J 19:632–638

Savransky V, Nanayakkara A, Li J et al. (2007) Chronic intermittent hypoxia induces atherosclerosis. Am J Respir Crit Care Med 175:1290–1297

Scharf SM, Iqbal M, Keller C et al. (2002) Hemodynamic characterization of patients with severe emphysema. Am J Respir Crit Care Med 166:314–322

Schuster DP (2007) The opportunity and challenges of developing imaging biomarkers to study lung function and disease. Am J Respir Crit Care Med 176:224–230

Shapiro BP, McGoon MD, Redfield MM (2007) Unexplained pulmonary hypertension in elderly patients. Chest 131:94–100

Siafakas NM, Anthonisen NR, Georgopoulos D (2004) Acute exacerbations of chronic obstructive pulmonary disease. Marcel Dekker, New York - Basel

Sin DD, Man SFP (2005) Chronic obstructive pulmonary disease as a risk factor for cardiovascular morbidity and mortality. Proc Am Thorac Soc 2:8–11

Sin DD, Wu LL, Man SFP (2005) The relationship between reduced lung function and cardiovascular mortality. A population-based study and a systematic review of the literature. Chest 127:1952–1959

Soliman A, Shanoudy H, Liu J et al. (1999) Increased prevalence of patent foramen ovale in patients with severe chronic obstructive pulmonary disease. J Am Soc Echocardiogr 12:99–105

Stewart BF, Siscovick D, Link BK et al. (1997) Clinical factors associated with calcific aortic valve disease. J Am Coll Cardiol 29:630–634

Thabut G, Dauriat G, Stern JB et al. (2005) Pulmonary hemodynamics in advanced COPD candidates for lung volume reduction surgery or lung transplantation. Chest 127:1531–1536

Van der Linden J, Bergman P, Hadjinikolaou L (2007) The topography of aortic atherosclerosis enhances its precision as a predictor of stroke. Ann Thorac Surg 83:2087–2092

Van der Woude HJ, Zaagsma J, Postma DS et al. (2005) Detrimental effects of β-blockers in COPD. A concern for nonselective β-blockers. Chest 127:818–824

Visontai Z, Lenard Z, Karlocai K, Kollai M (2000) Assessment of the viscosity of the pulmonary artery wall. Eur Respir J 16:1134–1141

Vizza CD, Lynch JP, Ochoa LL, Richardson G, Trulock EP (1998) Right and left ventricular dysfunction in patients with severe pulmonary disease. Chest 113:576–583

Vonk-Noordegraaf A, Marcus JT, Holverda S et al. (2005) Early changes of cardiac structure and function in COPD patients with mild hypoxemia. Chest 127:1898–1903

Weitzenblum E, Chaouat A (1998) Right ventricular function in COPD. Chest 113:567–568

Weitzenblum E, Chaouat A (2005) Severe pulmonary hypertension in COPD. Is it a distinct disease? Chest 127:1480–1482

Working Group Report (1998) How to diagnose diastolic heart failure. Eur Heart J 19:990–1003

Wright JL, Levy RD, Churg A (2005) Pulmonary hypertension in chronic obstructive pulmonary disease: current theories of pathogenesis and their implications for treatment. Thorax 60:605–609

Yamato H, Sun JP, Churg A, Wright JL (1997) Guinea pig pulmonary hypertension caused by cigarette smoke cannot be explained by capillary bed destruction. J Appl Physiol 82:1644–1653

Immunologic Lung Disease

12

Delphine Gamondès and Didier Revel

CONTENTS

12.1 Introduction

Immunologic lung disease regroups several entities with unknown origin, with pathophysiology involving an auto-immune process, and lesions (infiltrates or necrosis) that are often related to small- or medium-size vessels (vascularitis) and a biological profile with some immunological alterations, such as circulating immune complexes, antibodies, etc. Besides the lung, they can involve with a particular predilection the joints, the kidneys, the skin, the brain and, more particularly, the cardiovascular system. The prognosis is variable from one entity to the other, but the cardiovascular system is a major target in terms of life prognosis.

D. Gamondès, MD
Department of Thoracic and Cardiovascular Radiology, University Hospital Louis Pradel, 69006 Lyon, France
D. Revel, MD
Department of Radiology, Hôpital Cardio-vasculaire, Louis Pradel, 28 Avenue Doyen Lépine, 69677 Bron Cédex, France

In this chapter we will concentrate on the more frequent systemic lung disease with cardiac involvement (pericarditis, myocarditis, valvular abnormalities) and in particular ischemic coronary events occurring very often at a younger age than in the normal population. The contribution of MDCT combining a lung parenchymal study with an examination of the cardiovascular system during the same procedure will be discussed.

12.2 Pulmonary Manifestations of Systemic Disease

Lung involvement in systemic disease may be a manifestation of the underlying pathological process, may be a complication of the underlying disease or may be related to the treatment. Imaging and in particular CT (HRCT) play a central role for the evaluation of lung involvement especially when clinically suspected. This aspect, which is beyond the scope of this chapter, has been extensively covered over the last 10 or 15 years in the international literature.

HRCT has several established roles:

- It may demonstrate subtle findings of pathology when the chest radiograph appears normal in patient studied for immunologic lung disease.
- It may participate in narrowing the differential diagnosis in case of overlapping immunologic syndrome.
- It may help to assess the treatment response by acquiring comparative examinations during follow-up.

Aside from the well-established role of HRCT in studying lung parenchyma in these various disorders, the recently proposed technological development of multidetector CT with ECG gating allows the combination of lung parenchyma and heart study during the same examination.

12.3 Cardiac Involvement in Systemic Immunologic Diseases

It is now well know that the heart is a frequent target of several systemic autoimmune diseases with associated lung involvement. The more frequently encountered entities are in particular systemic lupus erythematosus (SLE), rheumatoid arthritis (RA) and progressive systemic sclerosis (PSS) (Roman and Salmon 2003), although cardiac involvement could also be observed during several vasculitis such as Churg-Strauss syndrome (CSS) (Pela 2006).

Cardiac involvement is considered common with a variable frequency from one entity to the other and is given a high rank among the causes of morbidity and mortality. There is a common finding among all these systemic auto-immune diseases; regarding cardiac disease, all structures of the heart may be involved (Table 12.1).

12.3.1 Pericardial Disease

Pericardial disease, as a manifestation of serositis, is the most clinical cardiovascular manifestation (20 to 50%) (Cervera et al. 1992; Sturfelt et al. 1992) of SLE. Pericardial effusions may occur in the setting of active disease, but may be asymptomatic (Doherty and Siegel 1985). In case of mild pericardial effusions, typical electrocardiographic changes may be absent. Thus, the detection of a small amount of serositis with MDCT may be easier than with echocardiography (Fig. 12.1). In systemic sclerosis, limited to cutaneous disease, including CREST syndrome and diffuse cutaneous disease in which organ involvement (kidneys, lung, etc.) may be seen, pericardial disease is characterized histologically by chronic inflammatory changes. However, clinically important pericardial disease appears to be very rare (Hara 1990).

12.3.2 Valvular Heart Disease

Systemic auto-immune diseases are often complicated by structural of functional valvular abnormalities. Echocardiographic studies as well as autopsy

Table 12.1. Cardiac manifestations of several systemic diseases

Disease	Involvement frequency %		Pericardium	Endocardium valve	Myocardium	Coronary artery
	Clinical	Anatomical				
Systemic lupus erythematosus (SLE)	30–60		++	++	+	+
Progressive systemic sclerosis (PSS)	7–15	50–70	+	0	++	++
Rheumatoid arthritis (RA)	1–10	30–50	++	+	0	+/–
Ankylosing spondylitis	40		+/-	++ (AI)	+	0
Systemic vasculitis						
- Behcet	2–6	16	+	+/–	0	+
- Wegener and Chug-Strauss	10–15	6–44	++	+/–	+/-	++
- Takayasu	72		0	++ (AI)	++	+/–

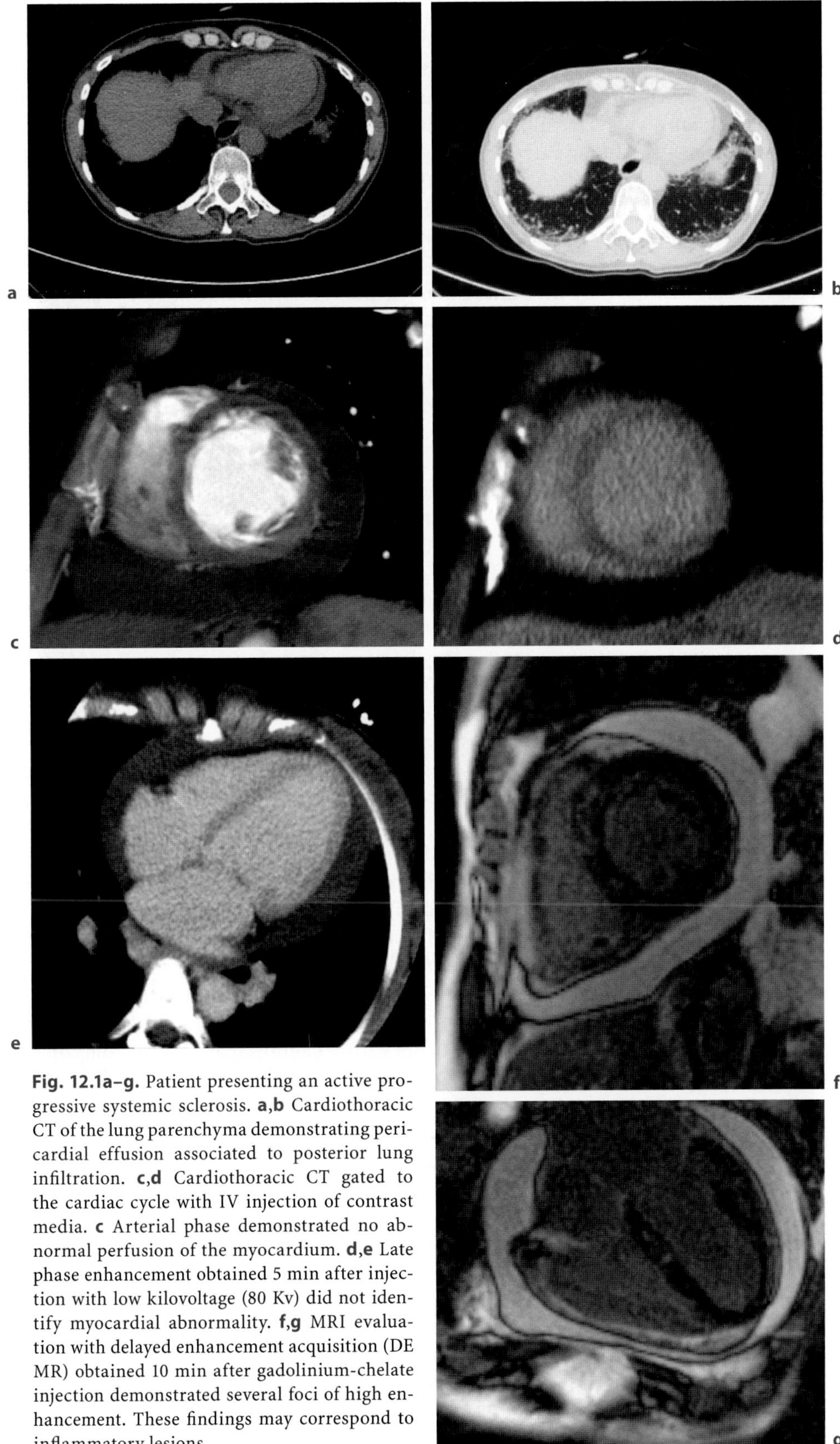

Fig. 12.1a–g. Patient presenting an active progressive systemic sclerosis. **a,b** Cardiothoracic CT of the lung parenchyma demonstrating pericardial effusion associated to posterior lung infiltration. **c,d** Cardiothoracic CT gated to the cardiac cycle with IV injection of contrast media. **c** Arterial phase demonstrated no abnormal perfusion of the myocardium. **d,e** Late phase enhancement obtained 5 min after injection with low kilovoltage (80 Kv) did not identify myocardial abnormality. **f,g** MRI evaluation with delayed enhancement acquisition (DE MR) obtained 10 min after gadolinium-chelate injection demonstrated several foci of high enhancement. These findings may correspond to inflammatory lesions

reports reveal abnormalities in up to 70% of patients with rheumatoid arthritis. These involvements have been described as "nonspecific endocarditis" with valvular inflammation and fibrosis with thickening and calcific changes detected more frequently at the base of the valve and in the valve ring (Fig. 12.2).

MDCT with reconstruction oriented along the valve anatomy is very powerful to detect these changes and in particular to characterize the calcific deposition. These changes may frequently result in mild valvular insufficiency with minimal or no hemodynamic modifications. Rheumatoid arthritis patients mostly have single valve involvement, but any of the valves may be affected. However, the mitral valve is the most frequently affected, followed by the aortic, tricuspid and pulmonic valves. In patients with systemic lupus erythematosus (SLE), valvular abnormalities have been demonstrated in up to 50% of patients. It is usually a non-specific thickening of the mitral and aortic valves (Roldan et al. 1996).

The most characteristic valvular abnormality of SLE is Libman-Sacks endocarditis, which appears as non-infectious verrucous valvular vegetations, most commonly on the mitral valve. MDCT may demonstrate the verrucae in the recess between the ventricle wall and posterior valve leaflet, but also on either surface of the valve, the commissures and the ring with appropriate anatomical plane reconstruction with thin sections (Fig. 12.2).

Although there is no specific treatment for valve disease in SLE, Libman-Sacks endocarditis should be a diagnosis of exclusion. Infective endocarditis or antiphospholipid antibody syndrome could be associated with valvular lesions in SLE merit specific treatment. Following the American Heart Association guidelines, bacterial endocarditis prophylaxis should be taken into account for SLE patients with valvular heart disease, even in absence of nodules. Indications for surgical interventions for valvular heart disease do not differ from those applied in the general population (Roman and Salmon 2007).

12.3.3 Myocardial Disease and Coronary Artery Disease

It is now well known that premature coronary heart disease is a major determinant of morbidity and mortality in patients with SLE and PSS. This is less true for patients with RA. Atherosclerosis occurs prematurely in patients with SLE and PSS and appears independent of traditional risk factors for cardiovascular disease. A recent study (Espaile 2001) suggested that SLE may be atherogenic through chronic activation of the immune system.

This premature development of atherosclerotic coronary artery disease has been demonstrated in autopsy (Bulkley 1975), mortality and population-based observational studies in SLE. MDCT may allow easy detection of coronary artery calcification clearly indicating in young patients that premature atherosclerosis occurs in SLE as a consequence of the disease itself.

Myocarditis is difficult to detect clinically. However, it is usually associated with active disease (myositis and serositis) (Borenstein et al. 1978). During lupus myocarditis, impaired left ventricle systolic function and segmental wall notion abnormalities may be observed and could be reversed by aggressive immunosuppressive therapy (Law et al. 2005).

These considerations may justify the evaluation of global and segmental left ventricle and right ventricle function during an MDCT examination of the chest in patients presenting an active phase of the disease or during the resolving phase.

In PSS, myocardial disease may be multifactorial. An autopsy study performed at Johns Hopkins Hospital suggested the existence of "primary" myocardial disease with focal areas of contraction band necrosis, reperfusion lesion and fibrosis in both ventricles despite patent epicardial coronary arteries (Bulkley 1976).

Myocardial disease may include segmental wall motion abnormalities and impaired coronary flow reserve in the absence of epicardial coronary artery disease. The existence of microvascular disease, including spasm, limits the contribution of MDCT to right ventricle and left ventricle function assessment up to now.

In the future, the development of MDCT technology allowing the study of myocardial tissue repeatedly with some pharmacological stress (such as in nuclear medicine or with MRI or myocardial contrast echocardiography) may be promising to detect microvascular alterations during these pathologies (Turiel et al. 2005).

The right ventricle may also be abnormal in systemic sclerosis, even in the absence of pulmonary hypertension, likely due to microvascular disease. This situation may also benefit from right ventricle function evaluation with MDCT. Potential explana-

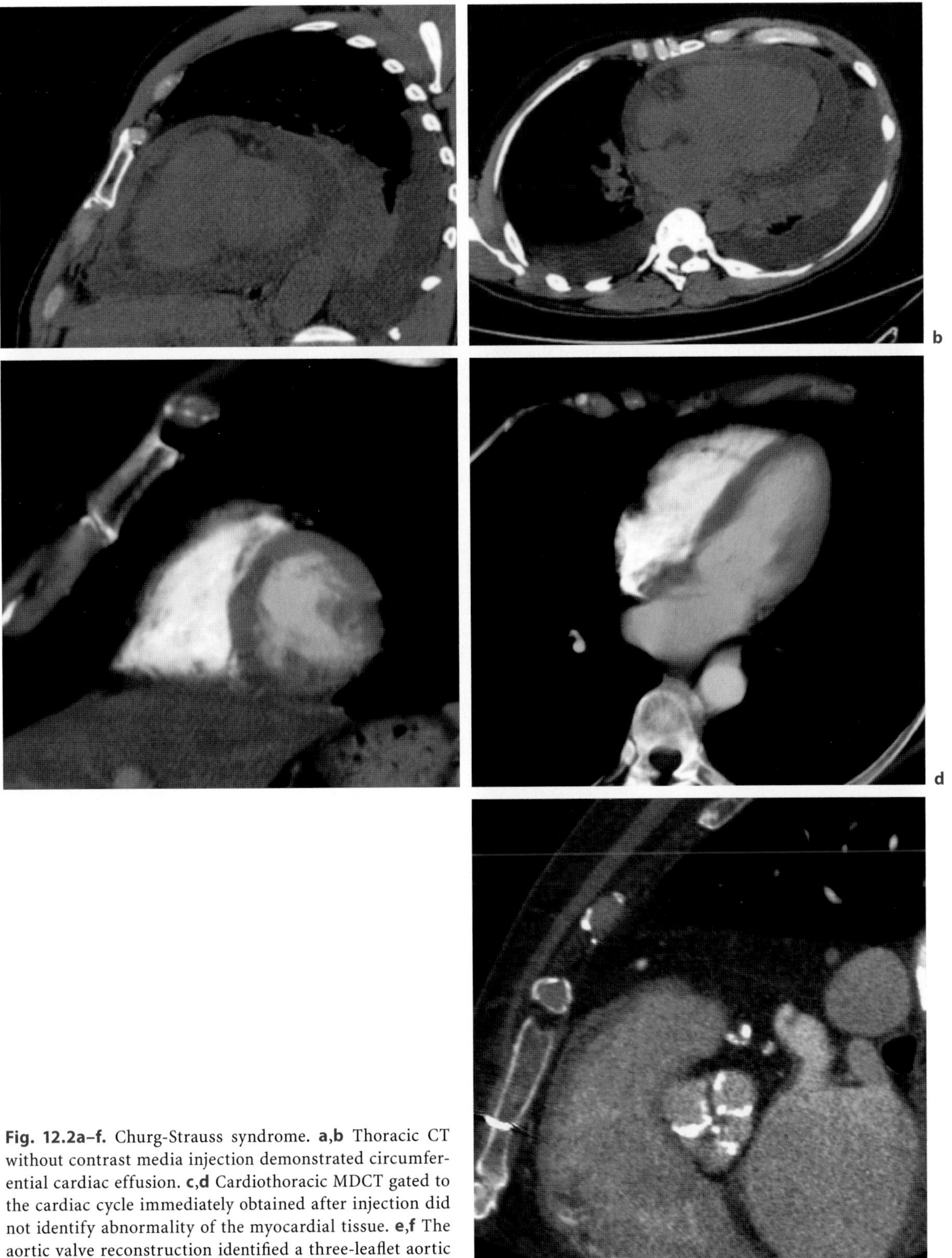

Fig. 12.2a–f. Churg-Strauss syndrome. **a,b** Thoracic CT without contrast media injection demonstrated circumferential cardiac effusion. **c,d** Cardiothoracic MDCT gated to the cardiac cycle immediately obtained after injection did not identify abnormality of the myocardial tissue. **e,f** The aortic valve reconstruction identified a three-leaflet aortic valve with calcifications

tions of SLE that may facilitate the atherosclerotic process include corticosteroid use, renal disease with hypertension and the presence of antiphopholipid antibodies. The corticosteroids largely used in these rheumatoid diseases probably have a role in the atherosclerosis observed (Manzi and Wasco 2006).

Although there are interesting parallels between the pathogenesis of SLE and RA and atherosclerosis (premature atherosclerosis at the microvascular level), a direct link between these inflammation-mediated disease and the inflammatory process underlying atherogenesis is still under investigation. The contribution of MDCT to the assessment of the myocardial involvement of these inflammatory diseases is still limited, although there are some early reports showing interesting findings in case of acute myocarditis with low kilovoltage acquisition. However, no particular study has already demonstrated myocardial involvement with MDCT. This evaluation today refers to MRI with late-enhancement acquisition after gadolinium-chelate intravenous injection (Figs. 12.1f–g, 12.3).

12.4 Conclusions

Cardiac complications of immunologic lung diseases are quite polymorphic. Their frequency, period of appearance during these different diseases, the type of lesions observed and the incidence on the prognosis are very variable from one entity to the other. However, knowing the kind of lesions that could be encountered justifies the use of cardiothoracic imaging as a comprehensive non-invasive modality to evaluate the involvement of the lung parenchyma as well as the cardiac system during the first evaluation and the follow-up under treatment of these pathological situations.

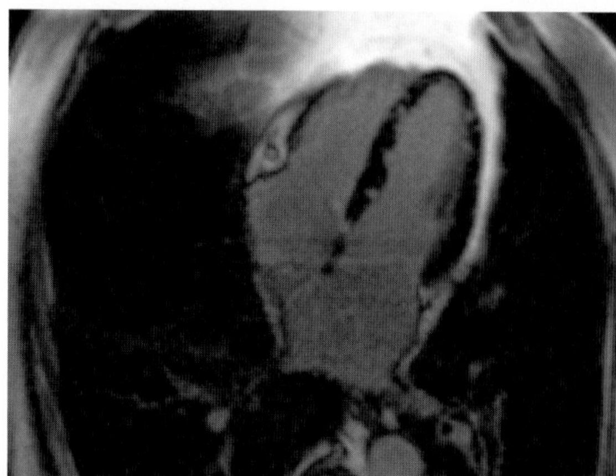

Fig. 12.3. Churg-Strauss syndrome. Cardiac MRI with a late-enhancement acquisition performed 10 min after gadolinium-chelate IV injection demonstrated several foci of high signal intensity on the septum demonstrating myocarditis with a preserved left ventricular function

References

Borenstein DG, Fye WB, Arne TT et al. (1978) The myocarditis of systemic lupus erythematosus: association with myositis. Ann Intern Med 89:619–624

Bulkley BH, Ridolfi KL, Salyer WR et al. (1976) Myocardial lesions of progressive systemic sclerosis: a cause of cardiac dysfunction. Circulation 53:483–490

Bulkley BH, Roberts WC (1995) The heart in systemic lupus erythematosus and the changes induced in it by corticosteroid therapy: a study of 36 necropsy patients. Am J Med 58:243–264

Cervera R, Font J, Pare C et al. (1992) Cardiac disease in systemic lupus erythematosus: prospective study of 70 patients. Ann Rheum Dis 51:156–159

Doherty NE and Siegel RJ (1985) Cardiovascular manifestations of systemic lupus erythematosus. Am Heart J 110:1257–1265

Espaile JM, Abrahamowicz M, Grodzicky T et al. (2001) Traditional Framingham risk factors fail to fully account for accelerated atherosclerosis in systemic lupus erythematosus. Arthritis Rheum 44:2331–2337

Hara KS, Ballard DJ, Ilstrup PM et al. (1990) Rheumatoid pericarditis: clinical features and survival. Medicine 69:81–91

Law WG, Thong BY, Lian TY et al. (2005) Acute lupus myocarditis: clinical features and outcome of an oriented case series. Lupus 14:827–831

Manzi S, Wasko MCM (2006) Inflammation-mediated rheumatic diseases and atherosclerosis. Ann Rheum Dis 59:321–325

Pela G, Tirabassin G, Pattoneri P et al. (2006) Cardiac involvement in the Chirg-Strauss syndrome. Am J Cardiol 97:1519–1524

Roldan CA, Shively BK, Crawford MH (1996) An echocardiographic study of valvular heart disease associated with systemic lupus erythematosus. N Engl J Med 335:1424–1430

Roman MJ, Salmon JE (2007) Cardiovascular manifestations of rheumatologic diseases. Circulation 116:2346–2355

Roman MJ, Shanker BA, Davis A et al. (2003) Prevalence and correlates of accelerated atherosclerosis in systemic lupus erythematosus. N Engl J Med 349:2399–2406

Sturfelt G, Eskilsson J, Nivel O et al. (1992) Cardiovascular disease in systemic lupus erythematosus: a study of 75 patients from a defined population. Medicine 71:216–223

Turiel M, Peretti R, Sarzi-Puttini P et al. (2005) Cardiac imaging techniques in systemic autoimmune diseases. Lupus 14:727–731

Sleep-Related Hypoventilation/Hypoxemic Syndromes (SRHH)

13

Jacques Rémy and Nunzia Tacelli

CONTENTS

13.1 Classification

These syndromes are attributable to disturbances of the ventilatory drive or of the respiratory mechanics. A contemporary review has recently been published (Casey et al. 2007). Its contents are briefly summarized.

J. Rémy, MD, Professor
N. Tacelli, MD
C.H.R.U. de Lille, Hôpital Calmette, Boulevard du Prof. J. Leclercq, 59037 Lille Cédex, France

13.1.1 Idiopathic Sleep-Related Non-Obstructive Alveolar Hypoventilation

Idiopathic sleep-related non-obstructive alveolar hypoventilation is a central hypoventilation without known neurological disease, such as tumors, malformations, infections, stroke or neurosurgical procedures.

13.1.2 Neuro-Muscular and Chest Wall Disorders

SRHHs due to neuro-muscular and chest wall disorders include the following.

13.1.2.1 Obesity-Hypoventilation Syndrome (OHS)

Most cases are associated with obstructive sleep apnea syndrome (OSAS). The prevalence of OSAS in otherwise healthy adults is 5–10%. OSAS is characterized by recurrent episodes of partial or complete obstruction of the upper airways during sleep with a consequent hypoxia. Sleep apnea is defined as episodes of obstructive apnea-hypopnea during sleep, with daytime sleepiness and altered cardio-pulmonary function (Strollo and Rogers 1996). Obesity-hypoventilation syndrome is defined as the association of obesity (body mass index $\geq$30 kg/m^2) and awake chronic hypercapnia. When hypercapnia is detected, chest imaging helps to exclude other respiratory causes (severe COPD, infiltrative lung disease, chest wall disorders). Comorbidities reported in this syndrome are hypertension with a prevalence of 70%, heart failure 30% and significant pulmonary hypertension 30% (Mokhlesi and Tulaimat 2007).

13.1.2.2
Neuro-Muscular Disorders

Neuro-muscular disorders include amyotrophic lateral sclerosis, spinal cord injury, diaphragmatic paralysis, myasthenia gravis, Eaton-Lambert syndrome, toxic and metabolic myopathies. Chest wall disorders include kyphoscoliosis, ankylosing spondylitis, trauma and chronic pleural disease.

13.1.3
COPD and Bronchial Asthma

SRHH is due to lower airways obstruction, including COPD and bronchial asthma.

13.1.4
Pulmonary or Lung Vascular Disorders

SRHH can be due to pulmonary or lung vascular disorders, which can worsen during sleep. These include cystic fibrosis, interstitial lung disease, hypersensitivity pneumonitis, PHT and hemoglobinopathies.

13.1.5
Congenital Central Alveolar Hypoventilation Syndrome

Congenital central alveolar hypoventilation syndrome is typically a pediatric disease.

Sleep-disorder breathing (SDB) is quantified as the average number of apnea-hypopnea events per hour of sleep during polysomnographic registration using the apnea-hypopnea index (AHI). Most of the reviews and articles acknowledge a relationship between the severity of SDB and cardiovascular disease. In addition, obesity and its cardiovascular risks are a major determinant of SDB. For patients with AHI values considered as normal or mildly elevated, there is also a modest to moderate effect of SDD on cardio-vascular disorders (Shahar et al. 2001). Whatever the CT examination performed, with or without contrast medium injection, in a patient with or suspected of having a SDB, and in terms of public health importance, having a look at the heart and great vessels is highly advised.

13.2
Systemic Vascular Disease and Sleep-Disorder Breathing

13.2.1
Early Signs of Atherosclerosis

Early signs of atherosclerosis are detected in middle-aged patients with OSAS who are free of hypertension and diabetes (Drager et al. 2005). They are detected on echo by alterations of mechanical properties of the large arteries. Measurements are performed on the right common carotid artery 1 cm below its bifurcation. They include intima-media thickness (IMT), lumen size, distensibility and plaque detection defined as a localized thickening of the artery wall greater than 1.2 mm. Carotid artery dilatation is a compensatory mechanism of early atherosclerosis and is explained by vascular remodeling aimed at preserving luminal diameter during plaque development (Drager et al. 2005). When acquired on CT with cardiac gating, aortic distensibility can also be measured from changes in aortic diameter during heart cycles. Clinical applications of this technique include cardio-vascular diseases and estimation of left ventricular afterload (Zhang et al. 2007). Arterial stiffness reduces the distensibility and is a risk marker of atherosclerosis.

The mechanisms of early atherosclerosis in OSAS not related to age, hypertension, diabetes mellitus, hypercholesterolemia and smoking are not precisely known. Two hypotheses can be kept in mind: the first one is that systemic inflammation plays a role. C-reactive protein, interleukins 6 and 18 might be associated with the progression of atherosclerosis (Minoguchi et al. 2005), as in COPD patients. These biological markers of inflammation should be known before choosing the acquisition protocols for COPD and SRHH disorders. The second hypothesis is that hypoxia plays a role. Chronic intermittent hypoxia and an atherogenic diet in wild-type mice, highly resistant to atherosclerosis, lead to atherosclerosis in the aortic origin and descending aorta. The same species does not have atherosclerosis when submitted to a high-cholesterol diet or when exposed to chronic intermittent hypoxemia without this atherogenic diet (Savransky et al. 2007).

The consequences of arterial stiffness and systemic hypertension impact on the left ventricle. From an echocardiographic study and after exclusion of patients aged >60 years, having diabetes mellitus, secondary hypertension, cerebrovascular, aortic and cardiac diseases, renal failure, arythmia, smoking and using of non-steroidal antiinflammatory drugs, anticoagulants and statins (Drager et al. 2007), the following conclusions can be drawn: OSAS without systemic hypertension is associated with early signs of left heart remodeling including increased left atrial diameter and interventricular septal thickness, increased ventricular posterior wall thickness, LV mass index and LV hypertrophy. The coexistence of OSAS and systemic hypertension has an addictive effect on arterial stiffness and left heart remodeling.

13.2.2 Sleep-Disordered Breathing and Prevalent Stroke

There is a significant association between sleep-disordered breathing and prevalent stroke, independent of potential confounding factors (Arzt et al. 2005).

13.3 SRHH and Cardiac Diseases

The pathophysiology of the cardiovascular consequences of normal sleep and OSAS has recently been analyzed in a state-of-the-art article (Leung and Bradley 2001). The prevalence of left and right ventricular hypertrophy is high in OSAS (Noda et al. 2006).

13.3.1 LV Remodeling

LV remodeling pathophysiology is multifactorial, including: hypoxia, cyclic increases in blood pressure at the end of apnea, increased arterial stiffness and systemic hypertension. Alterations in pulse-wave velocity contribute to LV afterload. LA enlargement is frequent in OSAS, and it is a risk factor for atrial fibrillation. In patients with non-ischemic dilated cardiomyopathy, OSAS often exists, and its presence is associated with an increased prevalence of left ventricular hypertrophy that predominates on the interventricular septum (Usui et al. 2006).

13.3.2 Ischemic Heart Disease

OSAS predisposes to myocardial ischemia during sleep. It can be asymptomatic. Conversely, among patients with coronary artery disease, those with OSAS have a higher mortality. Non-invasive screening of asymptomatic coronary artery disease is highly recommendable.

13.3.3 Congestive Heart Failure (CHF)

This risk exceeds that of other cardiovascular diseases. CHF can also contribute to the development of OSAS. Acute left ventricular failure during sleep, with nocturnal pulmonary edema, can be seen.

13.3.4 Pulmonary Hypertension (PHT) and RV Dysfunction

Of the patients with OSAS, 15–20% has resting awake PHT (Pinet and Orehek 2005). The main mechanism is hypoxia-induced pulmonary vasoconstriction. The others are hypercapnia, acidosis, transmission to the pulmonary vessels of left ventricular dysfunction and exaggerated negative intrathoracic pressure against the occluded upper airway during apnea (Bradley 1992). The consequences of PHT on RV function have already been reviewed in the COPD chapter. Briefly, the increased pulmonary artery pressure increases right ventricular afterload, which induces a leftward shift of the interventricular septum (Usui et al. 2006). OSAS-induced PHT is generally moderate.

13.3.5 Patent Foramen Ovale (PFO)

The prevalence of PFO is higher in patients with OSAS than in the normal population of the same age: 69% versus 17% according to Shanoudi et al. (1998). The pathophysiology is simple: during apnea-hypopnea noctural episodes, obstruction of the upper airways can act as Valsalva and Müller maneuvers as the patient expires and inspires against the upper airway obstacle (Pinet and Orehek 2005). Consequently, elevated pressures in the right cardiac cavities are comparable to those obtained during the Valsalva maneuver of transoesophageal echocardiography. A right-to-left shunt through the PFO can ensue. According to the level and nycthemeral variation of PHT, this shunt, responsible for a hypoxemia, can be observed in the awake state or during sleeping. As previously mentioned, the PFO can be detected on CT with an appropriate acquisition technique.

References

Arzt M, Young T, Finn L et al. (2005) Association of sleep-disordered breathing and the occurrence of stroke. Am J Respir Crit Care Med 172:1447–1451

Bradley TD (1992) Right and left ventricular function impairment and sleep apnea. Clin Chest Med 13:459–479

Casey KR, Cantillo KO, Brown LK (2007) Sleep-related hypoventilation/hypoxemic syndromes. Chest 131:1936–1948

Drager LF, Bortolotto LA, Lorenzi MC et al. (2005) Early signs of atherosclerosis in obstructive sleep apnea. Am J Respir Crit Care Med 172:613–618

Drager LF, Bortolotto LA, Figueiredo AC et al. (2007) Obstructive sleep apnea hypertension and their interaction on arterial stiffness and heart remodeling. Chest 131:1379–1386

Leung RST, Bradley TD (2001) Sleep apnea and cardiovascular disease. Am J Respir Crit Care Med 164:2147–2165

Minoguchi K, Yokoe T, Tazaki T et al. (2005) Increased carotid intima-media thickness and serum inflammatory markers in obstructive sleep apnea. Am J Respir Crit Care Med 172:625–630

Mokhlesi B, Tulaimat A (2007) Recent advances in obesity hypoventilation syndrome. Chest 132:1322–1336

Noda A, Okada T, Yasuma F et al. (2006) Cardiac hypertrophy in obstructive sleep apnea syndrome. Chest 107:1538–1544

Pinet C, Orehek J (2005) CPAP suppression of awake right-to-left shunting through patent foramen ovale in a patient with obstructive sleep apnea. Thorax 60:880–881

Savransky V, Nanayakkara A, Li J et al. (2007) Chronic intermittent hypoxia induces atherosclerosis. Am J Respir Crit Care Med 175:1290–1297

Shahar E, Whitney CW, Redline S et al. (2001) Sleep-disordered breathing and cardiovascular disease. Am J Respir Crit Care Med 163:19–25

Shanoudy H Soliman A, Raggi P et al. (1998) Prevalence of patent foramen ovale and its contribution to hypoxemia in patients with obstructive sleep apnea. Chest 113:91–96

Strollo PJJ, Rogers RM (1996) Obstructive sleep apnea. N Engl J Med 334:99–104

Usui K, Parker JD, Newton GE (2006) Left ventricular structural adaptations to obstructive sleep apnea in dilated cardiomyopathy. Am J Respir Crit Care Med 173:1170–1175

Zhang J, Fletcher JG, VrtiskaTJ et al. (2007) Large-vessel distensibility measurement with electrocardiographically gated multidetector CT: Phantom study and initial experience. Radiology 245:258–266

Medical Applications of Integrated Cardiothoracic Imaging

Thoracic Consequences of Cardiac Diseases

Imaging Findings Associated with Left-Sided Cardiac Dysfunction

14

Nicola Sverzellati and David M. Hansell

CONTENTS

Abstract

Computed tomography (CT) has provided new insights into the alterations that occur in the lungs in patients with cardiac disease. In this chapter the emphasis is on the imaging features associated with left sided-cardiac dysfunction, particularly the spectrum of thin-section CT thoracic abnormalities. Some controversial entities such as "cardiac asthma" and the chronicity of the pulmonary changes are discussed. The new perspective of integrating pulmonary and cardiac information provided by multidetector-row CT (MDCT) is also considered.

14.1 Introduction

The pulmonary manifestations of heart disease are diverse. The chest radiograph has historically been the mainstay in understanding the complex interaction between the heart and the lungs, and it remains a vital tool for understanding pulmonary complications of left heart disease. The relationship between cardiac hemodynamics and the chest radiograph in patients with left-sided cardiac failure has been well documented over the years (Milne et al. 1973; Pistolesi et al. 1985). In this context, the chest radiograph is not passé, but still useful. In addition to its lower dose and cost, an important advantage of the chest radiograph over CT is the facility of examining patients in the erect position, which provides more reproducible and pathophysiologic insights into a patient's hemodynamic status.

CT findings in the lungs of patients with heart disease have received relatively little attention. Nevertheless, CT is more sensitive to small changes in lung water content than chest radiography and may be helpful

N. Sverzellati, MD
Department of Clinical Sciences, Institute of Radiology, University of Parma, Via Gramsci 14, 43100 Parma, Italy
D. M. Hansell, MD, FRCP, FRCR
Department of Radiology, Royal Brompton Hospital, Sydney Street, London, SW3 6NP, UK

in diagnosing unrecognized pulmonary edema, or in differentiating edema from other disease processes in patients who have multiple medical problems (Goodman 1996). As CT plays a greater role in the imaging of intensive-care patients, radiologists are often called to interpret the common CT features associated with left-sided cardiac dysfunction. Furthermore, in order to avoid misdiagnosis it is also important to be aware of some confusing patterns associated with left-sided heart failure as, in clinical practice, an uncommon pattern of edema may be more common than an obscure interstitial lung disease.

14.2 Functional Consequences of Left-Sided Cardiac Dysfunction

Elevated pressures in the pulmonary microvasculature are usually due to left-sided cardiac failure, with elevated left atrial pressures transmitted in a retrograde direction into the pulmonary circulation. Left cardiac failure has many causes: it arises as a consequence of an abnormality in cardiac structure, function, rhythm or a combination. Ventricular dysfunction accounts for the majority of cases and results mainly from myocardial infarction, hypertension or, in many cases, both. Degenerative valve disease and cardiomyopathy are also frequent causes of left-sided heart failure (Figueroa and Peters 2006).

As pulmonary venous pressure rises, so do pulmonary capillary and arterial pressures. A rise in pulmonary venous pressure firstly increases the pulmonary blood volume through vessel distension and recruitment. At higher filling pressures, fluid may begin to cross the microvascular barrier. If the pressure increase is sufficient to exceed the rate of clearance of filtrate, pulmonary edema ensues. The filtrate accumulates in the interstitial spaces of the lung, first in the loose peribronchovascular tissues, in the interlobular septa and ultimately in the alveolar septa (Hughes 2005). It is thought that the fluid moves from the pulmonary interstitial spaces (i.e., subpleural space) across the visceral pleura. Fluid accumulates in the pleural space when the rate of entry exceeds the capacity of the lymphatics in the parietal pleura to remove the fluid (Wiener-Kronish 1993). Both pleural space and peribronchovascular tissue can be thought of as acting as a sump or safety valve to prevent an excessive rise in interstitial pressure, which would flood the alveoli with edema fluid and impair gas exchange (Hughes 2005).

The effects on the lung vary according to the severity of venous pressure elevation and the chronicity of the condition. For example, a previously healthy individual may develop pulmonary edema when the pulmonary capillary wedge pressure reaches only 25 mmHg, whereas a patient with longstanding congestive heart failure is symptom-free and without significant pulmonary edema at a filling pressure of 40 mmHg. The reason for this apparent paradox lies in a variety of adaptations that occur in the lung that has been exposed to chronically elevated filling pressures (Gelhbach and Geppert et al. 2002). These adaptations essentially consist of both hypertrophic and fibrotic changes in the pulmonary vessels, lymphatics, interstitium and alveolar walls (Haworth et al. 1988). Chronic left-sided cardiac dysfunction may also result in pulmonary arterial hypertension and right ventricular failure. Predictably, patients with chronic left-sided heart failure often exhibit a restrictive ventilatory defect, whereas airflow obstruction is a more frequent finding associated with acute failure (Light and George 1983; Johnson et al. 2001). The type of ventilatory deficit is variable because of differing contributions from edema, pleural effusions, vascular engorgement, raised airways resistance and respiratory muscle weakness.

A rise in airway resistance is often present, but not severe. The term "cardiac asthma" is used to describe the shortness of breath and the wheezing that can be heard on auscultation in patients with left-sided heart failure. This is likely due to airway wall edema or the effects of the increased bronchial venous pressure resulting in reflex bronchoconstriction (Bernard et al. 1995; Hwang et al. 2001). A few studies also report increased methacoline hyper-responsiveness in patients with congestive heart failure, in smokers and nonsmokers alike (Cabanes et al. 1989; Rolla et al. 1993). However, the degree of bronchial hyperreactivity that occurs in patients with heart failure is a matter of speculation.

14.3 Vascular Changes

The signs of raised pulmonary venous pressure on chest radiography are well known. Signs of vascular redistribution (from bases to apex), namely balanced flow or inverted flow, often suggest elevation of the pulmonary venous pressure. Both vascular dilation and redistribution are likely more appreciable in chronic or at least subacute left heart dysfunction (Morgan and Goodman 1991; Ketai 1998). The ratio of the diameter of adjacent pulmonary arteries and bronchi seen end-on, particularly at the level of the upper lobes, aids in determining whether vessels are abnormally enlarged (Woodring 1991). The measurement of the width of the so-called vascular pedicle (the superior mediastinum just above the aortic arch) is used to assess the patients' intravascular volume status and is mostly helpful when comparison radiographs are available (Ely 2002).

Chest radiographic signs of raised venous pressure have to be interpreted with care, as many factors may influence them. Assessment of early and subtle signs is prone to significant interobserver variation, and evaluation should be attempted only when patients are fully upright, films are exposed on inspiration, and lung bases are normal (i.e., simple atelectasis or pneumonia can result in blood flow cephalization).

Some CT vascular changes mirror the radiographic ones in patients with left-sided heart failure. Herold et al. (1992), using HRCT in a pig model, showed that acute fluid overload causes a 20% increase in arterial size, a 33% increase in venous size and a gravity-dependent increase in parenchymal attenuation. Although the increased artery/bronchus ratio is generally regarded as a reliable sign of abnormal vascular dilatation, minor discrepancies to this rule are frequently encountered due to prevailing physiologic conditions and artifacts, such as motion, or the orientation of the vessels in relation to the plane of CT section. Vascular dilatation is easiest to recognize in the perihilar regions, where arterial and bronchial diameters can be compared. However, it is not possible with high-resolution CT (HRCT) to reliably separate vascular dilatation from perivascular thickening due to interstitial edema, although the latter is more likely when the adjacent bronchial wall appears thickened. Maximum intensity projection (MIP) reformations of variable thickness are theoretically suitable for assessing the size and location of vessels, including both the pulmonary arteries and veins (Beigelman et al. 2005), but unfamiliarity with this rudimentary post-processing means that is not a maneuver that is often used in clinical practice (Fig. 14.1).

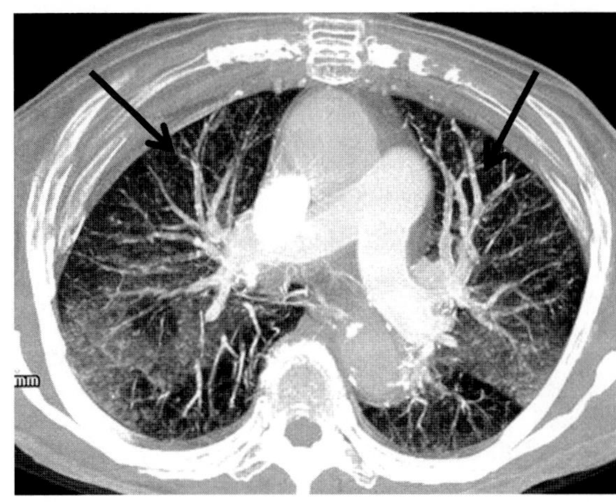

Fig. 14.1. Recurrent cardiogenic edema in a 67-year-old man. Coronal MIP image (10-mm-thick slab) shows bilateral ground-glass opacities in the upper lobes. The anterior (non-dependent) vessels (*arrows*) appear conspicuous and more dilated than those in the more dependent lung

Vascular dilatation may be observed in association with other HRCT abnormalities, before the development of frank pulmonary edema. Although not systematically documented, it is likely that the earliest detectable findings associated with enlarged vessels are scant interlobular septal thickening and ground-glass opacities. Smooth septal lines are often limited to the level of the pulmonary apices and may be contributed to by engorged septal veins (Storto et al. 1995). It has been shown in dogs that the increased venous pressure leads to ground-glass opacity before a significant increase in extravascular lung water (Scillia et al. 1999). It is possible that increased blood volume is the cause of ground-glass opacity on HRCT, or that ground glass opacity reflects very subtle interstitial edema (Hedlund et al. 1984; Herold et al. 1992; Scillia et al. 1999).

In patients with left-sided heart failure, centrilobular artery branches may appear prominent (Storto et al. 1995), and vessels may become more visible at the periphery of the lung, and non-gravity-dependent vessels may enlarge disproportionately, reflecting the process of "cephalization" seen on the chest radiograph (Goodman 1996) (Fig. 14.1). An accepted explanation for the redistribution of pulmonary blood flow is that of West and associates (1965), who suggested that the development of dependent edema may form a perivascular cuff, which acts as a buffer between the vessels and the distending forces being transmitted through the lungs, with resultant redistribution of blood flow (Hansell et al. 2005).

However, no information is available about the relationship between the hemodynamic measurements and vessel changes on CT in human subjects with left-sided heart failure. It is likely that such relationships are perturbed because of several factors, such as the tempo of the disease and lag phenomenon between hemodynamic and CT changes.

HRCT has not been reported as demonstrating signs of small airways disease ascribable to left-sided heart failure. Clearly there are difficulties in obtaining CT expiratory scans in ill patients. Nevertheless, Ribeiro et al. (2006) reported in most (67%) patients with left ventricular failure a mosaic attenuation pattern that may be, at least, suggestive of a component of small airways obstruction (Fig. 14.3).

14.4 Bronchial Changes

When edema collects in the peribronchovascular interstitial space, so-called "peribronchial cuffing" is seen on chest radiography (Don and Johnson 1977). This increase in the thickness is only readily evident in bronchi seen end-on, but it may be also evident along the posterior wall of the bronchus intermedius on the lateral chest radiograph (Schnur et al. 1981). Peribronchovascular thickening, readily seen on CT, corresponds to the peribronchial cuffing seen on chest radiography. Bronchial wall thickening is mostly evident at the level of subsegmental and segmental bronchi (Figs. 14.2, 14.3). Its high prevalence on CT is in contrast with the relatively low prevalence (10–35%) of the clinical features of "cardiac asthma" (Jorge et al. 2007), although previously some authors have suggested a relationship between the two (Hwang et al. 2001; Hunt et al. 2001).

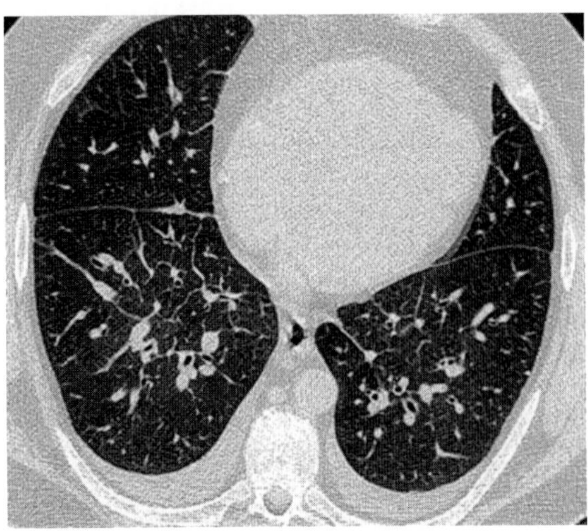

Fig. 14.2. Early interstitial edema. HRCT illustrates peribronchial thickening, diffuse increase in attenuation of the lung parenchyma, a few prominent interlobular septa and bilateral pleural effusion

14.5 Predominantly Interstitial Edema

On CT, interstitial pulmonary edema is usually seen as a combination of thickened interlobular septa, bronchovascular thickening and ground-glass opacities.

Thickened interlobular septa are due to fluid trasudate expanding the interlobular septa. Peripheral thickened interlobular septa on CT correspond to the Kerley lines A and B seen on the chest radiograph. In both the peripheral and the central lung regions, smooth thickened septa outlining one or more adjacent pulmonary lobules can be seen as polygonal arcades; these can be bilateral and diffuse, but occasionally focal and unilateral. In many cases bilateral thickened interlobular septa constitute the predominant CT sign of interstitial edema (Fig. 14.4). The absence of distortion of lung parenchyma and

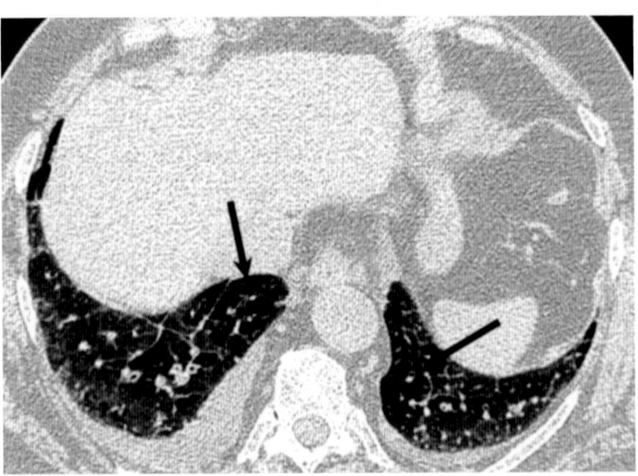

Fig. 14.3. Mosaic attenuation pattern in a patient with the clinical features on auscultation of "cardiac asthma" due to acute left ventricular failure. *Grey areas* are made of a few thickened interlobular septa, peribronchial thickening and ground glass, whereas there is mild dilatation of some of the bronchi within the decreased attenuation of the lung (*arrows*). Bilateral pleural effusion is also present

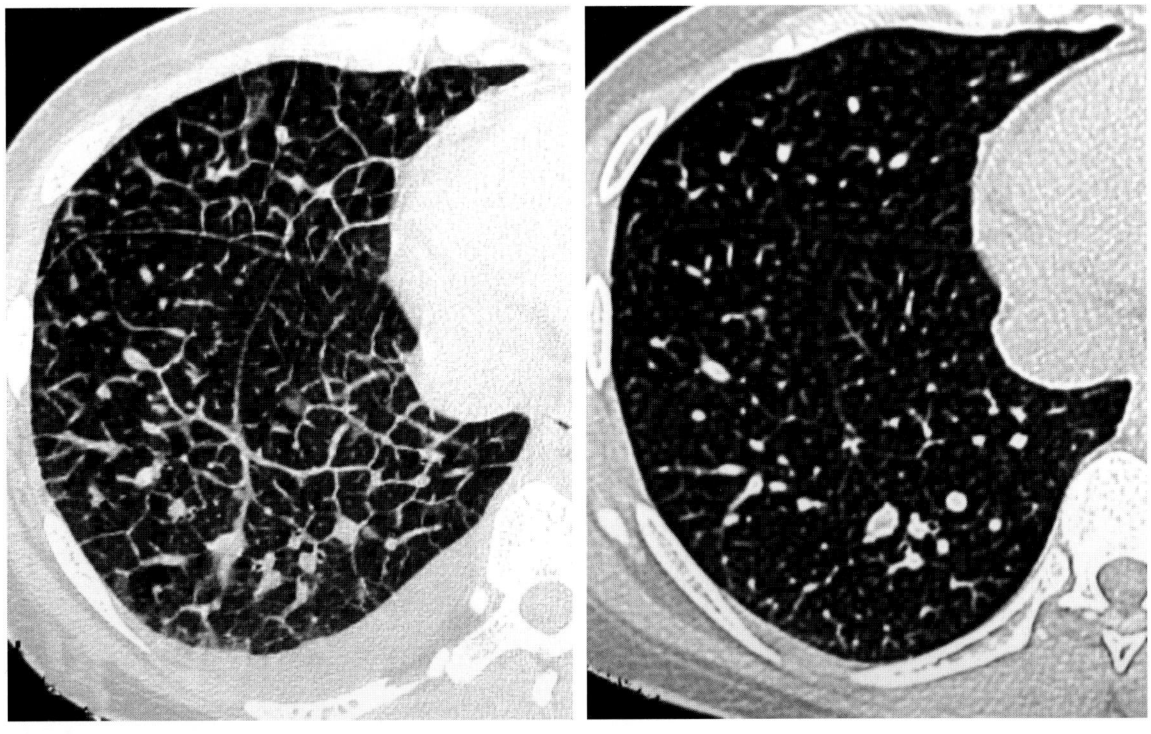

Fig. 14.4. a Acute interstitial edema characterized by diffuse smooth interlobular septal thickening and pleural effusion. **b** Follow-up CT after treatment demonstrates resolution of these abnormalities

the more linear, smooth septal thickening, despite extensive involvement, helps to differentiate cardiogenic interstitial edema from lymphangitis carcinomatosa, sarcoidosis and other interstitial lung diseases, which generally have associated findings, in addition to more irregular septal thickening.

One of the most consistent plain radiographic findings with pure interstitial edema, especially when follow-up films are available, is the lack of clarity of the intrapulmonary and hilar vessels (hilar haze) due to surrounding edema (Pistolesi and Giuntini 1978). This feature is also seen on HRCT, which may show central ground-glass opacification and somewhat indistinct central vascular margins. CT studies of experimental hydrostatic pulmonary edema in animals support the concept that edema tends to involve the peribronchovascular interstitium before affecting the interlobular septa (Forster et al. 1992). However, human lungs have relatively well-developed interlobular septa, whereas dog lungs show an almost complete lack of septa (Todo and Herman 1986; Forster et al. 1992). Thus, thickening of the interlobular septa, of the bronchovascular and subpleural interstitium, and thickening of the bronchovascular core structures in the pulmonary lobule may apparently occur simultaneously.

Accumulation of fluid in the loose connective tissue beneath the visceral pleura may be seen as thickening of the fissures and vertical lamellar opacities in the costophrenic angles. It is the lamellar shape with shadow conforming to the pleural boundary that suggests pulmonary rather than pleural fluid (Hansell et al. 2005). On HRCT, transient subpleural curvilinear opacities, possibly representing engorged lymphatics, have been described in patients with left-ventricular failure (Arai et al. 1990).

Ground-glass opacification is one of the most common findings, reflecting thickened (i.e., edematous) alveolar walls and intralobular interstitium. Ground-glass is often patchy in distribution (Fig. 14.5). When diffuse and uniform, ground-glass opacification may be a source of diagnostic uncertainty, as it is often contributed to by underinflation owing to an inability to hold breath at full inspiration (Dalal and Hansell 2006). Superimposition of interlobular and intralobular may result in a "crazy paving" pattern (Fig. 14.6a).

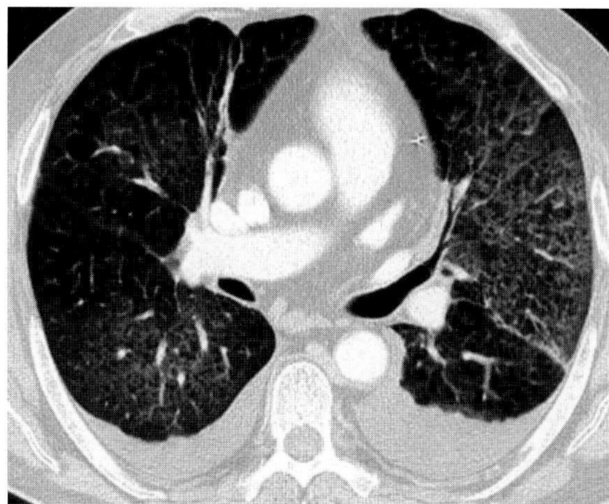

Fig. 14.5. A patient with acute left ventricular failure. Standard CT shows patchy areas of ground-glass opacity superimposed on a background of centrilobular emphysema, giving an unusual texture to the abnormal lung. There are bilateral pleural effusions

14.6 Alveolar Edema

If pulmonary edema is severe enough to flood the alveoli, bilateral, patchy or widespread "fluffy" lung opacities may become evident on chest radiography. These airspace shadows tend to coalesce into frank consolidation.

Ground-glass opacification, crazy paving pattern and consolidation are the typical CT findings associated with advanced alveolar edema (Fig. 14.6a,b). The extent of dense air-space opacification versus "ground-glass" opacification depends on the amount of gas displaced by the edema and atelectasis (Goodman 1996).

It has been postulated that the ventral-dorsal density gradient increases with time, because edema tends to distribute in the lower and central lung zones. However, it is now clear that distribution of pulmonary edema is much more variable than previously thought. For instance, distribution may be the result of the net effect of some opposing forces, such as the gravity and the augmented ventilatory movements in lower zones that promote the removal of fluid through the lymphatics (Müller et al. 2003). In most patients pulmonary edema has a diffuse and random distribution, with some lobes more severely affected than others. Occasionally, edema has a perihilar predominance relatively sparing the peripheral zones, producing the so-called "bat's wing" appearance (Fig. 14.7). Several theories have been proposed to explain the pathophysiology of the bat's wing appearance (Fleischner 1967; Gluecker et al. 1999), which, incidentally, is not specific and may be encountered in other diseases (e.g., pulmonary alveolar proteinosis and pulmonary hemorrhage).

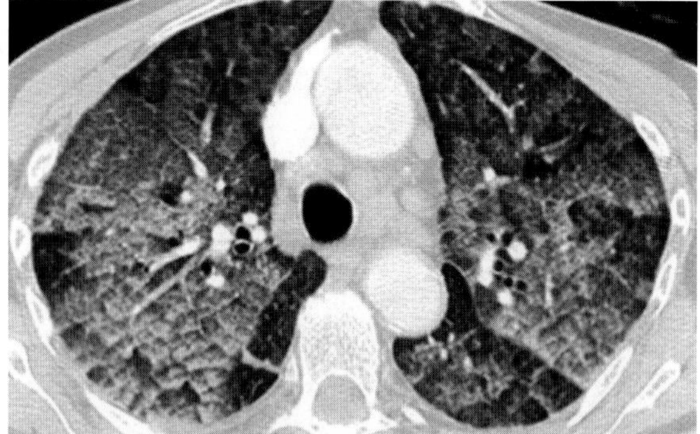

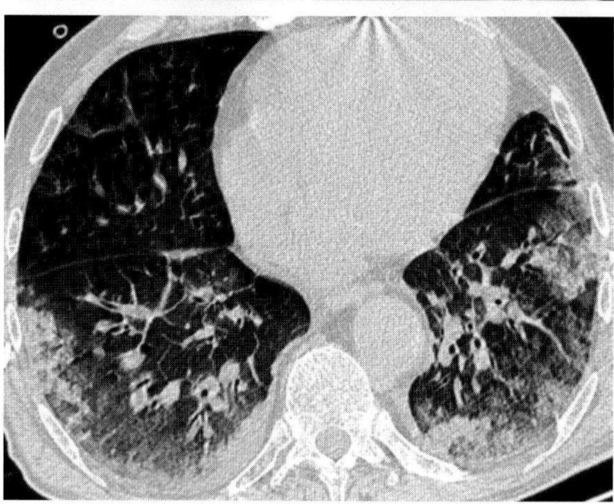

Fig. 14.6a,b. Two examples of alveolar edema. **a** CT shows extensive bilateral opacity with a more geographic distribution. A fine reticular pattern with interlobular as well as intralobular septal thickening superimposed on the ground-glass opacity (crazy-paving pattern). Enlarged mediastinal lymph nodes are also present. **b** In this case, thin-section CT demonstrates airspace consolidation mainly distributed in the dependent zones, with ground-glass opacities, interlobular septal thickening and enlarged vessels

Many factors modify the usual (if there is such a thing) distribution of pulmonary edema. Underlying diseases, such as fibrosis or pulmonary emphysema, may shift edema to more normally perfused areas. In those cases in which the edema is unilateral, it has an unexpected predisposition for the right lung, mostly in edema associated with mitral regurgitation (Gurney and Goodman 1989). Moreover, the position of the patient also influences the fluid distribution as edema will concentrate in the dependent lung.

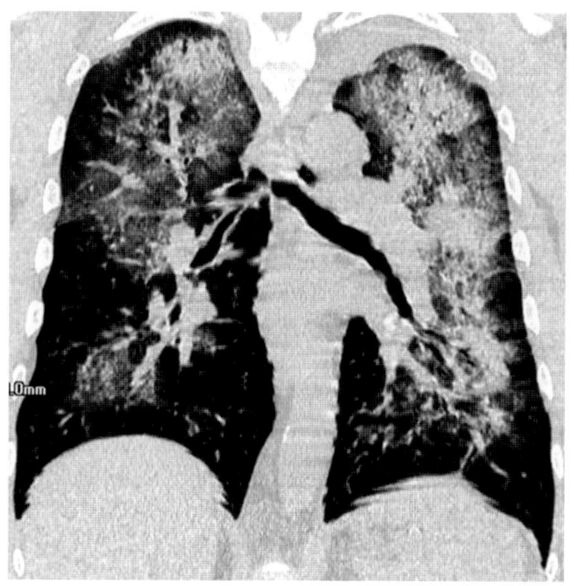

Fig. 14.7. Acute edema caused by myocardial infarction. Coronal reformation shows bilateral perihilar consolidation and ground-glass opacity giving the so-called "bat's wing" appearance

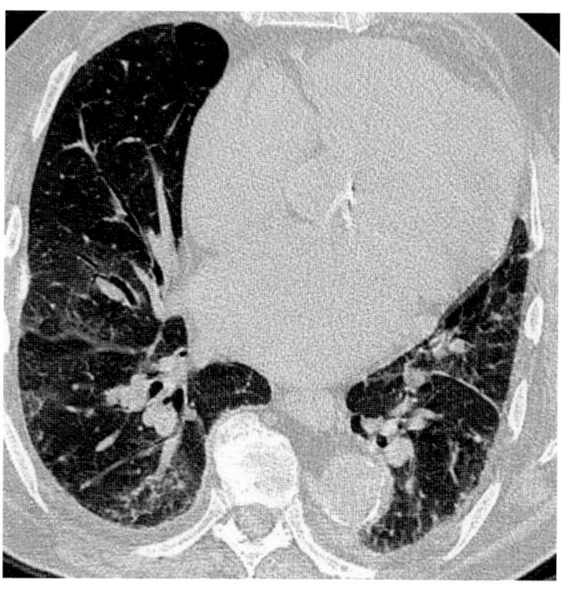

Fig. 14.8. A patient with a chronic left cardiac failure. Patchy ground-glass opacities and a few septal lines with markedly dilated left atrium are consistent of mild interstitial edema

14.7 Chronic Heart Failure

The clinical features of left-sided heart failure are traditionally divided in two phases: acute and chronic. Although significant clinical and radiological overlap can occur, the spectrum of CT features differs between the phases. In cases of chronically elevated pulmonary venous hypertension, CT features of interstitial changes (caused by proliferation of connective tissue, organization of interstitial edema, etc.) might be expected, given the reported pathologic findings (Haworth et al. 1988), but this is poorly documented in the literature (Fig. 14.8). Cardiomegaly and pleural thickening may be present, sometimes with thickening of interlobular septa, but without evident vascular changes and pulmonary edema. More rarely, hemosiderosis from microvascular hemorrhage may be visible on HRCT as small nodules, and hyperattenuating nodules may reflect focal ossification, but this is very rare in practice (Delaunois 2006).

14.8 Distinction between Cardiogenic and Non-Cardiogenic Pulmonary Edema

In the setting of left-sided cardiac failure, pulmonary edema is often called cardiogenic or high-pressure pulmonary edema. However, cardiogenic pulmonary edema is not necessarily purely hydrostatic, in that capillary endothelium damage may occur [even without diffuse alveolar damage (DAD)], resulting in permeability edema. The classification system that has been advocated recognizes four categories: (1) hydrostatic edema; (2) permeability edema caused by DAD; (3) permeability edema without DAD; (4) mixed hydrostatic and permeability (Ketai and Godwin 1998; Gluecker et al. 1999).

However, the division of pulmonary edema into "cardiogenic" or "noncardiogenic," although sometimes elusive, is still convenient, since treatment options are so different. This distinction, either by chest radiography or by CT, is often difficult. A peripheral distribution of the opacities with normal heart size favors noncardiogenic over cardiogenic edema. Exaggerated gravity-dependent consolidation with air bronchogram is seen more commonly in permeability edema. In permeability edema, the segmental and subsegmental bronchi may be dilated within areas of ground-glass opacification, and so resemble "traction bronchiectasis" (Howling et al. 1998). By contrast, in permeability edema vessels may not be as conspicuously dilated, and diffuse septal thickening is less pronounced, whereas they are often the major feature associated with cardiogenic edema (Fig. 14.4).

Ancillary signs, such as the increased cardiothoracic ratio (>0.52) and widened vascular pedicle on chest radiography, are more suggestive of cardiogenic pulmonary edema (Thomason et al. 1998). In addition, pleural effusions in ARDS are generally smaller than those observed in left-sided heart failure.

14.9 Pleural Effusion

Pleural effusions accompanied by cardiomegaly on chest radiography are very suggestive of congestive heart failure. Congestive heart failure is by far the most common cause of transudative pleural effusion (Figs. 14.2–14.5). Pleural fluid accumulates in patients with congestive heart failure when they have left-sided ventricular failure rather than elevated right-sided pressure (Wiener-Kronish et al. 1985, 1987). Porcel and Vives (2006) reviewed the radiographic sidedness of 444 effusions due to heart failure reported in five studies. Of the effusions, 69% were bilateral, 21% were unilateral on the right, and 9% were unilateral on the left. Of the bilateral pleural effusions, most were similarly sized, but either side can be larger.

14.10 Ancillary Abnormalities

Half of the patients with congestive heart failure have enlarged mediastinal lymph nodes on CT, without evidence of other disease (Slanetz et al. 1998; Lewin et al. 2000; Erly et al. 2003; Chabbert et al. 2004). The frequency of enlarged lymph node seems to correlate with the severity of the left heart failure (Slanetz et al. 1998; Chabbert et al. 2004). The most frequent sites for mediastinal lymphadenopathy on CT are the subcarinal, paratracheal and precarinal regions. It has been shown that most (64%) of these enlarged lymph nodes regress after initiation of treatment for cardiac failure (Chabbert et al. 2004) (Fig. 14.9).

Further mediastinal abnormalities can be recognized on CT, likely caused by diffuse fluid infiltration into the mediastinal fat due to elevated hydrostatitic pressure (Slanetz et al. 1998). The prevalence of haziness of mediastinal fat has been reported to be between 10 and 33% of patients with left-sided heart failure (Slanetz et al. 1998; Chabbert et al. 2004). Diffuse mediastinal enlargement has been documented, although significant enlargement is certainly a rare occurrence (Miller et al. 2000). As an

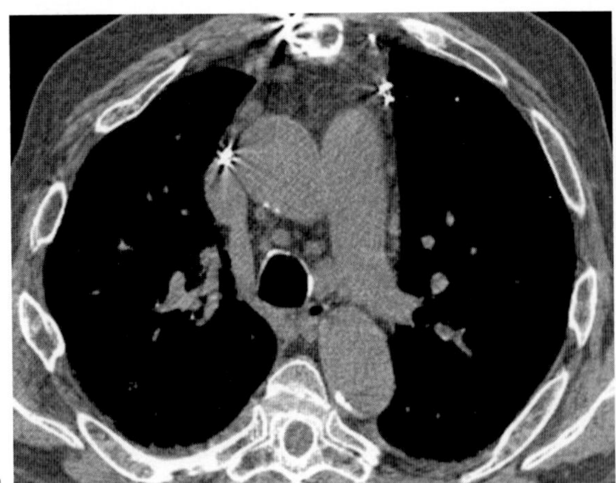

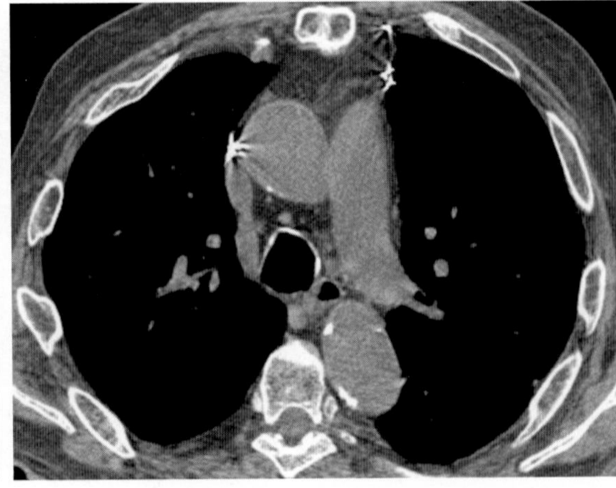

Fig. 14.9a,b. CT obtained in a patient with congestive heart failure due to ischemia. **a** Above the carina, CT shows both enlarged mediastinal lymph nodes and prominent/hazy anterior mediastinal fat. **b** Follow-up CT after treatment shows regression of these signs

aside, tracheal narrowing has also been described in sheep models of cardiogenic edema, and the degree of narrowing has been shown to correlate with the severity of pulmonary edema (Snapper et al. 1999).

14.11 Cardiothoracic Imaging: An Integrated Approach

CT examination of the thorax is often requested for the investigation of disorders that may have an important underlying cardiac cause (Bruzzi et al. 2006). Furthermore, the presence of significant cardiac disease is often underappreciated by the referring clinician (and reporting radiologist). Improvements in CT scanner technology, namely the development of multidetector CT scanners with high temporal and spatial resolution, now provide images during routine chest CT examinations that are much less degraded by cardiac motion artifacts and that allow detailed evaluation of both the lung parenchyma and the heart. This opportunity is particular useful in the setting of left-sided heart failure, as it may improve the detection of a cardiac disease component particularly in difficult scenarios, such as in cases of coexisting diseases, ambiguous pulmonary findings or previously unsuspected cardiac disease (e.g., cardiomyopathy). Many supporting findings, such as cardiomegaly and pericardial abnormalities, can be depicted on routine thoracic CT even without the recourse to the contrast medium administration and ECG gating (Fig. 14.8). For instance, in the presence of CT signs of cor pulmonale with normal-sized left cardiac chambers, interlobular septal thickening and ground-glass opacities are more suggestive of pulmonary veno-occlusive disease rather than pure interstitial edema (Frazier et al. 2007). However, it has to be recognized that CT features of pulmonary edema can be observed without cardiomegaly, for example, in acute left-cardiac dysfunction. The use of contrast-enhanced CT may lift the veil on important underlying causes of pulmonary edema, such as left atrial myxoma and cor triatriatum. Left-cardiac functional evaluations are also now feasible, and it has been recently shown that if the patient has a right-to-left ventricular transit time of contrast medium of more than 10.5 s, left ventricular failure can be diagnosed with a very high positive predictive value (Vanhoenacker and Van Hoe 2007). Further parameters such as ejection fraction, end diastolic volume and cardiac output can also be calculated with the addition of the ECG gating, and it is likely that with further software development such measurements will become more or less routine.

References

Arai K, Takashima T, Matsui O et al. (1990) Transient subpleural curvilinear shadow caused by pulmonary congestion. J Comput Assist Tomogr 14:87–88

Beigelman-Aubry C, Hill C, Guibal A et al. (2005) Multidetector row CT and postprocessing techniques in the assessment of diffuse lung disease. Radiographics 25:1639–1652

Bernard GR, Pou NA, Coggeshall JW et al. (1995) Comparison of the pulmonary dysfunction caused by cardiogenic and noncardiogenic pulmonary edema. Chest 108:798–803

Bruzzi JF, Rémy-Jardin M, Delhaye D et al. (2006) When, why, and how to examine the heart during thoracic CT: Part 2, clinical applications. AJR Am J Roentgenol 186:333–341

Cabanes LR, Weber SN, Matran R et al. (1989) Bronchial hyperresponsiveness to methacholine in patients with impaired left ventricular function. N Engl J Med 320:1317–1322

Chabbert V, Canevet G, Baixas C et al. (2004) Mediastinal lymphadenopathy in congestive heart failure: a sequential CT evaluation with clinical and echocardiographic correlations. Eur Radiol 14:881–889

Dalal PU, Hansell DM (2006) High-resolution computed tomography of the lungs: the borderlands of normality. Eur Radiol 16:771–780

Delaunois LM (2006) Cardiovascular diseases: congenital, cardiogenic pulmonary oedema, mitral stenosis, chronic heart failure and myocardial infarction. Eur Resp Mon 34:290–306

Don C, Johnson R (1977) The nature and significance of peribronchial cuffing in pulmonary edema. Radiology 125:577–582

Ely EW, Haponik EF (2002) Using the chest radiograph to determine intravascular volume status: the role of vascular pedicle width. Chest 121:942–950

Erly WK, Borders RJ, Outwater EK (2003) Location, size, and distribution of mediastinal lymph node enlargement in chronic congestive heart failure. J Comput Assist Tomogr 27:485–489

Figueroa MS, Peters JI (2006) Congestive heart failure: Diagnosis, pathophysiology, therapy, and implications for respiratory care. Respir Care 51:403–412

Fleischner FG (1967) The butterfly pattern of acute pulmonary edema. Am J Cardiol 20:39–46

Forster BB, Müller NL, Mayo JR et al. (1992) High-resolution computed tomography of experimental hydrostatic pulmonary edema. Chest 101:1434–1437

Frazier AA, Franks TJ, Mohammed TL et al. (2007) From the archives of the AFIP: pulmonary veno-occlusive disease and pulmonary capillary hemangiomatosis. Radiographics 27:867–882

Gehlbach BK, Geppert E (2004) The pulmonary manifestations of left heart failure. Chest 125: 669–682

Gluecker T, Capasso P, Schnyder P et al. (1999) Clinical and radiologic features of pulmonary edema. Radiographics 19:1507–1531

Goodman LR (1996) Congestive heart failure and adult respiratory distress syndrome. New insights using computed tomography. Radiol Clin North Am 34:33–46

Gurney JW, Goodman LR (1989) Pulmonary edema localized in the right upper lobe accompanying mitral regurgitation. Radiology 171:397–399

Hansell, DM, Armstrong P, Lynch DA et al. (2005). Pulmonary edema. In: Hansell DM, Armstrong P, Lynch DA et al. (eds) Imaging of diseases of the chest. Elsevier Mosby, Philadelphia, pp 401–406

Haworth SG, Hall SM, Panja M (1988) Peripheral pulmonary vascular and airway abnormalities in adolescents with rheumatic mitral stenosis. Int J Cardiol 18:405–416

Hedlund LW, Vock P, Effmann EL et al. (1984) Hydrostatic pulmonary edema. An analysis of lung density changes by computed tomography. Invest Radiol 19:254–262

Herold CJ, Wetzel RC, Robotham JL et al. (1992) Acute effects of increased intravascular volume and hypoxia on the pulmonary circulation: assessment with high-resolution CT. Radiology 183:655–662

Howling SJ, Evans TW, Hansell DM (1998) The significance of bronchial dilatation on CT in patients with adult respiratory distress syndrome. Clin Radiol. 53:105–109

Hughes JMB (2005) Pulmonary complications of heart disease. In: Mason RJ, Murray JF, Broaddus VC et al. (eds) Murray and Nadel's textbook of respiratory medicine, 4th edn, vol 2. Elsevier Saunders, Philadelphia, pp 2200–2222

Hunt SA; American College of Cardiology; American Heart Association Task Force on Practice Guidelines (Writing Committee to Update the 2001 Guidelines for the Evaluation and Management of Heart Failure) (2005) ACC/AHA 2005 guideline update for the diagnosis and management of chronic heart failure in the adult: a report of the American College of Cardiology/American Heart Association Task Force on Practice Guidelines (Writing Committee to Update the 2001 Guidelines for the Evaluation and Management of Heart Failure). J Am Coll Cardiol 46:e1–82

Hwang YS, Lefferts PL, Snapper JR (2001) Correlation between increased airway responsiveness and severity of pulmonary edema. Pulm Pharmacol Ther 14:47–53

Johnson BD, Beck KC, Olson LJ et al. (2001) Pulmonary function in patients with reduced left ventricular function. Chest 120:1869–1876

Jorge S, Becquemin MH, Delerme S et al. (2007) Cardiac asthma in elderly patients: incidence, clinical presentation and outcome. BMC Cardiovasc Disord 14:7:16

Ketai LH, Godwin JD (1998) A new view of pulmonary edema and acute respiratory distress syndrome. J Thorac Imaging 13:147–171

Lewin S, Goldberg L, Dec GW (2000) The spectrum of pulmonary abnormalities on computed chest tomographic imaging in patients with advanced heart failure. Am J Cardiol 86:98–100

Light RW, George RB (1983) Serial pulmonary function in patients with acute heart failure. Arch Intern Med 143:429–433

Milne EN (1973) Correlation of physiologic findings with chest roentgenology. Radiol Clin North Am 11:17–47

Morgan PW, Goodman LR (1991) Pulmonary edema and adult respiratory distress syndrome. Radiol Clin North Am 29:943–963

Müller NL, Fraser RS, Lee KS et al. (2003) Pulmonary edema. In: Müller NL, Fraser RS, Lee KS et al. (eds) Diseases of the lung. Lippincott Williams & Wilkins, Philadelphia, pp 255–266

Pistolesi M, Giuntini C (1978) Assessment of extravascular lung water. Radiol Clin North Am 16:551–574

Pistolesi M, Miniati M, Milne EN et al. (1985) The chest roentgenogram in pulmonary edema. Clin Chest Med 6:315–344

Porcel JM, Vives M (2006) Distribution of pleural effusion in congestive heart failure. South Med J 99:98–99

Ribeiro CMC, Marchiori E, Rodrigues R et al. (2006) Hydrostatic pulmonary edema: high-resolution computer tomography aspects. J Bras Pneumol 32:515–522

Rolla G, Bucca C, Brussino L et al. (1993) Bronchodilating effect of ipratropium bromide in heart failure. Eur Respir J 6:1492–1495

Schnur MJ, Winkler B, Austin JH (1981) Thickening of the posterior wall of the bronchus intermedius. A sign on lateral radiographs of congestive heart failure, lymph node enlargement, and neoplastic infiltration. Radiology 139:551–559

Scillia P, Delcroix M, Lejeune P et al. (1999) Hydrostatic pulmonary edema: evaluation with thin-section CT in dogs. Radiology 211:161–168

Slanetz PJ, Truong M, Shepard JA et al. (1998) Mediastinal lymphadenopathy and hazy mediastinal fat: new CT findings of congestive heart failure. AJR Am J Roentgenol 171:1307–1309

Snapper JR, Trochtenberg DS, Hwang YS et al. (1999) Effect of pulmonary edema on tracheal diameter. Respiration 66:522–527

Storto ML, Kee ST, Golden JA et al. (1995) Hydrostatic pulmonary edema: high-resolution CT findings. AJR Am J Roentgenol 165:817–820

Thomason JW, Ely EW, Chiles C (1998) Appraising pulmonary edema using supine chest roentgenograms in ventilated patients. Am J Respir Crit Care Med157:1600–1608

Todo G, Herman PG (1986) High-resolution computed tomography of the pig lung. Invest Radiol 21:689–696

Vanhoenacker PK, Van Hoe LR (2007) A simple method to estimate cardiac function during routine multi-row detector CT exams. Eur Radiol 17:2845–2851

West JB, Dollery CT, Heard BE (1965) Increased pulmonary vascular resistance in the dependent zone of the isolated dog lung caused by perivascular edema. Circ Res 17:191–206

Woodring JH (1991) Pulmonary artery-bronchus ratios in patients with normal lungs, pulmonary vascular plethora, and congestive heart failure. Radiology 179:115–122

Wiener-Kronish JP, Broaddus VC (1993) Interrelationship of pleural and pulmonary interstitial liquid. Annu Rev Physiol 55:209226

Wiener-Kronish JP, Matthay MA, Callen PW et al. (1985) Relationship of pleural effusions to pulmonary hemodynamics in patients with congestive heart failure. Am Rev Respir Dis 132:1253–1256

Wiener-Kronish JP, Goldstein R, Matthay RA et al. (1987) Lack of association of pleural effusion with chronic pulmonary arterial and right atrial hypertension. Chest 92:967–970

Medical Applications of Integrated Cardiothoracic Imaging

MDCT Management of Ambiguous Symptoms

Evaluation of Chest Pain, Hemoptysis and Dyspnea

15

Seung Min Yoo and Charles S. White

CONTENTS

S. M. Yoo, MD, PhD
C. S. White, MD
Department of Diagnostic Radiology University of Maryland Medical Center, 22 S Greene Street, Baltimore, MD 21201, USA

Remarkable advances in multidetector CT (MDCT) technology have facilitated accurate evaluation of coronary artery disease in a noninvasive manner. Recent studies indicate that MDCT can replace the radionuclide stress test in the evaluation of some patients who present to the emergency department with acute chest pain, and normal or nonspecific ECG results and normal initial serum cardiac biomarkers. The potential of MDCT to identify and exclude other urgent causes of acute chest pain, such as the acute aortic syndrome and pulmonary embolism, as well as acute coronary syndrome, suggests that MDCT may be a primary imaging modality for the evaluation of acute chest pain. MDCT for the evaluation of hemoptysis can provide not only a localization and source of hemoptysis, but also identification of the culprit artery responsible for triggering hemoptysis. The ability of MDCT to scan the entire chest with thin collimation and within a single breath hold can offer a comprehensive assessment in the evaluation of dyspnea. In addition to axial images, post-processing techniques, such as maximal and minimal intensity projection images, provide valuable additional information for the evaluation of dyspnea.

15.1 Evaluation of Chest Pain

15.1.1 Introduction of Chest Pain

Acute chest pain is the second most common presentation to the emergency department (ED), trailing only acute abdominal pain (McCaig and Nawar 2006). Emergent and life-threatening causes of chest pain include acute coronary syndrome (ACS), acute aortic syndrome (AAS), pulmonary embolism (PE), tension pneumothorax and esophageal rupture. Nonemergent causes of chest pain comprise disorders of musculoskelectal origin, gastrointestinal origin and psychological disorders, such as panic disorder (Ringstrom and Freedman 2006). One of the major challenges for ED physicians remains distinguishing urgent causes of chest pain from nonemergent etiologies, with the goal of a precise diagnosis. This chapter will focus on the role of multidetector CT (MDCT) in the assessment of life-threatening causes of acute chest pain, especially ACS and AAS. The discussion about nonurgent causes of chest pain is beyond the scope of this chapter.

15.1.2 Acute Coronary Syndrome (ACS)

15.1.2.1 Introduction of ACS

Acute coronary syndrome is comprised of ST segment elevation myocardial infarction (STEMI), non-ST segment elevation myocardial infarction (NSTEMI) and unstable angina (UA). Typically, chest pain caused by ACS is characterized by substernal heaviness or tightness with or without radiation of pain to the neck or arm. However, atypical presentations of ACS, such as epigastric pain, stabbing chest pain, isolated dyspnea without chest pain and pleuritic chest pain, are not rare. Diagnosis of ACS is straightforward in patients with typical substernal chest pain, electrocardiographic changes such as ST segment elevation and elevated serum cardiac biomarkers. MDCT currently plays no role in the evaluation of these patients. Immediate reperfusion therapy is mandatory to salvage viable myocardium, obviating further noninvasive diagnostic testing (Pollack and Gibler 2001; Braunwald et al. 2002).

The number of ED visits and hospitalizations in the United States due to chest pain annually approximates 5 million and 2 million, respectively (McCaig and Burt 2004). However, only one third of those who are admitted eventually prove to have ACS. Although most ED physicians and cardiologists have adopted a low threshold for hospital admission, the rate of missed diagnosis of ACS, which results in inappropriate discharge, is still substantial, accounting for approximately 2–5% of overall ACS. Notably, approximately one fourth of patients improperly discharged with ACS die (Goldman et al. 1996; Lee and Goldman 2000; Lee et al. 1987; Pope et al. 2000; Kaul et al. 2004). Thus, it is not surprising that misdiagnosis of ACS is the most common cause of malpractice among ED physicians in the US. One report suggested that the failure to detect ST segment elevation by ED physicians might be an important cause of inappropriate discharge in patients with ACS (Pope et al. 2000). However, most improper discharges of ACS patients appear to be associated with nonspecific symptoms, normal or nonspecific ECG results, and negative serum cardiac biomarkers. Because the heart, lung, esophagus and aorta share some afferent visceral nerve fibers, it is often difficult to distinguish ACS from other disease entities based solely on symptoms (Ringstrom and Freedman 2006). In addition, the results of ECG are often nonspecific, and serum cardiac biomarkers, such as creatine kinase MB isoenzyme (CK–MB isoenzyme) and cardiac troponins, might not be useful in patients who present to ED less than 4–5 h after symptomatic onset (Achar et al. 2005; Scirica and Morrow 2003).

Due to substantial advances in hardware and computer software technology, including ECG-gating, imaging of the entire heart is now possible with 64-slice MDCT with submillimeter scan collimation during a single breath hold. The increasing spatial and temporal resolution of MDCT has facilitated its use for the evaluation of cardiac diseases, especially coronary artery disease. Several recent reports suggest that 64-slice MDCT can provide excellent correlation with the results of invasive angiography in the evaluation of significant coronary arterial stenosis with sensitivity and specificity values of 83%–99% and 86%–98%, respectively (Mollet et al. 2005; Morgan-Hughes et al. 2005; Raff et al. 2005). The main coronary CTA finding of ACS is severe coronary artery stenosis caused by a non-calcifed atherosclerotic plaque with or without a calcified component (Fig. 15.1a,b).

More recent MDCT innovations include dual-source technology and whole heart coverage. Dual source technology employs two tubes placed 90 degrees from one another to maximize temporal resolution. Whole-heart coverage consists of at least 16 cm of longitudinal coverage such that the heart can be scanned in a single rotation. Each strategy is useful to reduce coronary artery motion and improve image quality.

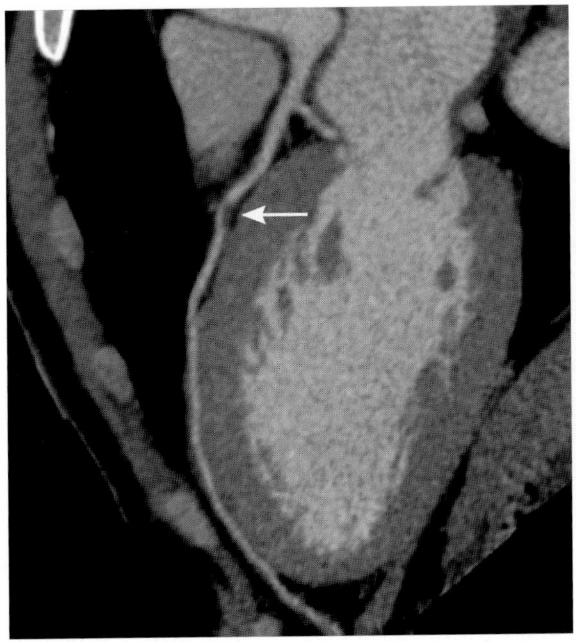

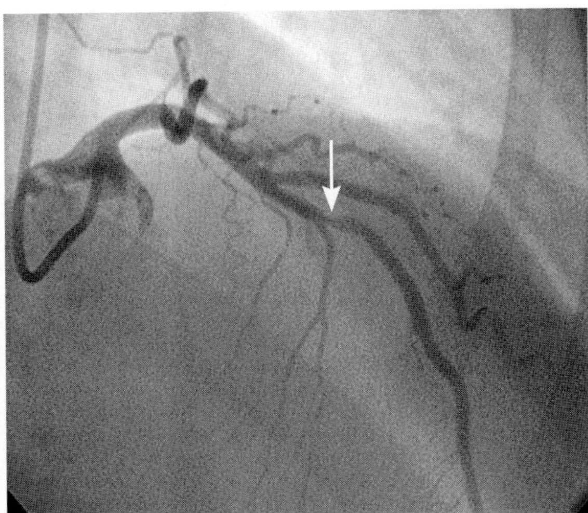

Fig. 15.1a,b. Coronary artery stenosis. **a** Curved multiplanar reformatted image of two-chamber view shows approximately 50–70% stenosis (*arrow*) in mid left anterior descending artery. **b** Coronary angiogram of left anterior oblique view in a same patient shows an excellent correlation (*arrow*) with **a**

15.1.2.2
MDCT Technique in the Evaluation of ACS

In general, there are two types of cardiac evaluation protocols used in the ED setting: dedicated coronary CT angiography (CTA) and the "triple rule out" MDCT protocol. Dedicated coronary CTA requires a limited field of view in order to increase spatial resolution. The triple rule out designation refers to simultaneous assessment of the coronary arteries, pulmonary arterial bed and aorta. The extent of the scan for triple rule out MDCT protocol ranges from above the aortic arch to the adrenal gland, whereas that of dedicated coronary CTA covers the aortic root to the base of the heart.

Certain prerequisites are required to obtain an optimal coronary CTA examination in the acute setting. Judicious shaving of the chest in hirsute patients is necessary to allow the ECG leads to adhere firmly. Although recent MDCT scanners may permit diagnostic images even if the heart rate exceeds 65 beats per minute, a target heart rate of less than 65 beats per minute is desirable to maintain optimal image quality (Giesler et al. 2002; Shim et al. 2005). Beta blocker is administered via an intravenous (5–20 mg of metoprotolol) or oral route (50 mg) before the cardiac MDCT examination unless there are contraindications such as asthma or high-grade AV block. Short acting nitroglycerin (0.4 mg) can also be administered via a sublingual route in order to dilate the coronary arteries. Contraindications for the administration of nitroglycerin include hypotension and recent usage of sidenafil citrate. The administration of a calcium channel-blocking agent may be an alternative to beta blockers in patients with asthma.

Breathing cooperation of patients is another important prerequisite for obtaining high quality images. The importance of explaining proper breath-holding and potential reactions to contrast injection (i.e., prior explanation of possible effects such as heating sensation, nausea and tingling sense) cannot be overemphasized. Multi-phasic injection of contrast followed by a saline chaser is performed to reduce the overall amount of contrast material used and to reduce the concentration of contrast material in the right ventricle or superior vena cava, which can hinder precise evaluation of the right coronary artery. A test injection or bolus tracking method is required to determine the optimal starting time of MDCT scanning. It is necessary to tailor the method of MDCT examination based on patient weight. In obese patients, thicker collimation, more radiation dose, a slower gantry rotation time and higher contrast volume may improve imaging quality. Renal insufficiency (creatinine level >1.5 mgL^{-1}), allergy to contrast materials, severe arrhythmia and hemodynamic instability are contraindications for coronary CTA. To reduce the possibility of renal injury, hydration is recommended prior to contrast injection.

15.1.2.3
Role of MDCT in the Evaluation of ACS

The major role of MDCT in the triage of ACS is currently restricted to evaluation of low-risk patients. Low-risk patients are those with nonspecific or negative ECG results and normal initial serum cardiac biomarkers without hypotension or rales on lung examination suggestive of pump failure. In this group of patients, the risk of a short-term major adverse cardiac event is relatively low (Goldman et al. 1996; Reilly et al. 2002). Such patients are typically admitted in order to rule out ACS, and the current strategy consists of serial ECGs, serum cardiac biomarkers for 12–24 h and stress testing, often with an exercise test, such as single-photon emission computed tomography (SPECT) or, less frequently, positron-emission tomography (PET).

Recent reports suggest that 64-slice MDCT may be an appropriate substitute for radionuclide perfusion imaging in the evaluation of low- to intermediate-risk patients with acute chest pain (Gallagher et al. 2007; Goldstein et al. 2007). A single center, randomized controlled study compared a 64-slice MDCT protocol with a standard protocol using radionuclide stress test in the evaluation of low-risk patients with acute chest pain. Ninety-nine and 98 patients were randomly assigned to separate MDCT and standard protocols, respectively. In patients with MDCT showing significant coronary stenosis (>70%), an invasive coronary angiogram was performed in follow-up. If only minimal coronary stenosis (≤25%) or a low calcium score (≤100 Agatston U) was found, patients were discharged home without further workup (Fig. 15.2a,b,c). If there was borderline coronary artery stenosis (26%–70%), a calcium score greater than 100 Agatston U or a non-diagnostic scan (e.g., motion due to blurring), patients underwent a follow-up radionuclide stress test. MDCT was successful in excluding or establishing coronary disease as the cause of acute chest pain in 75% of patients. In the remaining 25% patients, an additional radionuclide stress test was required due to indeterminate coronary stenosis or non-diagnostic imaging quality. Importantly, the study showed that the 64-slice MDCT protocol has a potential to lower overall costs and reduce triage time in the evaluation of acute chest pain in selected patients as compared with the standard protocol. However, the study also demonstrated clearly some drawbacks associated with the use of the 64-slice MDCT protocol. In particular, the lack of physiologic information about indeterminate coronary artery stenosis and suboptimal CT examinations may lead to further testing and exposure to radiation (Goldstein et al. 2007). Possible options to avoid additional radiation exposure from radionuclide stress testing include the use of MRI or stress echocardiography. Improvements in the MDCT technology will likely decrease the frequency of indeterminate examinations and may permit routine assessment of myocardial perfusion to provide a functional correlate in patients with indeterminate coronary lesions.

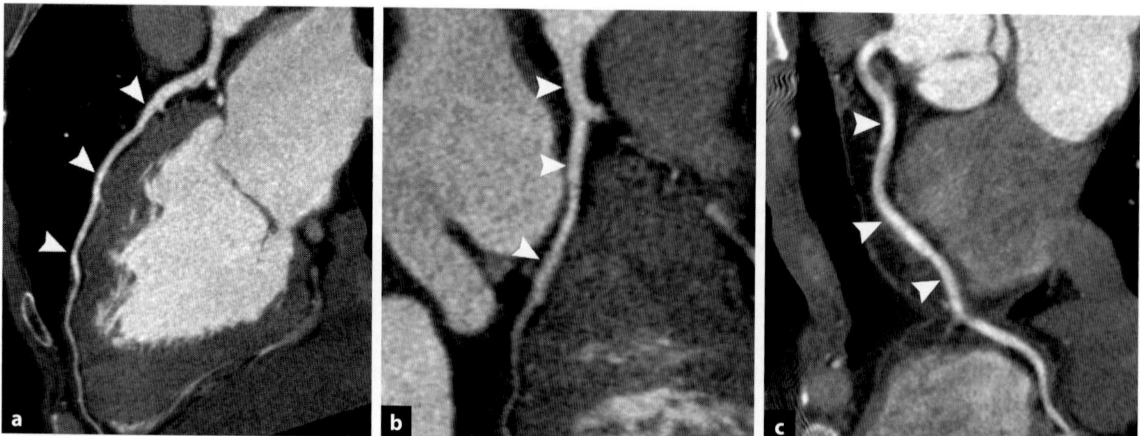

Fig. 15.2a–c. Normal coronary CTA. **a–c** Three curved multiplanar reformatted images show normal left anterior descending artery, left circumflex and right coronary arteries (*arrowheads*), respectively. Negative coronary CTA in a patient presenting to the emergency department with acute chest pain virtually excludes acute coronary syndrome

15.1.2.4 Limitations and Prospective of MDCT in the Evaluation of ACS

It is important to understand the strengths and weaknesses of the competing protocols used to evaluate acute chest pain in the ED: the comprehensive or triple rule-out MDCT protocol and dedicated coronary CTA protocol. The comprehensive MDCT protocol has the potential to exclude three life-threatening thoracic diagnoses (i.e., ACS, PE, and AAS) in one scan. A pilot study suggested that the triple rule-out MDCT protocol might be a valuable method to identify or exclude cardiac etiologies of acute chest pain in low-risk patients who present to ED. Moreover, this protocol could assess extracardiac causes of acute chest pain that could not be evaluated by the radionuclide stress test or stress echocardiography (White et al. 2005). However, the triple rule-out MDCT protocol also has drawbacks. When compared with dedicated coronary CTA, it necessitates a wider volume of coverage, broader field of view and prolonged contrast injection. Therefore, an increase in radiation dose, decrease of imaging resolution and higher risk for renal injury may be associated with this protocol.

There are varied opinions about which study protocol, a dedicated coronary CTA or triple rule out MDCT, is appropriate to evaluate acute chest pain in the ED. From a practical standpoint, many ED physicians would be hesitant to rely on a dedicated coronary CTA protocol to assess acute chest pain in the setting of a nonspecific initial evaluation because they could not completely exclude the possibility of AAS or PE as a cause of acute chest pain. In general, the dedicated coronary CTA protocol is the choice for elective situations such as the evaluation of stable angina as an outpatient. However, if there is low probability for PE based on clinical grounds and supported by a negative D dimmer test, dedicated coronary CTA appears to have a valuable role, because higher quality images of the coronary arteries can be obtained. To date, no study has been performed that directly compares the two protocols (Table 15.1).

Both dedicated and comprehensive coronary CTA protocols have potential limitations. The triple rule-out MDCT protocol is not ideal to exclude AAS. Many triple rule-out MDCT protocols do not include a precontrast scan, and thus it may be difficult to diagnose intramural hematoma (IMH). Typical MDCT findings of IMH are high attenuation and thickening of the involved aortic wall on precontrast CT imaging. A non-contrast scan is acquired for calcium scoring at many centers, and this may be useful to assess the unenhanced aorta for evidence of IMH. An additional difficulty is that the full extent of aortic dissection (AD) cannot be determined using a triple rule-out MDCT protocol because the abdomen and pelvis are not routinely imaged. This problem can be remedied by adding a protocol for a non-ECG gated scan of the abdomen and pelvis that is activated only if the initial triple rule-out scan is suspicious for AD.

An additional challenge is the need to provide off-hour service of MDCT (i.e., 24/7/365 coverage) to the ED. Currently, complete off-hour service of MDCT is not available in most hospitals. Several options exist to address this important issue. Remote reading by radiologists skilled in cardiac imaging is available. A less costly option is to train on-call residents or fellows to read cardiac CTA during off hours. A preliminary interpretation for definitely negative or positive cardiac CTA cases would permit early triage in targeted patients with acute chest pain. Based on the current literature, it is likely that more than 50% of patients could be triaged in this manner. For equivocal cardiac CTA studies, final triage would be delayed until the next morning until the study is re-

Table 15.1. Comparison of sample ED chest pain 64-slice MDCT protocols

Protocol	Dedicated CTA	Triple rule out
Field of view	220	400
Thickness (mm)	0.67	0.9
Increment (mm)	0.33	0.45
Direction	Cephalad-caudal	Caudal-cephalad
Time (s)	9–10	15–18
Z axis coverage	Aortic root–cardiac base	Aortic arch–adrenal gland

viewed by a cardiothoracic radiologist and cardiology consultant (White et al. 2005).

Another important issue to be addressed is the radiation dose of cardiac CT. Radiation dosage reported in recent studies of 64-slice MDCT coronary CTA is 9.6 to 15.2 mSv in men and 13.5 to 21.4 mSv in women. Radiation dosage of 64-slice MDCT coronary CTA tends to be higher than that of 16-slice MDCT coronary CTA because the thinner collimation of 64-slice MDCT requires a higher radiation dosage per slice to maintain the same signal-to-noise ratio (Thompson and Cullom 2006). On the other hand, competing imaging modalities, such as radionuclide perfusion test or conventional angiography, also have substantial radiation doses (Rohe et al. 1995). The expected risk of radiation-induced cancer is higher for the triple rule-out MDCT protocol. Therefore, a dedicated cardiac CTA study would be preferred in young patients with acute chest pain and low risk. One method to mitigate the amount of radiation exposure is to use a tube modulation technique in which radiation dose is automatically lowered during systolic phase. One report suggests that a reduction in radiation dose up to 44% is possible by using automatic tube current modulation (Poll et al. 2002). Another possible option is to use a prospective gating technique that reduces radiation dose substantially by imaging only a part of the cardiac cycle, usually diastole. Disadvantages of prospectively gated CT include the lack of functional information because images are not obtained in systole and the inability to obtain adequate image quality if the heart rate exceeds 70 beats per minute.

Overall, MDCT evaluation of patients with acute chest pain has multiple advantages compared with other diagnostic modalities. Radionuclide stress testing has both limited spatial resolution and longer image acquisition times compared with coronary CTA. In addition, the department of nuclear medicine is rarely located close to the ED. Moreover, radionuclide stress testing lacks the ability to evaluate extra-cardiac abnormalities that may cause acute chest pain.

In the future, if MDCT attains the same spatial resolution as conventional angiography (0.2×0.2×0.2 mm) and scanning time becomes faster, MDCT may provide a road map prior to percutaneous coronary intervention in more patients with ACS. On the basis of coronary MDCT findings, interventional cardiologists may perform selective percutaneous coronary intervention, reducing the time of the interventional procedure and frequency of complications. The decision to use MDCT in higher risk patients with acute chest pain may ultimately be a balance between the ability to gather rapid noninvasive information and the imperative to intervene quickly.

15.1.3 Acute Aortic Syndrome (AAS)

15.1.3.1 Introduction of Acute Aortic Syndrome (AAS)

AAS includes aortic dissection (AD), intramural hematoma (IMH) and penetrating atherosclerotic ulcer (PAU). In addition to AAS, traumatic aortic pseudoaneurysm and ruptured aortic aneurysm are also life-threatening aortic diseases. Differentiation among AD, IMH and PAU is difficult, if not impossible, based solely on clinical presentation because of overlapping symptoms (i.e., severe ripping or tearing back pain). MDCT has become the imaging modality of choice in the evaluation of potential AAS (Castarner et al. 2003; Chung et al. 1996; Sebastia et al. 1999). Recently, IMH and PAU have been identified with increasing frequency due to advances in cross-sectional imaging, especially MDCT. Because the different forms of AAS have varying prognoses and therapeutic strategies, distinction of these entities on the basis of imaging studies is vital.

15.1.3.2 Aortic Dissection (AD)

AD may result from an intimal tear of the aortic wall. Less frequently, bleeding of the Vasa vasorum may be a cause of AD. Hypertension is the most important risk factor for AD (Masuda et al. 1992). Other risk factors include Marfan's syndrome, cystic medial degeneration of the aorta, blunt trauma, a bicuspid aortic valve and previous surgery of the thoracic aorta (De Sanctis et al. 1987; Larson and Edwards 1984).

A dedicated MDCT protocol for AD extends from the thoracic inlet to the level of iliac arteries and includes pre-contrast scanning in order to exclude the possibility of IMH. The typical MDCT finding of AD after administration of contrast material is the presence of an intimal flap (Fig. 15.3a,b). The Stanford classification is used to categorize AD. Stanford type A is defined by an intimal flap that affects the ascending aorta or arch, whereas a Stanford type B dissection involves only the descending aorta. The term intimal flap is a misnomer. Because the rupture of AD extends along the outer one third of the aortic media, the detached flap is thicker than that of the intima and includes a part of the media. Thus, the outer wall of a false lumen opposite to the intimal flap consists only of adventitia and the outer one third of media. This explains why aortic rupture occurs so frequently through the outer wall of the false lumen.

The location of the entry and re-entry tears, differentiation between true and false lumen, the extent of dissection and the presence or absence of side-branch compromise or combined rupture should be evaluated while interpreting MDCT images of AD. Information about the location of the entry tear is important to decide on a treatment option.

The differentiation between the false and true lumen is usually not difficult on MDCT. The diameter of the false lumen is usually larger than that of true lumen (i.e., larger lumen sign) because the intraluminal pressure of the former is often higher than that of the latter. In determining which lumen is true or false, a lumen with a beak and an acute angle between the flap and aortic wall is indicative of the false lumen on MDCT images (Fig. 15.3a). The "cobweb" sign is also a marker of the false lumen and is a less frequent finding. A cobweb comprises small linear structures extending from the aortic wall to the flap and indicates incomplete tearing of muscle fibers in the dissected aortic wall (Lee et al. 1997; LePage et al. 2001; Williams et al. 1994). Another important finding, particularly in type B dissections, is direct continuation of the uninvolved portion of aorta with the true lumen on MDCT. The differentiation between the true and false lumen may be more apparent on coronal or sagittal reformatted MDCT images (Fig. 15.3b).

Information about the extent of AD is also essential to determine the appropriate treatment option. ADs involving the ascending aorta (i.e., Stanford type A) should be treated surgically. Up to 90% with this type of dissection who are treated conservatively die within 3 months due to aortic rupture or obstruction of the side branches, such as coronary, brachiocephalic or visceral arteries (Anagnostopoulos et al. 1972). By contrast, AD involving only the descending aorta is usually managed with medical therapy. However, evidence of ischemia of the legs (e.g., decreased femoral pulse, leg pain or discoloration of lower extremity) or abdominal viscera (e.g., renovascular hypertension, renal failure or ischemic bowel disease) and signs of impending rupture of the aorta (e.g., persistent severe pain, hypotension and hemothorax) are considered surgical indications in this type of AD.

There are two varieties of side-branch compromise related to AD: static obstruction and dynamic obstruction. Static obstruction results from direct extension of an intimal flap through the origin of the involved arterial branch. By contrast, dynamic obstruction is caused by the slit-like narrowing of the true lumen secondary to the intense pressure difference existing between the true and false lumens, thus rendering a more distal aortic branch of

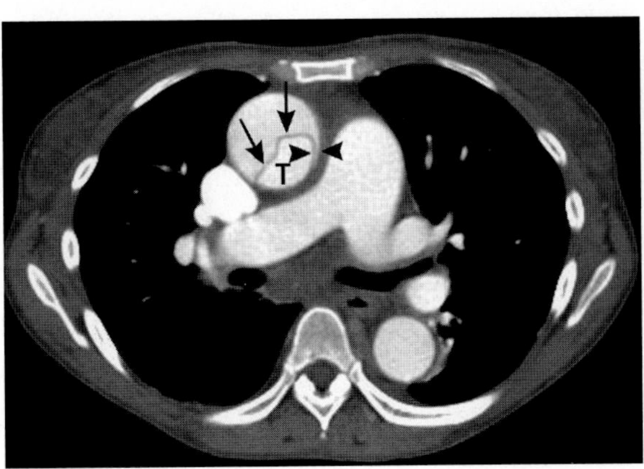

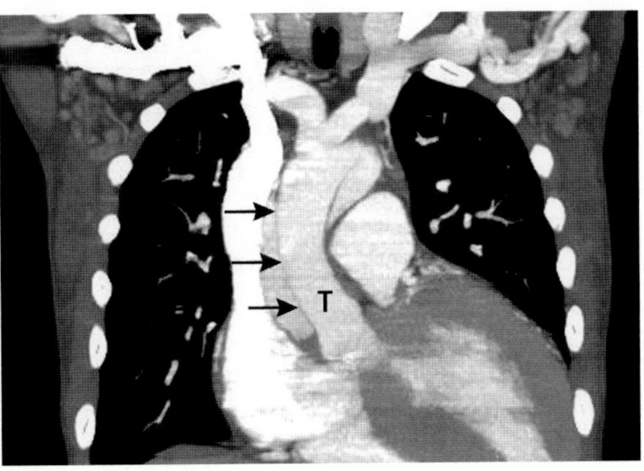

Fig. 15.3a,b. Stanford type A aortic dissection. **a** Intimal flap (*arrows*) and beak sign (*arrowheads*) indicating false lumen are noted on CT image at the level of main pulmonary artery, consistent with AD of Stanford type A. The diameter of true lumen (*T*) is smaller than that of false lumen. **b** The extent of intimal flap (*arrows*) is more clearly defined on the coronal reformatted maximal intensity projection image. The continuation of true lumen (*T*) with left ventricle on this image helps differentiate it from the false lumen

dynamic obstruction ischemic. The treatment approach to static and dynamic obstruction is quite different. Static obstruction is relieved by an endovascular stent placed in the true lumen of the involved artery, whereas dynamic obstruction is corrected by fenestration aimed at equalization of luminal pressure. If there is persistent luminal stenosis after fenestration, the deployment of an aortic stent should be considered in cases of the dynamic obstruction (Nienaber and Eagle 2003).

Aortic regurgitation complicating AD is optimally evaluated with transesophageal echocardiogram or MRI, but ECG-gated MDCT can also identify aortic regurgitation on the basis of poor leaflet coaptation.

15.1.3.3 Intramural Hematoma (IMH)

IMH is most likely caused by spontaneous bleeding of the vasa vasorum. It is postulated to be a variant of AD (Yamada et al. 1988). In some instances, it may also represent an earlier phase of classic AD (Nienaber et al. 1995).

Although the lack of an intimal tear is a typical feature of IMH, it is often difficult to differentiate IMH from thrombosed AD associated with a tiny intimal tear or PAU from a tiny or healed ulcer. However, the true lumen of a thrombosed AD can be compressed by the high pressure in the false lumen, whereas the residual aortic lumen of IMH tends to preserve its round shape. Most importantly, MDCT obtained without contrast enhancement shows typical high attenuation within the aortic wall, indicating intramural hematoma formation (Fig. 15.4a,b). Because the CT findings of IMH after contrast enhancement are easily misinterpreted as aortic thrombus, thorough and careful investigation of the pre-contrast CT image should be performed to look for the telltale finding of high attenuation in the aortic wall in patients with a clinical suspicion of AAS. Although IMH tends to involve a longer extent along the normal aortic wall, and aortic thrombus usually involves a shorter extent in a dilated aorta, it may be difficult to distinguish IMH from aortic thrombus based only on post-contrast MDCT findings.

The outcome of IMH varies. It may progress to overt AD, pseudoaneurysm or rupture (Castaner et al. 2003). Complete resolution of IMH is also possible. A greater maximal thickness of IMH on axial CT scan has been reported as a predictor of progression of IMH to overt AD. In one study, mean maximal thickness of IMH was 16.4 ± 4.4 mm in those who progressed to overt AD, whereas it was 10.5±3.8 mm in those who did not (Choi et al. 2001). Fundamentally, therapy for IMH is similar to classic AD, but the overall prognosis tends to be better in IMH, presumably because some resolve spontaneously (Song et al. 2001). It is controversial whether IMH involving the ascending aorta that lacks signs suggesting impending rupture (e.g., hemopericardium, hemothorax or hemodynamic instability) requires surgical intervention (Maraj et al. 2000; Song et al. 2001; Sueyoshi et al. 1997).

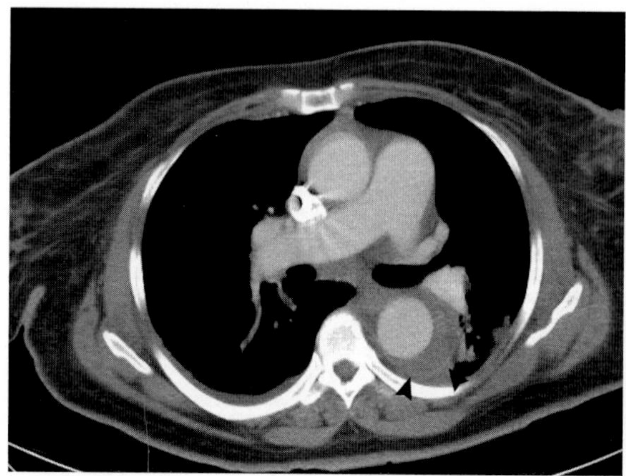
a

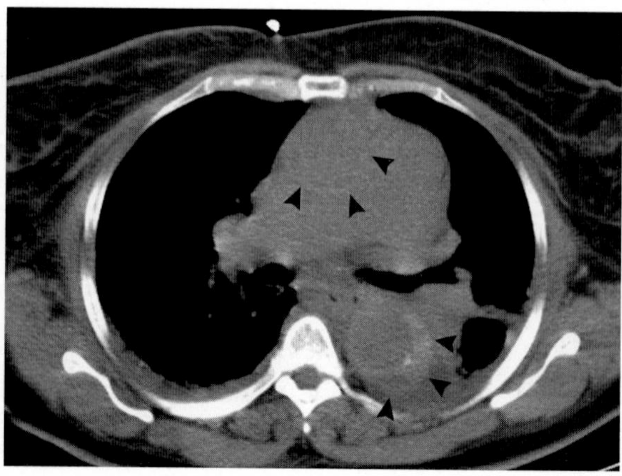
b

Fig. 15.4a,b. Intramural hematoma. **a** Wall thickening of descending aorta (*arrowheads*) and questionable wall thickening of ascending aorta are seen on CT image obtained after enhancement at the level of main pulmonary artery. Small bilateral pleural effusions and mediastinal hemorrhage are also demonstrated. **b** Typical crescent high attenuation (*arrowheads*) of intramural hematoma is noted in the wall of ascending and descending aorta on the pre-contrast CT image at almost the same level as **a**

15.1.3.4
Penetrating Atherosclerotic Ulcer (PAU)

By definition, PAU is an ulcer that extends through the internal elastic lamina of the aortic wall and into the media. PAU frequently occurs in the descending aorta of elderly patients with hypertension and advanced atherosclerosis. The most important predisposing factor is atherosclerosis. Hematoma in the adjacent aortic wall is frequently associated with PAU (Stanson et al. 1986; Welch et al. 1990).

Fibrotic change caused by severe atherosclerosis around the PAU tends to hinder the propagation of AD along the aortic wall and formation of re-entry tear (Roberts 1981). Therefore, thrombosed AD is more frequently encountered in the patients with PAU on CT scan than non-thrombosed AD. Other complications of PAU include aortic rupture and pseudoaneurysm. Because atherosclerotic change generally spares the ascending aorta, PAU is less likely to cause type A dissection (Hirst et al. 1958). By contrast, in AD confined to the descending aorta, especially thrombosed AD in elderly patients, PAU may be a predisposing condition.

The characteristics of PAU should be distinguished from those of an atheromatous ulcer on MDCT. MDCT findings of PAU are characterized by extension of the ulcer beyond the expected margin of aortic wall (Fig. 15.5a,b) with or without hematoma formation beneath the ulcer (Chiles and Carr 2005).

It is important to realize that the initial CT findings of PAU (i.e., the size or shape of the ulcer) are not useful for prognosis (Hayashi et al. 2000). Therefore, close follow-up CT is necessary to determine the appropriate treatment of PAU. Surgery is typically reserved for patients with ongoing chest pain or signs of impending rupture.

However, PAU frequently occurs in advanced age and may be associated with various comorbidities such as diabetes mellitus, pulmonary function abnormality or decreased cardiac function. If operative intervention proves necessary, severe atherosclerotic change of the aortic wall adjacent to PAU requires a more extensive resection of the aortic wall compared with surgery for AD. As a result, the rate of complications, such as postoperative spinal cord injury, heart failure, renal failure or respiratory failure, is higher after the surgery for PAU than for AD (Levy et al. 1999). Therefore, percutaneous interventional procedures, such as the use of an aortic stent, may be a good alternative to treat patients with a high probability of postoperative complication.

15.1.3.5
Traumatic Aortic Pseudoaneurysm

The most frequent location of traumatic aortic rupture or pseudoaneurysm is the aortic isthmus (Fig. 15.6a,b). Most injuries are secondary to traffic accidents or falls. It is possible to miss a small traumatic aortic tear

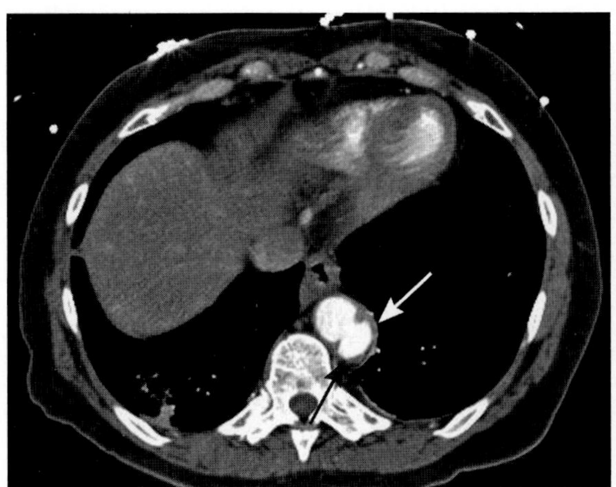

a

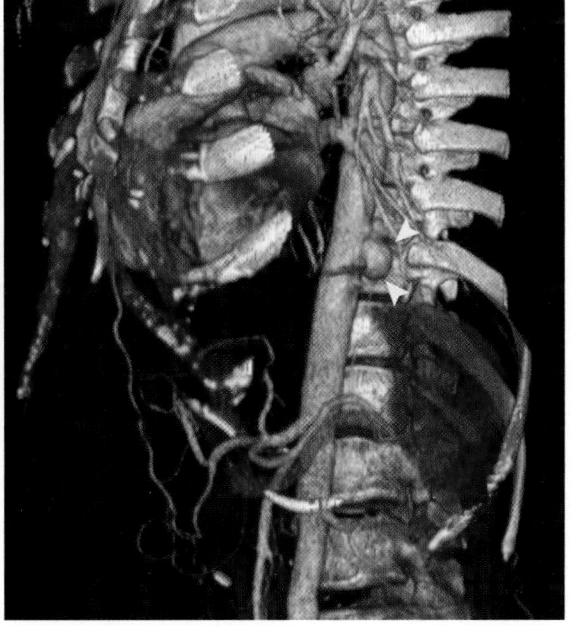

b

Fig. 15.5a,b. Penetrating aortic ulcer. **a** Axial CT image obtained after administration of contrast material at the level of lung base shows a large saccular penetrating aortic ulcer (*arrows*) in distal thoracic aorta. **b** Volume-rendered image in the same patient shows a saccular aneurysm (*arrowheads*) in distal thoracic aorta

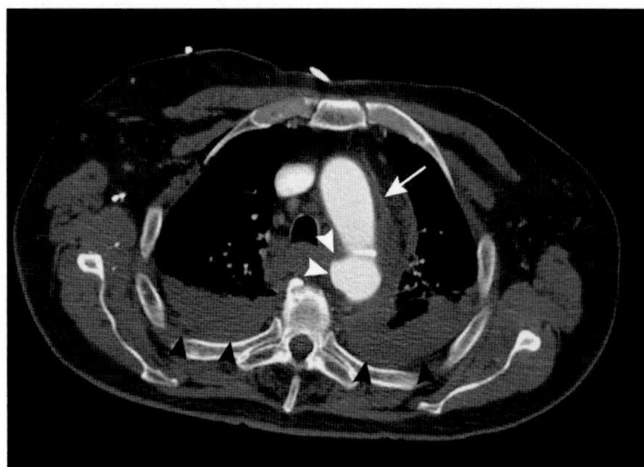

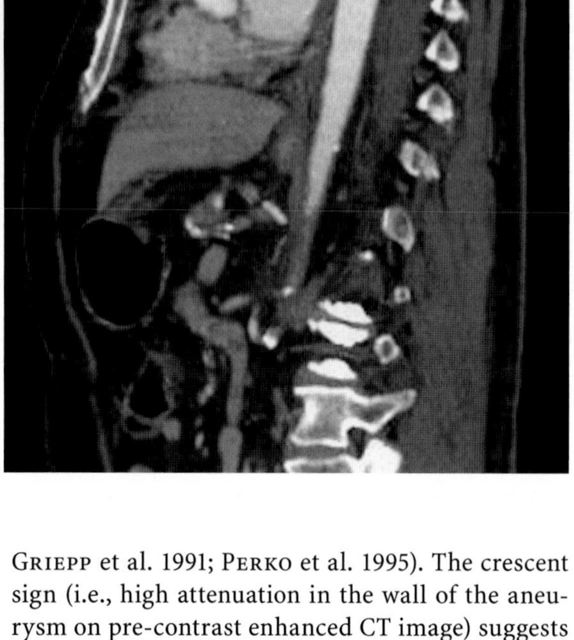

Fig. 15.6a,b. Traumatic aortic pseudoaneurysm. **a** Mild irregular bulging contour (*white arrowheads*) is noted at the aortic isthmus on CT image obtained after contrast administration at the level of aortic arch, suggesting the diagnosis of traumatic aortic pseudoaneurysm in a patient with an appropriate history. Mediastinal soft tissue density (*arrow*), which is consistent with mediastinal hemorrhage, and bilateral pleural effusions (*black arrowheads*) are also noted. **b** Oblique sagittal reformatted maximal intensity projection image more clearly shows traumatic aortic pseudoaneurysm (*arrowheads*)

if only the axial CT images are reviewed. Thus, sagittal or coronal maximal intensity projection (MIP) images of the aortic arch are valuable to facilitate the diagnosis. A useful secondary finding is localization of mediastinal fluid or hemorrhage adjacent to or surrounding the proximal descending aorta.

15.1.3.6 Ruptured Aortic Aneurysm

The most common cause of aortic aneurysm is atherosclerosis. The predominant site of an atherosclerotic aneurysm is the proximal descending aorta. Other causes of aortic aneurysm include infection (i.e., mycotic aneurysm), Marfan's syndrome or other connective tissue disease, poststenotic dilatation from aortic stenosis and trauma.

Aortic aneurysm is often conventionally defined by a diameter of more than 5 cm. Aortic aneurysm is frequently asymptomatic and discovered incidentally. Rarely, vague chest pain may be produced by compression of adjacent structures. Aortic aneurysm more than 6 cm in diameter is associated with an increased risk for rupture. An increase in size of aortic aneurysm of more than 0.5 cm in diameter on annual follow-up CT also represents an increased risk of rupture (Dapunt et al. 1994; Hirose et al. 1995; Griepp et al. 1991; Perko et al. 1995). The crescent sign (i.e., high attenuation in the wall of the aneurysm on pre-contrast enhanced CT image) suggests an impending rupture of an aortic aneurysm. It represents an intramural hemorrhage or hemorrhage of mural thrombus caused by ongoing dissection through mural thrombus or the aneurysmal wall (Gonsalves 1999). Hemothorax, hemopericardium and hemomediastinum can also indicate a ruptured aortic aneurysm. A rupture of aortic aneurysm with hemomediastinum, hemopericardium or hemothorax cannot be discriminated from aortic rupture secondary to PAU based on MDCT findings alone.

15.2 Evaluation of Hemoptysis

15.2.1 Introduction to Hemoptysis

Hemoptysis is a nonspecific symptom, but it is a potentially life-threatening event, and a serious underlying disease may manifest in this way. Numerous disease processes are associated with hemoptysis.

Pulmonary causes are most common and include lung cancer, infection, bronchiectasis, chronic bronchitis or mycetoma. Detailed description of these entities is beyond the scope of this chapter.

The capabilities of current-generation MDCT to scan the entire thorax with submillimeter collimation within a single breath hold and to perform three-dimensional reconstructions isotropically make MDCT the study of choice for the evaluation of patients with hemoptysis.

15.2.2 Technical Aspects and Role of MDCT in the Evaluation of Hemoptysis

The scanning range of MDCT for the evaluation of hemoptysis includes the area from the lower neck to the level of renal arteries in order to identify non-bronchial systemic collateral arteries or an ectopic origin of bronchial artery as a source of hemoptysis (Bruzzi et al. 2006). Both a rapid injection rate of high density contrast (i.e., more than 4 mLs^{-1}) and the selection of an appropriate scanning time supported by a bolus tracking method are necessary to obtain optimal enhancement of both systemic arteries and the pulmonary artery. The other technical aspects of MDCT in the evaluation for hemoptysis are similar to those for routine chest MDCT.

The primary role of MDCT in the evaluation of patients with massive hemoptysis differs from that of evaluation of patients with blood-tinged sputum or a small amount of hemoptysis. The major role of MDCT in the latter is to elucidate the cause of bronchial bleeding, whereas in the former the goal is to localize the culprit artery to be embolized during invasive angiography.

MDCT findings of hemoptysis include ground-glass attenuation and consolidation with or without atelectasis secondary to endobronchial obstruction due to a blood clot. If theses findings are unilateral, localization of the origin of hemoptysis may prove to be straightforward (Khalil et al. 2007) (Fig. 15.7a). On MDCT, active bronchial bleeding may manifest as direct spillage of contrast material into a larger airway, such as the trachea or a bronchus. However, this is an unusual finding because the rate of most bronchial bleeding is insufficient to be detected on MDCT.

The source of hemoptysis can be divided into bronchial arteries, non-bronchial systemic collateral arteries, pulmonary artery or a combination of the above. Hemoptysis due to bronchial arterial bleeding is most common (Yoon et al. 2003). Normal bronchial arteries usually originate from the descending thoracic aorta at the level of or slightly below the tracheal bifurcation (Remy-Jardin et al. 2004) (Fig. 15.7c). Variation in the origin and the number of bronchial arteries is well documented. Although hemoptysis arising from a normal-sized bronchial artery is possible, a bronchial artery with a diameter of 1.5 mm or more should be considered as abnormal and be treated by embolotherapy. The enlarged bronchial artery often is identified on MDCT as a cluster of dot-like structures posterior to the major bronchi, demonstrating strong contrast enhancement (Fig. 15.7b,d). The proximal portion of bronchial artery is readily identified on axial MDCT (Fig. 15.7c). However, its entire course is better elucidated on coronal or sagittal reformatted MIP images. Interventional radiologists can use information about the location of the origin and number of bronchial arteries and about the presence or absence of systemic collateral arteries as a roadmap prior to bronchial artery embolization. An aberrant origin of the bronchial artery is present in up to 30% of bronchial arteries (Khalil et al. 2007). The excellent axial resolution and robust three-dimensional post-processing capability of MDCT enable precise depiction of the aberrant origin of bronchial arteries (Yoon et al. 2005).

In addition, evaluation of non-bronchial systemic collateral arteries can routinely be performed with three-dimensional MDCT reconstruction techniques, such as MIP and volume rendering. Therefore, conventional aortography to determine the culprit non-bronchial systemic collateral artery is frequently not necessary (Remy-Jardin et al. 2004). Non-bronchial systemic collateral arteries contributing to hemoptysis can be suspected on CT if there is pleural thickening greater than 3 mm and pleural opacities with high attenuation, suggesting non-bronchial systemic collateral arteries. The origin of non-bronchial systemic collateral arteries is classified based on the involved lobe; in an upper lobe lesion, the subclavian artery or its branches (e.g., internal mammary artery, thyrocervical trunk and lateral thoracic artery), axillary artery or intercostal artery are culprit arteries; in a lower lobe lesion, the inferior phrenic artery, hepatic artery, gastric or intercostals artery are sources of bronchial bleeding (Moore et al. 1986; Yu-Tang Goh et al. 2002; Sellars and Belli 2001; Swanson et al. 2002; Wong et al. 2002).

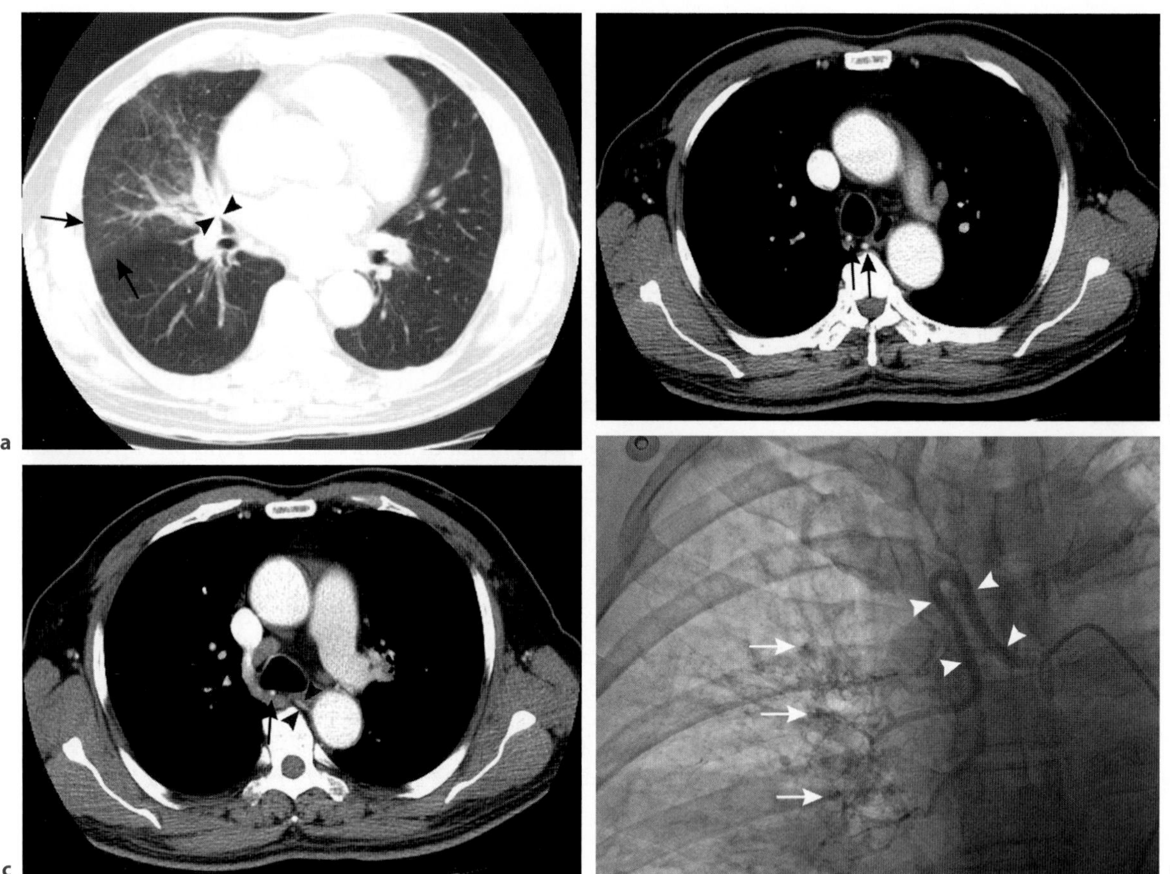

Fig. 15.7a–d. Hemoptysis caused by an enlarged bronchial artery. **a** CT image on lung window settings at the level of right middle lobe bronchus shows right middle lobe bronchus narrowing (*arrowheads*) caused by anthracofibrosis and ground-glass attenuation (*arrows*) in right middle lobe, consistent with aspirated blood in a patient with history of hemoptysis. **b** CT image on mediastinal window setting obtained at the level of aortopulmonary window after contrast administration shows two strongly enhancing dots (*arrows*) behind the trachea, indicating enlarged bronchial artery in the same patient as **a**. **c** CT image on mediastinal window settings obtained at the main pulmonary artery level after contrast administration shows the proximal (*arrowheads*) and more distal (*arrow*) bronchial artery. **d** Left bronchial angiogram also shows an enlarged bronchial artery (*arrowheads*) with hypervascularity in its distal portion (*arrows*)

Pseudosequestration is a rare condition characterized by systemic arterial supply into the lung instead of the pulmonary artery with normal bronchial connections. It can be complicated by hemoptysis. MDCT can provide a confident diagnosis of pseudosequestration by using multiplanar reformatted images and three-dimensional volume rendering (Bruhlmann et al. 1998; Chabbert et al. 2002).

Hemoptysis in patients with PE is associated with pulmonary infarction. Careful evaluation of the entire pulmonary arterial tree is necessary to exclude PE in patients who presented with hemoptysis and pleural-based wedge-shaped opacities on CT (Fig. 15.8). High pressure perfusion by a bronchial artery into the necrotic, infarcted area may result in hemoptysis in patients with PE.

Underlying causes of hemoptysis mainly originating from the pulmonary artery include postcapillary pulmonary hypertension (e.g., mitral stenosis, pulmonary venoocclusive disease, fibrosing mediastinitis or cardiogenic pulmonary edema), pulmonary arteriovenous malformation and pulmonary artery aneurysm due to infection or vasculitis. Postcapillary pulmonary hypertension secondary to longstanding pulmonary venous hypertension in mitral stenosis may cause pulmonary hemorrhage due to pulmonary capillary oozing. Pulmonary arteriovenous malformation is characterized by a strong enhancing mass with a feeding artery or arteries and a draining vein or veins on contrast-enhanced MDCT (Fig. 15.9).

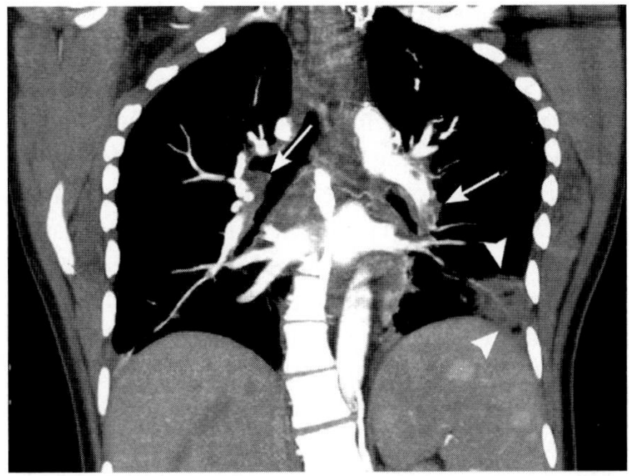

Fig. 15.8. Hemoptysis caused by pulmonary embolism with pulmonary infarction. Coronal maximal intensity projection MDCT image shows multiple pulmonary emboli in both pulmonary arteries (*arrows*) and peripheral wedge-shaped opacity (*arrowheads*) in the left lower lobe, consistent with pulmonary infarction

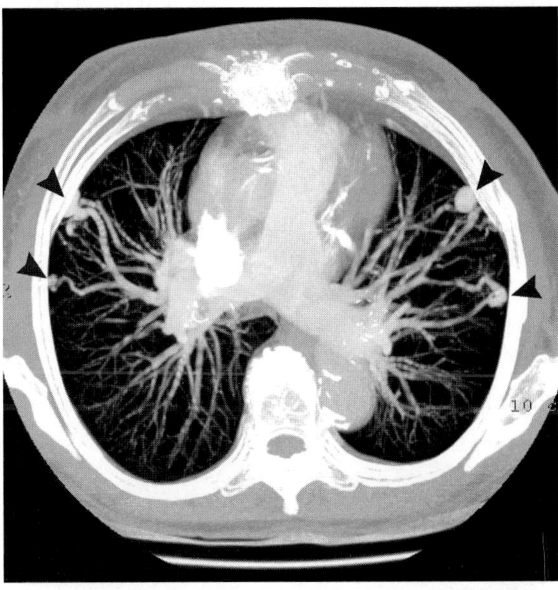

Fig. 15.9. Multiple pulmonary arteriovenous malformations. Multiple pulmonary arteriovenous malformations (*arrowheads*) are noted in the right middle and lingular segment on maximal intensity projection axial CT image at the level of main pulmonary artery

Recognition of a pulmonary arteriovenous malformation is essential to avoid performing a biopsy on what otherwise may appear to be a solitary pulmonary nodule. Another rare cause of pulmonary arterial bleeding is pulmonary arterial aneurysm. Rasmussen's aneurysm is caused by direct invasion of the pulmonary arterial wall by adjacent tuberculous infection. Pulmonary arterial aneurysm is also a complication in patients with Behcet's syndrome, a vasculitis characterized by orogenital ulcer, ocular involvement and other systemic manifestations.

The prevalence of hemoptysis of unknown origin ranges from 3% to 42% (Hirshberg et al. 1997; Boulay et al. 2000; Hiyama et al. 2002; Herth et al. 2001). However, most reports have not included MDCT as an investigational tool for hemoptysis so the true frequency is uncertain. In some instances, spread of aspirated blood into the alveolar spaces or airway may mask an otherwise detectable underlying disease process, leading to a diagnosis of cryptogenic hemoptysis even on MDCT. Therefore, a follow-up MDCT performed a few weeks after the initial episode may be valuable to avoid overlooking a discrete underlying cause.

15.3 Evaluation of Dyspnea

15.3.1 Overview of Dyspnea

The etiology of dyspnea is varied. Dyspnea is most commonly caused by pleuropulmonary and cardiovascular disorders. Rarely, it results from anemia, metabolic conditions (e.g., acidosis), upper airway obstruction (e.g., relapsing polychondritis), psychiatric problems (e.g., hyperventilation syndrome, anxiety and panic disorder), neuromuscular disease (e.g., amyotrophic lateral sclerosis, myasthenia gravis and Guillain-Barre syndrome) or diaphragmatic disorders (e.g., diaphragmatic rupture). These rare causes of dyspnea of non-cardiac and pleuropulmonary origin should be suspected in cases with severe dyspnea but a normal chest MDCT. Dyspnea of pleuropulmonary causes can be further divided into those caused by airway obstruction (e.g., asthma or chronic obstructive pulmonary disease), a pulmonary parenchymal abnormality (e.g., idiopathic pulmonary fibrosis, pulmonary tuberculosis or chronic parenchymal sarcoidosis) or pleural disease (e.g., pleural effusion or pleural fibrosis). With careful history taking, physical examination and other clinical data, a detailed evaluation of the heart as well as abnormalities of lung parenchyma as visualized on MDCT can determine the origin of dyspnea.

15.3.2 Technical Aspects and Role of MDCT in the Evaluation of Dyspnea

Fast gantry rotation time and use of current-generation MDCT scanners enable precise evaluation of patients with dyspnea within a single breath hold in most situations. In patients with severe dyspnea, it is useful to initiate CT scanning from lung bases because the upper lobes tend to be less affected by respiratory motion. In addition to rapid acquisition of thin-slice images on MDCT, robust three-dimensional reconstruction techniques, such as MIP and minimal intensity projection (MinP), permit MDCT to play a vital role in the evaluation of dyspnea. In a MIP image, the voxel with the highest attenuation value is used to represent the attenuation value of the entire set of voxels projected within a reformatted thickness, whereas in MinP image, the voxel with the lowest attenuation value is utilized. The MinP technique has shown benefit in increasing the sensitivity in the detection of minute traction bronchiolectasis, thus confirming the presence of a combined fibrotic process. In addition, this approach is useful to differentiate bronchiolitis obliterans from emphysema (Beigelman-Aubry et al. 2005). In contrast to emphysema, there is no evidence of architectural distortion of lung parenchyma on CT in patients with bronchiolitis obliterans (Fig. 15.10a,b).

Among causes of dyspnea of cardiovascular origin, only pulmonary edema and PE are discussed briefly in this chapter. Typical MDCT findings of pulmonary edema include thickening of interlobular and peribronchovascular interstitium, perihilar ground-glass opacities or consolidation, enlargement of the pulmonary veins and left ventricle, and bilateral pleural effusions. MIP imaging can optimize the visualization of enlarged pulmonary veins in the evaluation of patients with pulmonary edema, thus helping to distinguish pulmonary edema from the other disease entities (Beigelman-Aubry et al. 2005) (Fig. 15.11a,b). An accurate ejection fraction to evaluate systolic function can be calculated with ECG-gated MDCT.

The sudden onset of dyspnea with or without chest pain is another scenario that suggests the diagnosis of PE. The typical CT findings of PE are filling defects of low attenuation within the lumen of the enhanced pulmonary arteries (Fig. 15.12a,b). In the setting of PE, associated findings of right ventricular enlargement and straightening or bowing of the ventricular septum toward the left ventricle (Fig.15.12b) due to severe pulmonary arterial hypertension portend a poor prognosis (Oliver et al. 1998; Reid and Murchison 1998). In patients with suspected PE, MDCT can provide alternative diagnoses for dyspnea, including pneumonia, pulmonary edema, pericardial effusion and pleural effusion, an advantage over ventilation perfusion scanning (Chiles and Carr 2005).

In summary, there are a large number of diseases that cause chest pain, hemoptysis and dyspnea. Remarkable advances in MDCT, including EDG gating and the availability of a wide variety of reconstruction options, make this technique a powerful tool for achieving a precise diagnosis.

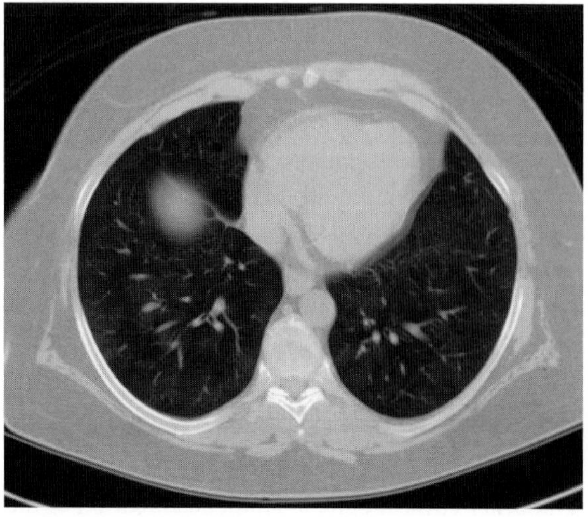

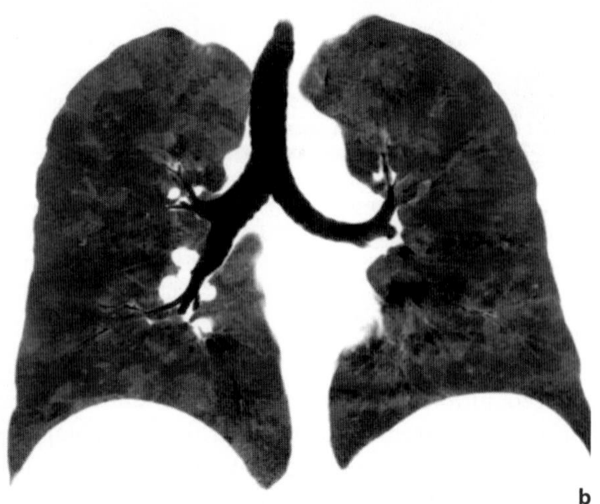

Fig. 15.10a,b. Bronchiolitis obliterans. **a** Axial CT image at the level of lung base shows diffuse multifocal mosaic attenuation, suggesting small airway disease. **b** Coronal minimal intensity projection CT image of the same patient shows clearly diffuse mosaic attenuations without any architectural distortion, consistent with bronchiolitis obliterans

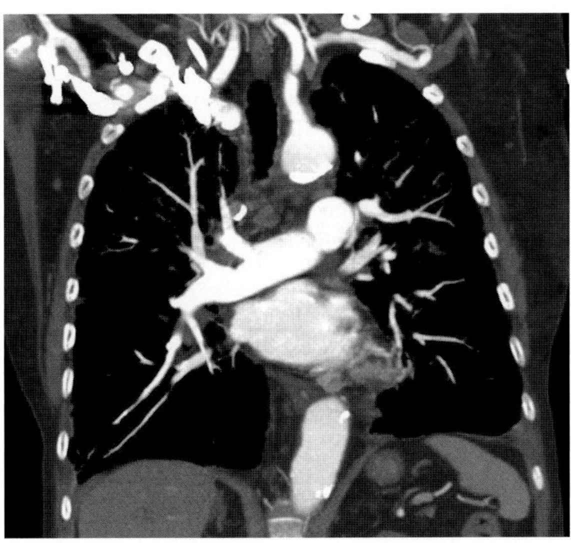
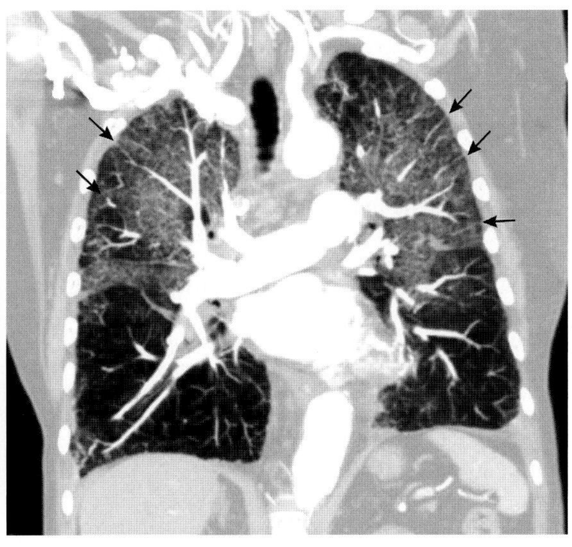

Fig. 15.11a,b. Pulmonary edema. **a** Coronal reformatted CT image in a patient with dyspnea shows no evidence of PE. **b** Coronal maximal intensity projection image of lung window setting at the same level as **a** shows enlarged pulmonary veins (*arrows*) secondary to pulmonary congestion and ground-glass attenuation mainly involving both upper lobes. Mild blunting of both cardiophrenic angles is also noted. These findings suggest pulmonary edema as the main cause of this patient's dyspnea

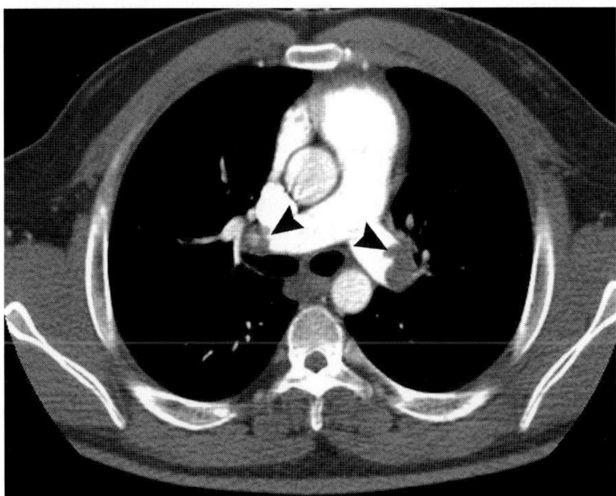
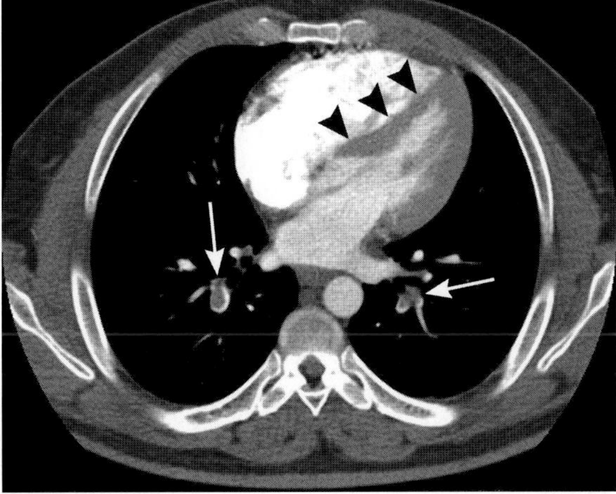

Fig. 15.12a,b. Pulmonary embolism with right ventricular strain. **a** Pulmonary emboli (*arrowheads*) are seen in right and left pulmonary artery on axial CT image obtained after enhancement at the level of bifurcation of main pulmonary artery. **b** Pulmonary emboli (*arrows*) are also noted in segmental pulmonary arteries of both lower lobes on axial CT image obtained after contrast administration at the level of left ventricle. Straightening of the interventricular septum (*arrowheads*) and mild right ventricular enlargement are demonstrated secondary to pulmonary hypertension

References

Achar SA, Kundo S, Norcross WA (2005) Diagnosis of acute coronary syndrome. Am Fam Physician 72:119–126

Anagnostopoulos CE, Prabhakar MJ, Kittle CF (1972) Aortic dissections and dissecting aneurysms. Am J Cardiol 30:263–273

Beigelman-Aubry C, Hill C, Guibal A et al. (2005) Multidetector row CT and postprocessing techniques in the assessment of diffuse lung disease. Radiographics 25:1639–1652

Boulay F, Berthier F, Sisteron O et al. (2000) Seasonal variation in cryptogenic and noncryptogenic hemoptysis hospitalizations in France. Chest 118:440–444

Braunwald E, Antman EM, Beasley JW et al. (2002) ACC/AHA 2002 guideline update for the management of patients with unstable angina and non-ST-segment elevation myocardial infarction–summary article: a report of the American College of Cardiology/American Heart Association task force on practice guidelines (Committee on the Management of Patients With Unstable Angina). J Am Coll Cardiol 40:1366–1374

Bruhlmann W, Weishaupt D, Goebel N et al. (1998) Therapeutic embolization of a systemic arterialization of lung without sequestration Eur Radiol 8:355–358

Bruzzi JF, Remy-Jardin M, Delhaye D et al. (2006) Multidetector row CT of hemoptysis. Radiographics 26:3–22

Castaner E, Andreu M, Gallardo X et al. (2003) CT in non-traumatic acute thoracic aortic disease: typical and atypical features and complications. Radiographics 23:S93–S110

Chabbert V, Doussau-Thuron S, Otal P et al. (2002) Endovascular treatment of aberrant systemic arterial supply to normal basilar segments of the right lower lobe: case report and review of the literature. Cardiovasc Intervent Radiol 25:212–215

Chiles C, Carr JJ (2005) Vascular diseases of the thorax: evaluation with multidetector CT. Radiol Clin North Am 43:543–569

Choi SH, Choi SJ, Kim JH et al. (2001) Useful CT findings for predicting the progression of aortic intramural hematoma to overt aortic dissection. J Comput Assist Tomogr 25:295–299

Chung JW, Park JH, Im JC et al. (1996) Spiral CT angiography of the thoracic aorta. Radiographics 16:811–824

Dapunt OE, Galla JD, Sadeghi AM et al. (1994) The natural history of thoracic aortic aneurysms. J Thorac Cardiovasc Surg 107:1323–1333

De Sanctis RW, Doroghazi RM, Austen WG et al. (1987) Aortic dissection. N Engl J Med 317:1060–1067

Gallagher MJ, Ross MA, Raff GL et al. (2007) The diagnostic accuracy of 64-slice computed tomography coronary angiography compared with stress nuclear imaging in emergency department low-risk chest pain patients. Ann Emerg Med 49:125–136

Giesler T, Baum U, Ropers D et al. (2002) Noninvasive visualization of coronary arteries using contrast enhanced multidetector CT: influence of heart rate on image quality and stenosis detection. AJR Am J Roentgenol 179:911–916

Goldman L, Cook EF, Johnson PA et al. (1996) Prediction of the need for intensive care in patients who come to the emergency departments with acute chest pain. N Engl J Med 334:1498–1504

Goldstein JA, Gallagher MJ, O'Neill WW et al. (2007) A randomized controlled trial of multi-slice coronary computed tomography for evaluation of acute chest pain. J Am Coll Cardiol 49:863–871

Gonsalves CF (1999) The hyperattenuating crescent sign. Radiology 211:37–38

Griepp RB, Ergin MA, Lansman SL et al. (1991) The natural history of thoracic aortic aneurysms. Semin Thorac Cardiovasc Surg 3:258–265

Hayashi H, Matsuoka Y, Sakamoto I et al. (2000) Penetrating atherosclerotic ulcer of the aorta: imaging features and disease concept. Radiographics 20:995–1005

Herth F, Ernst A, Becker HD (2001) Long-term outcome and lung cancer incidence in patients with hemoptysis of unknown origin. Chest 120:1592–1594

Hirose Y, Hamada S, Takamiya M (1995) Predicting the growth of aortic aneurysms: a comparison of linear vs exponential models. Angiology 46:413–419

Hirshberg B, Biran I, Glazer M et al. (1997) Hemoptysis: etiology, evaluation, and outcome a tertiary referral hospital. Chest 112:440–444

Hirst AE, Johns VJ Jr, Kime SW Jr (1958) Dissecting aneurysm of the aorta: a review of 505 cases. Medicine 37:217–279

Hiyama J, Horita N, Shiota Y et al. (2002) Cryptogenic hemoptysis and smoking. Chest 121:1375–1376

Kaul P, Newby LK, Johnson PA et al. (2004) International differences in evolution of early discharge after acute myocardial infarction. Lancet 363:511–517

Khalil A, Fartoukh M, Tassart M et al. (2007) Role of MDCT in identification of the bleeding site and the vessels causing hemoptysis. AJR Am J Roentgenol 188:117–125

Larson EW, Edwards WD (1984) Risk factors for aortic dissection: a necropsy study of 161 cases. Am J Cardiol 53:849–855

Lee DY, Williams DM, Abrams GD (1997) The dissected aorta: part II. Differentiation of the true from the false lumen with intravascular US. Radiology 203:32–36

Lee TH, Goldman L (2000) Evaluation of the patient with acute chest pain. N Engl J Med 342:1187–1195

Lee TH, Rouan GW, Weisberg MC et al. (1987) Clinical characteristics and natural history of patients with acute myocardial infarction sent home from the emergency room. Am J Cardiol 60:219–224

LePage M, Quint LE, Sonnad SS et al. (2001) Aortic dissection: CT features that distinguish true lumen from false lumen. AJR Am J Roentgenol 177:207–211

Levy JR, Heiken JP, Gutierrez FR (1999) Imaging of penetrating artheroslerotic ulcers of the aorta. AJR Am J Roentgenol 173:151–154

Maraj R, Perkpattanapipat P, Jacobs LE et al. (2000) Meta-analysis of 143 reported cases of aortic intramural hematoma. Am J Cardiol 86:664–668

Masuda Y, Takanashi K, Takasu J et al. (1992) Expansion rate of thoracic aortic aneurysms and influencing factors. Chest 102:461–466

McCaig LF, Burt CW (2004) National Hospital Ambulatory Medical Care Survey: 2002 emergency department summary. Adv Data 340:1–34

McCaig LF, Nawar EW (2006) National Ambulatory Medical Care Survey: 2004 emergency department summary. Adv Data 372:1–29

Mollet NR, Cademartiri F, van Mieghem CA et al. (2005) High-resolution spiral computed tomography coronary angiography in patients referred for diagnostic conventional coronary angiography. Circulation 112:2318–2323

Moore LB, Mcwey RE, Vujic I (1986) Massive hemoptysis: control by embolization of the thyrocervical trunk. Radiology 161:173–174

Morgan-Hughes GJ, Roobottom CA, Owens PE et al. (2005) Highly accurate coronary angiography with submillimeter, 16-slice computed tomography. Heart 91:308–313

Nienaber CA, Eagle KA (2003) Aortic dissection: new frontiers in diagnosis and management: Part II: therapeutic management and follow-up. Circulation 108:772–778

Nienaber CA, Von Kodolitsch Y, Peterson B et al. (1995) Intramural hemorrhage of the thoracic aorta. Diagnostic and therapeutic implications. Circulation 92:1465–1472

Oliver TB, Reid JH, Murchison JT (1998) Interventricular septal shift due to massive pulmonary thromboembolism shown by CT pulmonary angiography: an old sign revisited. Thorax 53:1092–1094

Perko MJ, Norgaard M, Herzog TM et al. (1995) Unoperated aortic aneurysm: a survey of 170 patients. Ann Thorac Surg 59:1204–1209

Poll LW, Cohnen M, Brachten S et al. (2002) Dose reduction in multi-slice CT of the heart by use of ECG-controlled tube current modulation ("ECG pulsing"): phantom measurements. Rofo 174:1500–1505

Pollack CV Jr, Gibler WB (2001) 2000 ACC/AHA guidelines for the management of patients with unstable angina and non-ST-segment elevation myocardial infarction: a practical summary for emergency physicians. Ann Emerg Med 38:229–240

Pope JH, Aufderheide TP, Ruthazer R et al. (2000) Missed diagnoses of acute cardiac ischemia in emergency department. N Engl J Med 342:1163–1170

Raff GL, Gallagher MJ, O'Neill WW et al. (2005) Diagnostic accuracy of noninvasive coronary angiography using 64-slice spiral computed tomography. J Am Coll Cardiol 46:552–557

Reid JH, Murchison JT (1998) Acute right ventricular dilatation: a new helical CT sign of massive pulmonary embolism. Clin Radiol 53:694–698

Reilly BM, Evans AT, Schaider JJ et al. (2002) Impact of a clinical decision rule on hospital triage of patients with suspected acute cardiac ischemia in the emergency department. JAMA 288:342–350

Remy-Jardin M, Bouaziz N, Dumount P et al. (2004) Bronchial and nonbronchial systemic arteries at multidetector row CT angiography: comparison with conventional angiography. Radiology 233:741–749

Ringstrom E, Freedman J (2006) Approach to undifferentiated chest pain in the emergency department: a review of recent medical literature and published practice guidelines. Mt Sinai J Med 73:499–505

Roberts WC (1981) Aortic dissection: anatomy, consequences, and causes. Am Heart J 101:195–214

Rohe RC, Thomas SR, Stabin MG et al. (1995) Biokinetics and dosimetry analysis in healthy volunteers for a two-injection (rest-stress) protocol of the myocardial perfusion imaging agent technetium 99m-labeled Q3. J Nucl Cardiol 2:395–404

Scirica BN, Morrow BA (2003) Troponins in acute coronary syndromes. Semin Vasc Med 3:363–374

Sebastia C, Pallisa E, Quiroga S et al. (1999) Aortic dissection: diagnosis and follow-up with helical CT. Radiographics 19:45–60

Sellars N, Belli AM (2001) Nonbronchial collateral supply from the left gastric artery in massive haemoptysis. Eur Radiol 11:76–79

Shim SS, Kim Y, Lim SM (2005) Improvement of image quality with beta-blocker premedication on ECG-gated 16-MDCT coronary angiography. AJR Am J Roentgenol 184:649–654

Song JK, Kim HS, Kang DH et al. (2001) Different clinical features of aortic intramural hematoma versus dissection involving the ascending aorta. J Am Coll Cardiol 37:1604–1610

Stanson AW, Kazmier FJ, Hollier LH et al. (1986) Penetrating atherosclerotic ulcers of the thoracic aorta: natural history and clinicopathologic correlations. Ann Vasc Surg 1:15–23

Sueyoshi E, Matsuoka Y, Sakamoto I et al. (1997) Fate of intramural hematoma of the aorta: CT evaluation. J Comput Assist Tomogr 21:931–938

Swanson KL, Jonhson M, Prakash UB et al. (2002) Bronchial artery embolization: experience with 54 patients. Chest 121:789–795

Thompson RC, Cullom SJ (2006) Issues regarding radiation dosage of cardiac nuclear and radiography procedures. J Nucl Cardiol 13:19–23

Welch TJ, Stanson AW, Sheedy PF et al. (1990) Radiologic evaluation of penetrating aortic atherosclerotic ulcer. Radiographics 10:675–685

White CS, Kuo D, Kelemen M et al. (2005) Chest pain evaluation in the emergency department: can MDCT provide a comprehensive evaluation? AJR Am J Roentgenol 185:533–540

Williams DM, Joshi A, Dake MD et al. (1994) Aortic cobwebs: an anatomic marker identifying the false lumen in aortic dissection–imaging and pathologic correlation. Radiology 190:167–174

Wong Ml, Szkup P, Hopley MJ (2002) Percutaneous embolotherapy for life-threatening hemoptysis. Chest 121:95–102

Yamada T, Tada S, Harada J (1988) Aortic dissection without intimal rupture: diagnosis with MR imaging and CT. Radiology 168:347–352

Yoon W, Kim YH, Kim JK et al. (2003) Massive hemoptysis: prediction of nonbronchial systemic arterial supply with chest CT. Radiology 227:232–298

Yoon YC, Lee KS, Jeong YJ et al. (2005) Hemoptysis: bronchial and nonbronchial systemic arteries at 16-detector row CT. Radiology 234:292–298

Yu-Tang Goh P, Lin M, Teo N et al. (2002) Embolization for hemoptysis: a 6-year review. Cardiovasc Intervent Radiol 25:17–25

Medical Applications of Integrated Cardiothoracic Imaging

Evaluation of Asymptomatic Cardiac Diseases

Lesions of Proximal Coronary Arteries

16

Filippo Cademartiri, Ludovico La Grutta, Anselmo Alessandro Palumbo, Erica Maffei, and Nico R. Mollet

CONTENTS

F. Cademartiri, MD, PhD
Department of Radiology, Azienda Ospedaliero, University of Parma, Via Gramsci 14, 43100 Parma, Italy
and
Department of Radiology and Cardiology, Erasmus Medical Center, Dr. Molewaterplein 60, 3015 GD Rotterdam, The Netherlands
L. La Grutta, MD
Department of Radiology and Cardiology, Erasmus Medical Center, Dr. Molewaterplein 60, 3015 GD Rotterdam, The Netherlands
and
Department of Radiology, University of Palermo, Italy
A. A. Palumbo, MD
Department of Radiology, Azienda Ospedaliero, University of Parma, Via Gramsci 14, 43100 Parma, Italy
and
Department of Radiology and Cardiology, Erasmus Medical Center, Dr. Molewaterplein 60, 3015 GD Rotterdam, The Netherlands
E. Maffei, MD
Department of Radiology, Azienda Ospedaliero, University of Parma, Via Gramsci 14, 43100 Parma, Italy
N. R. Mollet, MD, PhD
Department of Radiology and Cardiology, Erasmus Medical Center, Dr. Molewaterplein 60, 3015 GD Rotterdam, The Netherlands

16.1 Introduction

Coronary artery disease (CAD) remains the leading cause of death in the Western world. Conventional coronary angiography (CCA) is the gold standard method for evaluation of the vascular lumen and provides excellent results in demonstrating stenotic lesions of CAD. However, it is an invasive procedure with a small risk of fatal events. Furthermore, CCA is a lumen-oriented technique that does not permit a direct visualization and evaluation of the coronary artery wall. The characterization of coronary plaques without a significant lumen narrowing is also not feasible with CCA. This information is relevant since the comparison of angiographic studies of coronary arteries performed before and after non-fatal myocardial infarction has shown that 49% of the pre-existing lesions before MI was <50% of stenosis (Fishbein and Siegel 1996). The detection of vulnerable atherosclerotic plaques within the wall of the coronary arteries could represent a key factor for the prevention of acute events (Naghavi et al. 2003). Hence, it appears that some potentially dangerous lesions are often non-occlusive and thus difficult to diagnose with CCA. In the early stages the sequence of CAD is predictable, specific, uniform and asymptomatic; advanced lesions may progress in different morphogenetic stages, resulting in various lesion types and clinical syndromes. Therefore, patients with CAD may be asymptomatic due to the presence of non-significant stenosis (<50% lumen) or collateral circle blood supply. Furthermore, associated diseases such as diabetes may hide clinical symptoms of CAD.

Non-invasive coronary artery imaging challenges any diagnostic modality, because the coronary arteries are small and tortuous, while cardiac contraction and respiration cause motion artifacts. The availability of ECG-gated CT scanners with improved spatial and temporal resolution has allowed the evaluation of coronary arteries lumen and wall. The present chapter summarizes the current state of technology and clinical relevance of cardiac CT, with a special emphasis on coronary and non-coronary applications.

16.2 CT Coronary Angiography Technique

Electron beam CT firstly permitted the examination of moving structures, such as coronary arteries, but its spatial resolution allowed exploring only the proximal portion of the coronary arteries. The main application for this technique was the quantification of coronary calcifications (calcium score). The development of CT scanner technology brought more than a single row of detectors (2, 4, 16 and 64 detector rows) to systems and equipped them with faster gantry rotation speed. The resulting improvement in temporal and spatial resolution has placed multislice CT coronary angiography (MSCT-CA) in the field of cardiac clinical applications. With 64-slice CT scanners a high temporal resolution has been achieved by combining a fast gantry rotation speed (330 ms) with a "half scan" reconstruction algorithm that provides a temporal resolution of half the rotation time (165 ms) in the center area of the scanning field of view (Leschka et al. 2005; Raff et al. 2005; Mollet et al. 2005a; Leber et al. 2005; Ropers et al. 2006; Schuijf et al. 2006; Ong et al. 2006). The recently introduced dual-source CT (DSCT) scanner is characterized by two X-ray tubes and two corresponding detectors mounted into the rotating gantry with an angular offset of 90°. Regarding cardiac imaging capabilities, the new scanner system offers a high temporal resolution of 83 ms that is independent of the heart rate of the patient (Weustink et al. 2007; Leber et al. 2007; Scheffel et al. 2006).

Angiographic studies of coronary arteries are performed with a bolus of 80–100 ml contrast material with high iodine concentration (350–400 mg of Iodine per ml) injected through the brachial vein (flow rate of 4–5 ml/s). Bolus tracking technique is used to synchronize the arrival of contrast in the coronary arteries with the initiation of the scan.

The scan parameters for 64-slice CT coronary angiography (based on Sensation 64®, Siemens, Germany) are: individual detector width 0.6 mm, gantry rotation time 330 ms, effective temporal resolution 165 ms, kV 120, eff. mAs 600–700, feed/rotation 3.84 mm (11.6 mm/s; pitch factor 0.2) and scan direction cranio-caudal. The acquisition time takes 10–12 s.

The electrocardiographic (ECG) track is acquired during the scan, and afterwards the image reconstruction is performed with retrospective gating. After acquisition of the CT data the operator may set the reconstruction window at any point within the cardiac cycle by selecting the motionless dataset throughout the entire R-R interval. For these reasons, retrospective ECG gating is the standard scanning and reconstruction technique in cardiac MSCT, although the prospective ECG triggering may obtain data during a pre-selected phase of the cardiac cycle resulting in a significantly lower radiation exposure.

Reconstruction is performed with 0.6/0.75-mm effective slice thickness, medium-smooth to medium-sharp convolution algorithm and the field of view as small as possible to cover the heart and vessels of interest. The reconstructed contiguous axial slices are stacked in a volume to generate a 3D dataset from which any plane can be created. Currently, MIP (maximum intensity projection), MPR (multiplanar reformatting), cMPR (curved multi-planar reformatting) and VRT (volume-rendering technique) are the tools employed to obtain a diagnostic three-dimensional view of the coronary artery tree. Furthermore, datasets obtained with a large FOV were reviewed in mediastinal and lung windows to display incidental extra-coronary findings.

16.3 Diagnostic Performance and Applications

The results reported are robust in the field of coronary artery stenosis detection. Studies with 64-slice CT and DSCT demonstrated a high diagnostic accuracy and negative predictive value for the detection of >50% coronary artery stenosis in selected patient populations. The negative predictive value is between 96% and 100% in all major CT series published (Table 16.1) (Leschka et al. 2005; Raff et al. 2005; Mollet et al. 2005a; Leber et al. 2005; Ropers et al. 2006; Schuijf et al. 2006; Ong et al. 2006; Weustink et al. 2007; Leber et al. 2007; Scheffel et al. 2006). Hence, MSCT-CA may be used to ex-

Table 16.1. Diagnostic performance of 64-slice and dual-source CT coronary angiography as compared to conventional coronary angiography to detect significant (≥50 lumen diameter reduction) coronary stenoses on a per-segment analysis

	Pop. (n)	Excl. (%)	Sens. (%)	Spec. (%)	PPV (%)	NPV (%)
LESCHKA et al. (2005)	67	0	94	97	87	99
RAFF et al. (2005)	70	12	86	95	66	98
MOLLET et al. (2005)	52	0	99	95	76	99
LEBER et al. (2006)	55	0	76	97	75	97
ROPERS et al. (2006)	81	4	93	97	56	100
SCHUIJF et al. (2006)	60	1.4	85	98	82	99
ONG et al. (2006)	134	9.7	82	96	79	96
WEUSTINK et al. (2007)	77	0	95	95	75	99
LEBER et al. (2007)	88	1.3	94	99	81	99
SCHEFFEL et al. (2006)	30	0	96	97	86	99

Abbreviations: Number of patients enrolled (Pop.); number of excluded segments or branches in percentage (Excl.); sensitivity (Sens.), specificity (Spec.), positive (PPV) and negative predictive value (NPV) regarding the detection of significant coronary stenosis

clude the presence of significant stenosis in patients with low-intermediate pre-test probability because of the high negative predictive value. In these settings, the proper use of MSCT-CA would be after an inconclusive or borderline stress test or in patients with atypical chest pain. MSCT-CA has a negative predictive value of 100% in patients with stable angina (MOLLET et al. 2004). The recent guidelines on stable angina of the European Society of Cardiology have added CT to the diagnostic algorithm and, with a low level of evidence (IIB), suggest that the technique may be employed in patients with low to intermediate risk and with inconclusive stress test results or inability to undergo stress testing (FOX et al. 2006).

Based on current appropriateness criteria, major coronary MSCT-CA applications are: detection of CAD in patients with chest pain syndrome and uninterpretable or equivocal stress test (exercise, perfusion or stress echo), evaluation of patients with chest pain syndrome and intermediate pre-test probability of CAD with equivocal ECG or unable to exercise, evaluation of acute chest pain in patients with intermediate pre-test probability of CAD with negative ECG and serial cardiac enzymes, and detection of congenital heart disease including anomalies of coronary arteries, great vessels and cardiac chambers and valves (Figs. 16.1–16.3) (HENDEL et al. 2006).

Given the high sensitivity and negative predictive value of the technique, MSCT-CA could represent an alternative to CCA in asymptomatic patients with dilated cardiomiopathy of unknown origin and prior to cardiac valve surgery or transplant and major non-coronary cardiac surgery (MEIJBOOM et al. 2006).

MSCT-CA may be a possibility to rule out in-stent restenosis in selected cases (e.g., large-diameter stents in a proximal vessel segment, low and stable heart rate, and absence of excessive image noise). MSCT-CA may be also useful in very selected patients in whom only bypass graft assessment is necessary (e.g., failed visualization of a graft in invasive angiography) (HENDEL et al. 2006).

16.4 MSCT Coronary Plaque Imaging

There is growing interest concerning the ability of MSCT-CA to detect and possibly quantify and characterize non-calcified non-significant coronary atherosclerotic plaques. The identification of high-risk plaques and related risk stratification are currently the subject of much debate and research (SCHROEDER et al. 2001; LEBER et al. 2004; ACHENBACH et al. 2004).

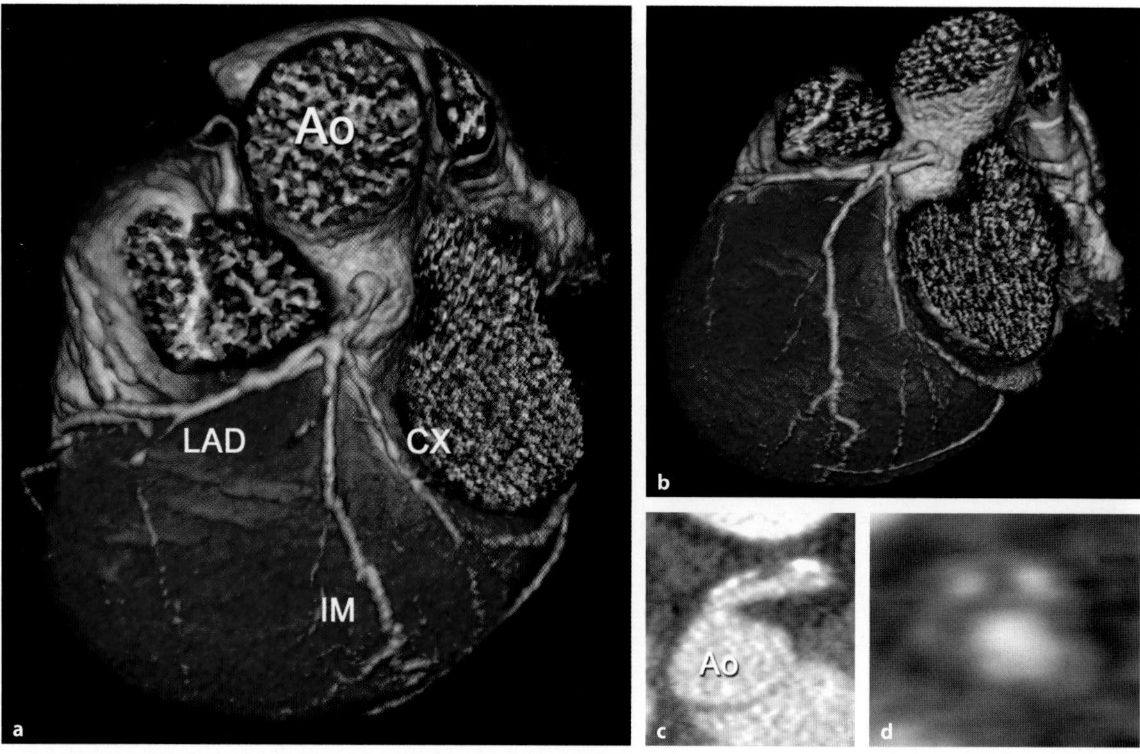

Fig. 16.1a–d. Example of patient with atypical chest pain + dyspnea (55-year-old female) and diffuse coronary atherosclerosis. The three-dimensional volume-rendering images (**a,b**) show diffuse irregularities of the coronary artery tree and an anatomical variant of left coronary anatomy (trifurcation with an intermediate branch). Beside the diffuse atherosclerosis in this patient, the multiplanar reformat (**c,d**) shows a very proximal border-line lesion (~50%) of the left main carrying a mixed eccentric plaque with positive remodeling. *Ao* = ascending aorta; *CX* = left circumflex; *LAD* = left anterior descending; *IM* = intermediate branch

Non-invasive MSCT-CA provides unique in-vivo information regarding coronary plaques (anatomical distribution throughout the coronary tree, number of diseased coronary segments, extent of vessel wall remodelling and shape) (Table 16.2) (Mollet et al. 2005b). It has been reported that MSCT-CA has the potential to detect coronary plaques (calcified, non-calcified and mixed plaques), quantify their volumes and eventually characterize their composition, based on the X-ray attenuating features of each structure measured in Hounsfield units (HU). Therefore, the overall plaque burden assessment using MSCT-CA represents an advance on the established calcium quantification approach. Firstly, Schroeder et al. (2001) showed a correlation between the echogenicity of plaques with intravascular ultrasound as compared to the CT attenuation values measured in HU. The CT attenuation resulted in 14±26 HU for soft (i.e., predominantly lipid) plaques, 91±21 HU for intermediate (i.e., predominantly fibrous) plaques and 419±194 HU for calcified plaques. Leber et al. (2004) showed that lesion echogenicity correlates well with MSCT attenuation measurements in coronary plaque. MSCT correctly classified 78% of sections containing hypoechoic plaque areas (soft plaques), 78% of sections containing hyperechoic plaque areas (fibrous plaques) and 95% of sections containing calcified plaque tissue. However, a sub-classification between lipid and fibrous plaques appears difficult, since a substantial overlap of density between hypoechoic (lipid-rich) and hyperechoic (fibrous) plaques was observed in the same study. Moreover, a sensitivity of only 53% to detect non-calcified plaque is reported (Achenbach et al. 2004). Leber et al. compared the predominant extent and composition of coronary atherosclerosis (i.e., coronary plaque burden) using MSCT-CA in patients with acute myocardial infarction and stable angina. Non-calcified plaques were more represented in patients with acute myocardial infarction as compared to patients with stable angina (Leber et al. 2003). One analysis of 100 patients who were followed for 16 months after MSCT-CA

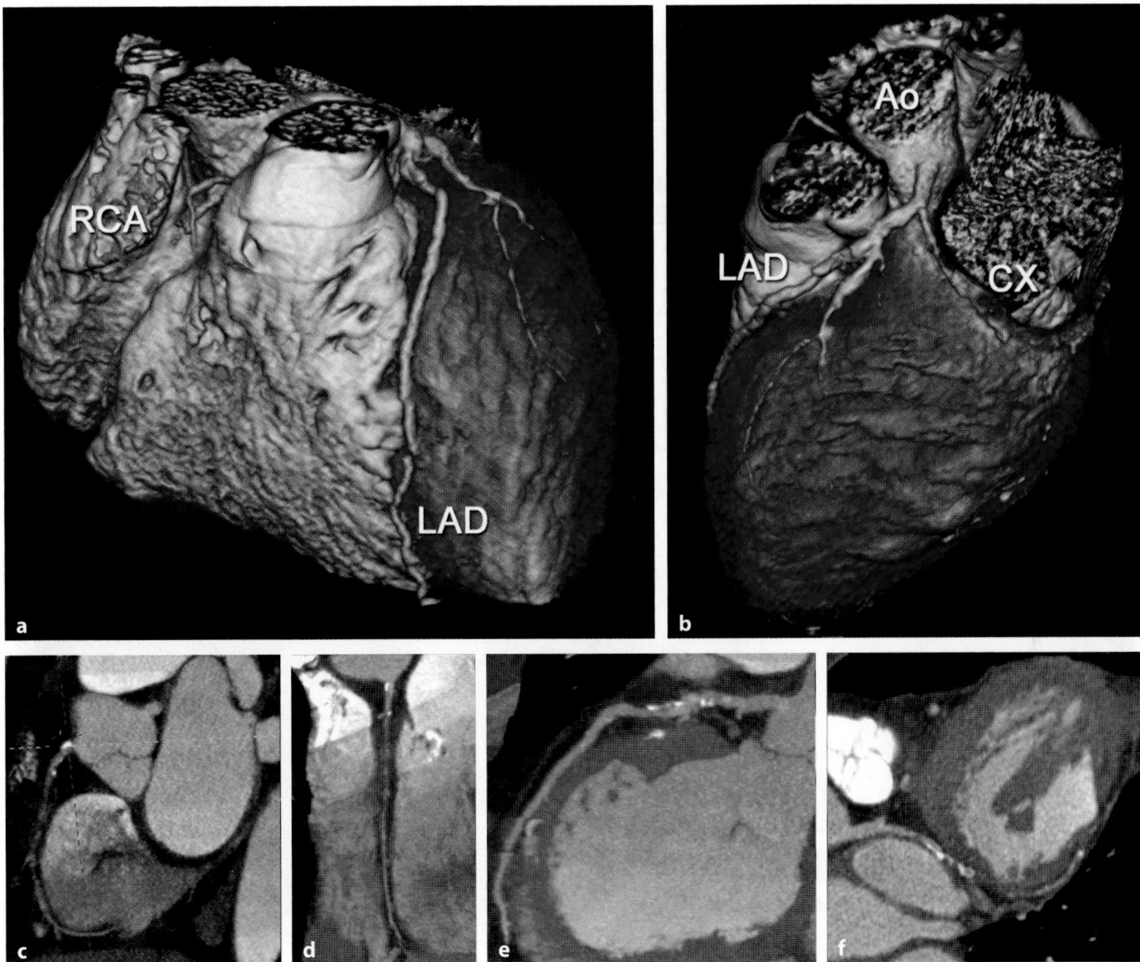

Fig. 16.2a–f. Example of patient with typical chest pain (58-year-old male) and severe diffuse coronary atherosclerosis. The three-dimensional volume-rendering images (**a**,**b**) show diffuse irregularities of the coronary artery tree. The multiplanar reformat (**c**-**f**) shows a proximal chronic total occlusion of the RCA (**c**,**d**), a proximal atherosclerosis of the LAD <50% and a chronic total occlusion of middle tract of CX. Underlying this disorder there is a dilated cardio-myopathy with reduced ejection fraction of the left ventricle, secondary to chronic heart disease. *Ao* = ascending aorta; *CX* = left circumflex; *LAD* = left anterior descending; *RCA* = right coronary artery

demonstrated a higher cardiovascular event rate in patients with non-obstructive plaque detected by MSCT compared with individuals without any plaque (Pundziute et al. 2007). Although these initial observations suggest that there may be a potential value of plaque imaging by MSCT-CA for risk prediction in asymptomatic high-risk individuals, several limitations must be taken into account. The reliable visualization of coronary plaque requires the highest image quality, which requires contrast agent and high radiation exposure. The substantial radiation exposure precludes unlimited re-investigations in asymptomatic individuals (i.e., assessment of coronary atherosclerosis progression and regression).

16.5 Non-Coronary Applications

Functional parameters, such as left and right ventricular end-diastolic and end-systolic volumes, stroke volume, ejection fraction and myocardial mass, can be calculated from MSCT-CA datasets. Although CT imaging allows accurate assessment of left and right ventricular function, CT examinations in most cases will not be performed specifically for that purpose. Other diagnostic tests without radiation exposure (i.e., magnetic resonance imaging) or need for contrast injection (i.e., echocardiography) are the methods of choice. However, it should be

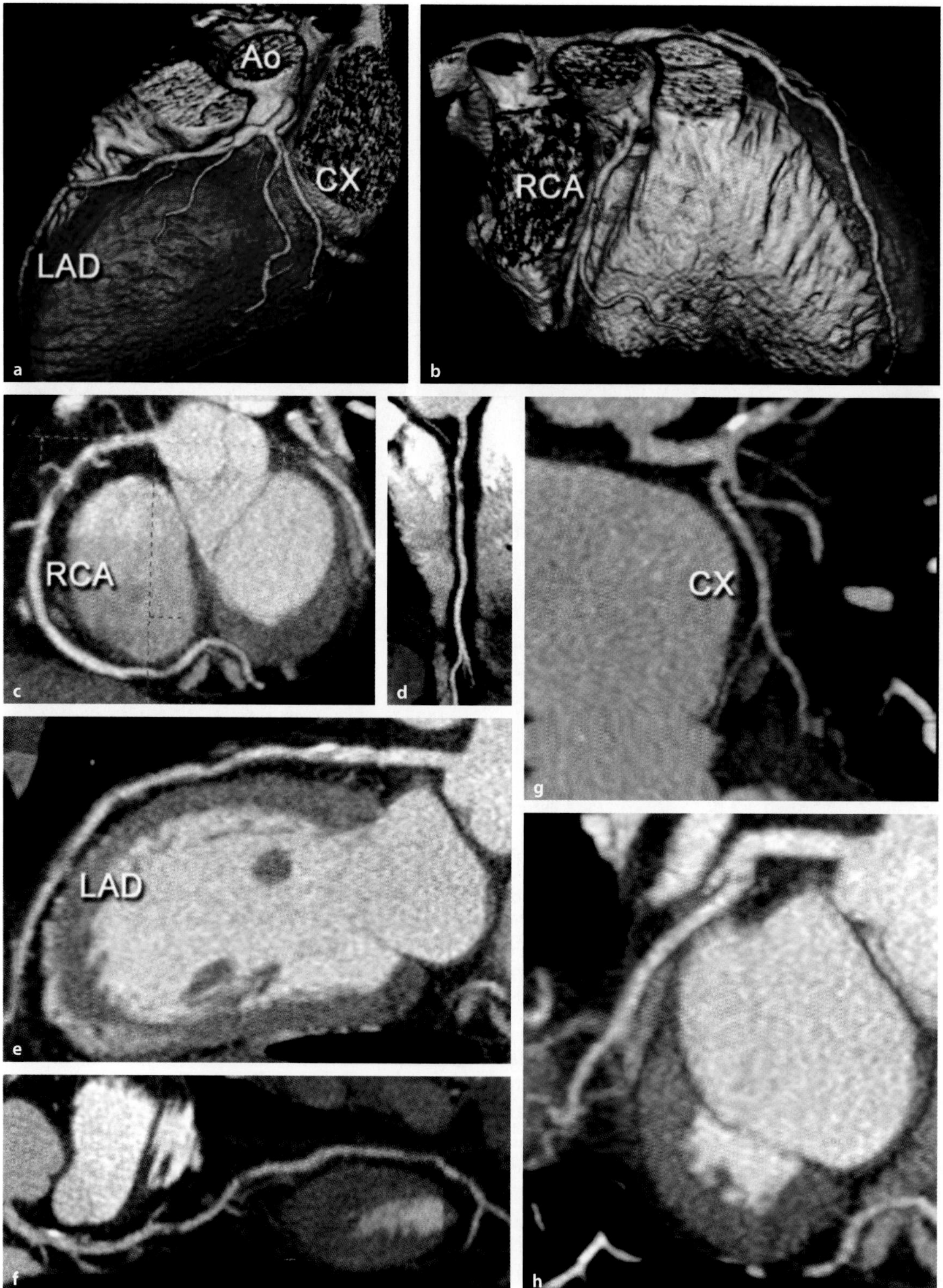

Fig. 16.3a–h. Example of patient with typical chest pain (66-year-old female) and mild diffuse coronary atherosclerosis. The three-dimensional volume-rendering images (**a**,**b**) show some degree of coronary atherosclerosis. The multiplanar reformat (**c**–**h**) shows a proximal long significant (> 50%) lesion of the RCA (**c**,**d**) due to a mixed plaque. Also, in the LAD there was proximal atherosclerosis with < 50% stenosis. The small CX, instead, does not show significant coronary plaque burden. *Ao* = ascending aorta; *CX* = left circumflex; *LAD* = left anterior descending; *RCA* = right coronary artery

Table 16.2. MSCT parameters in plaque imaging

Parameter	Type
Size	Lumen narrowing approach (obstructive ≥50%; non-obstructive <50%) Plaque-oriented quantitative approach (thickness; volume)
Characterization (Hounsfield unit)	Calcified plaques (calcium scoring software) Mixed plaques Non-calcified plaques
Remodeling index	Positive remodeling (outward expansion of the coronary vessel wall) Negative remodeling (shrinking of the coronary vessel wall)
Shape	Concentric plaques Eccentric plaques
Plaque burden	Anatomical distribution of plaques Plaque size Plaque tissue characterization Remodeling index

noted that ventricular function is additional information that can be obtained from standard MSCT-CA (Hendel et al. 2006).

The wide availability of MSCT scanners has led to a constant increase of cardiac studies throughout the world. It is remarkable that incidental pathological changes in organs and structures, which were not the target of the examination, are frequently reported. Sometimes these extra-cardiac collateral findings revealed during MSCT-CA are of major importance for the patient's health and correct diagnostic workup. Therefore, MSCT-CA datasets obtained with a large FOV should be reviewed in mediastinal and lung windows, in order to exhaustively report the investigation (Cademartiri et al. 2007). Still, limited clinical data have documented that MSCT allows assessment of myocardial viability by studying "late enhancement" in a similar fashion as magnetic resonance imaging (Mahnken et al. 2005).

The assessment of aortic or mitral valves using MSCT is also feasible with good diagnostic accuracy when other more commonly used methods, such as echocardiography and magnetic resonance imaging, fail to provide all relevant information. MSCT is also the test of choice to know the exact anatomy of the coronary veins before cardiac resynchronization therapy. MSCT also may be used to display left atrium and pulmonary veins prior to invasive electrophysiology procedures or in the follow-up after pulmonary vein ablation (Hendel et al. 2006).

Other non-coronary applications are the evaluation of cardiac masses (tumor or thrombus) and the evaluation of aortic (thoracic aneurysm or dissection, follow-up of prosthetic aortic valves) and pulmonary disease (embolism). However, in such applications a description of relevant CAD should be reported since heart and coronary arteries are included in the CT ECG-gated acquisition of the thorax. In this setting, a report of significant lesions of proximal coronary arteries is suggested.

16.6 Triple Rule-Out of Cardiothoracic Diseases

Acute chest pain represents a frequent cause for admission in the emergency department. Diagnosing the cause of acute chest pain in the emergency department remains a formidable task because of extensive etiology that ranges from benign (e.g., pneumonia, pneumothorax, pericarditis, esophagitis and gastritis) to potentially lethal pathologies (e.g., pulmonary embolism, myocardial infarction and aortic dissection). These pathologies may also be associated with similar clinical symptoms. The emergency physician has several elements (history, physical examination, ECG, chest X-ray, cardiac enzymes and D-dimers) to address the patient with the correct diagnosis. Nevertheless, it is hard to select the appropriate one for an early and accurate diagnosis. Some myocardial infarctions may not show any significant rise of markers in the first 6 h and not-conclusive ECG. The D-dimers may facilitate the diagnosis of pulmonary embolism; however, these markers are not specific, and only a negative value may exclude a thromboembolic event. The American College of Radiology appropriateness criteria on acute chest pain call for use of ECG and serum cardiac markers as first diagnostic approach (Stanford et al. 2000). Further diagnostic steps, depending on the patient's history, are chest X-ray, ventilation-perfusion scintigraphy, resting myocardial perfusion scanning, echocardiography, CT and angiography. However, the investigation can be time-consuming and expensive; furthermore, some diseases are associated with sudden death. Therefore, a fast one-stop shop examination is highly desirable to reduce the time and the cost of diagnostic workup.

The latest 64-slice CT scanners may rapidly acquire the entire thoracic volume with high resolution, thus allowing evaluation in the same time as coronary arteries, thoracic aorta and pulmonary arteries (Fig. 16.4) (Johnson et al. 2007). This "triple rule-out" scan could provide a faster approach to the

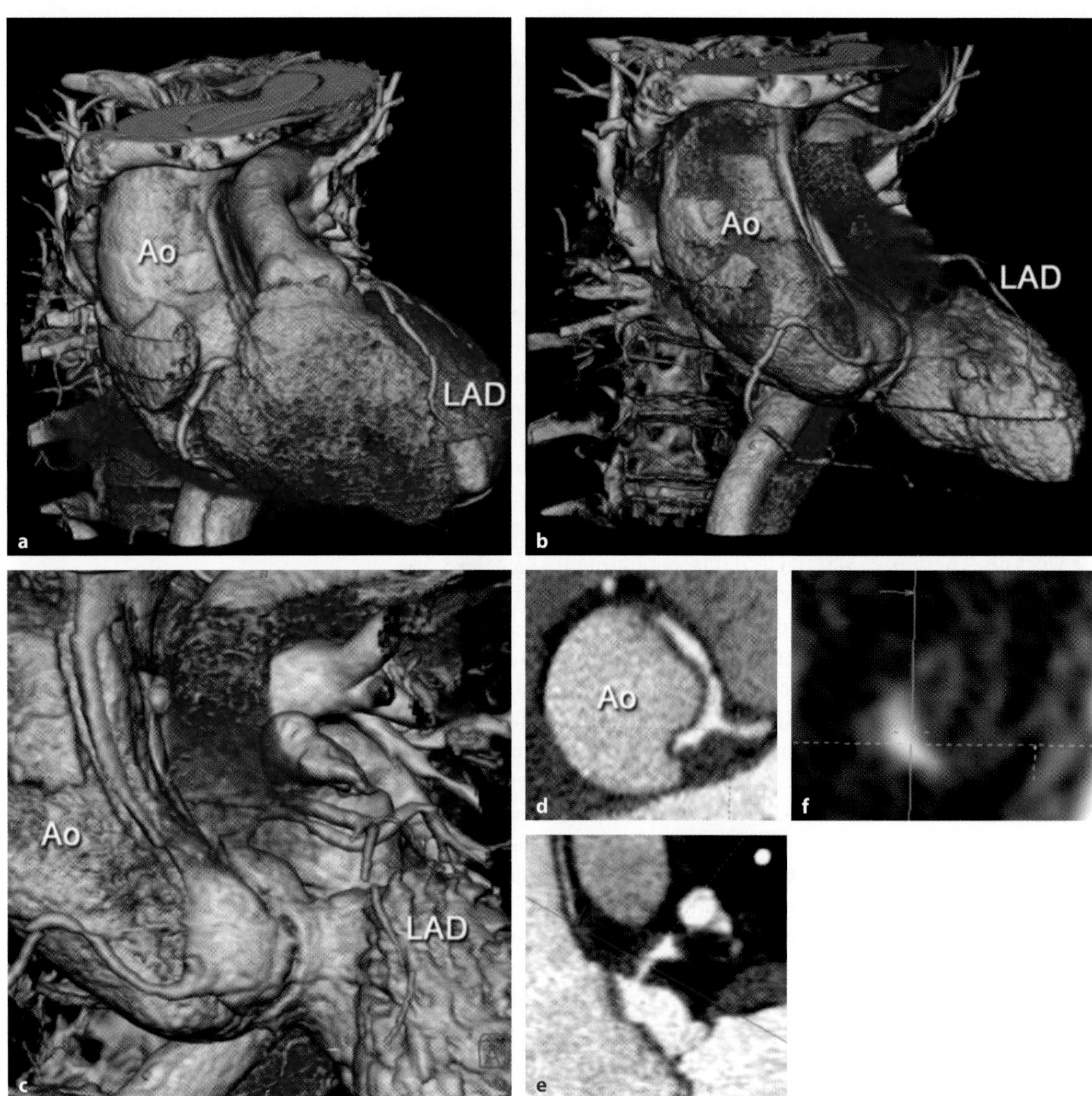

Fig. 16.4a–f. Example of patient with acute type A dissection of the thoracic aorta (62-year-old female). The three-dimensional volume-rendering images (**a–c**) show the intimal flap in the ascending aorta. The multiplanar reformat (**d–f**) shows the involvement of the left main (proximal lesion), which is dissected by the aortic tear causing a >50% stenosis. *Ao* = ascending aorta; *CX* = left circumflex; *LAD* = left anterior descending

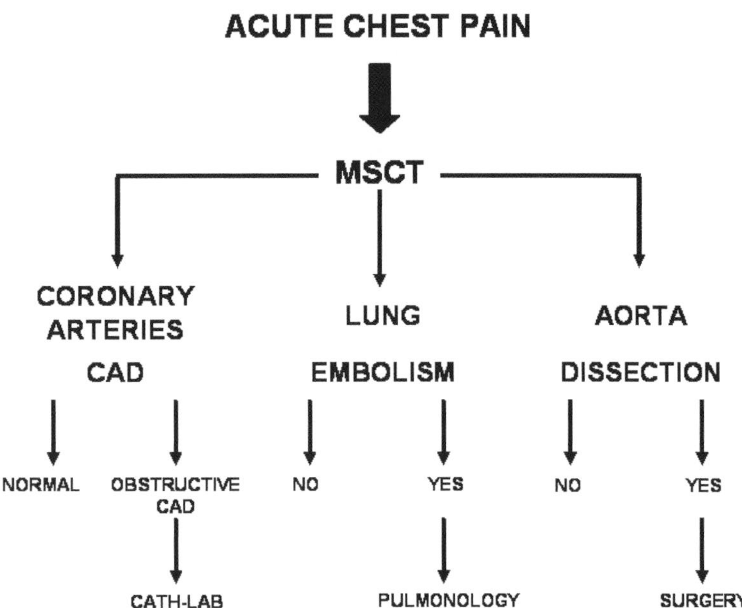

Fig. 16.5. Triple rule-out algorithm in acute chest pain

triage of acute chest pain (Fig. 16.5). This test may, thus, help to significantly reduce charges and length of hospitalization (Hoffmann et al. 2006; Savino et al. 2006).

Furthermore, if CT scanners with cardiac state-of-the-art capabilities will be installed in the emergency department, the early diagnosis of acute coronary syndromes with still negative enzymes and non-diagnostic ECG alterations also would be allowed.

A careful selection of patients and a strong co-operation with cardiologists and emergency physicians are mandatory. Patients with frankly benign symptoms and with a low likelihood of lethal acute conditions should be addressed to hospitalization or discharge after the observation time. Patients with a high likelihood of acute myocardial infarction (ECG changes, positive cardiac markers) do not need further investigations and may be addressed to the Cath-Lab rather than MSCT. Patients may undergo MSCT if the origin of chest pain is unclear, with negative or not conclusive ECG, and equivocal clinical findings. Then, MSCT is considered appropriate in patients with intermediate pre-test probability of CAD when ECG and cardiac enzymes are negative, while its role is uncertain in patients with low or high pre-test probability of CAD. MSCT is considered appropriate for the evaluation of aortic and pulmonary disease, while its role should be more deeply investigated for the "triple rule-out" purpose of excluding obstructive CAD, aortic dissection and pulmonary embolism in patients with acute chest pain (Hendel et al. 2006). In this setting, the performances still needs to be prospectively confirmed in larger groups of patients. However, the selection of patient candidates for MSCT should remain strictly based on clinical evidence in order to avoid an unjustified risk of ionizing radiation, especially in young patients.

In conclusion, since the advent of MSCT scanners with their improved spatial and temporal resolution, CT coronary angiography has been gradually evolving as a promising non-invasive method for the assessment of patients with CAD. ECG-gated MSCT could represent a logistically feasible and a promising comprehensive method for evaluating cardio-thoracic diseases. Hence, fast developments and robust results of MSCT scanner technology have led to a pivotal role to play for heart and coronary artery imaging in thoracic radiology.

References

Achenbach S, Moselewski F, Ropers D et al. (2004) Detection of calcified and noncalcified coronary atherosclerotic plaque by contrast-enhanced, submillimeter multidetector spiral computed tomography: a segment-based comparison with intravascular ultrasound. Circulation 109:14–17

Cademartiri F, Malagò R, Belgrano M et al. (2007) Spectrum of collateral findings in multislice CT coronary angiography. Radiol Med (Torino) 112:937–948

Fishbein MC, Siegel RJ (1996) How big are coronary atherosclerotic plaques that rupture? Circulation 94:2662–2666

Fox K, Garcia MA, Ardissino D et al. (2006) Guidelines on the management of stable angina pectoris: executive summary: the Task Force on the Management of Stable Angina Pectoris of the European Society of Cardiology. Eur Heart J 27:1341–1381

Hendel RC, Patel MR, Kramer CM et al. (2006) CCF/ACR/SCCT/SCMR/ASNC/NASCI/ SCAI/SIR 2006 appropriateness criteria for cardiac computed tomography and cardiac magnetic resonance imaging: a report of the American College of Cardiology Foundation Quality Strategic Directions Committee Appropriateness Criteria Working Group, American College of Radiology, Society of Cardiovascular Computed Tomography, Society for Cardiovascular Magnetic Resonance, American Society of Nuclear Cardiology, North American Society for Cardiac Imaging, Society for Cardiovascular Angiography and Interventions, and Society of Interventional Radiology. J Am Coll Cardiol 48:1475–1497

Hoffmann U, Pena AJ, Moselewski F et al. (2006) MDCT in early triage of patients with acute chest pain. AJR Am J Roentgenol 187:1240–1247

Johnson TR, Nikolaou K, Wintersperger BJ et al. (2007) ECG-gated 64-MDCT angiography in the differential diagnosis of acute chest pain. AJR Am J Roentgenol 188:76–82

Leber AW, Knez A, White CW et al. (2003) Composition of coronary atherosclerotic plaques in patients with acute myocardial infarction and stable angina pectoris determined by contrast-enhanced multislice computed tomography. Am J Cardiol 91:714–718

Leber AW, Knez A, Becker A et al. (2004) Accuracy of multidetector spiral computed tomography in identifying and differentiating the composition of coronary atherosclerotic plaques: a comparative study with intracoronary ultrasound. J Am Coll Cardiol 43:1241–1247

Leber AW, Knez A, von Ziegler F et al. (2005) Quantification of obstructive and nonobstructive coronary lesions by 64-slice computed tomography: a comparative study with quantitative coronary angiography and intravascular ultrasound. J Am Coll Cardiol 46:147–154

Leber AW, Johnson T, Becker A et al. (2007) Diagnostic accuracy of dual-source multi-slice CT-coronary angiography in patients with an intermediate pretest likelihood for coronary artery disease. Eur Heart J 28:2354–2360

Leschka S, Alkadhi H, Plass A et al. (2005) Accuracy of MSCT coronary angiography with 64-slice technology: first experience. Eur Heart J 26:1482–1487

Mahnken AH, Koos R, Katoh M et al. (2005) Assessment of myocardial viability in reperfused acute myocardial infarction using 16-slice computed tomography in comparison to magnetic resonance imaging. J Am Coll Cardiol 45:2042–2047

Meijboom WB, Mollet NR, Van Mieghem CA et al. (2006) Pre-operative computed tomography coronary angiography to detect significant coronary artery disease in patients referred for cardiac valve surgery. J Am Coll Cardiol 48:1658–1665

Mollet NR, Cademartiri F, Nieman K et al. (2004) Multislice spiral computed tomography coronary angiography in patients with stable angina pectoris. J Am Coll Cardiol 43:2265–2270

Mollet NR, Cademartiri F, van Mieghem CA et al. (2005a) High-resolution spiral computed tomography coronary angiography in patients referred for diagnostic conventional coronary angiography. Circulation 112:2318–2323

Mollet NR, Cademartiri F, Nieman K et al. (2005b) Noninvasive assessment of coronary plaque burden using multislice computed tomography. Am J Cardiol 95:1165–1169

Naghavi M, Libby P, Falk E et al. (2003) From vulnerable plaque to vulnerable patient: a call for new definitions and risk assessment strategies: Part I. Circulation 108:1664–1672

Ong TK, Chin SP, Liew CK et al. (2006) Accuracy of 64-row multidetector computed tomography in detecting coronary artery disease in 134 symptomatic patients: influence of calcification. Am Heart J 151:1323–1326

Pundziute G, Schuijf JD, Jukema JW et al. (2007) Prognostic value of multislice computed tomography coronary angiography in patients with known or suspected coronary artery disease. J Am Coll Cardiol 49:62–70

Raff GL, Gallagher MJ, O'Neill WW et al. (2005) Diagnostic accuracy of noninvasive coronary angiography using 64-slice spiral computed tomography. J Am Coll Cardiol 46:552–557

Ropers D, Rixe J, Anders K et al. (2006) Usefulness of multidetector row spiral computed tomography with 64×0.6-mm collimation and 330 ms rotation for the noninvasive detection of significant coronary artery stenoses. Am J Cardiol 97:343–348

Savino G, Herzog C, Costello P, Schoepf UJ (2006) Sixty-four-slice cardiovascular CT in the emergency department: concepts and first experiences. Radiol Med (Torino) 111:481–496

Scheffel H, Alkadhi H, Plass A et al. (2006) Accuracy of dual-source CT coronary angiography: First experience in a high pre-test probability population without heart rate control. Eur Radiol 16:2739–2747

Schroeder S, Kopp AF, Baumbach A et al. (2001) Noninvasive detection and evaluation of atherosclerotic coronary plaques with multislice computed tomography. J Am Coll Cardiol 37:1430–1435

Schuijf JD, Pundziute G, Jukema JW et al. (2006) Diagnostic accuracy of 64-slice multislice computed tomography in the non-invasive evaluation of significant coronary artery disease. Am J Cardiol 98:145–148

Stanford W, Levin DC, Bettmann MA et al. (2000) Acute chest pain–no ECG evidence of myocardial ischemia/infarction. American College of Radiology. ACR Appropriateness Criteria. Radiology 215 (Suppl):79–84

Weustink AC, Meijboom WB, Mollet NR et al. (2007) Reliable high-speed coronary computed tomography in symptomatic patients. J Am Coll Cardiol 50:786–794

Myocardial Infarction

17

Christoph R. Becker

CONTENTS

17.1 Introduction

Non-invasive imaging of the coronary arteries by CT has been the primary clinical focus for the last decade. Multi-detector row CT angiography of the coronary arteries has been compared to cardiac catheters in more than 40 papers for more than 2,500 patients. In patients particularly investigated by 64-slice CT, the sensitivity and specificity of detecting stenoses as compared to cardiac catheter are in the range of 98% and 92%, respectively (Janne d'Othee et al. 2007). CT scanning of the heart, however, not only provides information about the coronary arteries, but also about the valves and the myocardium. Coronary artery wall changes and plaques may either result in significant luminal narrowing or sudden occlusion of the coronary artery and therefore subsequently in changes of the myocardial blood flow.

Chronic myocardial ischemia with blood flow maintained above a certain threshold may result in loss of regular contractility, known as hibernating myocardium. Hibernating myocardium may regain its regular function if regular blood flow is restored. Acute myocardial ischemia on the other hand may result in stunned myocardium if perfusion is preserved above a certain threshold. However, if regular blood flow is restored, stunned myocardium may not regain its regular function although it is still viable. Reversible myocardial ischemia has best been detected by function or perfusion imaging under rest and exercise.

Conversely, irreversible myocardial damage with reduced perfusion below a certain threshold may result in the loss of cell membrane integrity and increased permeability of small vessels within the myocardium. In the early phase of myocardial infarction, an interstitial edema is followed by an invasion of inflammatory cells. Subsequently, necrotic infracted myocardium is replaced by fibrous or fatty tissue. Myocardial wall thinning is one of the indirect signs of chronic and healing myocardial infarction. In a longitudinal study in patients with myocardial infarction, the wall thickness of the myocardium decreased significantly in the area of the infarction over time (Masuda et al. 1984).

Patients presenting with acute chest pain and ST elevation in the ECG are obviously presenting with a myocardial infarction (ST-elevated myocardial infarction = STEMI). But even in the absence of a typical ECG sign, elevated cardiac enzymes may be indicative of an acute myocardial infarction (non ST-elevated myocardial infarction = NSTEMI). Ideally, any of these patients would undergo immediate revascularization to keep the extent of the infarction as small as possible. Patients with unstable angina (UA) may present without elevated ST segments or positive cardiac enzymes. In these patients it is mandatory to follow them in order to detect any later signs of myocardial infarction or to prove the evidence for coronary artery disease with subsequent exercise tests. In any of these scenarios of unstable

C. R. Becker, MD
Department of Clinical Radiology, Ludwig-Maximilians-University, Grosshadern Hospital, Marchioninistrasse 15, 81377 Munich, Germany

angina, CT may provide important information not only about the coronary arteries, but also about status of the myocardium.

17.2 Myocardial Perfusion Imaging

Well-established techniques such as single-photon emission tomography (SPECT) or positron emission tomography (PET) are commonly used to detect impaired blood flow in the myocardium. In the last decade, perfusion imaging of the myocardium has extensively been performed with MRI. The difference between stress and rest perfusion allows the calculation of the myocardial flow reserve and subsequently the determination of the hemodynamic relevance of a coronary artery lesion.

The pharmacological and physiological properties of contrast agent to determine the myocardial blood flow are principally the same for MRI and CT, respectively. Perfusion imaging by CT is a well-established technique for the assessment of stroke in the brain. The influx of contrast media in the cerebral arteries may be used to calculate the input function for the perfusion study. In principle, CT is the ideal method for perfusion imaging because of the linear relationship between contrast volume and X-ray attenuation. Myocardial perfusion imaging by CT is based on the dynamic visualization of contrast agent first pass through the cardiac chambers (Fig. 17.1). There are two techniques available for imaging the myocardial perfusion by CT: prospective ECG triggering and retrospective ECG gating, both without table movement during scanning. Prospective ECG triggering is the preferred method in order to reduce radiation exposure. Scanning should be performed every heartbeat to ensure sufficient temporal resolution for the evaluation. It is mandatory to inject a sharp and short contrast medium bolus that is immediately followed by a saline chaser bolus. The amount of contrast media should be in the order of magnitude of 40 ml highly concentrated (>350 mg/ml) contrast media, injected at high flow

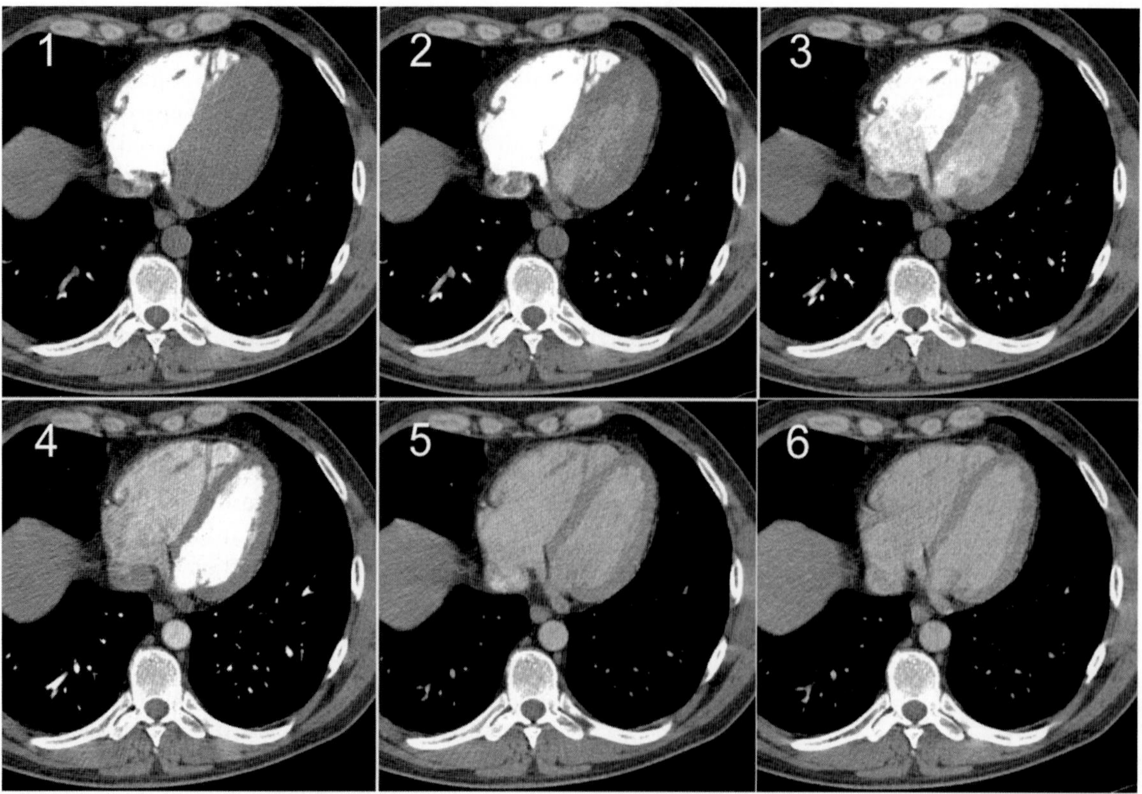

Fig. 17.1. Dynamic first-pass imaging of contrast media by MDCT performed at a certain level of the heart. A sharp contrast bolus has to be administered through a peripheral vein and followed by a saline chaser bolus

rate (>5 ml/s) through a peripheral vein. In order to keep the contrast bolus compact and to allow for adequate post-processing, the contrast media bolus should be followed with a reasonable amount of saline (>50 ml) injected with the same flow rate. Perfusion deficits in the axial slice can be assigned to a certain territory that belongs to one of three major vessels (Fig. 17.2).

The underlying basic principle of first-pass perfusion imaging is based on indicator dilution theory and the Stewart-Hamilton equation (MEIER and ZIERLER 1954):

Blood volume (BV) = blood flow (F) × mean transit time (MTT)

Quantitative myocardial perfusion (ml min-1 g-1) is defined as myocardial blood flow (ml min-1) per myocardial mass (g). However, for the use of the indicator dilution theory in clinical perfusion imaging in CT or MRI, a few assumptions have to be made concerning the contrast agent properties and bolus profiles (ZIERLER 2000).

Unfortunately, perfusion imaging of the heart is far more challenging than imaging of the brain because of the rapid cardiac and respiratory motion and the complex anatomy of the heart and its position within the chest. Furthermore, the huge amount of contrast media that arrives in the cardiac chambers frequently results in beam-hardening artifacts in particular in the sub-endocardial region and the apex, making perfusion assessment of these particular important segments impossible (Fig. 17. 3).

Therefore, successful perfusion studies of the myocardium have so far only been performed by multi-slice CT in animal models showing good correlation between perfusion deficits and microsphere-determined blood flow (HOFFMANN et al. 2004). Numerous data are available on perfusion imaging with multi-detector row CT in animals (GEORGE et al. 2006, 2007; LARDO et al. 2006). At present there are only very few data available on perfusion imaging of the myocardium by MDCT in humans. It has been shown in humans that the coronary perfusion reserve can be derived from MDCT data (Fig. 17.4). Using the Fermi function model, reasonable results concerning absolute blood flow quantification

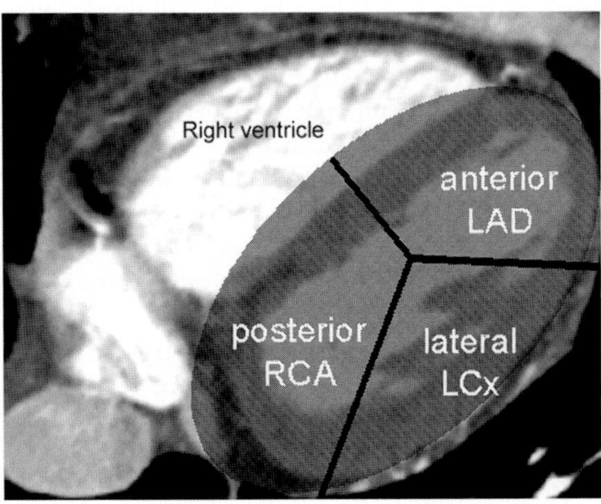

Fig. 17.2. In a dominant right coronary artery supplement type, certain territories of the myocardium can be assigned to one of the three major vessels

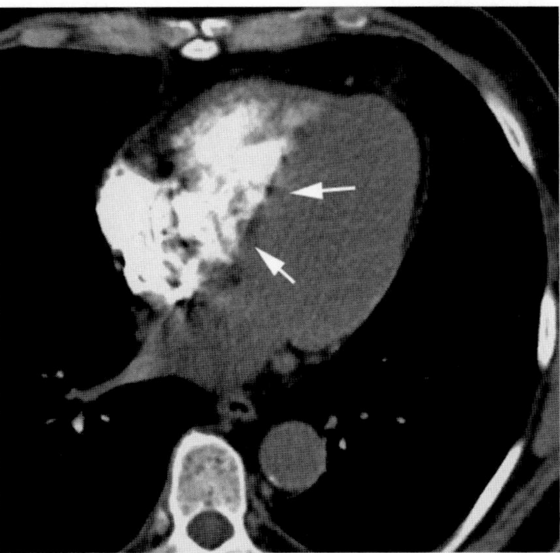

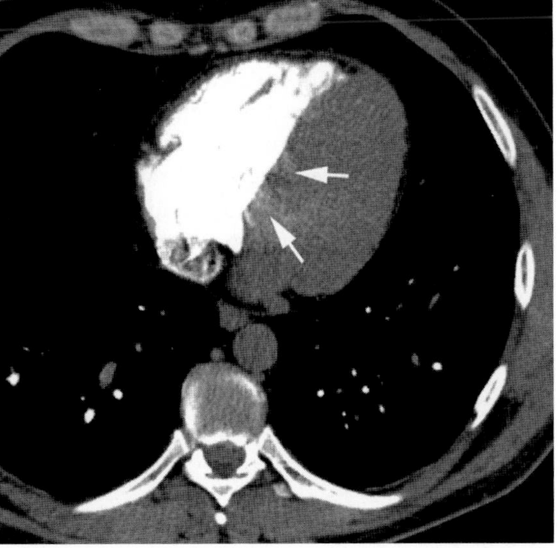

Fig. 17.3. Influx of contrast media during first pass may result in significant artifacts in particular in the area of the sub-endocardial region. Assessment of the myocardial perfusion can be substantially affected by this artifact

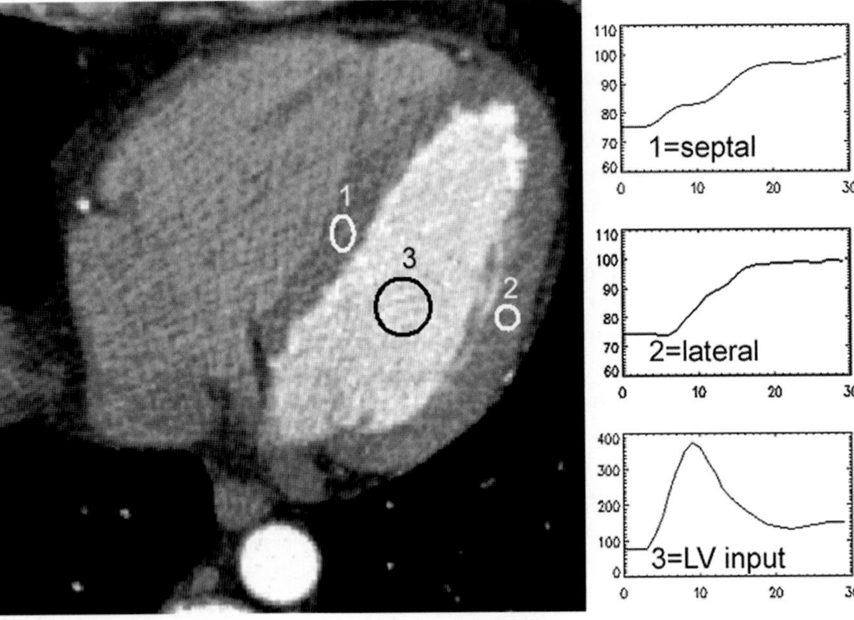

Fig. 17.4. Under certain circumstances myocardial perfusion can be derived from certain measurements using the Fermi function model as an assumption

can be achieved. The resulting perfusion values (0.73±0.2 ml/g/min) were well in the range of what is known for resting myocardium (Nikolaou et al. 2005). However, a broad application of this technique is prevented by the reasons discussed above.

A comprehensive perfusion study of the myocardium would require a measurement during, i.e., pharmacological stress. As any stress of the heart goes along with an increase of the heart rate, this would result in impaired image quality for the assessment of the coronary arteries by CT. Currently perfusion imaging of the myocardium would be limited to the range of the detector width, i.e., 4 cm in a 64-slice CT scanner. Complete coverage of the left ventricular myocardium is therefore not available yet. Furthermore, repeated X-ray scanning at the same location may result in a significant amount of radiation. For all the reasons mentioned above, myocardial perfusion imaging is still a topic of research and has not yet been applied routinely in clinical settings.

17.3 Viability imaging

Within recent years, a number of studies have focused on imaging of perfusion deficits by CT either in the first pass of the contrast media application or in the delayed phase, aiming at the visualization of non-vital myocardium. This approach of imaging represents more of a static snapshot of the blood volume distribution in the early phase and detection of interstitial leakage in the late phase rather than real perfusion imaging of the myocardium with assessment of the wash in and out of the contrast agent dependent on time.

Blood volume imaging may provide unspecific information about myocardial edema or infarction (Fig. 17.5), but may also be found in severe local ischemia without infarction or hypertrophic cardiomyopathy. Furthermore, myocardial enhancement depends on a variety of different independent factors, such as contrast protocol or cardiac output. Therefore, rather than defining absolute attenuation values, relative changes in the density may allow for discriminating infarcted from non-infarcted myocardium. If decreased attenuation and wall thinning are considered myocardial infarction signs in CT, the sensitivity and specificity of CT compared to MIR are 86% and 91%, respectively (Nikolaou et al. 2004). Consequently, it has been described that CT frequently underestimates the true extent of myocardial infarction (Schmermund et al. 1998). In principle, recent infarctions are more difficult to detect by CT than chronic infarction scars.

In several studies, a delayed contrast enhancement (5 to 10 min after first pass of contrast media) has been described predominantly in recent infarction, but also in some chronic infarction scars. Furthermore, CT similar to MRI may be able to detect the zone of microvascular obstruction in the sub-endocardial region (Fig. 17.6). However, because of the lower difference between the signal intensities of non-vital and vital myocardium, late myocardial enhancement cannot be detected that consistently by CT compared to MRI.

17.4 Myocardial Infarction Sequelae

By imaging the heart, MDCT provides comprehensive information about infarct-related findings, such as myocardial aneurysms, intramural calcifications, intra-cavitary thrombi or infarct involvement of the

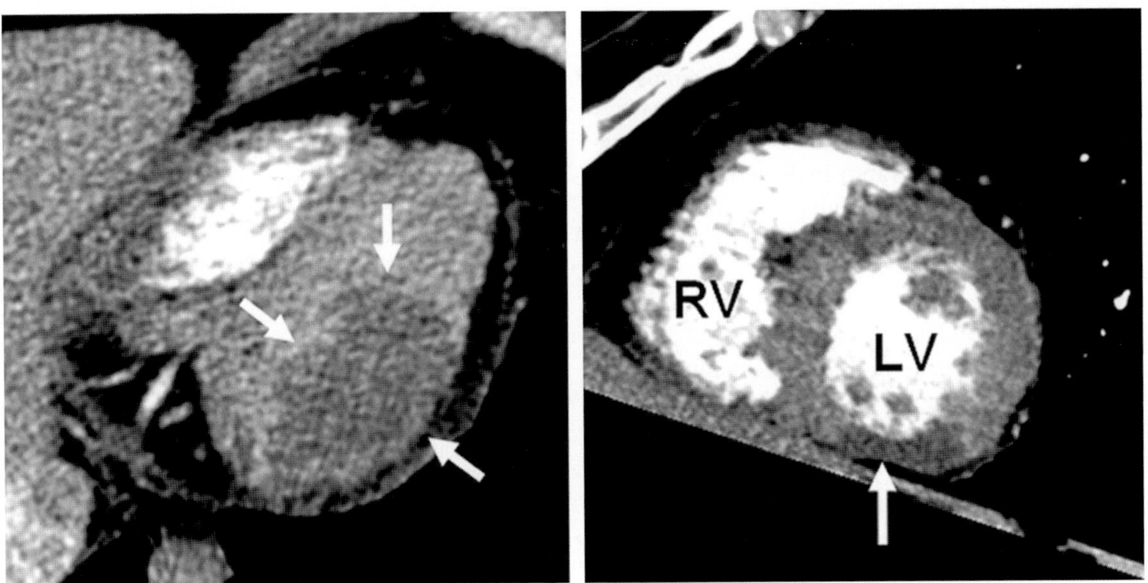

Fig. 17.5a,b. During the first pass of contrast media, myocardial infarction may already become visible. **a** Acute myocardial infarction with a region of hypo-attenuation (edema) in the posterior wall, most likely related to an occlusion of the circumflex artery or one of its side branches. **b** Chronic myocardial infarction scar with hypo-enhancement and thinning of the myocardial wall

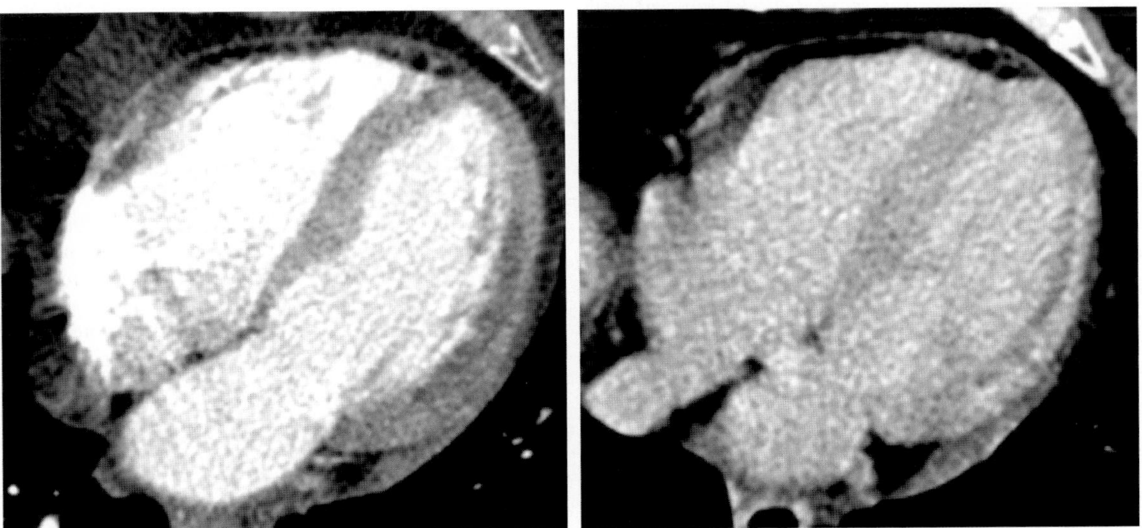

Fig. 17.6. First pass (*left*) and late myocardial enhancement scan (*right*) by MDCT. The sub-endocardial region of the lateral wall remains hypo-intense in both phases and therefore corresponds to the zone of micro-vascular obstruction. This zone is surrounded by a hyper-intense area of non-viable myocardium as seen in the delayed CT scan

papillary muscle. Catheter-based ventriculography on the first glance provides clinically relevant information about myocardial aneurysms and wall-motion abnormalities. The diagnostic criterion of myocardial pseudo-aneurysms is protrusion of the left ventricular wall, which can be detected by MDCT similarly to catheter angiography. MDCT, however, furthermore provides information about the myocardial wall and thereby allows differentiation between myocardial pseudo-aneurysms and diverticula (Ghersin et al. 2007).

Left ventricular thrombi are one of the most severe complications of myocardial infarction. MDCT seems to have the advantage over catheter angiography and echocardiography in detecting intra-cavitary thrombi. MDCT provides detailed information about the surface area and border between the thrombus and the myocardial wall (Fig. 17. 7). Free-floating or mural organized thrombi can clearly be distinguished by MDCT (Doepp et al. 2005).

Cardiac tamponade is a life-threatening condition that results from slow or rapid compression of the heart secondary to accumulation of fluid, pus, blood, gas or tissue within the pericardial cavity. MDCT is an excellent method to detect intramural calcification or pericardial effusion that might be the result of a myocardial infarction (Restrepo et al. 2007).

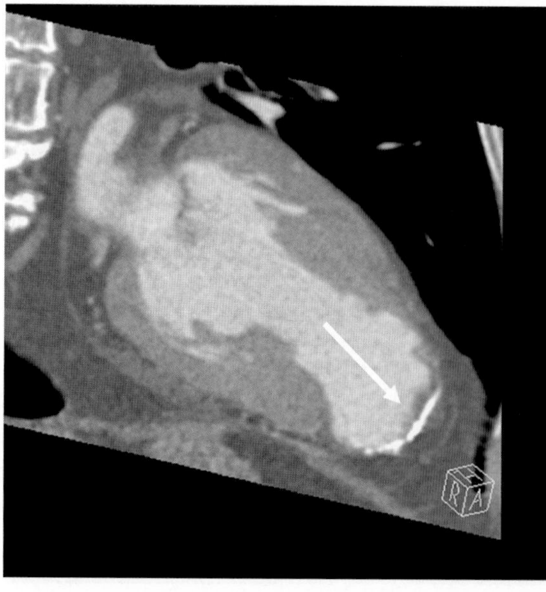

Fig. 17.7. Partially calcified thrombus formation in the apex of the left ventricle as a consequence of an anterior wall infarction and aneurysm in the apex of the heart

References

Doepp F, Sanad W, Schreiber SJ, Baumann G, Borges AC (2005) Left ventricular apical thrombus after systemic thrombolysis with recombinant tissue plasminogen activator in a patient with acute ischemic stroke. Cardiovasc Ultrasound 3:14

George RT, Silva C, Cordeiro MA et al. (2006) Multidetector computed tomography myocardial perfusion imaging during adenosine stress. J Am Coll Cardiol 48:153–160

George RT, Jerosch-Herold M, Silva C et al. (2007) Quantification of myocardial perfusion using dynamic 64-detector computed tomography. Invest Radiol 42:815–822

Ghersin E, Kerner A, Gruberg L, Bar-El Y, Abadi S, Engel A (2007) Left ventricular pseudoaneurysm or diverticulum: differential diagnosis and dynamic evaluation by catheter left ventriculography and ECG-gated multidetector CT. Br J Radiol 80:e209–211

Hoffmann U, Millea R, Enzweiler C et al. (2004) Acute myocardial infarction: contrast-enhanced multi-detector row CT in a porcine model. Radiology 231:697–701

Janne d'Othee B, Siebert U, Cury R, Jadvar H, Dunn EJ, Hoffmann U (2008) A systematic review on diagnostic accuracy of CT-based detection of significant coronary artery disease. Eur J Radiol 65:449–461

Lardo AC, Cordeiro MA, Silva C et al. (2006) Contrast-enhanced multidetector computed tomography viability imaging after myocardial infarction: characterization of myocyte death, microvascular obstruction, and chronic scar. Circulation 113:394–404

Masuda Y, Yoshida H, Morooka N, Watanabe S, Inagaki Y (1984) The usefulness of X-ray computed tomography for the diagnosis of myocardial infarction. Circulation 70:217–225

Meier P, Zierler KL (1954) On the theory of the indicator-dilution method for measurement of blood flow and volume. J Applied Physiol 6:731–744

Nikolaou K, Knez A, Sagmeister S et al. (2004) Assessment of myocardial infarctions using multidetector-row computed tomography. J Comput Assist Tomogr 28:286–292

Nikolaou K, Sanz J, Poon M et al. (2005) Assessment of myocardial perfusion and viability from routine contrast-enhanced 16-detector-row computed tomography of the heart: preliminary results. Eur Radiol 15:864–871

Restrepo CS, Lemos DF, Lemos JA et al. (2007) Imaging findings in cardiac tamponade with emphasis on CT. Radiographics 27:1595–1610

Schmermund A, Gerber T, Behrenbeck T et al. (1998) Measurement of myocardial infarct size by electron beam computed tomography: a comparison with 99mTc sestamibi. Invest Radiol 33:313–321

Zierler K (2000) Indicator dilution methods for measuring blood flow, volume, and other properties of biological systems: a brief history and memoir. Ann Biomed Eng 28:836–848

Aortic Bicuspidia, Silent Ductus Arteriosus

18

SALAH D. QANADLI and ELENA RIZZO

CONTENTS

18.1 Introduction

The bicuspid aortic valve (BAV) is the most common congenital cardiac anomaly, occurring in 1% to 2% of the general population (FEDAK et al. 2002). Although the physiopathology and natural history are not completely understood, the bicuspid aortic valve syndrome (BAVS) is a clinically challenging issue for physicians and more recently for radiologists. It has been demonstrated that the majority of patients with BAVS develop significant anatomic changes and complications that require specific treatment. Thus, recognition of the silent disease could have significant implications for patient management. This section will focus on anatomic features of the BAV, assessment of the bicuspidia, especially using relatively new cross-sectional modalities, and identification of cardiac and vascular complications.

S. D. QANADLI, MD
E. RIZZO, MD
Service de Radiologie, CHU Vaudois, 1011 Lausanne, Switzerland

18.2 Anatomy and Pathology of the Aortic Bicuspidia

The aortic valve is a complex structure communicating between the left-ventricle out-flow tract with the ascending aorta through the aortic root. Attached to the sinotubular junction of the aorta, typically the aortic valve contains three equal-size cusps (tricuspid valve). Each cusp has a semilunar leaflet (freely moving part). The commissure is commonly used to describe the peripheral part of apposition of leaflets and the annulus to describe their attachment to the proximal margin to the aortic root. During the cardiac cycle, the leaflets intersect at the center of the annulus at 120° angles in the diastolic phase (closed position) demonstrating complete coaptation and swing cranially in the systolic phase (open position), revealing a central typical triangular orifice. The BAV, characterized by only two cusps, is a result from abnormal fusion of cusps during valvulogenesis.

The BAV is currently regarded as having the most frequent aberrant cusps of the complex phenotypic continuum in the valvulogenesis process, which includes unicuspid valves (severe form), bicuspid valves (moderate form), tricuspid valves (normal), and the rare quadricuspid form (FERNANDEZ et al. 2000). The pathogenesis of aortic valve malformations is still debated. However, more recent evidence suggests genetic disorders that affect the extracellular matrix and the microfibrillar proteins as fibrillin and fibulin (Eisenberg et al. 1995; Epstein et al. 2000; Lee et al. 2000). In support of a genetic origin, BAV is associated with congenital abnormalities of the aorta (aortic coarctation and patent ductus arteriosus) and coronary arteries. Whether BAV can be considered as a hereditary anomaly is not clear. The high incidence of familial BAV (Huntington et al. 1997; Clementi et al. 1996) is compatible with autosomal dominant inherence with reduced penetrance.

18.3 Natural History of Aortic Bicuspidia

BAV is a common congenital disease that occurs in 1% to 2% of the population, compared with 0.8% for all other congenital cardiac diseases (Ward 2000). The incidence of clinically normally functioning BAV is 0.6% to 0.9% (Roberts 1970). The clinical profile of BAVS is heterogeneous with respect to morphological changes in the valve (raphé location, presence of calcifications) and valve function (normal function, stenosis or regurgitation) as well as clinical symptoms. Some patients remain asymptomatic and complication-free for a lifetime, while some have rapid and progressive valve dysfunction and aortic dilatation. However, the vast majority of patients develop complications requiring specific management. Considering that severe complications occur in more than one third of patients, the BAVS may be responsible for more mortality and morbidity than all congenital heart diseases combined (Ward 2000).

18.3.1 Valvular Complications

Valvular complications include aortic stenosis, regurgitation, and endocarditis. Aortic stenosis is the most frequent complication. Aortic stenosis results directly from the valve anatomy with asymmetrical cusps [stenosis is more rapid in asymmetrical cup shape (Ward 2000)] and premature morphological changes due to fibrosis, stiffening, and calcium deposits. The calcium deposit is an active process similar to the atherosclerotic plaque calcification that plays a significant role in the disease progression and complications (Mohler et al. 2001). Echocardiography studies have shown that calcifications are an important predictive factor of the clinical outcome (Bahler et al. 1999; Rosenhek et al. 2000). Regarding the BAV, recently, using multi-detector CT (MDCT), Ferda et al. (2007) observed no significant difference in the severity of valve calcifications between tricuspid and BAV in symptomatic patients with aortic valve stenosis. The incidence of aortic stenosis in patients with BAVS ranged from 15% to 71% (Ward 2000). The wide range is probably explained by the effect of age in the development of valve stenosis. Additionally, the risk of developing stenosis in the BAVS seems to be increased in patients with lipid profiles and those who smoke (Chan 2001).

Aortic regurgitation, a less frequent complication with an incidence of 1.5% to 3% (Ward 2000), usually results from prolapse of the larger cusp, fibrotic retraction of leaflets, dilatation of the aortic sinotubular junction, or combined mechanisms. Aortic regurgitation induced by the BAV usually occurs in younger patients than aortic stenosis (Pachulski et al. 1993) and is probably underestimated (Stefani et al. 2008). The aortic regurgitation may occur as an isolated pathology (Roberts et al. 1981) or in association with ascending aortic dilatation (Guiney et al. 1987), coarctation of the aorta, or infective endocarditis (Ward 2000).

Infective endocarditis is a severe complication that occurs in about one third of patients with BAVS, more frequently in those with regurgitation (Fedak et al. 2002). Infective endocarditis may induce cusp perforation and consequently aortic regurgitation. Subsequently, infective endocarditis is responsible for than 50% of severe aortic regurgitation in patients with BAVS (Roberts et al. 1981).

18.3.2 Vascular Complications

Vascular complications in patients with BAVS include ascending aortic aneurysms and aortic dissection. The mechanism of these complications and the relationship with BAVS remain controversial. Some argue there are proponent environmental causes of aortic dilatation due to post-valvular hemodynamic changes that trigger progressive dilatation. However, even if the latest mechanism may contribute to the acceleration of the dilatation process, an intrinsic defect in the aortic wall independent from the aortic valve function is regarded as the major factor inducing aortic dilatation in the BAVS (Keane et al. 2000; Nistri et al. 1999). Focal structural abnormalities have been identified within the aortic wall in patients with BAVS, such as matrix disruption and smooth muscle loss similar to those observed in firillin-1-deficient aorta and Marfan syndrome (Niwa et al. 2001; Fedak et al. 2003). The resulting degenerative process may induce weaknesses of the aortic wall that preclude dilatation, precursor to life-threatening events such as aortic rupture and dissection. Clinical findings in patients with the BAVS support associated intrinsic aortic wall disorder in patient with BAVS. Nistri et al. (1999) reported that the majority of young patients with normally functioning BAV have dilation of the ascending aorta on echocardiography. In addition, vascular complications occur also in patients in whom native BAV was replaced by prosthesis as reported by Yasuda et al. (2003).

18.4 Diagnostic Imaging

18.4.1 Assessment of the Aortic Valve

Echocardiography, including the transesophageal approach, is the main imaging modality used for aortic valve morphology and function (Hatle et al. 1980). Two views are usually used (long axis and short axis) for complete assessment (Fig. 18.1). To quantify the aortic area, two methods are used: the estimated area with a hemodynamic calculation based on the continuity equation and direct measurement by planimetry. Morphology and function of the aortic valve are well evaluated with MR. More recently, ECG-gated multi-detector CT has demonstrated a potential to visualize the valve anatomy as an integrated part not only of cardiac CT angiography, but also of thoracic CT angiography. Thus, the increasing application of ECG-gated thoracic CTs invites more extensive discussion of this point in order to prepare the radiologist for systematic evaluation of the aortic valve. Valve assessment requires no real specific acquisition parameters. Standard protocols using high resolution and optimal enhancement for coronary artery angiography, which have been described in previous chapters, are sufficient for aortic valve assessment. However, multiphase reconstructions are mandatory. The reconstruction interval is typically every 5% to 10% during the RR cycle. No clear evidence supports interest in shorter intervals, particularly in the assessment of the aortic valve. Caution should be taken to keep sufficient image quality during the systolic phase when the ECG-dose modulation program is applied, which may alter images in the systolic phase. The quality of aortic valve images during the cardiac cycle depends also on the heart rate, even with the latest CT scan generations. The aortic valve in the closed position is routinely well analyzed in the mid-diastole at 70% to 80% of the RR cycle. Due to the lack of temporal resolution in the current CT scanners, the open position is relatively instable during the temporal acquisition window in the systolic phase (Fig. 18.2). The open position is usually best visualized at 20% to 30% of the RR cycle. CT images provide morphologic analysis of the valve components. Using planimety with similar principles to echocardiography, additional information regarding the aortic valve function could be obtained (Fig. 18.3). A good correlation between the narrowest aortic valve area of the orifice at mid-systole and the aortic valve area obtained by transesophageal echocardiography has been reported (Alkhadi et al. 2006). Indirect estimation of the severity of the aortic stenosis could be provided by calcium quantification in the valve. The quantification method is similar to the one commonly used to calculate the coronary calcium score. Incomplete coaptation of valve leaflets in diastole is suggestive of aortic regurgitation. The regurgitant orifice could be quantified by planimetry. However, it is not indicative of regurgitation severity. The normal area of the aortic valve is subject to large inter-individual variations ranging from 2.5 to 6 cm^2 as recently established by the American College of Cardiology/American Heart Association (Bonow et al. 2006) (Table 18.1).

18.4.2 Bicuspid Valve Features

Post-mortem studies have identified three features that characterize the BAV: cusp asymmetry (inequality of cusp size), presence of a central raphé

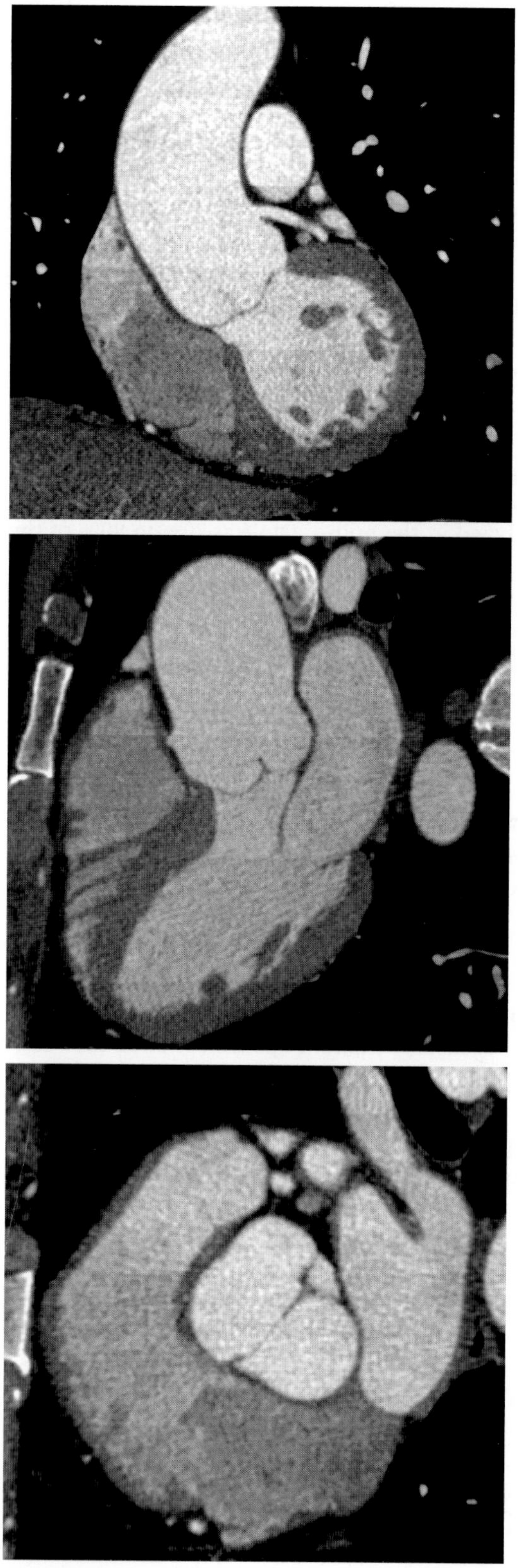

Fig. 18.1a–c. Enhanced ECG-gated multi-detector CT scan showing a bicuspid aortic valve in long axis view (**a**,**b**) and short axis view (**c**)

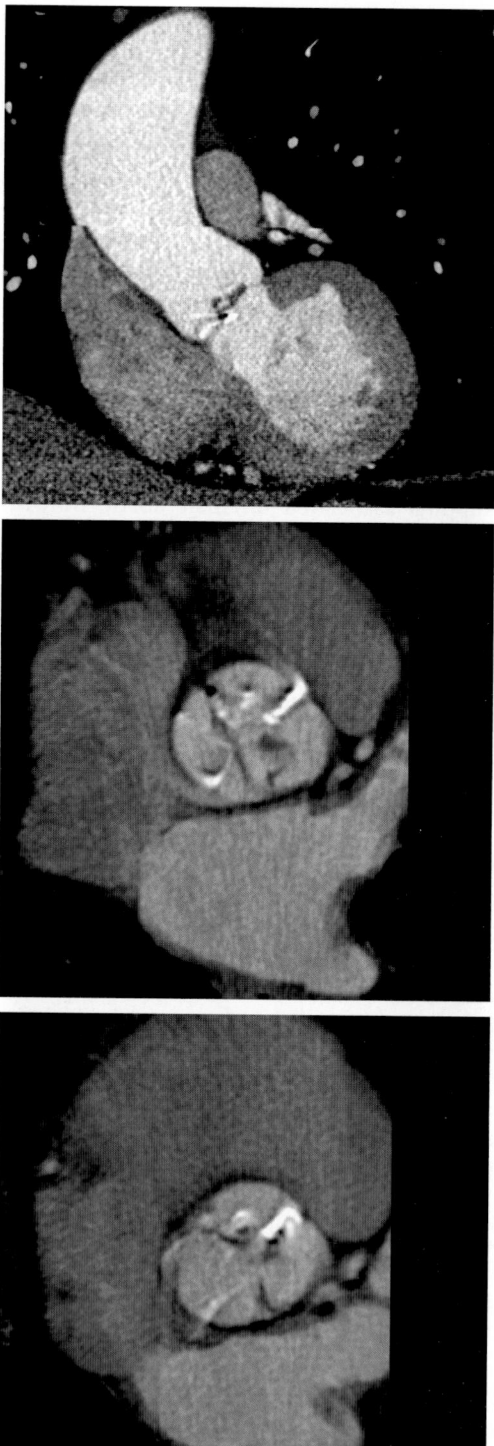

Fig. 18.2a–c. Enhanced ECG-gated CT in a 53-year-old obese women with aortic bicuspid valve with grade 2 calcifications and présence of raphé. The patient had a significant aortic stenosis and aneurysm of the ascending aorta. Note motion artifacts in the short axis views on the aortic valve

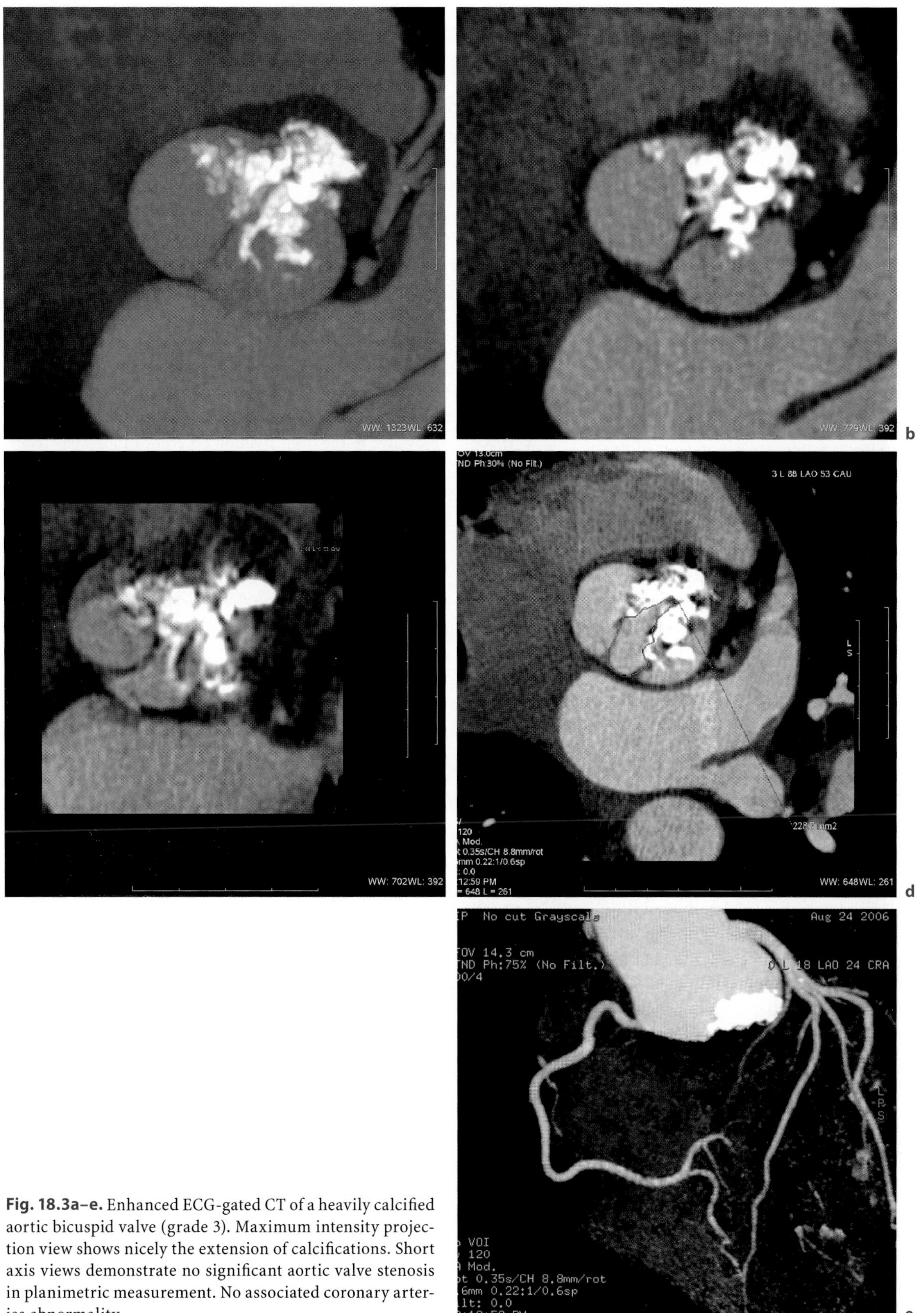

Fig. 18.3a–e. Enhanced ECG-gated CT of a heavily calcified aortic bicuspid valve (grade 3). Maximum intensity projection view shows nicely the extension of calcifications. Short axis views demonstrate no significant aortic valve stenosis in planimetric measurement. No associated coronary arteries abnormality

Table 18.1. Classification of aortic stenosis severity

	Valve area (cm^2)	Pressure gradient (mmHg)
Normal	2.5–6.0	
Mild	1.6–2.5	<25
Moderate	1.0–1.5	25–40
Severe	<1.0	>40

(ridge), and smooth cusp margins (Roberts et al. 1970). The raphé is usually located in the center of the larger cups. The smooth margins differentiate the BAV from an initially tricuspid valve with secondary fusion of two cusps as a result of inflammatory process. Orientation of cusps is equally reported in the antero-posterior and transverse axis (Roberts et al. 1970). Calcifications in the BAV are typically confined to the raphé and the base of the cusps. In contrast, calcifications are more extensive in post-inflammatory diseases, and margins are severely distorted and fused. Although the mechanism behind calcification development is not known, it has been demonstrated that calcifications increase with age.

By definition, diagnostic imaging, independent of the imaging modality, is based on the demonstration of two cusps and two commissures on a short-axis view of the aortic valve (Figs. 18.1, 18.4, 18.5). The BAV demonstrates a characteristic "fish mouth" sign in the open position on the short axis view that is different from the normal triangular orifice. Additional views could be obtained, especially on MDCT and MR as oblique sagittal or coronal views. More refinements in the BAV features include cusp redundancy, eccentric valve closure, and a single coaptation line between the cusps in the diastolic phase. The identification of fused commissure (raphé) is also important, particularly in MDCT (Fig. 18.2). It is also important to notice the orientation of the BAV, which may have some bearing on complication rates (Olson et al. 1984). Calcifications can be quantified using a semi-quantitative scale (Table 18.2) (Rosenhek et al. 2000) or quantitative methods based on determination of a score or calculation of volume (Cowell et al. 2003; Morgan-Hugues et al. 2003). Typical features of the BAV may be obscured by severe calcifications or cases of prominent raphé that could simulate a third coaptation line.

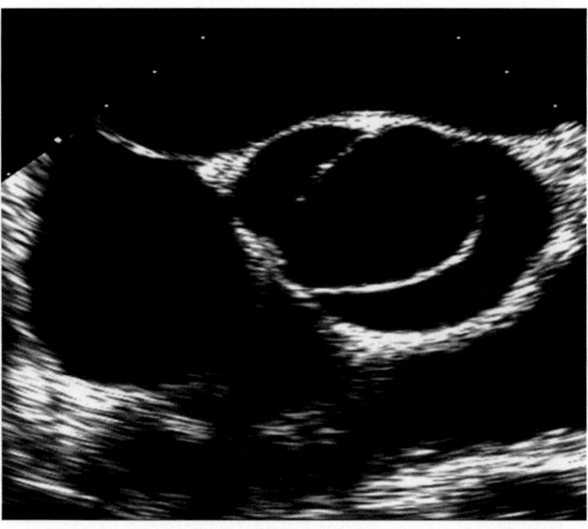

Fig. 18.4 Typical feature of "fish-mouth" sign of aortic bicuspid valve in the open position on echocardiography (courtesy of Dr. X. Jeanreneaud)

Table 18.2. Classification of aortic valve calcifications

	Calcifications
Grade 1 (mild)	Small isolated spots
Grade 2 (moderate)	Multiple large spots
Grade 3 (heavy)	Extensive

18.4.3 Screening of Valvular Complications

18.4.3.1 Aortic Valve Stenosis

It is interestingly to note that absence of clinical symptoms and absence of electrocardiograhic changes do not exclude severe stenosis (Khalid et al. 2006). Three methods can assess the aortic valve stenosis severity: the hemodynamic method using the continuity equation (echocardiography and MR), the morphologic method using the valve area measurement (echocardiography, CT, and MR), and quantification of valve calcifications (echocardiography and CT).

Electron-beam CT and, more recently, MDCT have evaluated the amount of calcifications in the aortic valve to predict the presence of a significant stenosis. Currently, the volumetric method used to quantify valve calcifications is derived from the score described initially for coronary arteries by

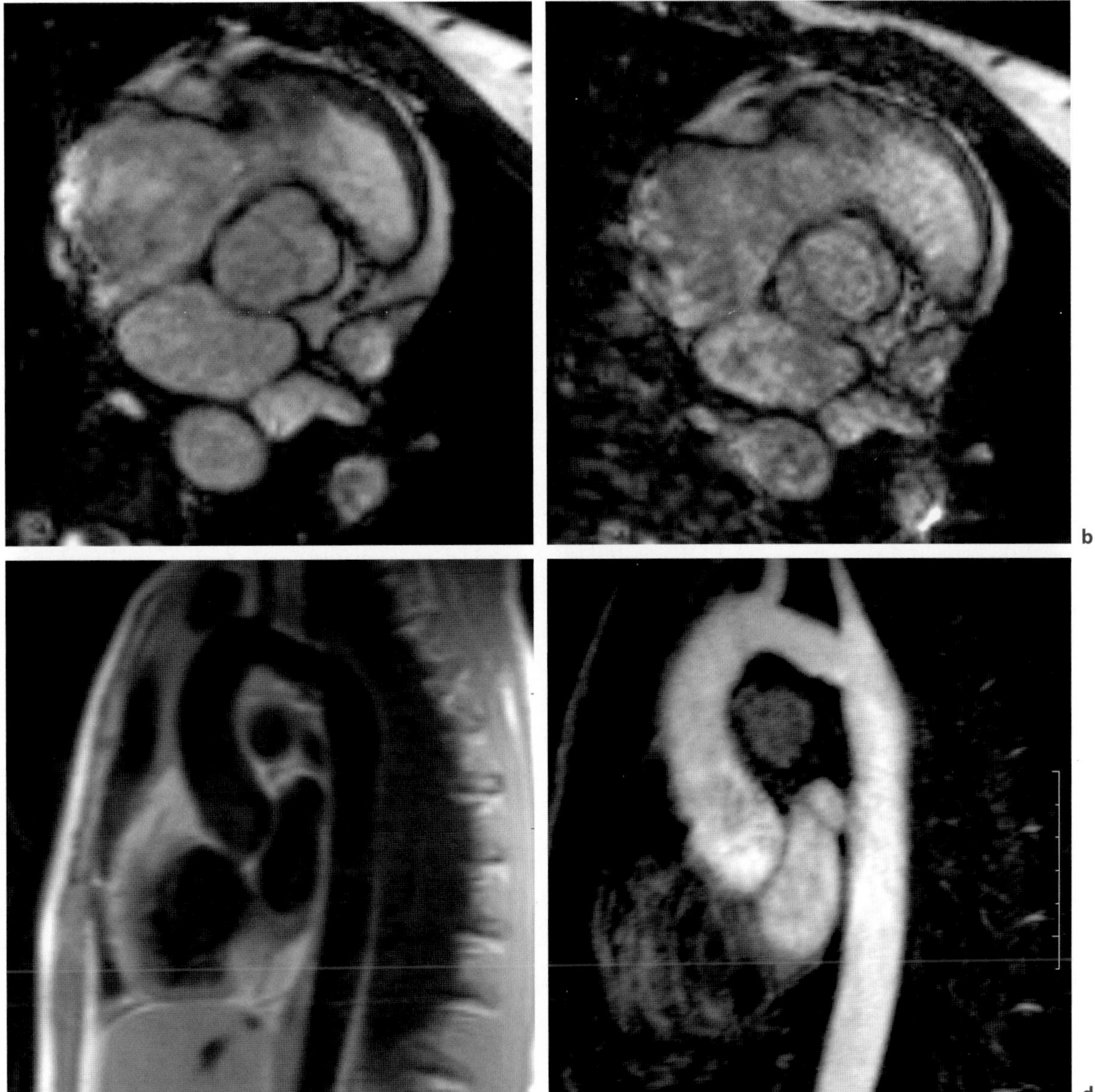

Fig. 18.5a–d. Postoperative assessment with MR of a 17-year-old woman with aortic bicuspid valve and aortic coarctation

Agatston et al. (1990). Budoff et al. (2002) reported very good reproducibility of CT using the volumetric method with an interscan variability of 6.2%, and interobserver and intraobserver variability of 5% and 1%, respectively. Compared to echocardiography, a volumetric score of more than 100 had a sensitivity of 100% and a specificity of 77% for identifying a significant aortic stenosis as reported by Yamamoto et al. (2003). More recent studies using MDCT have reported similar results (Cowell et al. 2003; Morgan-Hugues et al. 2003). It is therefore clinically relevant when identifying BAV with calcifications in CT to quantify these calcifications. ECG-gated images are, however, required for accurate quantification.

Valve area can be estimated either by the application of the continuity equation or by planimetry. Cine gradient echo imaging identifies valvular stenosis as signal void. Using cine MR images, Friederich et al. (2002) have reported good correlation (r=0.78) between direct measurement of valve area and cardiac catheterization findings, while Caruthers et al. (2003) found good agreement (r=0.83) between cine-MR and echocardiography regarding the valve area. MDCT demonstrates a high potential to provide comparable information (Alkadhi et al. 2006; Laissy et al. 2007). However, MDCT seems to overestimate the valve area compared to echocardiography (Laissy et al. 2007). This probably could be explained by the fact that the two techniques do not measure exactly the same parameter even if the planimery method is applied. Echocardiography measures a "hemodynamic" orifice, while MDCT provides a purely morphologic assessment. MR enables quantitative evaluation of the aortic valve stenosis with velocity mapping sequences. Good correlation has been shown between this technique and Doppler echocardiography and cardiac catheterization (Eichenberger et al. 1993). Looking at comparison of MDCT, cine MR imaging, transthoracic and transesophageal echocardiography in aortic valve area assessment, Pouleur et al. (2007) found high correlation of MDCT and cine MR (r=0.98), transthoracic echocardiography (r=0.96), and transesophageal echocardiography (r=0.98). However, even if the assessment of valve area needs no additional data set than those obtained for coronary arteries, MDCT using the current available techniques is still associated with a significant radiation dose ranging from 8.8 to 13.6 mSv (Alkadhi et al. 2007).

18.4.3.2 Aortic Valve Regurgitation

Echocardiography (Berkerdjian et al. 2005) and MR (Sechtem et al. 1988) are the best techniques to identify aortic valve regurgitation. Using MRI assessment of aortic valve regurgitation can be obtained by multiple techniques: a qualitative assessment of signal loss on cine MR images or a quantitative approach by measurement of ventricular volumes or by phase-contrast velocity mapping. The regurgitant volume can be quantified either as an absolute value or as regurgitant fraction. The regurgitant volume usually defines the severity of regurgitation. Table 18.3 outlines the severity classification as reported by Sechtem et al. (1988).

Table 18.3. Severity classification of aortic regurgitation

	Regurgitant fraction (%)
Mild	15–20
Moderate	20–40
Severe	>40

Recent evidence supports that the aortic valve regurgitation can be accurately analyzed by MDCT, not only to identify the regurgitation, but also to provide accurate quantification of the regurgitation severity by planimetric measurements of the regurgitant orifice. Measurements are done on the image on which the regurgitant orifice had the smallest diameter. Alkadhi et al. (2007) reported a good correlation of MDCT planimetric area and transesophageal echocardiography in detection and classifying aortic regurgitations.

18.4.4 Screening of Vascular Complications

Aortic dissection and aortic rupture are life-threatening complications of the BAVS that occur with acute symptoms. A more interesting complication is aortic dilatation associated with the BAV. Aortic dilatation is more frequent, occurring in 50–60% of patients with normally functioning BAV (Ward 2000). Screening of aortic dilatation is clinically relevant since it may affect patient management independently of valvular complications of the BAV (Figs. 18.2 and 18.6).

Diameters of the ascending aorta could be accurately measured by MDCT, especially on multiplanar reformations or center line-based reconstructions or by MR imaging and echocardiography. Monitoring of the aortic dilatation usually uses echocardiography.

Aortic repair of the ascending aorta is recommended more aggressively for patients with BAV (40 to 50 mm) than those with tricuspid valve (50 to 60 mm) (Burks et al. 1998). Prevention of aortic dilatation progression with beta-blockers is still debated, as well as the role of matrix metalloproteinase inhibitors and gene therapy (Fedak 2002).

18.4.5 Screening of Cardiac Complications

Left ventricle hypertrophy (in aortic valve stenosis) and left ventricle dimension and function are crucial in therapeutic decision making and should be an integrated part in the image analysis when BAV is identified. Left ventricular assessment could be obtained by echocardiography and MR and more recently by MDCT.

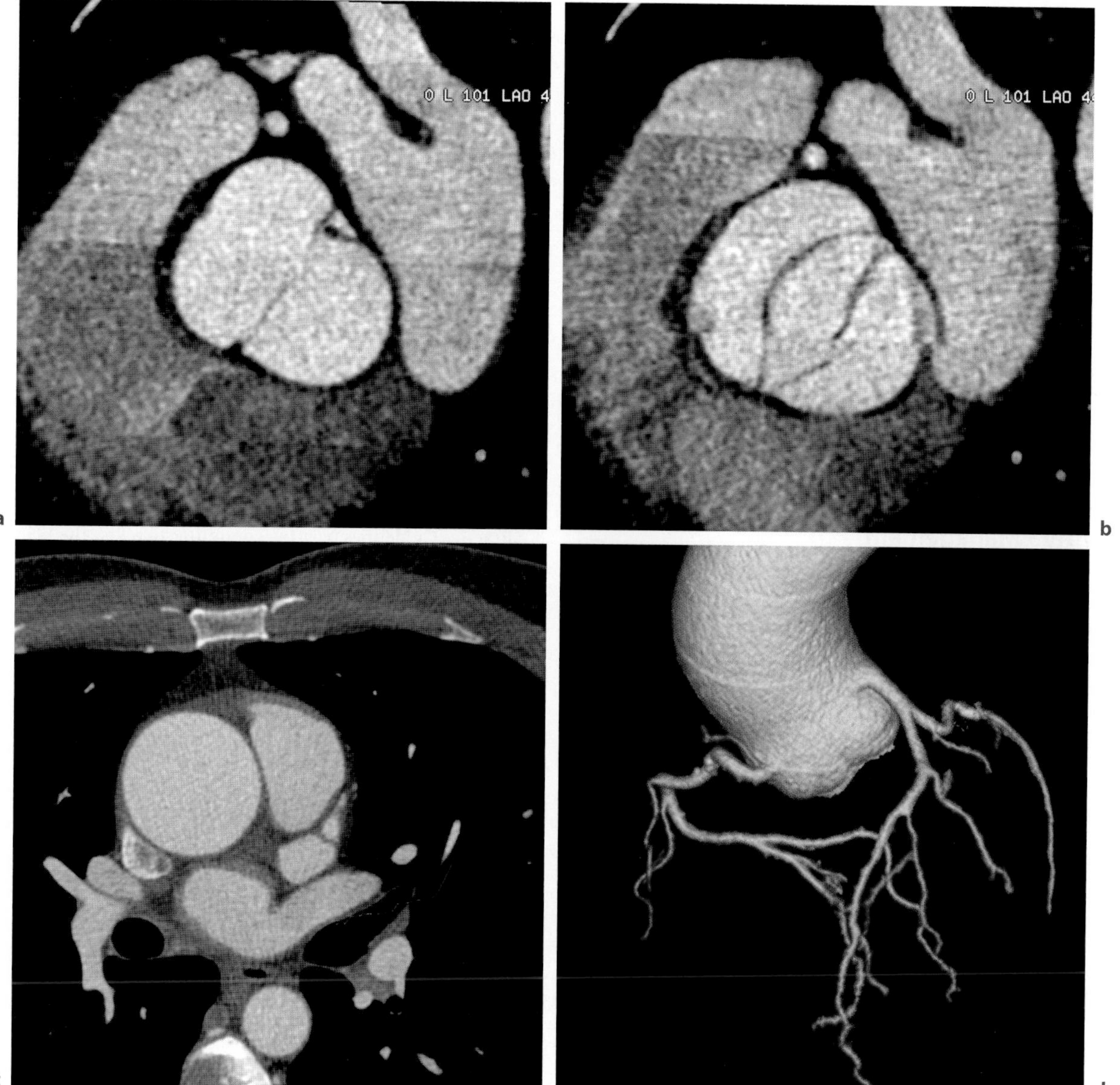

Fig. 18.6a–d. Enhanced ECG-gated CT in a 45-year-old man with bicuspid aortic valve. Non-calcified bicuspid aortic valve with no dysfunction detected at CT (and echocardiography) (**a**,**b**). Aneurysm of 52 mm of the ascending aorta (**c**). Normal coronary artery tree (**d**)

18.4.6 Screening of Associated Congenital Anomalies

Many cardiovascular anomalies could be associated with BAV. Two are of practical importance in the adult population: coarctation of the aorta and patent ductus arteriosis. Coarctation of the aorta occurs in 20–85% of patients with BAV (Stewart et al. 1993). MR and CT are helpful to screen and characterize associated aortic coarctation (Fig. 18.5).

The ductus arteriosis is defined as communication between the distal arch and the proximal left pulmonary artery. The clinical significance of patent ductus arteriosus in adult patients depends on the defect size and the resulting shunt. MDCT and MR could provide diagnosis and sizing of the patent ductus arteriosis, which facilitate therapeutic procedures, particularly those using percutaneous vaso-occlusion with coils or vascular plug devices.

The ductus arteriosis, even when clinically silent, may be associated with major complications. The first is infective endocarditis and the second aneurysmal formation. The incidence of aneurysms in the ductus arteriosis is not known, and its pathogenesis remains unclear. Aneurysms may result from infective endocarditis as mycotic false aneurysm or from the weakening of the aortic wall as previously discussed for the ascending aorta dilatation. The role of atherosclerosis is unclear. MDCT may be helpful in diagnosis and characterization of aneurysms of the ductus arteriosis.

18.5 BAVS Management

The generally accepted approach for BAVS with mild-to-moderate valvular dysfunction and normal left ventricle (dimensions and function) is regular monitoring with echocardiography (Fedak et al. 2002). However, early referral to surgery before significant deterioration of the cusps for successful valvular repair has been advocated by some authors (Ward 2000). Table 18.4 summarizes the current strategy for management of patients with BAVS.

Clinically silent BAV discovered on imaging investigations indicated for other settings should implicate complete characterization of the BAV and associated vascular lesions and ventricular consequences with the same imaging modality whenever possible (ECG-gated acquisition), especially in the era of extended non-invasive cardiac imaging including MR and CT.

Aortic dilatation should be monitored by echocardiography or MR. Due to its high spatial resolution and 3D imaging capabilities, CT should be indicated in cases of discrepancies or in the pre-therapy assessment.

References

Agatston AS, Janowitz WR, Hildner FJ, Zusmer NR, Viamonte M Jr, Detrano R (1990) Quantification of coronary artery calcium using ultrafast computed tomography. J Am Coll Cardiol 15:827–832

Alkadhi H, Desbiolles L, Husmann L et al. (2007) Aortic regurgitation: assessment with 64-section CT. Radiology 245:111–121

Alkadhi H, Wildermuth S, Plass A et al. (2006) Aortic stenosis: comparative evaluation of 16-detector row CT and echocardiography. Radiology 240:47–55

Bahler RC, Desser DR, Finkelhor RS, Brener SJ, Youssefi M (1999) Factors leading to progression of valvular aortic stenosis. Am J Cardiol 84:1044–1048

Bekeredjian R, Grayburn PA (2005) Valvular heart disease: aortic regurgitation. Circulation 112:125–134

Bonow RO, Carabello BA, Kanu C et al. (2006) ACC/AHA 2006 guidelines for the management of patients with valvular heart disease: a report of the American College of Cardiology/American Heart Association Task Force on Practice Guidelines (writing committee to revise the 1998 Guidelines for the Management of Patients With Valvular Heart Disease): developed in collaboration with the Society of Cardiovascular Anesthesiologists: endorsed by the Society for Cardiovascular Angiography and Interventions and the Society of Thoracic Surgeons. Circulation 114:e84–231

Budoff MJ, Mao S, Takasu J, Shavelle DM, Zhao XQ, O'Brien KD (2002) Reproducibility of electron-beam CT measures of aortic valve calcification. Acad Radiol 9:1122–1127

Burks JM, Illes RW, Keating EC, Lubbe WJ (1998) Ascending aortic aneurysm and dissection in young adults with bicuspid aortic valve: implications for echocardiographic surveillance. Clin Cardiol 21:439–443

Caruthers SD, Lin SJ, Brown P et al. (2003) Practical value of cardiac magnetic resonance imaging for clinical quantification of aortic valve stenosis: comparison with echocardiography. Circulation 108:2236–2243

Chan KL, Ghani M, Woodend K, Burwash IG (2001) Case-controlled study to assess risk factors for aortic stenosis in congenitally bicuspid aortic valve. Am J Cardiol 88:690–693

Clementi M, Notari L, Borghi A, Tenconi R (1996) Familial congenital bicuspid aortic valve: a disorder of uncertain inheritance. Am J Med Genet 62:336–338

Cowell SJ, Newby DE, Burton J et al. (2003) Aortic valve calcification on computed tomography predicts the severity of aortic stenosis. Clin Radiol 58:712–716

Eichenberger AC, Jenni R, von Schulthess GK (1993) Aortic valve pressure gradients in patients with aortic valve

Table 18.4. Clinical management of patient with BAVS (adapted from Fedak et al. 2002)

Criteria for clinical observation	Criteria for surgical repair
Mild to moderate aortic stenosis/aortic regurgitation	Severe aortic stenosis/aortic regurgitation
Normal left ventricle dimensions	Increased left ventricle size
Normal left ventricle function	Decreased left ventricle function
Absence of aortic dilatation	Aortic dilatation

stenosis: quantification with velocity-encoded cine MR imaging. AJR Am J Roentgenol 160:971–977

Eisenberg LM, Markwald RR (1995) Molecular regulation of atrioventricular valvuloseptal morphogenesis. Circ Res 77:1–6

Epstein JA (2000) Developmental cardiology comes of age. Circ Res 87:833–834

Fedak PW, de Sa MP, Verma S et al. (2003) Vascular matrix remodeling in patients with bicuspid aortic valve malformations: implications for aortic dilatation. J Thorac Cardiovasc Surg 126:797–806

Fedak PW, Verma S, David TE, Leask RL, Weisel RD, Butany J (2002) Clinical and pathophysiological implications of a bicuspid aortic valve. Circulation 106:900–904

Ferda J, Linhartova K, Kreuzberg B (2007) Comparison of the aortic valve calcium content in the bicuspid and tricuspid stenotic aortic valve using non-enhanced 64-detector-row-computed tomography with prospective ECG-triggering. Eur J Radiol. [Epub ahead of print]

Fernandez MC, Duran AC, Real R et al. (2000) Coronary artery anomalies and aortic valve morphology in the Syrian hamster. Lab Anim 34:145–154

Friedrich MG, Schulz-Menger J, Poetsch T, Pilz B, Uhlich F, Dietz R (2002) Quantification of valvular aortic stenosis by magnetic resonance imaging. Am Heart J 144:329–334

Guiney TE, Davies MJ, Parker DJ, Leech GJ, Leatham A (1987) The aetiology and course of isolated severe aortic regurgitation: a clinical, pathological, and echocardiographic study. Br Heart J 58:358–368

Hatle L, Angelsen BA, Tromsdal A (1980) Non-invasive assessment of aortic stenosis by Doppler ultrasound. Br Heart J 43:284–292

Huntington K, Hunter AG, Chan KL (1997) A prospective study to assess the frequency of familial clustering of congenital bicuspid aortic valve. J Am Coll Cardiol 30:1809–1812

Keane MG, Wiegers SE, Plappert T, Pochettino A, Bavaria JE, Sutton MG (2000) Bicuspid aortic valves are associated with aortic dilatation out of proportion to coexistent valvular lesions. Circulation 102:III35–39

Khalid O, Luxenberg DM, Sable C et al. (2006) Aortic stenosis: the spectrum of practice. Pediatr Cardiol 27:661–669

Laissy JP, Messika-Zeitoun D, Serfaty JM et al. (2007) Comprehensive evaluation of preoperative patients with aortic valve stenosis: usefulness of cardiac multidetector computed tomography. Heart 93:1121–1125

Lee TC, Zhao YD, Courtman DW, Stewart DJ (2000) Abnormal aortic valve development in mice lacking endothelial nitric oxide synthase. Circulation 101:2345–2348

Mohler ER 3rd, Gannon F, Reynolds C, Zimmerman R, Keane MG, Kaplan FS (2001) Bone formation and inflammation in cardiac valves. Circulation 103:1522–1528

Morgan-Hughes GJ, Villaquiran J, Roobottom CA, Ring NJ, Kuo J, Marshall AJ (2003) Calcified patent ductus arteriosus diagnosed following aortic valve replacement. Ann Thorac Surg 76:271–273

Nistri S, Sorbo MD, Marin M, Palisi M, Scognamiglio R, Thiene G (1999) Aortic root dilatation in young men with normally functioning bicuspid aortic valves. Heart 82:19–22

Niwa K, Perloff JK, Bhuta SM et al. (2001) Structural abnormalities of great arterial walls in congenital heart disease: light and electron microscopic analyses. Circulation 103:393–400

Olson LJ, Subramanian R, Edwards WD (1984) Surgical pathology of pure aortic insufficiency: a study of 225 cases. Mayo Clin Proc 59:835–841

Pachulski RT, Chan KL (1993) Progression of aortic valve dysfunction in 51 adult patients with congenital bicuspid aortic valve: assessment and follow up by Doppler echocardiography. Br Heart J 69:237–240

Pouleur AC, le Polain de Waroux JB, Pasquet A, Vanoverschelde JL, Gerber BL (2007) Aortic valve area assessment: multidetector CT compared with cine MR imaging and transthoracic and transesophageal echocardiography. Radiology 244:745–754

Roberts WC (1970) The congenitally bicuspid aortic valve. A study of 85 autopsy cases. Am J Cardiol 26:72–83

Roberts WC, Morrow AG, McIntosh CL, Jones M, Epstein SE (1981) Congenitally bicuspid aortic valve causing severe, pure aortic regurgitation without superimposed infective endocarditis. Analysis of 13 patients requiring aortic valve replacement. Am J Cardiol 47:206–209

Rosenhek R, Binder T, Porenta G et al. (2000) Predictors of outcome in severe, asymptomatic aortic stenosis. N Engl J Med 343:611–617

Sechtem U, Pflugfelder PW, Cassidy MM et al. (1988) Mitral or aortic regurgitation: quantification of regurgitant volumes with cine MR imaging. Radiology 167:425–430

Stefani L, Galanti G, Toncelli L et al. (2008) Bicuspid aortic valve in competitive athletes. Br J Sports Med 42:31–35; discussion 35

Stewart AB, Ahmed R, Travill CM, Newman CG (1993) Coarctation of the aorta life and health 20–44 years after surgical repair. Br Heart J 69:65–70

Ward C (2000) Clinical significance of the bicuspid aortic valve. Heart 83:81–85

Yamamoto H, Shavelle D, Takasu J et al. (2003) Valvular and thoracic aortic calcium as a marker of the extent and severity of angiographic coronary artery disease. Am Heart J 146:153–159

Yasuda H, Nakatani S, Stugaard M et al. (2003) Failure to prevent progressive dilation of ascending aorta by aortic valve replacement in patients with bicuspid aortic valve: comparison with tricuspid aortic valve. Circulation 108 Suppl 1:II291–294

Cardiac Calcifications

19

Annemarieke Rutten and Mathias Prokop

CONTENTS

A. Rutten, MD, PhD
M. Prokop, MD, PhD
Department of Radiology, University Medical Center Utrecht, Room E 01.123, P.O. Box 85500, 3508 GA Utrecht, The Netherlands

19.1 Introduction

Calcifications in the heart are frequent findings on chest CT that indicate abnormal processes, such as atherosclerosis, degenerative or reparative change of the affected structures. Calcifications in the coronary arteries are probably the most well known cardiac calcifications. They are an indirect indicator of the total amount of atherosclerotic plaque in the coronary arteries (Rumberger et al. 1995) and have been shown to be an independent risk factor for developing cardiovascular complications (Pletcher et al. 2004; Shaw et al. 2003; Taylor et al. 2005; Vliegenthart et al. 2005).

However, calcifications not only occur in the coronary arteries, but also in other cardiac structures, such as the valves, the ventricular wall or the pericardium. Many cardiac calcifications suggest an underlying disease: severe aortic valve calcifications, for example, are associated with a high probability for aortic stenosis (Koos et al. 2004). As a consequence, cardiac calcifications are an important incidental finding on chest CT scans; calcifications frequently indicate diseases that warrant further evaluation or treatment (Table 19.1).

19.2 Scanning Technique and Artifacts

Detection of cardiac calcifications is not limited to CT examinations that are targeted specifically to the heart. In fact, any general chest CT scan can detect and frequently correctly localize cardiac calcifications. Most cardiac calcifications are incidental findings that can be detected on non-contrast scans as well as contrast-enhanced scans. To be able to

Table 19.1. Cardiac calcifications: morphology and clinical significance by location

Location	Morphology	Clinical significance
Coronary arteries	Small and punctate ("calcified nodule") to large calcified plaques of several centimetres length (fibrocalcified plaque)	Coronary calcium increases the probability of significant coronary artery disease and is associated with increased cardiac morbidity and mortality
Valves	–	–
Aortic valve	Along commissural edges of leaflets, most on aortic side	Moderate to severe calcification is associated with aortic stenosis and increased mortality
Mitral valve	Annulus	Extensive calcification can lead to mitral regurgitation
	Leaflets	May indicate mitral sclerosis or stenosis
Myocardium	–	–
Ventricular wall	Thinned or aneurysmatic ventricular wall	Indicative of old transmural myocardial infarction or chronic Chagas' disease
	Interventricular septum	Occur with hyperparathyroidism
	Along inner border of ventricular wall	May indicate endomyocardial fibrosis, a rare cardiomyopathy
Papillary muscle	Extensive	Associated to ischemia, may lead to mitral valve malfunctioning
	Small, near apex	Common insignificant finding in elderly patients
Pericardium	Linear or plaque-like, usually over right ventricle, posterior surface left ventricle and atrioventricular groove	May indicate constrictive pericarditis
Calcified mass	–	–
Thrombus	In older thrombi, common at left ventricular apex (aneurysm); less common in left atrial appendage or region of turbulent blood flow	Cardiac thrombus increases stroke risk and embolism risk at cardioversion of atrial fibrillation
Myxoma	In heterogeneous low attenuation mass in left atrium	Benign neoplasm. Most common primary cardiac tumor
Fibroma	Dystrophic calcifications in homogeneous ventricular mass with soft-tissue attenuation	Extremely rare benign neoplasm
Osteosarcoma	Minimal speckles to dense deposits in low attenuation mass. Primary in left atrium, metastatic in right atrium	Primary cardiac osteosarcomas are aggressive and have poor prognosis

differentiate calcifications from contrast-opacified vascular lumen, a wide window setting is required (Fig. 19.1). There is a slight risk that minor calcifications are missed on contrast-enhanced scans if enhancement in the lumen is similar to the CT attenuation of a calcification. Apart from calcium scoring for the coronaries, missing such small calcifications is hardly clinically relevant.

A higher image quality is required for quantification of calcifications in the coronary arteries or for the precise localization of calcifications relative to the cardiac valves. For this purpose, ECG synchronization (prospective triggering or retrospective gating) is mandatory.

19.2.1 Non-Gated Acquisitions

Standard chest CT does not apply cardiac synchronization. Artifacts due to cardiac motion are therefore inevitable. The amount of artifact var-

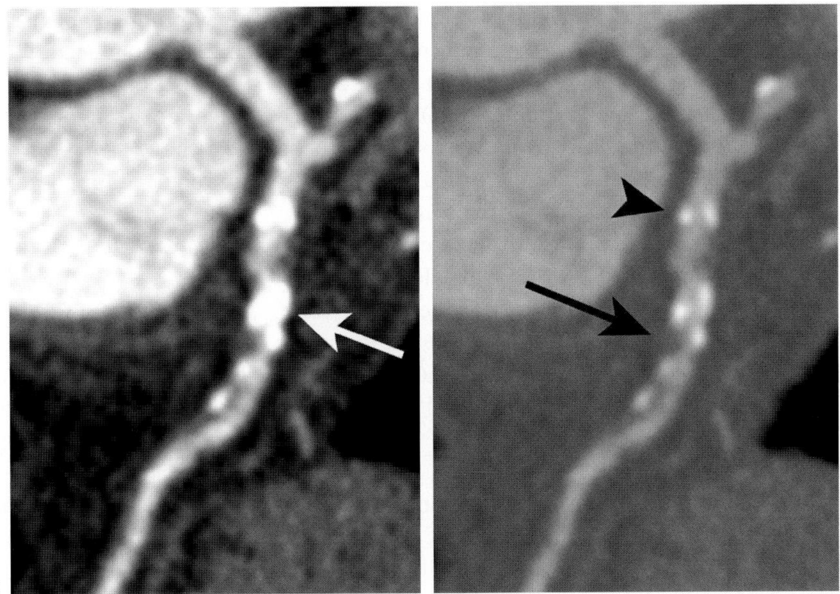

Fig. 19.1 a, b. Extensive calcification hampers stenosis evaluation in contrast-enhanced image (*white arrow*) (**a**). By widening the window width from 600 (**a**) to 1,500 (**b**), stenosis classification is improved. Stenosis classification is less influenced by presence of mixed plaques (*black arrow*) or of calcified nodules (*arrowhead*)

ies with the heart phase at which a certain slice has been acquired. Artifacts are most pronounced in mid systole during cardiac contraction and affect the right coronary more than other cardiac structures (Jahnke et al. 2006; Wang et al. 1999). Motion during mid diastole or end systole is least pronounced. Motion is less with reduced cardiac output. Scanners with faster rotation speed reduce artifacts during the phases with less cardiac motion but still suffer from artifacts during mid systole.

Motion artifacts vary periodically as a helical acquisition progresses through the chest. The length of these periods increases with faster scanners or slower heart rate. Since it depends on chance, it is impossible to predict whether a structure of interest will be displayed during a phase with reduced or pronounced artifact, even with fast scanners.

Non-gated acquisitions therefore can provide valuable cardiac information, but there is no guarantee that all structures can be evaluated completely. Motion will blur calcifications, induce streak artifacts and reduce the CT number of a calcification (Horiguchi et al. 2006; Rutten et al. 2008a). Very small calcifications may be lost, but larger calcifications will be detectable and can usually be correctly localized.

19.2.2 Prospective ECG Triggering

Prospective ECG triggering is based on a short scan during a pre-selected phase of the cardiac cycle with as little cardiac motion as possible (usually mid diastole). Prospective ECG triggering uses a partial scan technique with the shortest possible scan duration.

The resulting high temporal dose efficiency is the main advantage of prospective ECG triggering; depending on the implementation, up to 100% of the radiation dose given to the patient makes it into the image. However, the high dose efficiency comes at the price of less robustness against variations in heart rhythm. Since the precise timing of the ECG trigger has to be determined from the behavior of the heart rate during the previous beats, a sudden shortening of the RR interval, for example due to an extra systole or a sudden volume load due to contrast material injection, will lead to a suboptimum timing and may cause motion artifacts. For calcium scoring, however, the heart rate usually stays more stable than for coronary CTA because no contrast material is injected.

Prospective ECG-triggering is the only cardiac synchronization technique available with EBCT.

With the advent of MDCT, it still remains the technique recommended for calcium scoring by the American Heart Association (Budoff et al. 2006), but motion artifacts will be increased at higher heart rates and for scanners with a slower rotation speed. As the width of the detectors of modern scanners becomes wider, more of the heart can be imaged during one heartbeat, and fewer heartbeats are necessary to cover the full heart. With 16-cm-wide detectors (e.g., the new generation of 320-slice scanners), only one heartbeat is necessary to image the heart. Prospective triggering then will be the technique of choice because of its high dose efficiency and superior image quality.

Since prospective triggering uses a step-and-shoot (sequential) scanning mode, only multiples of the available section collimations can be reconstructed. This will not always make it possible for MDCT scanners to acquire the 3-mm-thick slices used for coronary calcium scoring with EBCT. As a result, 2.5-mm-thick sections will have to be used on many 4-, 16- or 64-slice scanners of various manufacturers (Table 19.2). Low heart rates will yield fewer motion artifacts and better reproducibility of calcium scores (Hong et al. 2003b). When calcium scores are only used for estimating cardiovascular risk, then beta blockade is usually not necessary. If follow-up scans are considered, however, a low heart rate is recommended. Depending on scanner speed the heart rate should be lower than 60–70 bpm, which may require beta blockade.

For calcium scoring, low-dose protocols are used. We vary tube current settings by patient size with mGy values ranging between 2.5 and 5.0 (Rutten et al. 2008b). Mean estimated radiation dose is below 1 mSv with this protocol.

Contrast-enhanced cardiac CT with prospective triggering is only recommended for 64-slice scanners or more. For this purpose, the thinnest possible collimation is used. This allows precise evaluation of the position of calcifications relative to coronaries, valves or the myocardium. However, low heart rates (less than 60–70 bpm, depending on scanner speed) are required for good results (Earls et al. 2008).

19.2.3 Retrospective ECG Gating

Retrospective ECG gating is based on a continuous data acquisition during all of the cardiac cycle. Retrospectively, the best phase for image reconstruction is chosen, and data from multiple heartbeats can be combined to increase temporal resolution well beyond that of partial scan techniques. Retrospective ECG gating is only available with MDCT.

The temporal resolution is the main advantage of retrospective ECG gating: depending on implementation, a temporal resolution of 50–100 ms can be obtained with modern scanners. Motion artifacts are minimized, which is why this technique has been the technique of choice for coronary CTA in the past. The retrospective choice of the optimum phase offers more robustness against variations in heart rhythm. However, the high temporal resolution comes at the price of very bad temporal dose efficiency. If the tube current remains constant during the cardiac cycle, then the temporal dose efficiency decreases with increasing temporal resolution. For an 85-ms temporal resolution at a heart rate of 60 bpm (RR interval 1,000 ms), for example, the temporal dose efficiency is only 85/1,000=8.5%. This means than over 90% of the dose is not used for image reconstruction. For this reason, retrospective ECG gating is usually combined with ECG tube current modulation, which reduces tube current to

Table 19.2. Suggested section collimation (N×SC) and reconstructed section thickness (SW) for prospective calcium scoring with typical scanners of the various manufacturers

Detector rows	General Electric		Philips		Siemens		Toshiba	
	N×SC	SW	N×SC	SW	N×SC	SW	N×SC	SW
4	4×2.5	2.5	4×2.5	2.5	4×2.5	2.5	4×3	3.0
16	16×1.25	2.5	16×1.5	3.0	16×1.5	3.0	8×3	3.0
64*	32×1.25	2.5	40×0.625	2.5	2×32×0.6	3.0	20×3	3.0
≥128*	–	–	2×128×0.625	3.0	2×128×0.6	3.0	320×0.5	3.0

*For cardiac CT angiography with prospective triggering the thinnest collimations are used

some 20% during those phases of the cardiac cycle that are not used for evaluation of the coronaries. Depending on heart rate, a dose reduction of up to 50% has been demonstrated without influencing calcium scores (Jakobs et al. 2002; Poll et al. 2002; Rutten et al. 2008a). Even with ECG tube current modulation, the required dose is well above that with prospective triggering.

For coronary calcium scoring, the higher temporal resolution of retrospective gating improves reproducibility and makes it a technique best suited when follow-up scans are intended. However, ECG dose modulation and low mAs technique are mandatory in order not to require excessive dose. For calcium scoring, protocols with lower dose than for coronary CTA are used (5–15 mGy depending on patient size).

Since retrospective gating uses a helical acquisition, any section thickness that is larger or equal to the collimation can be reconstructed. This makes it always possible to obtain 3-mm-thick sections for coronary calcium scoring.

Contrast-enhanced scans with retrospective ECG gating offer excellent coronary artery visualization, but also allow for reconstruction of multiple heart phases, which is mandatory for evaluating valvular motion or cardiac function. With prospective ECG triggering, only the pre-selected phase is acquired, which will make evaluation of cardiac function only possible if at least two scans per RR interval become possible with future scanner generations.

19.3 Coronary Calcifications

Coronary calcifications are caused by atherosclerosis and are not present in normal coronary arteries. Atherosclerosis is an active inflammatory process that induces calcification due to increased bone-regulatory protein expression (Goldbarg et al. 2007). Although calcifications represent only about 20% of total plaque burden, the amount of coronary calcification can be used as a measure of the extent of atherosclerotic disease (Rumberger et al. 1995). Coronary calcifications can be readily identified on any CT that includes the heart. However, ECG synchronization (prospective triggering or retrospective gating) improves quantification so that calcium scoring can be used not only to estimate the severity of arteriosclerosis, but also to monitor disease progression. While EBCT was the predominant technique in the 1990s, MDCT is the technique of choice today. Because of the best dose efficiency, guidelines of the American Heart Association recommend prospectively ECG-triggered scanning for calcium scoring (Budoff et al. 2006).

19.3.1 Basic Concepts of Calcium Scoring

CT scanning for quantification of coronary calcifications was originally performed with EBCT (Agatston et al. 1990). Scanning and quantification protocols still are related to the techniques first employed in the era of EBCT because the largest body of clinical data was acquired using this technique. Radiation dose with EBCT was limited and could not be adjusted to larger body habitus. This made it necessary to choose section thickness and thresholds for calcium detection appropriate to accommodate noise levels typically found with these scanners. As a consequence, scoring still is commonly performed on 3-mm-thick sections using a threshold for calcium detection of 130 HU, parameter settings that were found to be optimum for EBCT.

Calcium scoring always relies on two steps: identification of calcified plaques and quantification of these plaques. Coronary calcium is identified as any voxels along the coronaries with CT attenuation of 130 HU or above, a threshold that is two standard deviations above the CT attenuation of blood on EBCT in an average size patient. In addition, a minimum size of 2–4 pixels is used to distinguish true calcification from image noise. When comparing results from calcium scoring, however, it is important to know precisely how the scoring was performed previously since thinner sections, other thresholds (mainly 90 HU) and varying noise filters may be used.

Current calcium scoring software provided by the various CT or 3D workstation manufacturers highlights candidate voxels (above a certain threshold) and asks the user to identify calcified coronary plaques (Fig. 19.2). By clicking on a highlighted plaque, all voxels that are connected to it are marked using a region-growing algorithm. The software commonly allows users to assign a plaque to a specific coronary branch so that calcium scores for the various coronary branches can be calculated separately.

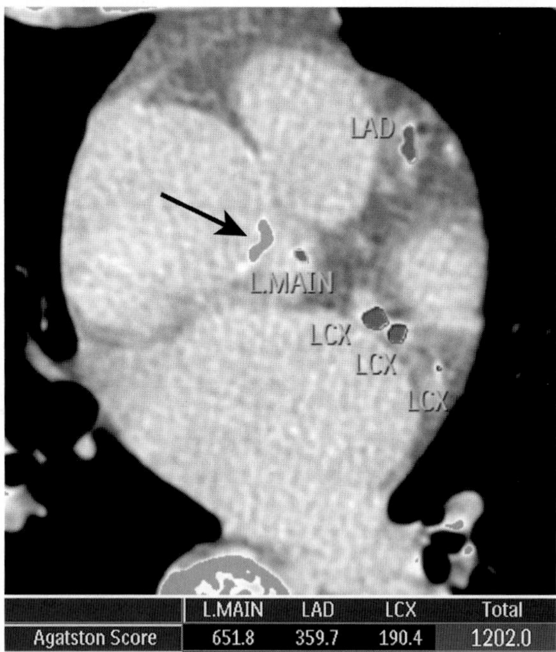

Fig. 19.2. Semi-automatic coronary calcium scoring software: an observer marks calcifications and assigns them to the main coronary arteries. The software automatically calculates the calcium score (here: Agatston score) per vessel and in total. Note that calcifications at the origin of the left main coronary artery (*arrow*) may cause inter-observer variability because they could be assigned to either the aorta or the coronaries

Quantification techniques also vary with respect to how they incorporate the CT attenuation of a calcified plaque. There are three main techniques, the Agatston score (Agatston et al. 1990), the volume score (Callister et al. 1998) and the mass score (Ulzheimer et al. 2003). The Agatston score uses a simple weighting factor that depends on the maximum CT number within the plaque, the volume score neglects CT numbers altogether (except for the threshold), and the mass score uses a continuous weighting factor and a calibration that allows for estimating the mass of calcium hydroxyapatite within a plaque.

19.3.2 Agatston Score

The Agatston score was the first technique for quantification of coronary calcium. The Agatston score is calculated by multiplying the plaque volume with a weighting factor that depends on the maximum CT number of this plaque. The weighting factor is 1 for a maximum CT number between 130 and 199 HU, 2 for numbers between 200 and 299 HU, 3 for numbers between 300 and 399 HU and 4 for maximum CT numbers above 400 HU. The scores of all individual plaques are summed to obtain the total Agatston score.

The Agatston score has been used for many clinical trials and is therefore the "classical" and most well-know calcium scoring algorithm. Most outcome data are based on EBCT studies using the Agatston score (Arad et al. 1996; Kondos et al. 2003; Secci et al. 1997; Shaw et al. 2003). EBCT scanning of the heart to determine the Agatston score was widely implemented for screening symptomatic and asymptomatic populations for the presence of coronary calcifications and for determination of the associated cardiovascular risk. It also allows for a simple categorization of results (Table 19.3) that facilitates clinical interpretation.

Because the weighting factors depend on *maximum* CT numbers within the plaques, however, the Agatston score is semi-quantitative and will vary abruptly if this maximum CT number changes due to a different choice of scanning or reconstruction parameters. For this reason, other scores have been developed that are supposed to suffer less from such effects and improve reproducibility.

19.3.3 Volume Score

Callister et al. (1998) described the calcium volume score to provide a continuous score and improve reproducibility. The same threshold of 130 HU is used. The volume of each calcified plaque is determined by isotropic interpolation. Usually Agatston and volume scores are in the same range.

The volume score has been around since the era of EBCT, but has not been too successful in substituting for the Agatston score. While it is slightly more reproducible, the improvement in reproducibility is not major, which is probably why it is still not widely used. Like the Agatston score the volume score is influenced by partial volume effects: as soon as the CT number of a portion of a plaque is reduced below the threshold level, it will not be counted. If the CT number is above the threshold, the voxel will be fully counted.

Table 19.3. Guidelines for interpretation of the Agatston score in asymptomatic patients (Rumberger et al. 1999). Adapted with permission from Mayo Clin Proc (1999) 74:243–252 Dowden Health Media

Agatston score	Plaque burden	Probability coronary artery disease	Cardiovascular risk	Treatment recommendation
0	None	Very low	Very low	Reassure
1–10	Minimal	Very unlikely	Low	Discuss primary prevention
11–100	Mild	Mild or minimal likely	Moderate	Counsel risk factor modification
101–400	Moderate	Highly likely	Moderately high	Institute risk factor modification; exercise testing
>400	Severe	Significant stenosis highly likely	High	Aggressive risk factor modification; exercise test or pharmacological stress test

Calcium mass score ≈ Agatston score × 0.83; volume score ≈ Agatston score

19.3.4 Mass Score

To compensate for partial volume effects, the mass score was developed (Ulzheimer et al. 2003). It uses a weighting factor that is proportional to the CT number and makes sure that voxels that are just above the threshold are counted less than voxels that are much denser. However, in order to qualify as a calcification, each voxel within a plaque still needs to have a CT number above a certain threshold, usually again 130 HU.

The calcium mass score is calibrated in milligram calcium hydroxyapatite. In order to do so, either a calibration phantom needs to be scanned together with the patient or a global calibration function needs to be provided by the scanner manufacturer that takes into account differences in patient size and resulting beam-hardening effects. Both techniques are not perfect: the calibration phantom is usually placed under the patient and thus does not fully represent the conditions within the heart of the patient, while a global calibration factor has to use calculations and no actual measurements to compensate for beam-hardening and other disturbing effects. The use of a threshold for identification of calcified plaques in addition hampers the full compensation of partial volume effects.

An international consensus group has chosen the coronary calcium mass as the standard measure for the quantification of coronary calcium because this measure is least influenced by technical factors and therefore has the best reproducibility (McCollough et al. 2003). The mass score is always substantially lower than the Agatston and volume score (Hong et al. 2004). With the increasing use of multidetector CT, the mass and volume scores are more frequently used, and outcome data are becoming available for these scores also.

19.3.5 Accuracy and Reproducibility of Calcium Scoring

Studies performed on coronary calcium phantoms could demonstrate that the mass score is less vulnerable to changes of scanning parameters than volume or Agatston score (Hong et al. 2003a). The main factors influencing accuracy and reproducibility are the partial volume effect, motion artifacts and image noise.

The influence of the partial volume effect is reduced by using thinner sections, overlapping images and a lower threshold. The use of a threshold for identification of calcified plaques makes full compensation of partial volume effects impossible, which is why also the mass score is not perfect. In theory, the mass score should be independent of slice thickness because thicker sections will lead to more partial volume effects that will cause a seemingly larger plaque volume, but also proportionally lower CT numbers. In practice, this effect is counteracted by the fact that all voxels with CT numbers below the threshold are neglected. This will always lead to a systematic increase in scores (mass as well as volume and Agatston scores) with thinner sections (Horiguchi et al. 2007).

Thinner sections and a lower threshold reduce partial volume effects, but negatively influence the effect of image noise: more noise will make it difficult to distinguish between true calcifications and pixels with a high CT number caused by noise (Fig. 19.3). Noise can be reduced by higher dose, but radiation dose is a limiting factor if calcium scoring is performed in asymptomatic individuals.

Motion leads to "smearing" of plaques (Fig. 19.4). The consequences are reduced CT numbers and apparently lower calcium content. However, the opposite may also happen: increased density areas may cause erroneously high calcium content. Good motion suppression is therefore mandatory. The best phases are centered on the mid diastole (70–80% of the RR interval) for low heart rates (< 60 bpm) and on

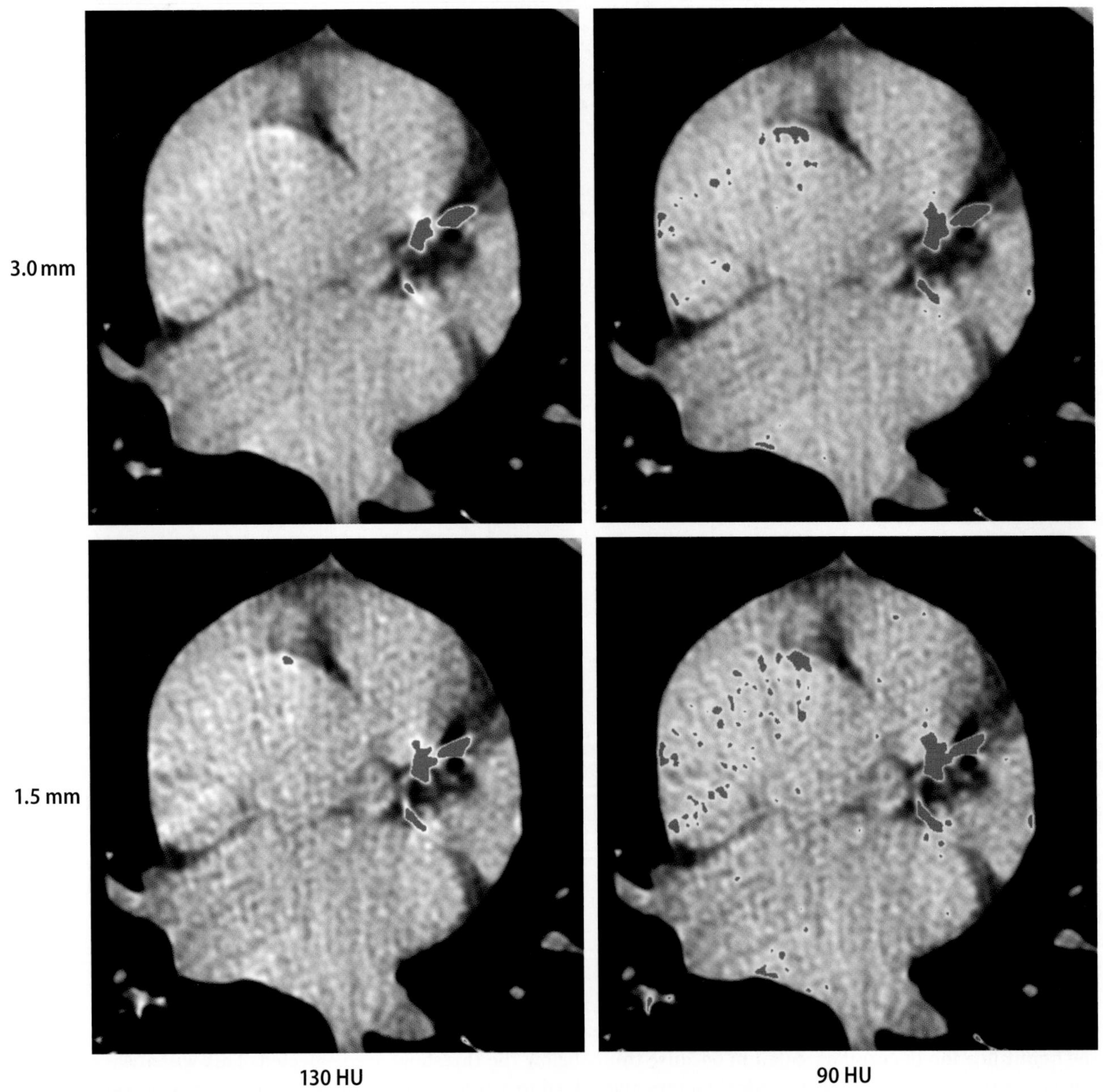

Fig. 19.3. Calcium scoring is usually performed on 3-mm slices at a 130 HU threshold (*upper left*). Decreasing slice thickness and/or threshold increases plaque size and noise unless radiation dose is increased

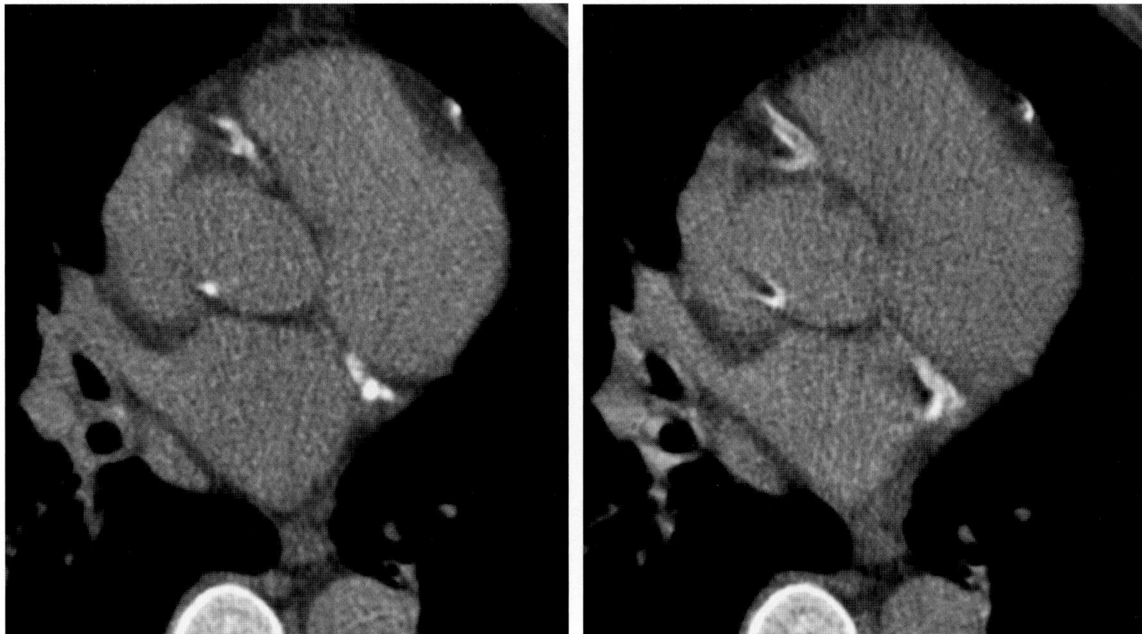

Fig. 19.4. Cardiac motion causes variation in calcium scores between phases of the RR interval. Cardiac motion generally causes a decrease in score because of blurring (*right image*) and thereby a decrease in density of the calcification compared to a motionless state (*left image*)

the end systole (around 40% of the RR interval) for high heart rates (> 80 bpm) (Rutten et al. 2008a). In the range between 60 and 80 bpm. either phase can yield the least artifacts.

Agatston scores obtained with EBCT suffered from an inter-scan variability between 15% and 49% (Devries et al. 1995; Wang et al. 1996, Yoon et al. 2000). Mean inter-scan variability for Agatston, volume and mass scores with prospectively ECG-triggered MDCT was 20%, 14% and 9%, respectively, in a study by Hong et al. (2003a). Multiple causes of inter-scan variability have been suggested, including cardiac motion artifacts, section thickness, scoring algorithm, choice of threshold, ECG-trigger timing and variation in starting position (Callister et al. 1998; Devries et al. 1995; Mao et al. 2001b, 2001a; Rutten et al. 2008a,b; Wang et al. 1996). At high heart rates (> 70 bpm) calcium scoring inter-scan variability increases since more cardiac motion artifacts are present in the images (Hong et al. 2003b).

Reproducibility is improved by scanning at a low heart rate (< 65 bpm), which requires beta-blockers if necessary. For prospective triggering, the choice of a rate-adapted ECG-trigger time point has been shown to improve inter-scan variability (Lu et al. 2002, Mao et al. 2001b). For this technique, the ECG-trigger time point is determined based on the patient heart rate before the start of the scan.

Small variations in scan starting position may explain a considerable amount of the inter-scan variability of the calcium score obtained from datasets with non-overlapping 3-mm-thick sections (Rutten et al. 2008b) because the starting position will affect partial volume effects for calcified plaques. For this reason, the best option to reduce inter-scan variability caused by partial volume effects is the use of overlapping reconstructions. However, on most current scanners this is only feasible if a retrospectively ECG-gated acquisition is performed.

19.3.6 Calcium Score and Cardiovascular Risk

The amount of coronary calcification is a measure of the extent of atherosclerotic disease (Rumberger et al. 1995). Multiple studies indicate that the calcium score can be used as a risk indicator for future *cardiac morbidity and mortality* in asymptomatic patient groups (Pletcher et al. 2004; Shaw et al. 2003, 2006; Taylor et al. 2005; Vliegenthart et al. 2004). This ability applies to both sexes (LaMonte et al. 2005) and different races (Detrano et al. 2008) and remains at high ages (Vliegenthart et al. 2002). Higher calcium scores are associated with a higher 10-year morbidity and mortality.

Studies have shown that calcium scores can either be used as an independent measure for *risk stratification* or on top of other measures such as the Framingham risk score (Budoff et al. 2007; Greenland et al. 2004). High calcium scores not only indicate a higher risk of future morbidity and mortality, but can also help in identifying *silent myocardial ischemia* in an asymptomatic patient group (He et al. 2000). Furthermore, *event-free survival after invasive coronary angiography* for the evaluation of chest pain was significantly lower with Agatston scores > 100 (Keelan et al. 2001).

Patients with *diabetes mellitus* tend to have higher calcium scores. In this patient group, it is the absence of calcifications that has predictive value since subjects without coronary calcifications have a low short-term risk of death even in the presence of diabetes mellitus (Raggi et al. 2004b).

In patients with *atypical chest pain* calcium scoring shows a high sensitivity (around 95%) for detecting coronary atherosclerosis at a low specificity (20%). Sensitivity drops to around 67% for the detection of hemodynamically significant coronary artery stenoses at an increased specificity of 80% (Herzog et al. 2004).

19.3.7 Guidelines for Interpretation and Use

Interpretation of coronary calcium scores is based on the presence of calcium, the absolute score and the score relative to an age- and sex-matched control. Presence of coronary calcification always indicates coronary arteriosclerosis. The more coronary calcifications are present, the higher the chance of a significant coronary artery stenosis. However, the location of calcifications and coronary stenoses are only loosely correlated (Kajinami et al. 1997). While massive calcifications may cause stenoses, not all stenoses occur in the regions of calcifications, but rather are caused by non-calcified plaques.

To simplify risk stratification, Rumberger defined five risk groups based on the absolute Agatston calcium score (Table 19.3) (Rumberger et al. 1999). Similar risk groups have not been determined for the volume and mass score, but Table 19.3 gives a rough guideline for transforming Agatston scores into volume and mass scores. Subjects with an Agaston score above 300 have been shown to have a hazard ratio of 6.84 (95% CI 2.93–15.99) for a major coronary event (myocardial infarction or death) and even 9.67 (95% CI 5.20–17.98) for any coronary event compared to subjects with a calcium score of 0 after adjustment for standard risk factors (Detrano et al. 2008).

Age- and sex-specific percentile scores are increasingly available from independent large population studies such as the MESA (Multi-Ethnic Study of Atherosclerosis) and the Heinz Nixdorf Recall Study (Bild et al. 2002; Schmermund et al. 2006b). The public websites of these studies provide online calculators to determine the age- and sex-specific percentile for an observed Agatston score (www.mesa-nhlbi.org and www.recall-studie.uni-essen.de). Such scores allow for assessing the risk of an individual relative to his or her peers and may provide an indicator for more aggressive risk management, medication or further testing. Using non-population based data (e.g., from self-referred patients) for determining percentile ranks results in an underestimation in the individual risk compared to using population-based data (Schmermund et al. 2006b).

While guidelines initially recommended against the use of the calcium score in risk prediction, more recent versions of several guidelines are no longer against its use. The Third National Cholesterol Education Program Adult Treatment Program (NCEP ATP III) as well as the Third Joint Task Force of European and other Societies of Cardiovascular Disease Prevention in Clinical Practice (European Society of Cardiology guidelines) and the American College of Cardiology Foundation Clinical Expert Consensus Task Force (ACCF/AHA guidelines) have suggested the use of coronary calcium scoring for further risk stratification (Greenland et al. 2007; National Cholesterol Education Program 2001). Such risk stratification should be performed on top of existing conventional risk scores [e.g. Framingham (USA), HeartScore (Europe)] (Graham 2006; National Cholesterol Education Program 2001).

Coronary calcium scoring is not recommended in asymptomatic subjects with a 10-year event risk of less than 10% or more than 20% because of the limited additional value of the results for determining optimal treatment. Subjects with two or more major risk factors and a 10–20% 10-year risk for hard cardiac events are considered at *moderately high risk* (previously intermediate risk). Coronary calcium scoring can be used in these subjects for confirmation or reclassification of the individual risk as derived from initial risk assessment.

A *calcium score of zero* confirms a low risk. Healthy lifestyle habits can be recommended. Reassessment in 5 years can be considered because the absence of coronary calcification does not entirely exclude the presence of coronary artery disease (Budoff et al. 2007).

Patients reclassified to a *high-risk group* based in the calcium score (≥75th percentile) are strongly advised to change their lifestyle. Drug treatment according to standard guidelines for primary prevention is advised.

Repeated calcium-scoring scans for monitoring treatment of coronary atherosclerosis is disputed because treatment with statins alone has not been able to attenuate coronary calcification progression in randomized studies (Redberg 2006; Schmermund et al. 2006a). However, progression of coronary calcifications may be a prognostic marker for the occurrence of a cardiovascular event: subjects with the greatest progression of coronary calcifications have the greatest risk for the occurrence of a cardiovascular event (Raggi et al. 2004a).

In patients presenting with *nonspecific chest pain in the emergency department*, the calcium score might be of use in selecting those eligible for further examinations (Greenland et al. 2007). Patients without any coronary calcifications are not recommended to undergo further cardiac workup. Their chance of a cardiac cause of their chest pain is exceedingly low. However, one has to keep in mind that a zero calcium score does not entirely exclude the presence of (stenotic) non-calcified plaques (Rubinshtein et al. 2007).

19.4 Aortic Valve Calcifications

Calcifications of the aortic valve are a common incidental finding on chest CT or calcium scoring scans in an elderly population. Aortic valve calcifications in a younger individual should raise the suspicion of a bicuspid aortic valve (Fig. 19.5). Aortic valve calcification can be found as an incidental finding in around 13–18% of multi-detector row CT scans; in around 5% of cases calcification is moderate or severe (Fig. 19.6) (Koos et al. 2006).

Identification of aortic valve calcifications is important because such calcifications are associated with aortic stenosis (Koos et al. 2004). Aortic valve calcifications are usually distributed along the commissural edges of the leaflets and occur most commonly on the aortic side of the aortic valve leaflets where flow is most turbulent. There is a good correlation between the extent of aortic valve leaflet calcification demonstrated by CT and the severity of aortic valve stenosis (Koos et al. 2006; Morgan-Hughes et al. 2003). Higher aortic valve calcium scores are associated with increased mean gradients across the aortic valve. Moderate or severe aortic valve calcification is a strong predictor for adverse clinical outcomes, such as aortic valve surgery or increased mortality (Rosenhek et al. 2000). Minor aortic valve calcification, on the other hand, is a common finding on CT and is generally of no significance.

The presence of cardiovascular risk factors or renal insufficiency is associated with a faster progression of aortic valve calcifications (Goldbarg et al. 2007). Despite multiple common risk factors for coronary artery disease and calcific aortic stenosis, however, only one-half of patients with severe calcific aortic stenosis have significant coronary artery disease, and most patients with coronary artery disease do not have aortic stenosis (Goldbarg et al. 2007).

Definite diagnosis of aortic valve stenosis, however, requires contrast-enhanced scans, preferably with ECG gating and systolic reconstructions. The CT diagnosis of aortic stenosis may be made if calcification of the aortic valve is combined with left ventricular hypertrophy and mild to moderate (post-stenotic) dilatation of the ascending aorta. Limited motion and reduced systolic aortic valve area directly prove aortic stenosis. The opening area of the valve can be used as a direct measure of the amount of stenosis.

19.5 Mitral Valve Calcifications

Mitral valve calcification can occur with rheumatic mitral valve stenosis or as a result of degeneration in elderly patients. Degenerative mitral valve calcification often involves the annulus and occasionally the leaflets (Fig. 19.7).

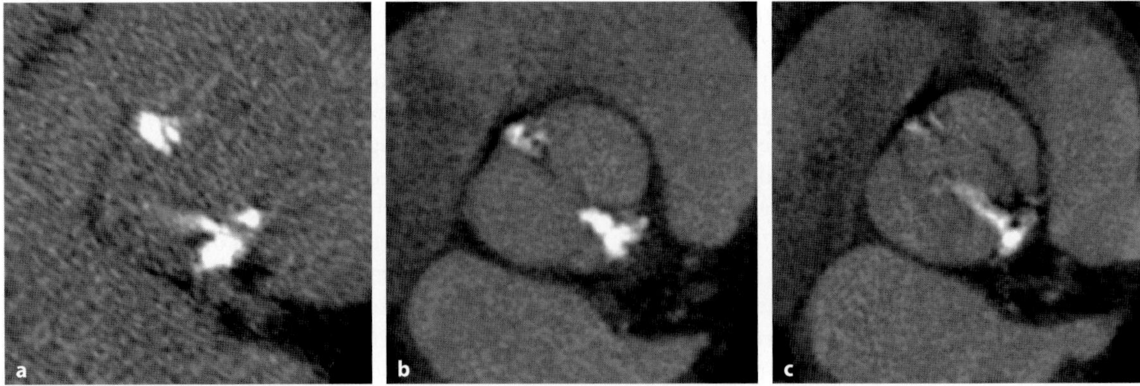

Fig. 19.5 a–c. Bicuspid aortic valve with early degenerative calcification that limits valve opening in a 44-year-old patient. Non-contrast-enhanced image (**a**) and contrast-enhanced images in diastole (**b**) and systole (**c**)

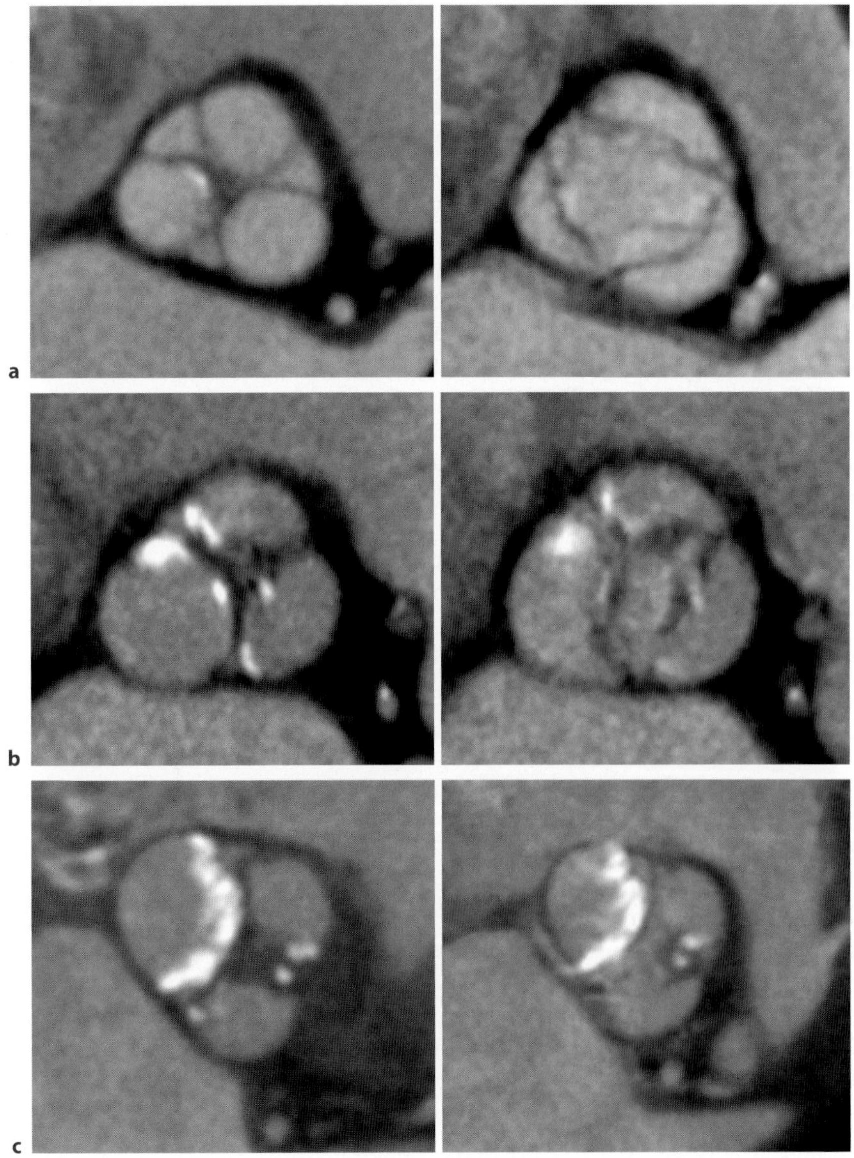

Fig. 19.6 a–c. Three degrees of calcification of the aortic valve in closed (*left*) and open condition (*right*): minor (**a**), moderate (**b**) and severe (**c**) (three different patients). Opening of the valve is severely limited with severe calcification compared to with minor calcification

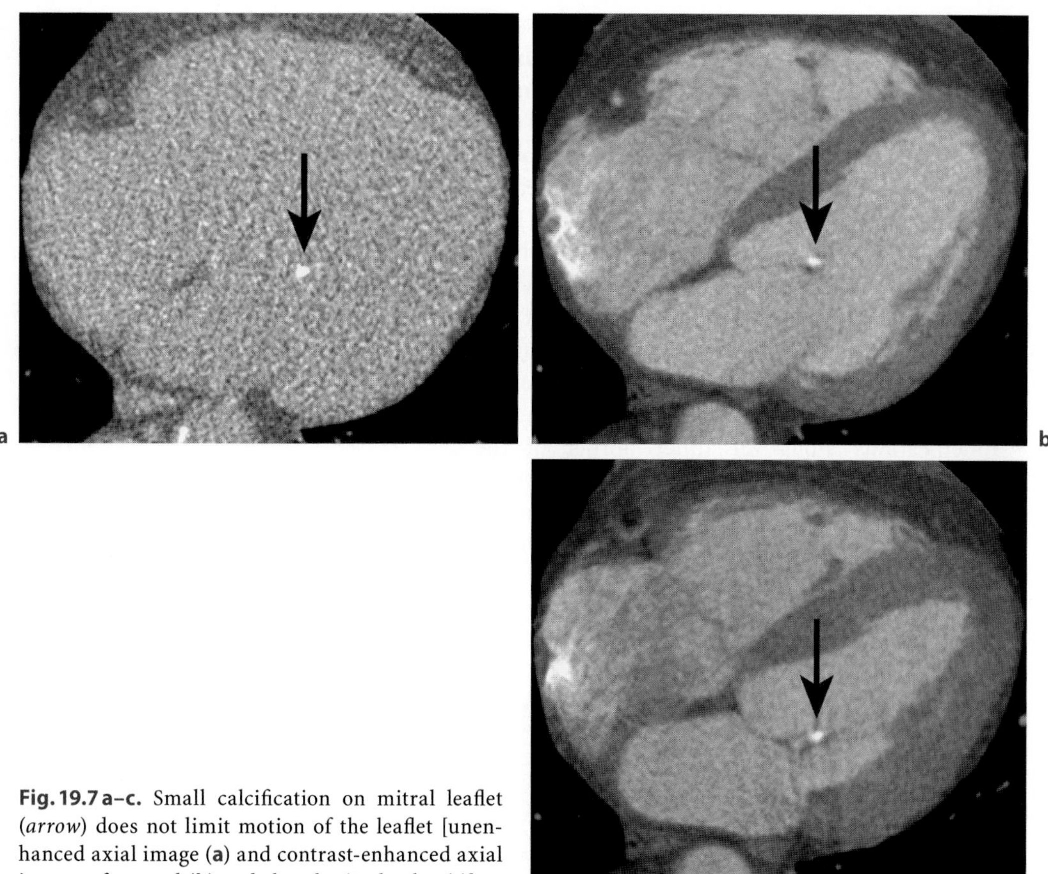

Fig. 19.7 a–c. Small calcification on mitral leaflet (*arrow*) does not limit motion of the leaflet [unenhanced axial image (**a**) and contrast-enhanced axial images of opened (**b**) and closed mitral valve (**c**)]

Extensive degenerative calcification of the *mitral valve annulus* can extend to the leaflets and limit their motility (Fig. 19.8). Mitral regurgitation can be the result. The association between mitral annulus calcification and mitral sclerosis and stenosis is less certain. There is an association between mitral annulus calcification and hypertrophic cardiomyopathy, atrial fibrillation, stroke, and coronary artery calcifications (Benjamin et al. 1992; Boon et al. 1997; Nair et al. 1983).

Leaflet calcification may cause fusion of the leaflets and, as a consequence, may lead to mitral stenosis. Mitral valve stenosis induces enlargement of the left atrium and increases the risk of atrial fibrillation and atrial thrombus formation. Calcifications of the *left atrial wall* are a rare consequence (Fig. 19.9).

19.6 Myocardial Calcifications

Calcifications in the myocardium are usually incidental findings on CT of the chest or cardiac CT. Locating a calcification in the ventricular wall or papillary muscles on a non contrast-enhanced scans is feasible, but localization is easier on contrast-enhanced scans.

19.6.1 Ventricular Wall Calcifications

Ventricular wall calcifications are rare and occur in a number of diseases, such as hyperparathyroidism, myocardial infarction and chronic Chagas' disease, a tropical parasitic disease. Myocardial infarction is by far the most common cause.

Calcifications in the presence of a left ventricular aneurysm may be the result of transmural myocardial infarction (Fig. 19.10) or chronic Chagas' disease. A ventricular aneurysm presents as a bulge in heart contour with marked localized thinning of the myocardium compared with adjacent areas. On gated contrast-enhanced scans, the aneurysmatic wall shows a paradoxical systolic expansion instead of contraction.

Patients with hyperparathyroidism have a high incidence of myocardial calcifications, mainly in the interventricular septum, along with valvular calcifications and an increased incidence of left ventricular hypertrophy. After parathyroidectomy the hypertrophy regresses, but calcifications persist (Stefenelli et al. 1993).

Calcifications along the inner border of the myocardium suggest *endomyocardial fibrosis* (Mousseaux et al. 1996). Endomyocardial fibrosis is a rare, severe and progressively restrictive form

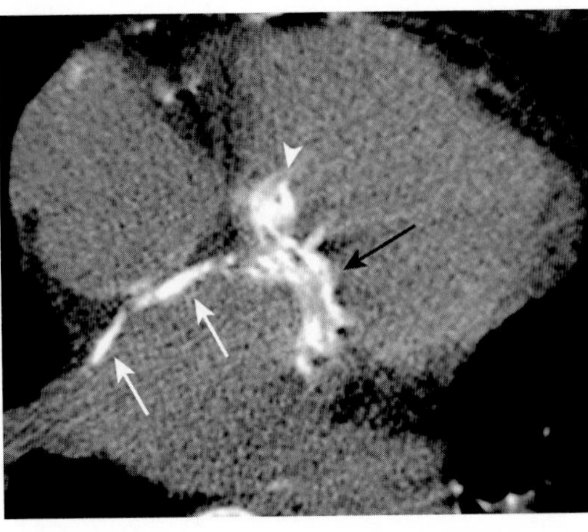

Fig. 19.9. Calcifications of left atrial wall (*white arrows*) in patient with artificial mitral (*black arrow*) and aortic valve (*white arrowhead*)

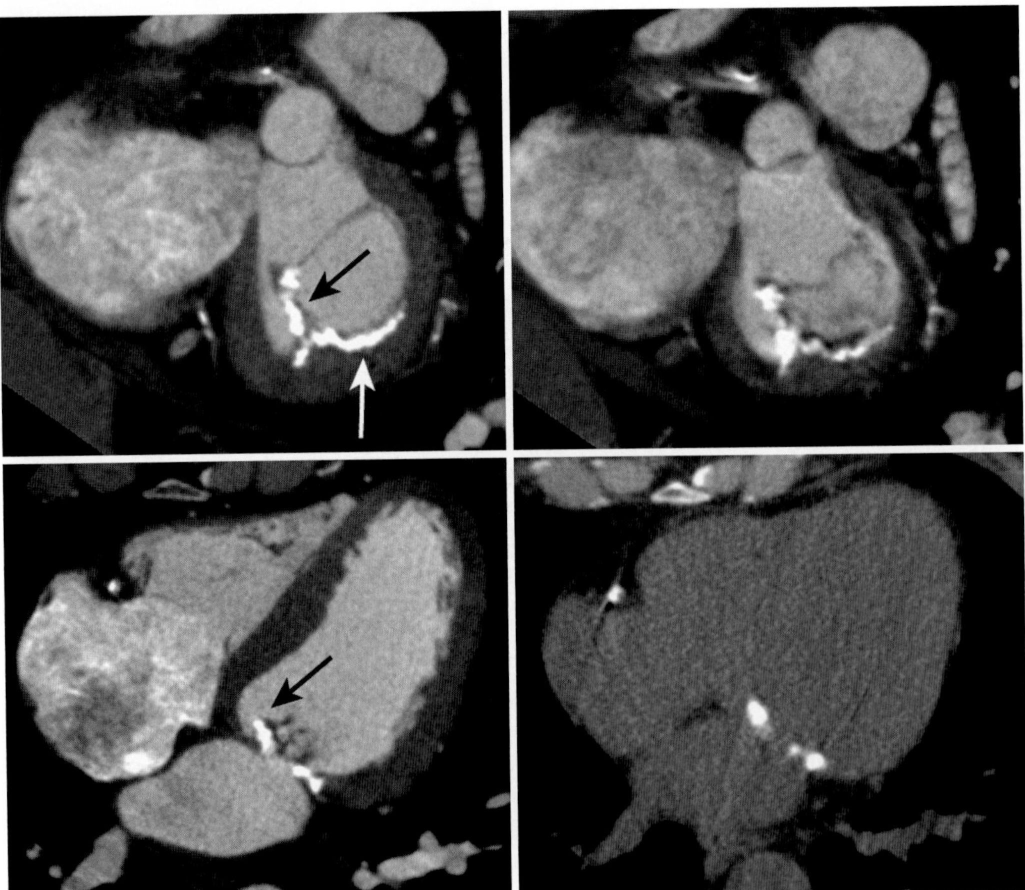

Fig. 19.8. Severe calcification of the mitral annulus (*white arrow*) limits movement of the mitral annulus during closure of the mitral valve (*upper right*), which induces mitral insufficiency. If calcification extends to the mitral leaflet (*black arrow*), limited motion of the leaflet can cause stenosis

of cardiomyopathy of unknown etiology. Marked fibrous endocardial thickening occurs of the inflow tract in one or both ventricles. It restricts ventricular filling and causes valvular incompetence due to fibrosis of chordae tendinae, papillary muscles and posterior atrioventricular valve cusps.

19.6.2 Papillary Muscle Calcifications

Small calcifications in the papillary muscles near the apex are common in elderly patients (Roberts 1986). Extensive calcifications of the papillary muscles are a rare finding, but can lead to malfunctioning of the mitral valve (Fig. 19.10) (Madu et al. 1997). Association has been found between papillary muscle calcification, mitral regurgitation and congestive heart failure (Come et al. 1982). Ischemia is a likely cause of papillary muscle calcification since an association between coronary artery disease and papillary muscle calcification has been described.

19.7 Pericardial Calcifications

Pericardial calcifications can be caused by injury (i.e., infarction, surgery, radiotherapy), infection, connective-tissue disease, uremia or occur idiopathically (Wang et al. 2003). Pericardial calcifications are associated with constrictive pericarditis,

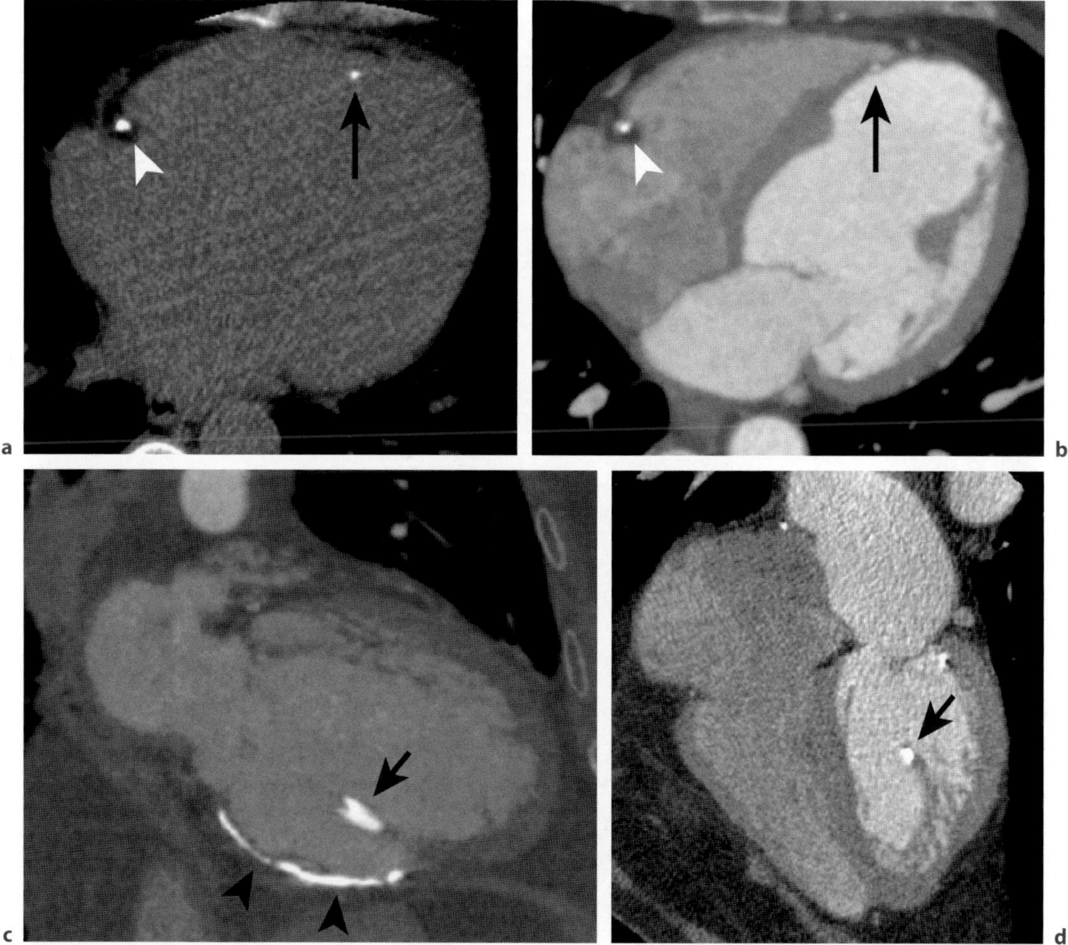

Fig. 19.10 a–d. Calcifications in a thin (**c**) or even aneurysmatic (**b**) ventricular wall after myocardial ischemia can be small (*large black arrow*) and more easily detected on unenhanced images (**a**), or completely line the scarred myocardium (*black arrowheads*). Papillary muscle calcification (*short arrow*) (**c**,**d**) is associated with myocardial ischemia. *White arrowheads* point at calcification in right coronary artery

but diagnosis of constrictive pericarditis requires additional signs of cardiac constriction.

Constrictive pericarditis is characterized by fibrous thickening of the pericardium, which leads to restriction of heart motion and decreased filling of the ventricular chambers. Abnormal thickening is indicated by a pericardial thickness of 4 mm or more. Extensive linear or plaque-like calcifications of the pericardium are common in constrictive pericarditis (Fig. 19.11). Calcifications occur especially over the right ventricle, the posterior surface of the left ventricle and in the atrioventricular groove.

CT signs of cardiac constriction include dilation of the SVC and IVC, reflux of contrast into the liver veins and coronary sinus, flattening right ventricle and bulging of intraventricular septum to the left. Associated ascites and pleural effusion are an indication of decompensated right heart failure. If no symptoms of cardiac constriction are present, pericardial thickening and calcification are not diagnostic of constrictive pericarditis, but indicate an increased risk of developing constrictive pericarditis in the future.

19.8 Calcified Masses

Calcifications due to cardiac masses are a rare. Cardiac masses that occasionally contain calcifications are either neoplasms or thrombi. Because calcifications are an important feature for the differential diagnosis of cardiac neoplasms, pre-contrast CT can offer additional information over echocardiography or MRI. Pre-contrast CT is followed by ECG-synchronized contrast-enhanced acquisitions to better determine extent and morphology of the mass. Echocardiography, however, remains the primary imaging modality, while MRI offers excellent soft-tissue contrast and delineation of the intra- and extracardiac extent of the lesion.

19.8.1 Cardiac Thrombus

Thrombi are the most common intracardiac masses and may occasionally contain calcifications (Tatli et al. 2005). Common locations for intracardiac thrombi are the left atrial appendage and the left ventricular apex. The latter commonly occurs in the presence of an akinetic, aneurysmatic left ventricular apex after myocardial infarction. Regions of turbulent blood flow, for example in valvular disease, are also common sites. While most thrombi are not mobile, the presence of thrombus, primarily in the left atrial appendage, puts patients at high risk for stroke and embolism at cardioversion of atrial fibrillation.

Calcifications are a sign of older, organizing thrombi. They most frequently occur in the region of the ventricular apex (Fig. 19.12). On pre-contrast CT, calcifications at a short distance from the left

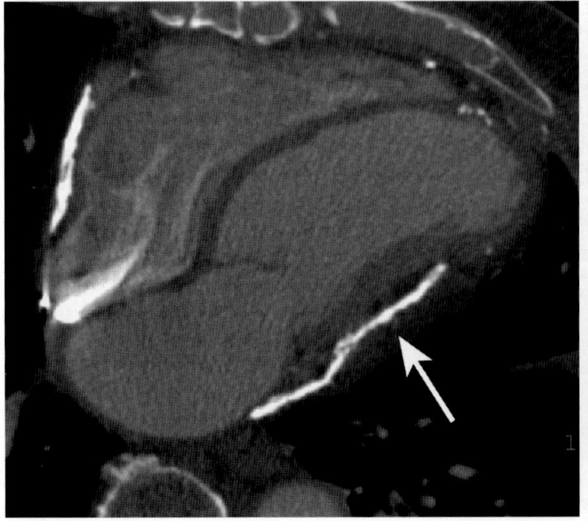
a

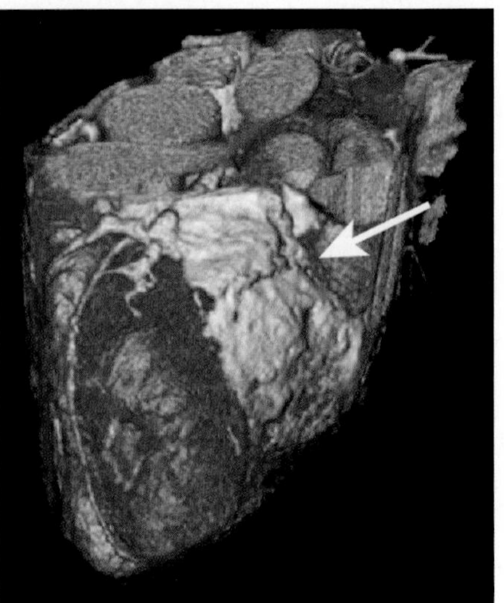
b

Fig. 19.11 a, b. Extensive linear pericardial calcification (*arrow*) in constrictive pericarditis that limits ventricular motion [axial contrast-enhanced image (**a**) and volume rendering of the heart (**b**)]

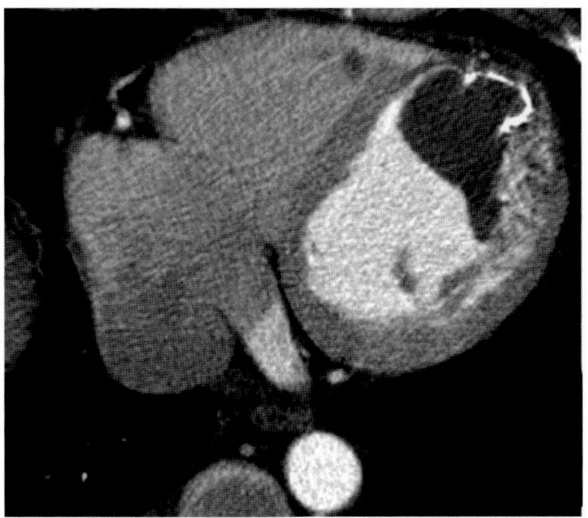

Fig. 19.12. Large thrombus with calcifications at left ventricular apex

ventricular apex may be the first sign of such a thrombus. They are rare incidental findings on calcium scoring scans or HRCT of the chest.

19.8.2 Cardiac Neoplasms–Overview

Primary cardiac neoplasms are rare (0.001–0.03% of patients in autopsy series) and more commonly benign than malign (Araoz et al. 2000). Metastases to the heart occur 20–40 times more often (Araoz et al. 1999). Although benign cardiac neoplasms do not metastasize, they do lead to morbidity and mortality by affecting blood flow and by inducing arrhythmias and emboli. Usually these benign neoplasms can be treated successfully.

Benign cardiac neoplasms that commonly contain calcifications are myxomas and fibromas. Calcifications are rare in papillary fibroelastomas and paragangliomas and do not occur in lipomas and lymphangiomas. Most malignant cardiac neoplasms do not contain calcifications. Calcification is typical in osteosarcomas and very rare in leiomyosarcomas. Calcification of a pericardial mass may suggest teratoma or old hematoma (Wang et al. 2003).

19.8.3 Cardiac Myxoma

Cardiac myxoma is the most common primary cardiac tumor. It is a benign neoplasm of unknown etiology that accounts for about 50% of the primary cardiac neoplasms. Myxomas typically occur in adulthood, with 90% of patients being between 30 and 60 years old. It is slightly more frequent in women than in men. In younger patients cardiac myxoma can be present as part of the autosomal dominant Carney complex (myxomas, hyperpigmented skin lesions and extracardiac neoplasms).

The tumor most frequently arises from a narrow stalk with a predilection for the interatrial septum (i.e., fossa ovalis) (Fig. 19.13). In 75–80% of cases it occurs in the left atrium. Occasionally the tumor prolapses through the cardiac valves. Myxoma has a heterogeneous low attenuation at CT that can contain cysts, necrosis and hemorrhage. Calcification is present in around 16% of myxomas.

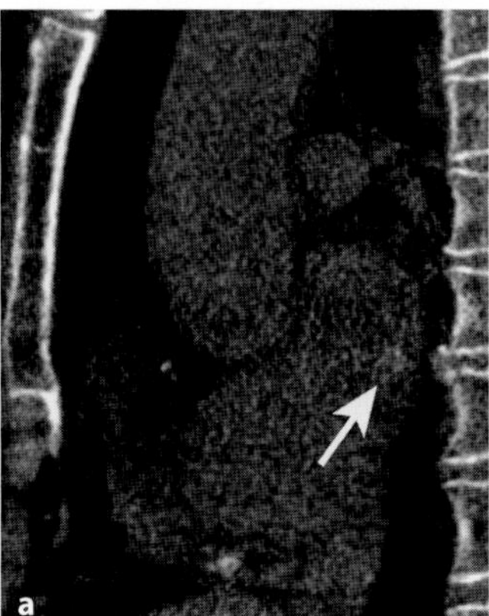

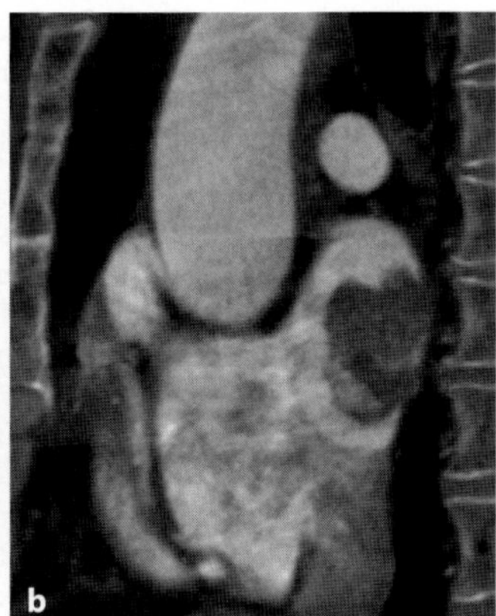

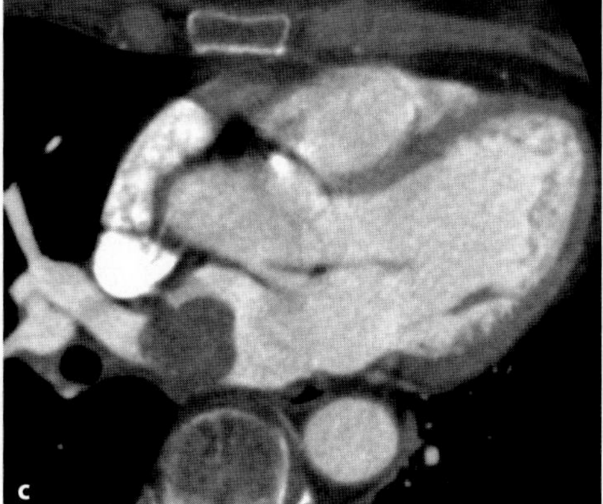

Fig. 19.13 a–c. Left atrial myxoma not visible on unenhanced image (**a**) except for small calcifications (*white arrow*) at the location of the mass in contrast-enhanced image (**b**). The myxoma typically arises from the atrial septum and in this case obstructs the orifice of a pulmonary vein (**c**)

19.8.4 Cardiac Fibroma

Cardiac fibroma (or fibromatosis, fibrous hamartoma, fibroelastic hamartoma) is a collection of fibroblasts interspersed among large amounts of collagen. It primarily occurs in infants and in utero and is extremely rare (100 cases since 1976). Fibromas appear as homogeneous masses with soft-tissue attenuation at CT. Often dystrophic calcifications are present. Mean diameter is about 5 cm, and the mass may either be sharply defined or infiltrative. The primary location is the ventricles, most commonly in the ventricular septum and left ventricular free wall. The ventricular cavity may be completely obliterated.

19.8.5 Cardiac Osteosarcoma

Osteosarcomas are a heterogeneous group of uncommon tumors that contain malignant, bone producing cells. Primary cardiac osteosarcomas most often occur in the left atrium, while metastatic osteosarcomas tend to occur in the right atrium. CT shows a low-attenuation mass with calcifications. Calcifications range from minimal speckles to dense deposits. In absence of dense calcifications, osteosarcomas may be mistaken for myxomas. The tumor has a broad base of attachment with an aggressive growth pattern such as invasion into the atrial septum or infiltrative growth along the epicardium. Primary cardiac osteosarcomas are often aggressive with poor prognosis.

References

Agatston AS, Janowitz WR, Hildner FJ et al. (1990) Quantification of coronary artery calcium using ultrafast computed tomography. J Am Coll Cardiol 15:827–832

Arad Y, Spadaro LA, Goodman K et al. (1996) Predictive value of electron beam computed tomography of the coronary arteries: 19-month follow-up of 1,173 asymptomatic subjects. Circulation 93:1951–1953

Araoz PA, Eklund HE, Welch TJ et al. (1999) CT and MR imaging of primary cardiac malignancies. Radiographics 19:1421–1434

Araoz PA, Mulvagh SL, Tazelaar HD et al. (2000) CT and MR imaging of benign primary cardiac neoplasms with echocardiographic correlation. Radiographics 20:1303–1319

Benjamin EJ, Plehn JF, D'Agostino RB et al. (1992) Mitral annular calcification and the risk of stroke in an elderly cohort. N Engl J Med 327:374–379

Bild DE, Bluemke DA, Burke GL et al. (2002) Multi-ethnic study of atherosclerosis: objectives and design. Am J Epidemiol 156:871–881

Boon A, Cheriex E, Lodder J et al. (1997) Cardiac valve calcification: characteristics of patients with calcification of the mitral annulus or aortic valve. Heart 78:472–474

Budoff MJ, Achenbach S, Blumenthal RS et al. (2006) Assessment of coronary artery disease by cardiac computed tomography: a scientific statement from the American Heart Association committee on cardiovascular imaging and intervention, council on cardiovascular radiology and intervention, and committee on cardiac imaging, council on clinical cardiology. Circulation 114:1761–1791

Budoff MJ, Shaw LJ, Liu ST et al. (2007) Long-term prognosis associated with coronary calcification: observations from a registry of 25,253 patients. J Am Coll Cardiol 49:1860–1870

Callister TQ, Cooil B, Raya SP et al. (1998) Coronary artery disease: improved reproducibility of calcium scoring with an electron-beam CT volumetric method. Radiology 208:807–814

Come PC, Riley MF (1982) M mode and cross-sectional echocardiographic recognition of fibrosis and calcification of the mitral valve chordae and left ventricular papillary muscles. Am J Cardiol 49:461–466

Detrano R, Guerci AD, Carr JJ et al. (2008) Coronary calcium as a predictor of coronary events in four racial or ethnic groups. N Engl J Med 358:1336–1345

Devries S, Wolfkiel C, Shah V et al. (1995) Reproducibility of the measurement of coronary calcium with ultrafast computed tomography. Am J Cardiol 75:973–975

Earls JP, Berman EL, Urban BA et al. (2008) Prospectively gated transverse coronary CT angiography versus retrospectively gated helical technique: improved image quality and reduced radiation dose. Radiology 246:742–753

Goldbarg SH, Elmariah S, Miller MA et al. (2007) Insights into degenerative aortic valve disease. J Am Coll Cardiol 50:1205–1213

Graham IM (2006) The importance of total cardiovascular risk assessment in clinical practice. Eur J Gen Pract 12:148–155

Greenland P, LaBree L, Azen SP et al. (2004) Coronary artery calcium score combined with Framingham score for risk prediction in asymptomatic individuals. JAMA 291:210–215

Greenland P, Bonow RO, Brundage BH et al. (2007) ACCF/AHA 2007. Clinical expert consensus document on coronary artery calcium scoring by computed tomography in global cardiovascular risk assessment and in evaluation of patients with chest pain: a report of the American College of Cardiology Foundation Clinical Expert Consensus Task Force (ACCF/AHA writing committee to update the 2000 expert consensus document on electron beam computed tomography) developed in collaboration with the Society of Atherosclerosis Imaging and Prevention and the Society of Cardiovascular Computed Tomography. J Am Coll Cardiol 49:378–402

He ZX, Hedrick TD, Pratt CM et al. (2000) Severity of coronary artery calcification by electron beam computed tomography predicts silent myocardial ischemia. Circulation 101:244–251

Herzog C, Britten M, Balzer JO et al. (2004) Multidetector-row cardiac CT: diagnostic value of calcium scoring and CT coronary angiography in patients with symptomatic, but atypical, chest pain. Eur Radiol 14:169–177

Hong C, Bae KT, Pilgram TK (2003a) Coronary artery calcium: accuracy and reproducibility of measurements with multi-detector row CT – assessment of effects of different thresholds and quantification methods. Radiology 227:795–801

Hong C, Bae KT, Pilgram TK et al. (2003b) Coronary artery calcium quantification at multi-detector row CT: influence of heart rate and measurement methods on interacquisition variability–initial experience. Radiology 228:95–100

Hong C, Pilgram TK, Zhu F et al. (2004) Is coronary artery calcium mass related to Agatston score? Acad Radiol 11:286–292

Horiguchi J, Fukuda H, Yamamoto H et al. (2006) The impact of motion artifacts on the reproducibility of repeated coronary artery calcium measurements. Eur Radiol 17:81–86

Horiguchi J, Matsuura N, Yamamoto H et al. (2007) Variability of repeated coronary artery calcium measurements by 1.25-mm- and 2.5-mm-thickness images on prospective electrocardiograph-triggered 64-slice CT. Eur Radiol 18:209–216

Jahnke C, Paetsch I, Achenbach S et al. (2006) Coronary MR imaging: breath-hold capability and patterns, coronary artery rest periods, and beta-blocker use. Radiology 239:71–78

Jakobs TF, Becker CR, Ohnesorge B et al. (2002) Multislice helical CT of the heart with retrospective ECG gating: reduction of radiation exposure by ECG-controlled tube current modulation. Eur Radiol 12:1081–1086

Kajinami MD, Seki MD, Takekoshi MD et al. (1997) Coronary calcification and coronary atherosclerosis: site by site comparative morphologic study of electron beam computed tomography and coronary angiography. J Am Coll Cardiol 29:1549–1556

Keelan PC, Bielak LF, Ashai K et al. (2001) Long-term prognostic value of coronary calcification detected by electron-beam computed tomography in patients undergoing coronary angiography. Circulation 104:412–417

Kondos GT, Hoff JA, Sevrukov A et al. (2003) Electron-beam tomography coronary artery calcium and cardiac events: a 37-month follow-up of 5,635 initially asymptomatic low- to intermediate-risk adults. Circulation 107:2571–2576

Koos R, Mahnken AH, Sinha AM et al. (2004) Aortic valve calcification as a marker for aortic stenosis severity: assessment on 16-MDCT. Am J Roentgenol 183:1813–1818

Koos R, Kuhl HP, Muhlenbruch G et al. (2006) Prevalence and clinical importance of aortic valve calcification detected incidentally on CT scans: comparison with echocardiography. Radiology 241:76–82

LaMonte MJ, FitzGerald SJ, Church TS et al. (2005) Coronary artery calcium score and coronary heart disease events in a large cohort of asymptomatic men and women. Am J Epidemiol 162:421–429

Lu B, Zhuang N, Mao SS et al. (2002) EKG-triggered CT data acquisition to reduce variability in coronary arterial calcium score. Radiology 224:838–844

Madu EC, D'Cruz IA (1997) The vital role of papillary muscles in mitral and ventricular function: echocardiographic insights. Clin Cardiol 20:93–98

Mao S, Bakhsheshi H, Lu B et al. (2001a) Effect of electrocardiogram triggering on reproducibility of coronary artery calcium scoring. Radiology 220:707–711

Mao S, Budoff MJ, Bakhsheshi H et al. (2001b) Improved reproducibility of coronary artery calcium scoring by electron beam tomography with a new electrocardiographic trigger method. Invest Radiol 36:363–367

McCollough CH, Ulzheimer S, Halliburton SS et al. (2003) A multi-scanner, multi-manufacturer, international standard for the quantification of CAC using cardiac CT (abstr). Radiology 229:630–631

Morgan-Hughes GJ, Owens PE, Roobottom CA et al. (2003) Three dimensional volume quantification of aortic valve calcification using multislice computed tomography. Heart 89:1191–1194

Mousseaux E, Hernigou A, Azencot M et al. (1996) Endomyocardial fibrosis: electron-beam CT features. Radiology 198:755–760

Nair CK, Aronow WS, Sketch MH et al. (1983) Clinical and echocardiographic characteristics of patients with mitral anular calcification: Comparison with age- and sex-matched control subjects. Am J Cardiol 51:992–995

National Cholesterol Education Program (2001) Executive summary of The Third Report of The National Cholesterol Education Program (NCEP) Expert Panel on detection, evaluation, and treatment of high blood cholesterol in adults (Adult Treatment Panel III). JAMA 285:2486–2497

Pletcher MJ, Tice JA, Pignone M et al. (2004) Using the coronary artery calcium score to predict coronary heart disease events: a systematic review and meta-analysis. Arch Intern Med 164:1285–1292

Poll LW, Cohnen M, Brachten S et al. (2002) Dose reduction in multi-slice CT of the heart by use of ECG-controlled tube current modulation ("ECG pulsing"): phantom measurements. Rofo Fortschr Geb Rontgenstr Neuen Bildgeb Verfahr 174:1500–1505

Raggi P, Callister TQ, Shaw LJ (2004a) Progression of coronary artery calcium and risk of first myocardial infarction in patients receiving cholesterol-lowering therapy. Arterioscler Thromb Vasc Biol 24:1272–1277

Raggi P, Shaw LJ, Berman DS et al. (2004b) Prognostic value of coronary artery calcium screening in subjects with and without diabetes. J Am Coll Cardiol 43:1663–1669

Redberg RF (2006) Coronary artery calcium: should we rely on this surrogate marker? Circulation 113:336–337

Roberts WC (1986) The senile cardiac calcification syndrome. Am J Cardiol 58:572–574

Rosenhek R, Binder T, Porenta G et al. (2000) Predictors of outcome in severe, asymptomatic aortic stenosis. N Engl J Med 343:611–617

Rubinshtein R, Gaspar T, Halon DA et al. (2007) Prevalence and extent of obstructive coronary artery disease in patients with zero or low calcium score undergoing 64-slice cardiac multidetector computed tomography for evaluation of a chest pain syndrome. Am J Cardiol 99:472–475

Rumberger JA, Brundage BH, Rader DJ et al. (1999) Electron beam computed tomographic coronary calcium scanning: a review and guidelines for use in asymptomatic persons. Mayo Clin Proc 74:243–252

Rumberger JA, Simons DB, Fitzpatrick LA et al. (1995) Coronary artery calcium area by electron-beam computed tomography and coronary atherosclerotic plaque area. A histopathologic correlative study. Circulation 92:2157–2162

Rutten A, Krul SP, Meijs MF et al. (2008a) Variability of coronary calcium scores throughout the cardiac cycle: implications for the appropriate use of electrocardiogram-dose modulation with retrospectively gated computed tomography. Invest Radiol 43:187–194

Rutten A, Isgum I, Prokop M (2008b) Coronary calcification: effect of small variation of scan starting position on Agatston, volume, and mass scores. Radiology 246:90–98

Schmermund A, Achenbach S, Budde T et al. (2006a) Effect of intensive versus standard lipid-lowering treatment with atorvastatin on the progression of calcified coronary atherosclerosis over 12 Months: a multicenter, randomized, double-blind trial. Circulation 113:427–437

Schmermund A, Mehlenkamp S, Berenbein S et al. (2006b) Population-based assessment of subclinical coronary atherosclerosis using electron-beam computed tomography. Atherosclerosis 185:177–182

Secci A, Wong N, Tang W et al. (1997) Electron beam computed tomographic coronary calcium as a predictor of coronary events: comparison of two protocols. Circulation 96:1122–1129

Shaw LJ, Raggi P, Callister TQ et al. (2006) Prognostic value of coronary artery calcium screening in asymptomatic smokers and non-smokers. Eur Heart J 27:968–975

Shaw LJ, Raggi P, Schisterman E et al. (2003) Prognostic value of cardiac risk factors and coronary artery calcium screening for all-cause mortality. Radiology 228:826–833

Stefenelli T, Mayr H, Bergler-Klein J et al. (1993) Primary hyperparathyroidism: Incidence of cardiac abnormalities and partial reversibility after successful parathyroidectomy. Am J Med 95:197–202

Tatli S, Lipton MJ (2005) CT for intracardiac thrombi and tumors. Int J Cardiovasc Imaging (formerly Cardiac Imaging) 21:115–131

Taylor AJ, Bindeman J, Feuerstein I et al. (2005) Coronary calcium independently predicts incident premature coronary heart disease over measured cardiovascular risk factors: mean three-year outcomes in the Prospective Army Coronary Calcium (PACC) project. J Am Coll Cardiol 46:807–814

Ulzheimer S, Kalender WA (2003) Assessment of calcium scoring performance in cardiac computed tomography. Eur Radiol 13:484–497

Vliegenthart R, Oudkerk M, Song B et al. (2002) Coronary calcification detected by electron-beam computed tomography and myocardial infarction. The Rotterdam Coronary Calcification Study. Eur Heart J 23:1596–1603

Vliegenthart R, Oei HH, van den Elzen APM et al. (2004) Alcohol cnsumption and cronary clcification in a gneral population. Arch Intern Med 164:2355–2360

Vliegenthart R, Oudkerk M, Hofman A et al. (2005) Coronary calcification improves cardiovascular risk prediction in the elderly. Circulation 112:572–577

Wang S, Detrano RC, Secci A et al. (1996) Detection of coronary calcification with electron-beam computed tomography: evaluation of interexamination reproducibility and comparison of three image-acquisition protocols. Am Heart J 132:550–558

Wang Y, Vidan E, Bergman GW (1999) Cardiac motion of coronary arteries: variability in the rest period and implications for coronary MR angiography. Radiology 213:751–758

Wang ZJ, Reddy GP, Gotway MB et al. (2003) CT and MR imaging of pericardial disease. Radiographics 23:S-67–S180

Yoon HC, Goldin JG, Greaser LE, III et al. (2000) Interscan variation in coronary artery calcium quantification in a large asymptomatic patient population. AJR Am J Roentgenol 174:803–809

Left Superior Vena Cava

20

Thierry Couvreur and Benoît Ghaye

CONTENTS

Summary

The left-sided superior vena cava (LSVC) is the most frequent abnormality of the systemic venous return, with prevalence of 0.1-0.5% in the general population and up to 12.9% in patients with congenital heart disease. The persistence of a LSVC results from failure of involution of the left anterior cardinal vein. Right-sided SVC and LSVC co-exist together in 80%–90% of cases. LSVC usually drains into a dilated coronary sinus, but it can also drain less frequently into the left atrium, and thus be responsible for a right-to-left shunt or even a left-to-right shunt with important clinical implications. MDCT is the method of choice to differentiate LSVC from other veins that may present with a vertical course through the left side of the mediastinum.

20.1 Introduction

The first description of a left-sided superior vena cava (LSVC) was reported by Le Cat in 1738 (cited in Harris 1960). LSVC is a not rare congenital abnormality of the systemic venous return that can have

T. Couvreur, MD
B. Ghaye, MD
Department of Medical Imaging, University Hospital of Liege, 4000 Liege 1, Belgium

various presentations and can be isolated or associated with congenital heart disease. The persistence of a LSVC results from failure of involution of the left anterior cardinal vein (CV) (Cha and Khoury 1972). In the past, this anomaly was usually detected incidentally during cardiac surgery or autopsy (Winter 1954). In most cases, LSVC has no consequence, but this variant is important to know in case of central venous catheter positioning, pacemaker insertion or cardiac surgery. LSVC is usually draining into a dilated coronary sinus (CS), but it can also drain less frequently into the left atrium, and thus be responsible for a right-to-left shunt or even a left-to-right shunt with important clinical implications.

20.2 Anatomy of Right Superior Vena Cava

The superior vena cava (SVC) drains the venous blood flow of the upper half of the body. The SVC is usually right-sided (RSVC) and receives its tributaries, namely the innominate veins, also called the brachiocephalic veins, behind the first right costal cartilage. Then it descends vertically along the right side of the mediastinum and terminates its course in the roof of the right atrium. The RSVC also drains the azygos arch in its medio-dorsal part, which contributes to draining the posterior part of the body (Godwin and Chen 1986; Jaafar et al. 1999).

RSVC measures approximately 7 cm in length and 1.5 cm in diameter, and is devoid of venous valves (Cormier et al. 1989). The intra-pericardial portion is about one-third of the vein course and measures around 2–3 cm (Herold et al. 2001). The ventral and lateral relations of the RSVC are to the pleura, thymus, right phrenic nerve and adjacent right lung. Posteriorly, it is related to the right brachio-cephalic artery, trachea, right main bronchus, right pulmonary artery and right superior pulmonary vein. Medially, the SVC is in contact with the ascending aorta. It is also bordered by lymph nodes (Cormier et al. 1989).

20.3 Embryology

20.3.1 Normal Development of RSVC

During the 4th week of embryological development, the venous system is formed by three pairs of veins draining into the sinus venosus (Fig. 20.1). They consist of the umbilical veins collecting the blood of the chorion, the vitelline veins collecting the blood of the yolk sac and primitive gut, and the common CVs collecting the blood of the embryo (Gensini et al. 1959; Kellman et al. 1988). At this time, the sinus venosus is connected to the primitive atrium via a central hole and is composed of a transversal part and two lateral horns (Lagrange et al. 2003). The latter forms the future systemic venous return through two common CVs, also called the ducts of Cuvier, which are formed by the junction of an anterior and a posterior CVs on each side (Gensini et al. 1959). Anterior CVs drain the venous blood flow from the cephalic region, whereas posterior CVs drain the caudal region of the embryo (Kellman et al. 1988). The sinus venosus will gradually merge

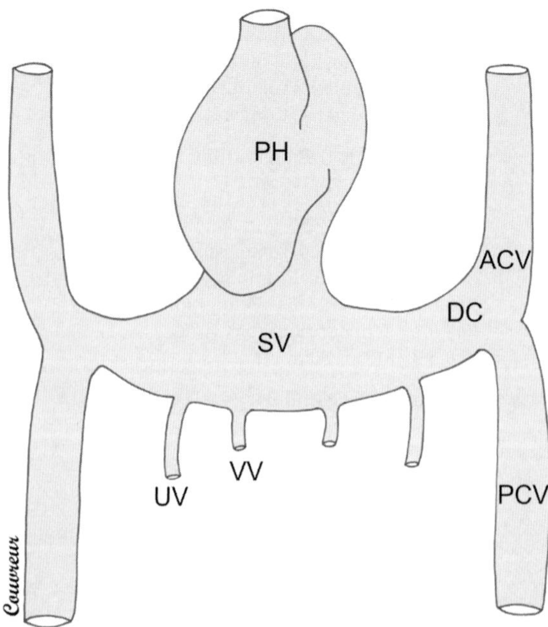

Fig. 20.1. Embryology during the 4th week. *ACV* anterior cardinal vein; *PCV* posterior cardinal vein; *DC* duct of Cuvier; *PH* primitive heart; *SV* sinus venosus; *UV* umbilical vein; *VV* viteline vein

with the right atrium, and the right horn widens. Then a caudal traction of the heart straightens the common CVs, with the consequence that the common CVs present as an extension of the anterior CVs (Lagrange et al. 2003).

During the 7th week of gestation, a transverse anastomosis between the right and the left anterior CVs develops and becomes the future left innominate vein (LIV) (Fig. 20.2) (Kellman et al. 1988; Cormier et al. 1989; Lagrange et al. 2003). As the LIV develops, the blood flow from the left side into the right duct of Cuvier progressively increases (Steinberg et al. 1953). This results in an increase in diameter of the right anterior CV, as the left anterior CV collapses caudally to LIV and eventually obliterates (Fig. 20.3) (Tak et al. 2002). According to Nsah et al. (1991), the mechanism of the obliteration could be initiated by an extrinsic compression of LSVC between the left atrium and the left hilum, whereas the RSVC is not subject to such a pressure.

The right duct of Cuvier and lower part of the right anterior CV will form the SVC, whereas the upper portion of the right anterior CV gives rise to the right innominate vein (Gensini et al. 1959; Kellman et al. 1988). On the left side, a small cranial portion of the left anterior CV persists and becomes the left superior intercostal vein, and a caudal remnant of the left duct of Cuvier forms the CS and the oblique vein of the left atrium or vein of Marshall (Cha and Khoury 1972; Page et al. 1990). The latter vein can involute and then forms the oblique ligament of Marshall (Cormier et al. 1989).

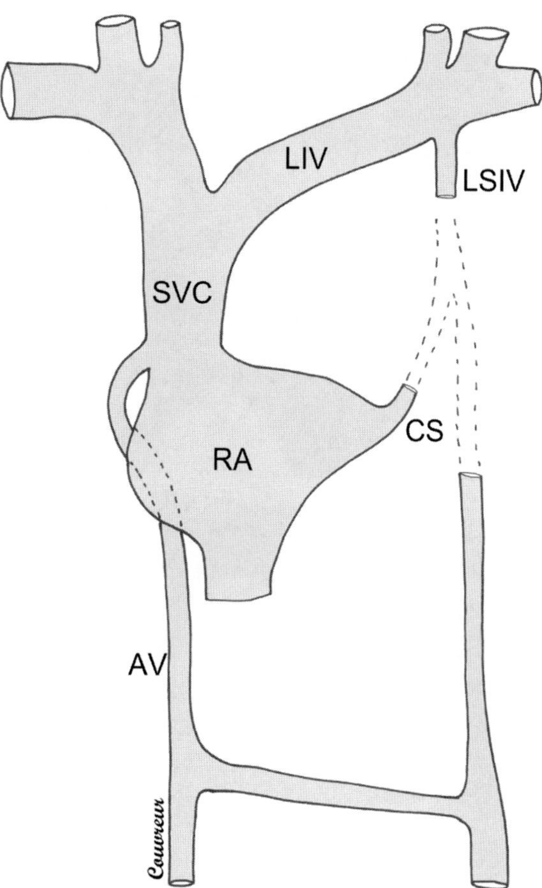

Fig. 20.3. Embryology at term. *SVC* superior vena cava; *RA* right atrium; *LIV* left innominate vein; *CS* coronary sinus; *LSIV* left superior intercostal vein; *AV* azygos vein

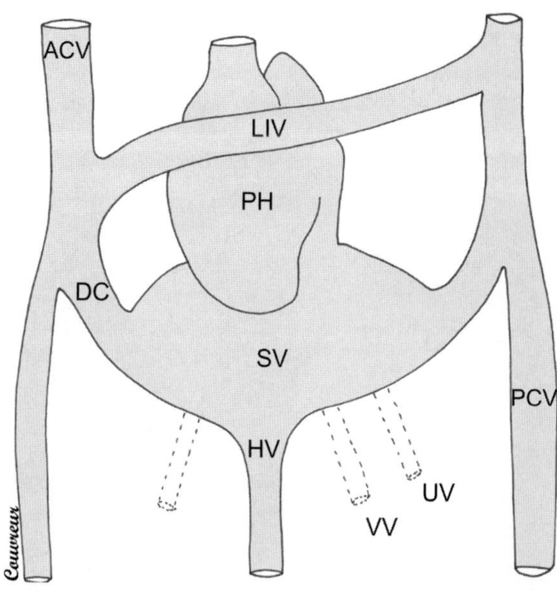

Fig. 20.2. Embryology during the 7th week: Straightening of ducts of Cuvier and development of transverse anastomosis. *ACV* anterior cardinal vein; *PCV* posterior cardinal vein; *DC* duct of Cuvier; *HV* hepatic vein; *LIV* left innominate vein; *PH* primitive heart; *SV* sinus venosus; *UV* umbilical vein; *VV* viteline vein

20.3.2 Persistence of LSVC

Persistence of LSVC results from the failure of involution of the left anterior CV, and usually drains into the right atrium via a dilated CS (Fig. 20.4) (Cha and Khoury 1972; Webb et al. 1982; Kellman et al. 1988; Tak et al. 2002). The lack of development of the LIV with the persistence of the LSVC as a consequence has been hypothesized (Steinberg et al. 1953). Nevertheless, the absence of the LIV cannot

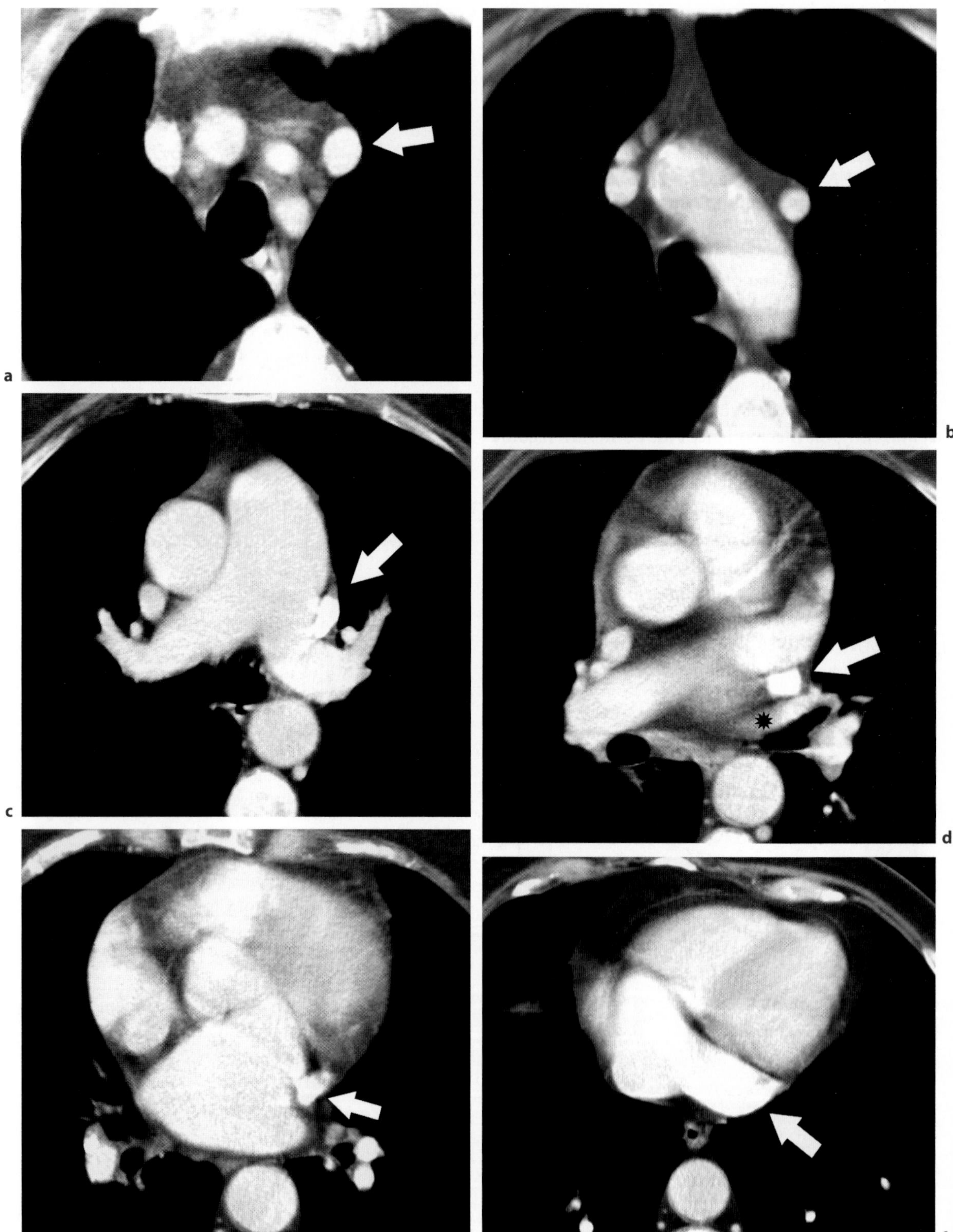

Fig. 20.4a–f. Normal course of LSVC in a patient with double SVC and without left innominate vein. LSVC (*arrows*) passes laterally to the aortic arch (**b**), in front of left pulmonary artery (**c**) and left superior pulmonary vein (*) (**d**), in the left atrioventricular groove (**e**), and finally drained into a dilated coronary sinus (**f**)

be considered as an explanation in all cases of LSVC. Ancel and Villemin (1908) have suggested complementary explanations that can be found in the transversal orientation of the LIV; i.e., when oblique downwards to the left, the LIV conducts the blood flow from the right to the left, thereby maintaining the function of the LSVC (Winter 1954). Other theories have been proposed, but none can reasonably explain all cases of LSVC (Winter 1954).

20.4 Presentation of LSVC

20.4.1 Prevalence

The LSVC is the most frequent abnormality of the systemic venous return, with prevalence in the general population of 0.1–0.5% (Bunger et al. 1981; Nsah et al. 1991; Tak et al. 2002). However, the real incidence of this anomaly is difficult to establish, considering the absence of symptom in the majority of cases (Cha and Khoury 1972; Cormier et al. 1989). The prevalence in patients with congenital heart disease is higher and is between 1.3 and 12.9% (Buirski et al. 1986; Hansell et al. 2004).

20.4.2 RSVC and LSVC

RSVC and LSVC coexist together in 80%–90% of cases (Figs. 20.4 and 20.5) (Webb et al. 1982; Jaafar et al. 1999). The RSVC drains normally, while LSVC enters the CS and drains into the right atrium (Cormier et al. 1989; Heye et al. 2007). When a LSVC coexists with a RSVC, the diameter of the left-sided vein rarely exceeds the right one and is frequently equal or sometimes smaller (Winter 1954). In 10–20%, the LSVC is unique without RSVC (single LSVC) with only a 0.1% incidence rate in the visceroatrial situs solitus, but up to 40% in abnormal situs (Fig. 20.6) (Webb et al. 1982; Jaafar et al. 1999; Heye et al. 2007).

20.4.3 LIV

The frequency of LIV between both SVCs varies from 35% (Kellman et al. 1988) to 60% (Winter 1954; Corbisiero et al. 2003). When present, LIV can be oriented downwards to the right, downwards to the left or horizontally. The size of both SVCs depends on their blood flows resulting from the orientation of the LIV. Additional cross-communication between SVCs can exist (Godwin and Chen 1986; Cormier et al. 1989).

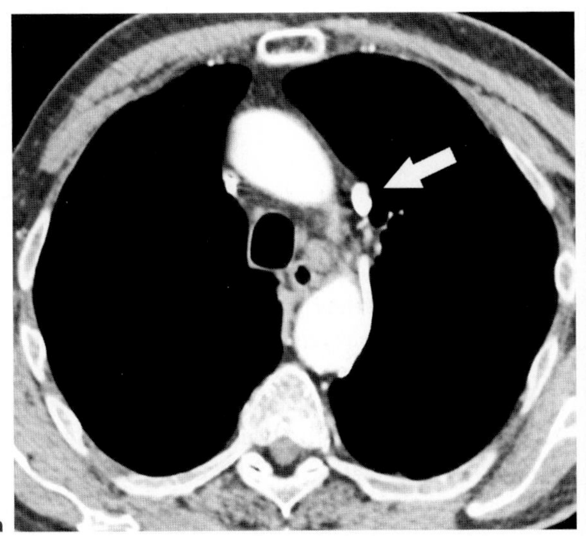
a

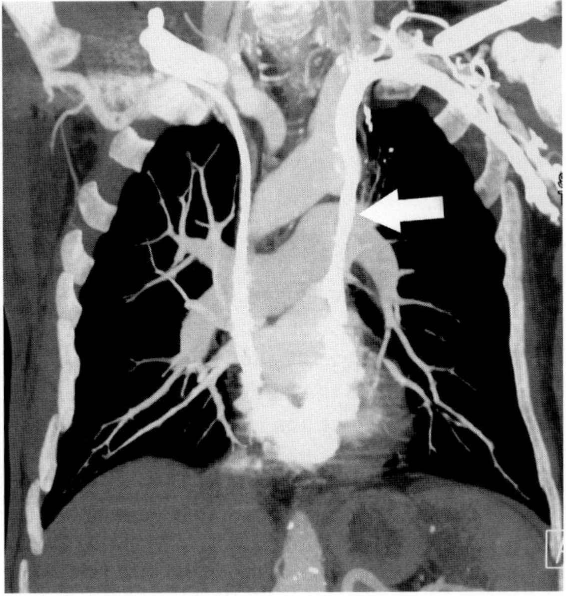
b

Fig. 20.5a,b. Double SVC. MIP CT projection shows RSVC and LSVC (*arrow*) draining into the right atrium

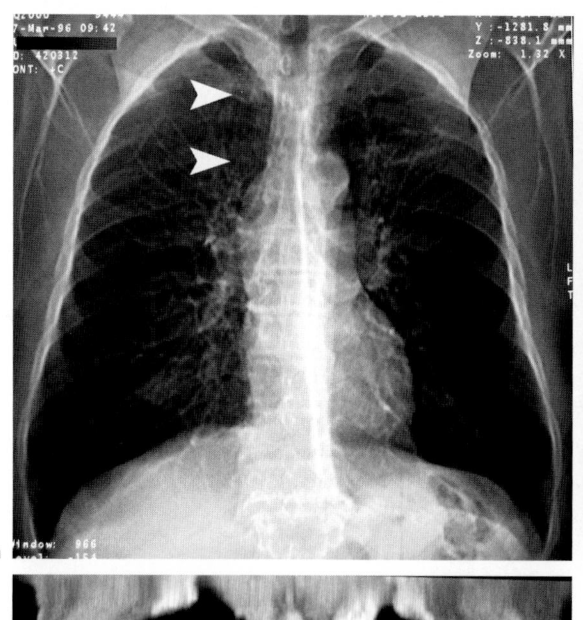

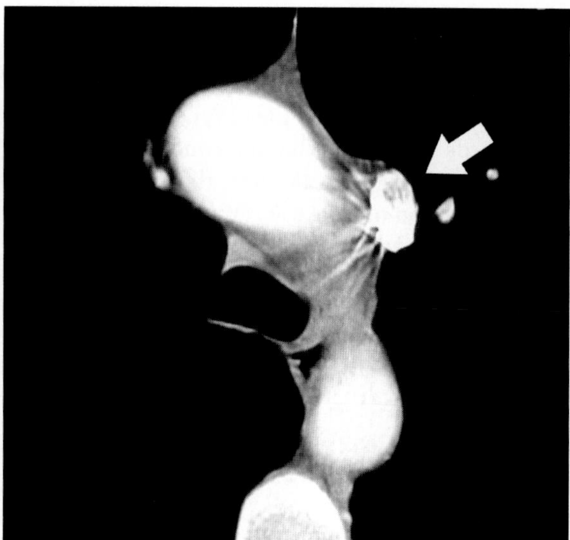

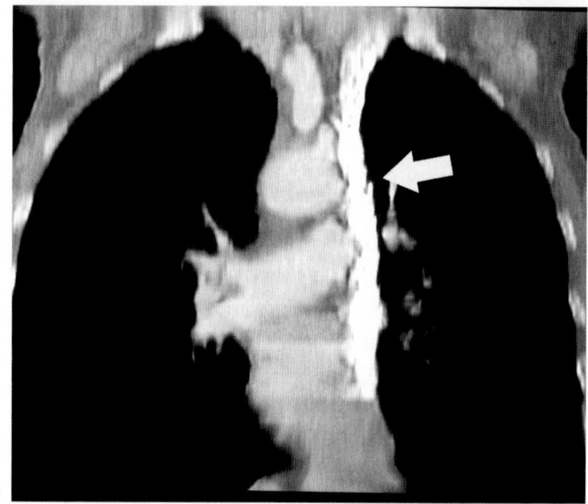

Fig. 20.6a–c. Single LSVC (*arrow*). Chest X-ray shows absence of RSVC shadow (*arrowheads*) in the right superior mediastinum. Correlations with frontal MPR CT reformat

20.4.4 Drainage

In 80-92% of cases, the RSVC drains into the right atrium, while the LSVC drains into the CS without hemodynamic consequences (Schummer et al. 2003; Ratliff et al. 2006). In 8–20% of cases, the LSVC drains into the left atrium and creates a right-to-left shunt, either through an unroofed CS (see below) or in a straight line into the roof of the left atrium (Soward et al. 1986; Leibowitz et al. 1992). The hemodynamic consequences of this shunt will depend on the existence of an associated RSVC and communication through the LIV between both SVCs (Dupuis et al. 1981) (Table 20.1).

20.4.5 Azygos System

In 25% of cases of LSVC, the left hemiazygos vein enters into the LSVC posteriorly, at the same level as the azygos arch on the right (Winter 1954). In case of single LSVC, the azygos system is often reversed, i.e., the azygos vein is left sided and the hemiazygos veins are on the right side, creating a complete situs inversus of the mediastinal venous system (Gris et al. 1995; Peltier et al. 2006). Nevertheless, inversion of the azygos system can also be found in a double SVC (Keyes and Keyes 1925).

Table 20.1. Classification of LSVC according to hemodynamic consequences

<table>
<tr><th colspan="5">Left superior vena cava</th></tr>
<tr><td colspan="3">No hemodynamic anomaly</td><td colspan="2">Hemodynamic anomalies</td></tr>
<tr><td colspan="3">LSVC without associated anomalies or shunt</td><td rowspan="3">Associated congenital anomalies</td><td rowspan="3">Anomalous drainage of LSVC into the left atrium</td></tr>
<tr><td colspan="2">Double SVC</td><td rowspan="2">Single LSCV</td></tr>
<tr><td>Anastomosis through LIV</td><td>No anastomosis</td></tr>
</table>

20.5 Anatomy of LSVC

The LSVC descends vertically, anteriorly and left to the aortic arch and the main pulmonary artery (Fig. 20.4). It is just medial to the left phrenic nerve and along the left mediastinal pleura. Caudally, the LSVC enters the pericardium, runs into the posterior atrio-ventricular groove and drains into the CS (Cha and Khoury 1972; Cormier et al. 1989). The latter is frequently enlarged, particularly when there is no LIV or RSVC, which can be due to either the increased blood flow into the CS or to regurgitant enlargement during atrial contraction (Winter 1954; Cormier et al. 1989).

20.6 Other Presentations of LSVC

20.6.1 Absence of Shunt

Cases of LSVC draining into an obliterated CS have been described, in which the blood flow is reversed and then directed upwards into the right atrium through the LIV and the RSVC (Winter 1954; Harris 1960; Sahinoglu et al. 1994; Muster et al. 1998; Bonnet 2003). Sahinoglu et al. (1994) have reported a case of a LSVC emptying into the upper branch of a double CS that was intramural, crossed the walls of the left and right atria and drained into the right atrium. The lower branch seemed to be a more normal CS and received all main cardiac veins.

Brickner et al. (1990) have reported a case of a left-sided inferior vena cava (IVC), which communicated with LSVC via a dilated hemiazygos vein. This LSVC emptied into a very large CS, while a large hepatic vein drained directly into the right atrium. Sakamoto et al. (1993) have reported a case of a LSVC not draining into the CS and without LIV. The LSVC drained into the RSVC through a transverse anastomosis between the two azygos systems. Taira and Akita (1981) have reported a case of aneurysm of the LSVC that was complicated with rupturing after thrombosis.

20.6.2 Right-to-Left Shunt

The drainage of a LSVC into the left atrium through an unroofed CS, which is an imperfect partitioning of the CS from the left atrium, is responsible for right-to-left shunt (Fig. 20.7) (Mazzucco et al.

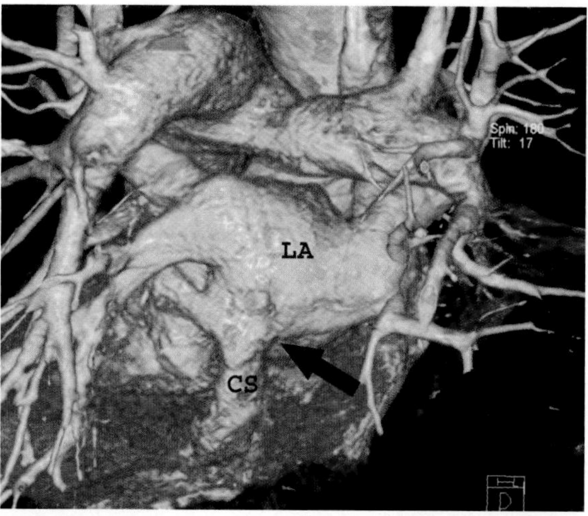

Fig. 20.7. Unroofed coronary sinus. Posterior-view volume-rendering CT reformat shows a defect of partitioning (unroofed coronary sinus) (*arrow*) between the left atrium (*LA*) and the coronary sinus (*CS*)

1990). A LSVC draining directly into the roof of the left atrium has also been described, either associated with a normally formed CS or without CS (Winter 1954; Wiles 1991). Absence of CS has been observed with or without associated congenital anomalies. In these cases, the coronary veins drain directly into a cardiac chamber through Thebesian veins (Muster et al. 1998). LSVC draining into the left superior pulmonary vein has also been described (Fig. 20.8) (McCotter 1916).

Dupuis et al. (1981) have reported a complex cardiopathy associated with an IVC continuation to the hemiazygos, draining into a LSVC and terminating in the left atrium. As a consequence, the entire venous return from the IVC and the LSVC drained into the left atrium.

20.6.3 Left-to-Right Shunt

Connection of LSVC with the left atrium can result in left-to-right shunt in some circumstances. Five cases demonstrated double SVCs with a large LIV, in which there was a higher mean pressure inside the left than in the right atrium. The blood flow was ascending from the left atrium into LSVC, passed through the LIV and the RSVC, and terminated into

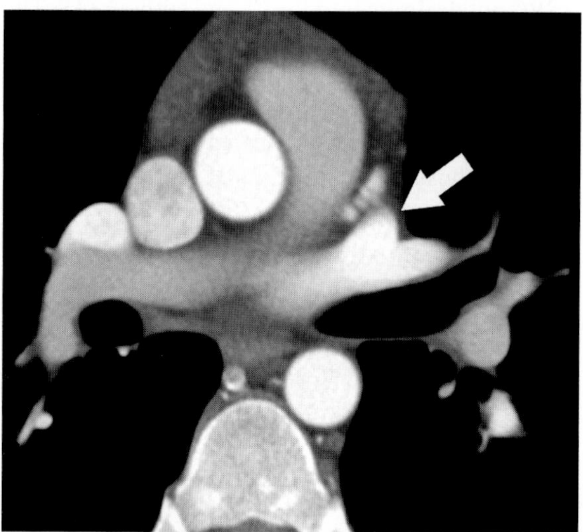

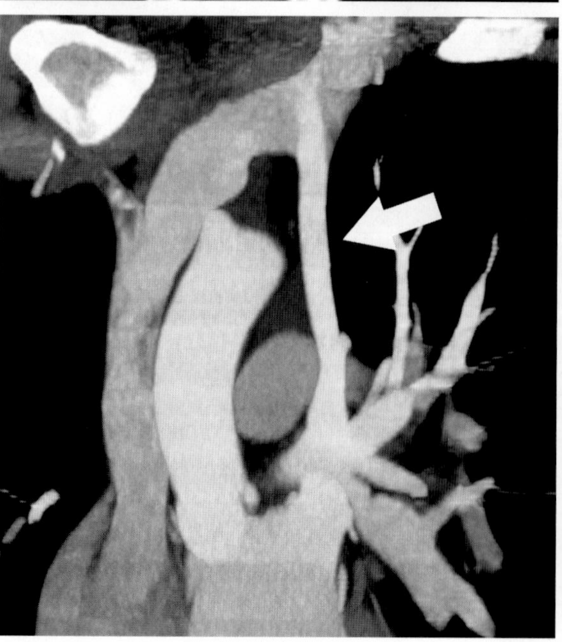

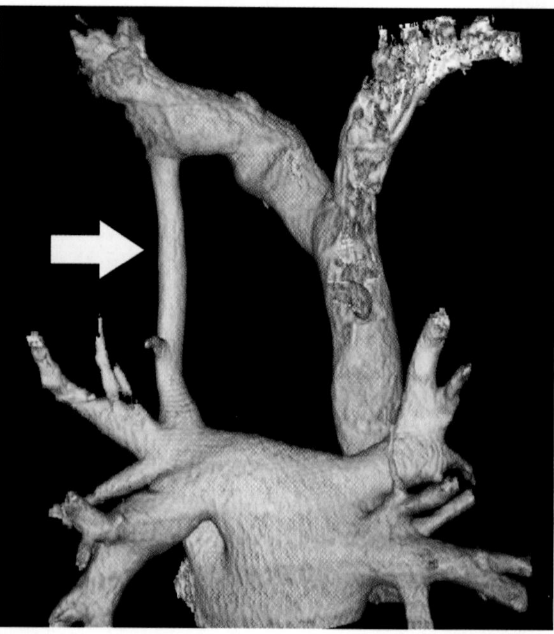

Fig. 20.8a–c. Double SVC with drainage of LSVC into the left atrium. The LSVC (*arrows*) drains directly in the left upper PV (**a**), resulting in R-to-L shunt. Frontal anterior-view MIP CT (**b**) and posterior-view volume-rendering CT (**c**) reformat. (Case courtesy of Dr. C. Deible and Dr. J. Lacomis, University of Pittsburg Medical Center, PA, USA)

the right atrium (Blank and Zuberbuhler 1968; Dupuis et al. 1981). Hipona (1966) has reported a case of an arteriovenous fistula between the posterior circumflex branch of the left coronary artery and a LSVC in a patient presenting with a cardiac murmur.

20.6.4 Complex Cases

Cases of LSVC draining into the right atrium, associated with a RSVC draining to the left atrium and potentially resulting in paradoxical emboli have been described (Rey et al. 1986; Pretorius and Gleeson 2004). Otherwise, the CS can be completely incorporated to the wall of the left atrium, producing a wide communication between both atria, and resulting in a left-to-right shunt associated with a right-to-left shunt due to the LSVC draining to left atrium (Mazzucco et al. 1990).

20.6.5 Associated Congenital Diseases

When found in the fetus or the newborn, persistence of LSVC should raise suspicions about potentially associated cardiac and extra-cardiac malformations, particularly in case of single LSVC (Godwin and Chen 1986; Heye et al. 2007) (Table 20.2). The most common associated cardiac anomalies are atrial septal defect (ASD) and ventricular septal defect (Cha and Khoury 1972; Postema et al. 2007). Tetralogy of Fallot, aortic coartaction, transposition of great vessels and anomalous connections of pulmonary veins have also been reported (Gensini et al. 1959; Heye et al. 2007). The most frequent associated extra-cardiac anomaly is esophageal atresia. Multi-organ syndromes have also been reported, including VACTERL or trisomy 21 (Postema et al. 2007).

20.7 Clinical Presentation

There is no clinical symptom in about 75% of cases with double SVC or single LSVC (Cormier et al. 1989). When the blood flow returns to the venous systemic circulation, there is no hemodynamic consequence (Gensini et al. 1959; Godwin and Chen 1986; Pahwa and Kumar 2003). In patients with associated congenital anomalies, the clinical, electrocardiographic and radiological findings are actually related to these associated abnormalities (Gensini et al. 1959).

When the LSVC drains into the left atrium, the patient can present with variable cyanosis, shortness of breath or pleuritic chest pain (Bonnet 2003;

Table 20.2. Congenital anomalies potentially associated with LSVC (Gensini et al. 1959; Cha and Khoury 1972; Bjerregaard and Laursen 1980; Postema et al. 2007)

Cardiac abnormality	Vascular abnormality
Atrial septal defect	Absent right superior vena cava
Atrioventricular septal defect	Anomalous pulmonary venous return
Bicuspid aortic valve	Aortic stenosis
Ventricular septal defect	Coarctation of aorta
Common atrioventricular canal	Persistent ductus arteriosus
Cor univentriculare	Pulmonary atresia
Dextrorotation of the heart	Transposition of the great arteries
Ebstein anomaly	Pulmonary stenosis
Levocardia	
Single atrium	**Multi-organ syndrome**
Tricuspid atresia	VACTERL association
Underdeveloped left ventricule	Eisenmenger's complex
Truncus arteriosus	Fibroelastosis
	Situs inversus
Abdominal abnormality	Tetralogy of Fallot
Esophageal atresia	Trisomy
Asplenia	
Partial transposition of the viscera	

Pretorius and Gleeson 2004). This anatomical presentation is frequently associated with an ASD (Mazzucco et al. 1990). When both SVCs coexist, they communicate through the LIV, and the cyanosis may or may not be present, depending on the volume and the direction of the blood flow through this anastomosis (Rey et al. 1986; Pretorius and Gleeson 2004). Persistent LSVC draining into the left atrium has the same risks as other right-to-left shunt anomalies, i.e., paradoxical embolism with stroke or intracranial abscess (Fig. 20.9) (Rey et al. 1986; Troost et al. 2006).

20.8 Imaging

20.8.1 X-Ray

Routine chest X-ray performed after insertion of a central venous catheter or cardiac pacemaker can suggest a diagnosis of LSVC (Fig. 20.10) (Heye et al. 2007). LSVC can also produce a widening of the left superior mediastinum or a crescentic vascular

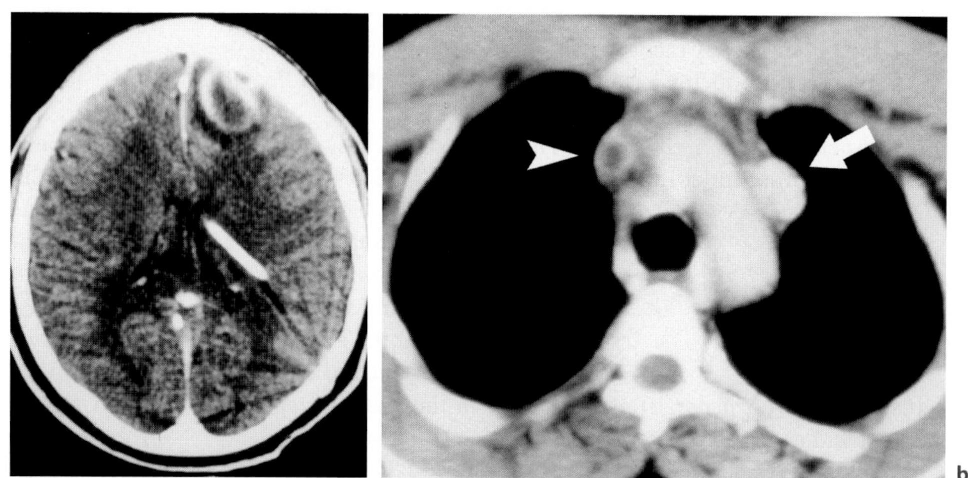

Fig. 20.9a,b. Paradoxical emboli. CT shows a left frontal brain abscess in a patient with double SVC. Note a clot in the RSVC (*arrowheads*). The LSVC (*arrow*) was draining into the left atrium and produced a R-to-L shunt, responsible for paradoxical emboli

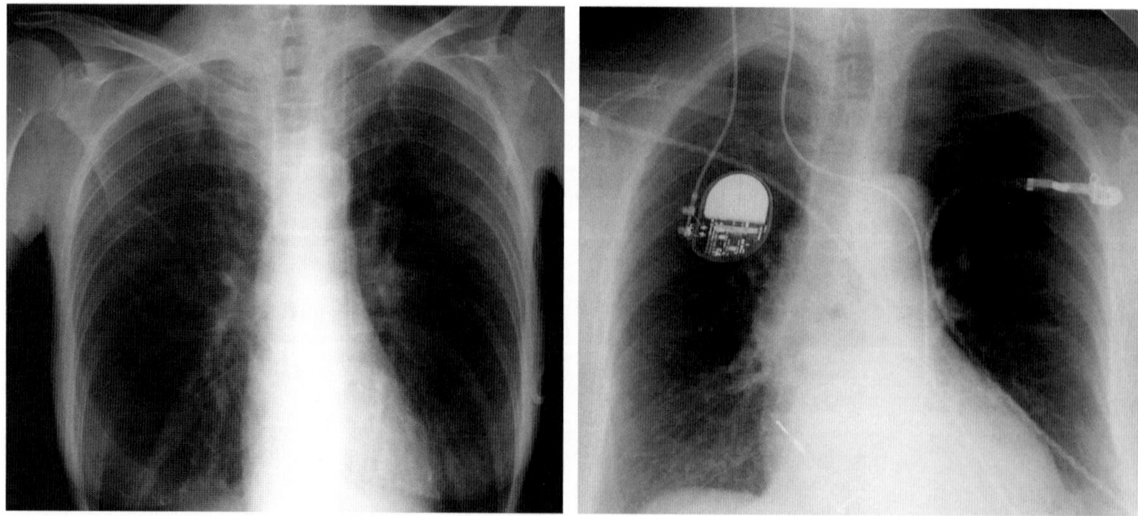

Fig. 20.10a,b. Intravascular material. Chest X-ray shows central venous catheter (**a**) and pacemaker (**b**) inside LSVC

shadow extending from the left superior margin of the aortic arch to the left clavicle (Jaafar et al. 1999; Ratliff et al. 2006). A widening of the aortic shadow or of the vascular pedicle, paramediastinal bulging under the aortic arch or a specific strip of low density along the upper left cardiac margin can also be observed (Cha and Khoury 1972; Sarodia and Stoller 2000; Pahwa and Kumar 2003). The RSVC opacity can also be missing in case of single LSVC (Fig. 20.6) (Lenox et al. 1980; Heye et al. 2007).

20.8.2 Computed Tomography

Non-enhanced acquisition can provide useful information, but definite visualization of the SVCs requires the use of intravenous contrast medium. The left mediastinal smooth tubular formation has a route that is symmetrical to the RSVC, descending on the lateral border of the aortic arch, and then joining the hilum ahead of the left main bronchus. Finally, the vein terminates into a dilated CS, but, since LSVC enters the pericardium, it may no longer be well visualized (Huggins et al. 1982; Jaafar et al. 1999; Peltier et al. 2006).

Contrast medium injection should be bi-brachial as often as possible. Otherwise, left-sided is preferentially used. To minimize artifacts of beam hardening and laminar flow, the volume of injected medium should be important (100–150 cc), with a low concentration and a flow of 2 ml/s (Lagrange et al. 2003). Thus, CM should be injected simultaneously in both arms by one injector through an Y-adapter at 4 ml/s (2 ml/s for each side). The contrast medium amount will be about 30–40 ml (300 mg I/ml) diluted in 80–120 ml of saline. Scanning should begin after 15 s, and a flush of additional saline can be administered after the acquisition.

Multiplanar reformatting at workstations offers an excellent opportunity to produce venography-like images and helps in the assessment of the anomaly using cine viewing, maximum intensity projection and volume-rendering techniques (Fig. 20.5) (Herold et al. 2001).

20.8.3 Other Explorations

20.8.3.1 Conventional Venography

Conventional venography has been the gold standard for diagnosis of LSVC before the advent of CT. Contrast medium has to be injected through a left venous access and the film taken in the antero-posterior position to demonstrate its drainage (Fig. 20.11) (Gensini et al. 1959). Nevertheless, contrast medium must be simultaneously injected through a bi-brachial access to investigate the entire upper systemic venous system.

20.8.3.2 Echocardiography

A dilated CS suggesting LSVC and sometimes the LSVC itself can be visualized at echocardiography (Ratliff et al. 2006; Heye et al. 2007). Contrast-enhanced echocardiography can be performed to explore a dilated CS and possibly associated cardiac abnormalities (Boussuges et al. 1997).

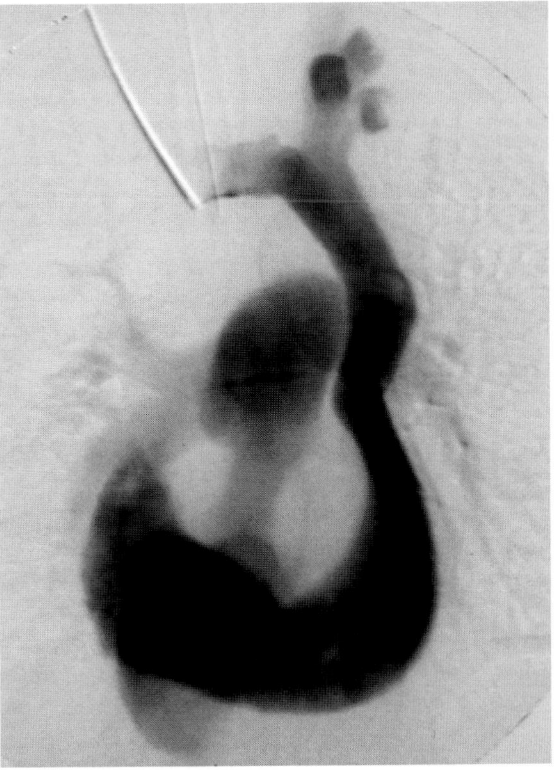

Fig. 20.11. Single LSVC. Single LSVC draining into coronary sinus on conventional venography

20.8.3.3 MRI

LSVC can be evidenced by MRI with or without the use of contrast medium (Fisher et al. 1985; Boussuges et al. 1997; Jaafar et al. 1999). MRI also supplies precise demonstration of the venous anomaly, flow direction, its drainage and associated cardiovascular malformations (Fisher et al. 1985; White et al. 1997).

20.9 Differential Diagnosis

20.9.1 Left Mediastinal Veins

LSVC must be distinguished from other veins that may present with a vertical course through the left side of the mediastinum (Figs. 20.12 and 20.13) (Gris et al. 1995):

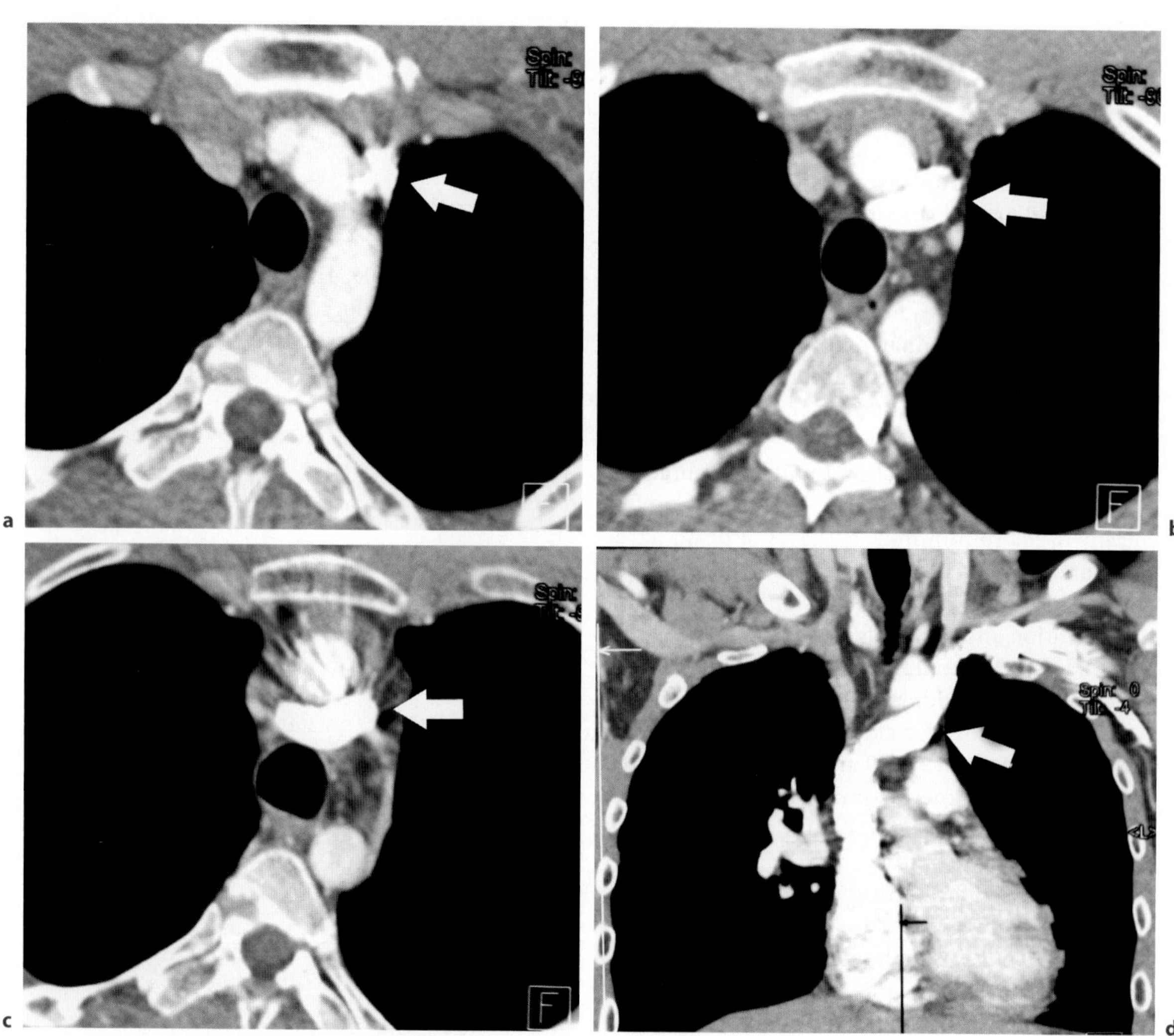

Fig. 20.12a–d. Infra-aortic left innominate vein. CT shows the left innominate vein (*arrows*) passing laterally to (**a**) and then below (**b**) the aortic arch, before joining the right innominate vein to form the SVC (**c**). Frontal MPR CT reformat (**d**)

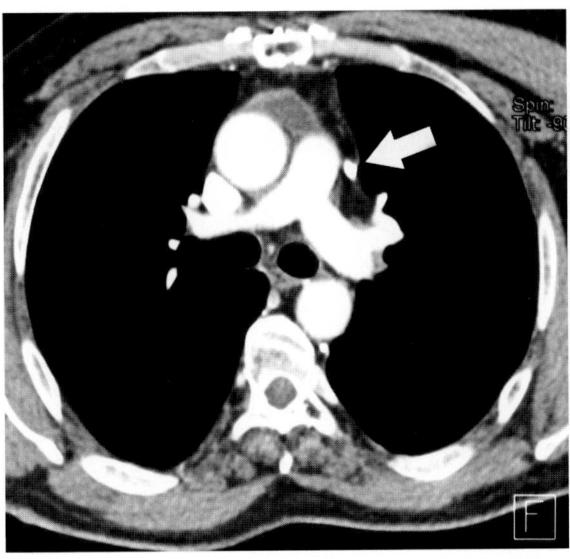

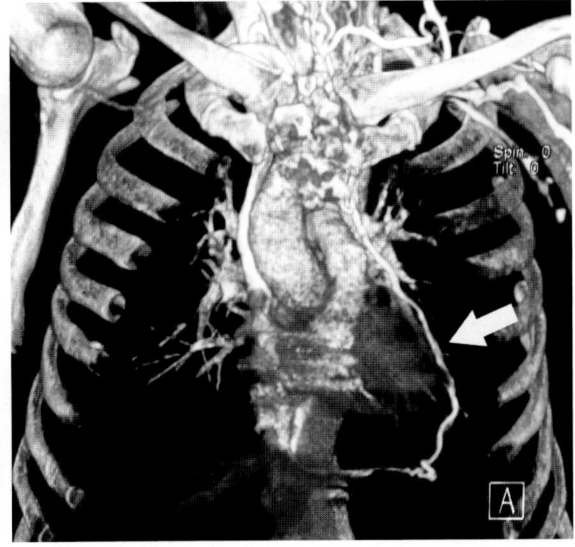

a b

Fig. 20.13a,b. Pericardiophrenic vein. CT shows a dilated pericardiophrenic vein (*arrow*) descending vertically into the left anterior mediastinum in a patient presenting with occlusion of the left innominate vein. Frontal volume-rendering CT reformat shows the usual course lateral to and below the left ventricle, and finally drainage into the IVC (**b**)

- Left vertical vein
- Left infra-aortic innominate vein
- Hemiazygo-caval continuation
- Dilated pericardiophrenic vein
- Dilated left superior intercostal vein

20.9.2 Left Vertical Vein

LSVC has not to be confused with a left vertical vein. Even if both veins may share some common embryologic origins, they should be differentiated in terms of anatomy and blood flow. The left vertical vein drains a partial or total anomalous pulmonary venous return into the LIV (see Chap. 21) (Cha and Khoury 1972; Cormier et al. 1989; Wiles 1991). Usually the blood flow in the left vertical vein is directed upwards, whereas in the LSVC the blood flow is directed downwards. Nevertheless, as previously mentioned, inversed blood flow in a LSVC has also been reported.

20.9.3 Anomalous Route of the Left Innominate Vein

The LIV can present with a more vertical course than usual and cross the mediastinum below the aortic arch (Fig. 20.12) (Bonnet 2003). Then the LIV joins the SVC between the azygos arch and the superior cavo-atrial junction. In most cases, the subaortic LIV runs anterior to the arterial ligament or a patent arterial duct (Mill et al. 1993). This anomaly is particularly found in association with the tetralogy of Fallot with a right aortic arch (Bonnet 2003).

20.9.4 Left Paramediastinal Catheter Position on Frontal Chest X-Ray

A lateral chest X-ray obtained during injection of contrast medium through the catheter is a fast, economical and reliable method for differentiating a correct position in a LSVC from a left-sided extravascular or an intravascular mal-positioning along the left border of the mediastinum (Schummer et al. 2003) (Table 20.3).

20.9.5 Dilated Coronary Sinus

The dilatation of the CS is frequent in presence of a LSVC, but can also be found in other anomalies (Table 20.4).

Table 20.3. Intravascular and extravascular positioning of catheters on the left side of the mediastinum (Marret et al. 2000; Kazerooni and Gross 2004; Konvicka and Villamaria 2005; Ratliff et al. 2006)

Intra-vascular positioning	Extra-vascular positioning
Left superior vena cava	Pleural space
Left superior intercostal vein	Pericardium
Left pericardiophrenic vein	Mediastinum
Left internal thoracic vein	
Left subclavian or carotid artery	
Descending thoracic aorta	
Left thymic vein	
Left-sided small mediastinal vein	
Thoracic duct	

Table 20.4. Differential diagnosis of dilated CS (Tak et al. 2002; Bonnet 2003)

LSVC
Isolated atresia or stenosis of the CS
Partial anomalous hepatic venous connection to CS
Partially unroofed CS
Anomalous pulmonary venous return to CS
Coronary arterio-venous fistula
Aneurysm of the CS

20.10 Complications and Implications

20.10.1 Clinical

The attitude to adopt towards a catheter localized in a LSVC remains controversial. Most authors suggest leaving the catheter in place, but others advise placing a new central venous catheter in another location (Marret et al. 2000). Furthermore, the placement of a central venous catheter, cardiac catheterization or cardiac pacemaker leads may pose difficulties when LSVC has not been suspected previously (Corbisiero et al. 2003; Schummer et al. 2003; Heye et al. 2007). Procedure of pacemaker leads implantation via the transvenous approach is more difficult and makes instability of leads more common (Corbisiero et al. 2003). Ineffective pacemaker activity up to sudden death has also been reported (Soward et al. 1986). A case of fatal perforation of the innominate vein by venous catheter has been described in a patient having a LSVC without RSVC (Schummer et al. 2003).

Occasionally LSVC can be associated with cardiac arrhythmia (ventricular fibrillation and conduction troubles), probably due to the stretching of the atrioventricular node and bundle of His, as consequences of the enlargement of the CS that is located just near the nodal tissue (Momma and Linde 1969; Lenox et al. 1980; Pugliese et al. 1984; Huang 1986; Page et al. 1990; Ratliff et al. 2006; Paval and Nayak 2007).

20.10.2 Cardiac Catheterism

During cardiac catheterization of patients with LSVC via the anomalous vein, chest pain, angina, increased risk of arrhythmia, cardiac arrest or even electrocardiographic changes consistent with myocardial ischemia have been reported (Colman 1967; Godwin and Chen 1986; Peltier et al. 2006). Such complications seem to occur with higher frequency than in the normal population with RSVC (Huggins et al. 1982). Supraventricular tachycardia has been reported in 38% of patients catheterized through a LSVC, compared to 7.9% in patients catheterized through a RSVC (Bunger et al. 1981). Rare cases of fatal outcome have been reported after repeated manipulations or vigorous effort during the cardiac catheterization (Gensini et al. 1959).

20.10.3 Surgical

LSVC is important to known before cardiothoracic surgery, as it requires special handling when a cardiopulmonary bypass or an intra-operative pacemaker implantation is necessary (Horwitz et al. 1973; Huggins et al. 1982; Heye et al. 2007). Appropriate cannulation techniques should be applied to eliminate the large amount of systemic venous blood that enters the heart through the CS (Schummer et al. 2003). Furthermore, the presence of anastomosis between both SVCs or the rare absence of the RSVC has to be investigated, otherwise ligation of the LSVC would result in a SVC syndrome (Schummer et al. 2003; Peltier et al. 2006). The retrograde cardioplegia through an unexpected LSVC can lead to inadequate myocardial perfusion and so be ineffective (Sarodia and Stoller 2000; Ratliff et al. 2006). The surgeon must also pay attention to cases of ostial atresia of the CS that drains the LSVC, which implies that the LSVC cannot be interrupted due to the risk of myocardial ischemia and necrosis (Sarodia and Stoller 2000).

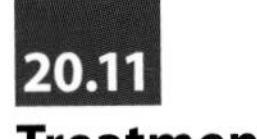

20.11 Treatment

20.11.1 LSVC into the Right Atrium

LSVC draining into right atrium is not a cyanogenous malformation and does not require surgery (Page et al. 1990). Catheter ablation using radiofrequency is possible and safe in patients with arrhythmia (Okishige et al. 1997). The region of the CS ostium and the postero-inferior area of Koch's triangle are suggested sites of successful ablation (Katsivas et al. 2006).

20.11.2 LSVC into the Left Atrium

Various surgical treatments have been described, based on associated vascular and cardiac anomalies. LSVC can be tunnelled into the right atrium together with a simultaneous closure of the ASD, or the LSVC can be reimplanted into the right atrium or the left pulmonary artery (Dupuis et al. 1981; Pugliese et al. 1984; Rey et al. 1986). Unroofed CS can be treated by a running suture (Mazzucco et al. 1990). The LSVC can be ligatured only in cases when a RSVC and a LIV co-exist. Nevertheless, in case of CS ostium atresia, the only outlet of the blood flow is the LSVC. Its ligation or division results in severe, acute coronary venous hypertension (Muster et al. 1998). Percutaneous closure of a persistent LSVC draining into the left atrium has been reported with occluder devices (Troost et al. 2006; Abadir et al. 2007). Heng and De Giovanni (1997) have reported a case of a large LSVC draining into an unroofed CS successfully occluded by a transcatheter delivery of a vena cava filter packed with detachable coils.

References

Abadir S, Bouzguenda I, Boudjemline Y et al. (2007) Percutaneous occlusion of a left superior vena cava draining into the left atrium: two case reports. Arch Mal Coeur Vaiss 100:470–473

Ancel P, Villemin F (1908) Sur la persistance de la veine cave supérieure gauche chez l'homme. J de l'anat 44:46–62

Bjerregaard P, Laursen HB (1980) Persistent left superior vena cava. Incidence, associated congenital heart defects and frontal plane P-wave axis in a paediatric population with congenital heart disease. Acta Paediatr Scand 69:105–108

Blank E, Zuberbuhler JR (1968) Left to right shunt through a left atrial left superior vena cava. Am J Roentgenol Radium Ther Nucl Med 103:87–92

Bonnet D (2003) Anomalies du retour veineux systémique. Encycl Méd Chir (Elsevier, Paris), Radiodiagnostic-Coeur-Poumon 32-016-A-15:1–4

Boussuges A, Ambrosi P, Gainnier M et al. (1997) Left-sided superior vena cava: diagnosis by magnetic resonance imaging. Int Care Med 23:702–703

Brickner ME, Eichhorn EJ, Netto D et al. (1990) Left-sided inferior vena cava draining into the coronary sinus via persistent left superior vena cava: case report and review of the literature. Cathet Cardiovasc Diagn 20:189–192

Buirski G, Jordan SC, Joffe HS et al. (1986) Superior vena caval abnormalities: their occurrence rate, associated cardiac abnormalities and angiographic classification in a paediatric population with congenital heart disease. Clin Radiol 37:131–138

Bunger PC, Neufeld DA, Moore JC et al. (1981) Persistent left superior vena cava and associated structural and functional considerations. Angiology 32:601–608

Cha EM, Khoury GH (1972) Persistent left superior vena cava. Radiologic and clinical significance. Radiology 103:375–381

Colman AL (1967) Diagnosis of left superior vena cava by clinical inspection, a new physical sign. Am Heart J 73:115–120

Corbisiero R, DeVita M, Dennis C (2003) Pacemaker implantation in a patient with persistent left superior vena cava and absent right superior vena cava. J Interv Card Electrophysiol 9:35–37

Cormier MG, Yedlicka JW, Gray RJ et al. (1989) Congenital anomalies of the superior vena cava: a CT study. Semin Roentgenol 24:77–83

Dupuis C, Pernot C, Rey C et al. (1981) Left superior vena cava communicating with the left atrium. Apropos of eight cases. Arch Mal Coeur Vaiss 74:507–516
Fisher MR, Hricak H, Higgins CB (1985) Magnetic resonance imaging of developmental venous anomalies. AJR Am J Roentgenol 145:705–709
Gensini GG, Caldini P, Casaccio F et al. (1959) Persistent left superior vena cava. Am J Cardiol 4:677–685
Godwin JD, Chen JT (1986) Thoracic venous anatomy. AJR Am J Roentgenol 147:674–684
Gris P, Wilmet B, Benchillal A et al. (1995) Persistent left superior vena cava. Apropos of two cases. Rev Pneumol Clin 51:33–35
Hansell DM, Armstrong P, Lynch DA et al. (2004) The normal chest. In: Hansell DM, Armstrong P, Lynch DA, McAdams HP (eds) Imaging of diseases of the chest, 4th edn, pp 27–67
Harris WG (1960) A case of bilateral superior venae cavae with a closed coronary sinus. Thorax 15:172–173
Heng JT, De Giovanni JV (1997) Occlusion of persistent left superior vena cava to unroofed coronary sinus using vena cava filter and coils. Heart 77:579–580
Herold CJ, Bankier AA, Fleischmann D (2001) Spiral CT of the superior vena cava. In: Remy-Jardin M, Remy J (eds) Spiral CT of the chest. Springer, Berlin Heidelberg New York, pp 265–281
Heye T, Wengenroth M, Schipp A et al. (2007) Persistent left superior vena cava with absent right superior vena cava: morphological CT features and clinical implications. Int J Cardiol 116:e103–105
Hipona FA (1966) Congenital coronary arterial fistula to a persistent left superior vena cava. Am J Roentgenol Radium Ther Nucl Med 97:355–358
Horwitz S, Esquivel J, Attie F et al. (1973) Clinical diagnosis of persistent left superior vena cava by observation of jugular pulses. Am Heart J 86:759–763
Huang SK (1986) Persistent left superior vena cava in a man with ventricular fibrillation. Chest 89:155–157
Huggins TJ, Lesar ML, Friedman AC et al. (1982) CT appearance of persistent left superior vena cava. J Comput Assist Tomogr 6:294–297
Jaafar S, Hennequin L, Fays J et al. (1999) Exploration de la veine cave supérieure et sa pathologie. Encycl Méd Chir (Elsevier, Paris), Radiodiagnostic–Coeur-Poumon 32-225-F-20:1–25
Katsivas A, Koutouzis M, Nikolidakis S et al. (2006) Persistent left superior vena cava associated with common type AV nodal reentrant tachycardia and AV reentrant tachycardia due to concealed left lateral accessory pathway. Int J Cardiol 113:E124–125
Kazerooni EA and Gross BH (2004) Cardiopulmonary Imaging. Lippincott, Williams and Wilkins, Philadelphia
Kellman GM, Alpern MB, Sandler MA et al. (1988) Computed tomography of vena caval anomalies with embryologic correlation. Radiographics 8:533–556
Keyes DC, Keyes HC (1925) A case of persistent of left superior vena cava with reversed azygos system. Anatom Record 31:23–26
Konvicka JJ, Villamaria FJ (2005) Images in anesthesia: anesthetic implications of persistent left superior vena cava. Can J Anaesth 52:805
Lagrange C, El Hajjam M, Pelage JP et al. (2003) Imagerie et angiographie interventionnelle de la veine cave supérieure. In: Jeanbourquin D (eds) Imagerie thoracique de l'adulte. Masson, Paris, pp 629–650
Leibowitz AB, Halpern NA, Lee MH et al. (1992) Left-sided superior vena cava: a not-so-unusual vascular anomaly discovered during central venous and pulmonary artery catheterization. Crit Care Med 20:1119–1122
Lenox CC, Zuberbuhler JR, Park SC et al. (1980). Absent right superior vena cava with persistent left superior vena cava: implications and management. Am J Cardiol 45:117–122
Marret E, Meunier JF, Dubousset AM et al. (2000) Diagnosis of a persistent left superior vena cava in the operating room during a central venous catheterization. Ann Fr Anesth Reanim 19:191–194
Mazzucco A, Bortolotti U, Stellin G et al. (1990) Anomalies of the systemic venous return: a review. J Card Surg 5:122–133
McCotter RE (1916) Three cases of the persistence of the left superior vena cava. Anatom Record 10:371–383
Mill MR, Wilcox BR, Detterbeck FC et al. (1993) Anomalous course of the left brachiocephalic vein. Ann Thorac Surg 55:600–602
Momma K, Linde LM (1969) Abnormal rhythms associated with persistent left superior vena cava. Pediatr Res 3:210–216
Muster AJ, Naheed ZJ, Backer CL et al. (1998) Is surgical ligation of an accessory left superior vena cava always safe? Pediatr Cardiol 19:352–354
Nsah EN, Moore GW, Hutchins GM (1991) Pathogenesis of persistent left superior vena cava with a coronary sinus connection. Pediatr Pathol 11:261–269
Okishige K, Fisher JD, Goseki Y et al. (1997) Radiofrequency catheter ablation for AV nodal reentrant tachycardia associated with persistent left superior vena cava. Pacing Clin Electrophysiol 20(Pt 1):2213–2218
Page Y, Tardy B, Comtet C et al. (1990) Venous catheterization and congenital abnormalities of the superior vena cava. Ann Fr Anesth Reanim 9:450–455
Pahwa R, Kumar A (2003) Persistent left superior vena cava: an intensivist's experience and review of the literature. South Med J 96:528–529
Paval J, Nayak S (2007) A persistent left superior vena cava. Singapore Med J 48:e90–93
Peltier J, Destrieux C, Desme J et al. (2006) The persistent left superior vena cava: anatomical study, pathogenesis and clinical considerations. Surg Radiol Anat 28:206–210
Postema PG, Rammeloo LA, van Litsenburg R et al. (2007) Left superior vena cava in pediatric cardiology associated with extra-cardiac anomalies. Int J Cardiol 121:17–18
Pretorius PM, Gleeson FV (2004) Case 74: right-sided superior vena cava draining into left atrium in a patient with persistent left-sided superior vena cava. Radiology 232:730–734
Pugliese P, Murzi B, Aliboni M et al. (1984) Absent right superior vena cava and persistent left superior vena cava. Clinical and surgical considerations. J Cardiovasc Surg (Torino) 25:134–137
Ratliff HL, Yousufuddin M, Lieving WR et al. (2006) Persistent left superior vena cava: case reports and clinical implications. Int J Cardiol 113:242–246
Rey C, Marache P, Manouvrier J et al. (1986) Double superior vena cava with drainage of the right superior vena cava

into the left auricle. Presentation as a cerebral abscess in an adult. Arch Mal Coeur Vaiss 79:1645–1648

Sahinoglu K, Cassell MD, Miyauchi R et al. (1994) Human persistent left superior vena cava with doubled coronary sinus. Ann Anat 176:451–454

Sakamoto H, Akita K, Sato K et al. (1993) Left superior vena cava continuing to the accessory hemiazygos without anastomosis with the coronary sinus. Surg Radiol Anat 15:151–154

Sarodia BD, Stoller JK (2000) Persistent left superior vena cava: case report and literature review. Respir Care 45:411–416

Schummer W, Schummer C, Frober R (2003) Persistent left superior vena cava and central venous catheter position: clinical impact illustrated by four cases. Surg Radiol Anat 25:315–321

Soward A, Ten Cate F, Fioretti P et al. (1986) An elusive persistent left superior vena cava draining into left atrium. Cardiology 73:368–371

Steinberg I, Dubilier W Jr, Lukas DS (1953) Persistence of left superior vena cava. Dis Chest 24:479–488

Taira A, Akita H (1981) Ruptured venous aneurysm of the persistent left superior vena cava. Angiology 32:656–659

Tak T, Crouch E, Drake GB (2002) Persistent left superior vena cava: incidence, significance and clinical correlates. Int J Cardiol 82:91–93

Troost E, Gewillig M, Budts W (2006) Percutaneous closure of a persistent left superior vena cava connected to the left atrium. Int J Cardiol 106:365–366

Webb WR, Gamsu G, Speckman JM et al. (1982) Computed tomographic demonstration of mediastinal venous anomalies. AJR Am J Roentgenol 139:157–161

White CS, Baffa JM, Haney PJ et al. (1997) MR imaging of congenital anomalies of the thoracic veins. Radiographics 17:595–608

Wiles HB (1991) Two cases of left superior vena cava draining directly to a left atrium with a normal coronary sinus. Br Heart J 65:158–160

Winter FS (1954) Persistent left superior vena cava; survey of world literature and report of 30 additional cases. Angiology 5:90–132

Partial Anomalous Venous Return

21

Benoît Ghaye and Thierry Couvreur

CONTENTS

B. Ghaye, MD
T. Couvreur, MD
Department of Medical Imaging, University Hospital of Liege, 4000 Liege 1, Belgium

Summary

Anomalous pulmonary venous returns (APVRs) are congenital malformations in which a portion or the entirety of the pulmonary veins drains into the right atrium or one of its tributaries, resulting in left-to-right (L-to-R) shunt. Partial APVR (PAPVR) is found in 0.4–0.7% of routine necropsy and in 10–15% of patients with atrial septal defect. PAPVRs occur on the right side twice as often as on the left. PAPVRs can be classified in four groups based on their drainage: into supracardiac veins (SVC, azygos vein, vertical vein, left SVC, etc.), into right atrium or coronary sinus, into infradiaphragmatic veins (IVC, portal vein, etc.), and as mixed patterns. PAPVRs may be completely asymptomatic and incidentally discovered, but some will present with large L-to-R shunt requiring surgery. MDCT is currently considered as a first-line technique in the work-up of PAPVRs, as it evidences the anomalous vein and its drainage and shows associated tracheobronchial, lung or vascular abnormalities.

21.1 Introduction

Congenital anomalies of the pulmonary veins (PV) can be conveniently classified into the following categories: (1) anomalous pulmonary venous return (APVR) with or without abnormal course in the lung, (2) anomalous pulmonary venous route without abnormal connection, or (3) abnormal venous diameters, including varicosities, stenoses, and atresia (Remy-Jardin and Remy 1999). This classification, however, fits with more complex congenital malformations if we accept overlapping conditions between categories.

Anomalies in central and pulmonary venous anatomy can result in significant cardiopulmonary abnormalities, including shunts and paradoxical emboli. Moreover, when unrecognised on preoperative chest CT, such variations can lead to intra- or postoperative complications (Galetta et al. 2006). APVRs are defined as congenital malformations in which a portion or the entirety of the pulmonary venous drainage drains into the right atrium or one of its tributaries instead of the left atrium, resulting in a L-to-R shunt. In partial anomalous pulmonary venous return (PAPVR), the shunt can vary from less than 10% when only a segmental PV is concerned to more than 75% when all but one lobes are involved (Fish et al. 1991).

The first report of APVR was made by Winslow as early as 1739 (cited in Brody 1942). PAPVRs represent 70% of all APVRs (Snellen et al. 1968). PAPVR is found in 0.4–0.7% of routine necropsy, in 10–15% of patients with atrial septal defect (ASD) and almost all patients with sinus venosus type of ostium secundum defect (Healey 1952; Blake et al. 1965; Gotsman et al. 1965; Kalke et al. 1967; Schatz et al. 1986). PAPVRs occur on the right side twice as often as on the left (Brody 1942).

Blake et al. (1965) and Snellen et al. (1968) described more than 30 patterns of APVRs. APVRs can be classified into four groups based on their drainage: (1) into supracardiac veins, (2) into the right atrium or coronary sinus, (3) into infradiaphragmatic veins, and (4) mixed patterns (Darling et al. 1957). APVRs are recognized with increasing frequency at chest or cardiac CTs and are probably more common than previously thought. MDCT is the method of choice in the assessment of congenital anomalies of the pulmonary venous return, enabling a non-invasive evaluation of the associated tracheobronchial, lung parenchyma and pulmonary arterial malformations in the same examination.

21.2 Embryology

21.2.1 Normal Development

PVs originate from a single common PV during the 4th week of gestation before the separation of the right and left atrium. The common PV progresses inside the dorsal mesenchyma of the mesocardium, bridging the heart and the mediastinum, towards concomitantly forming lung buds. The common PV ostium is then displaced to the left by the development of the left valve of the sinus venosus and is located on the left side of the septum primum initiating atrial septation. Subsequently, as the apex of the heart rotates to the left, the left atrium being placed into the dorsal midline position and the right atrium becoming anterior and further positioned to the right, the common PV is incorporated into the left dorsal atrium. This complex remodelling of the heart occurs until the 7th week of gestational age. Further incorporation is gained with continuous growth of the atrial chamber (Bliss and Hutchins 1995).

On the other hand, pulmonary venous blood is drained via the primitive pulmonary splanchnic plexus into the primordium of the systemic venous system, including the anterior and posterior cardinal veins (CVs) and the umbilicovitelline veins (Fig. 21.1). By the 4th week of gestation, connections develop between the common PV and the pulmonary venous plexus, while most connections with the splanchnic plexus, CVs and umbilicovitelline veins are lost (Healey 1952; Neill 1956; Zylak et al. 2002).

21.2.2 PAPVR

It is probable that multiple pathogenic mechanisms are needed to explain all anatomic variations of PAPVRs. First, failure of connections between the primitive pulmonary splanchnic plexus and the common PV may result in persistence of embryonic anastomosis between the primitive pulmonary splanchnic plexus and the CVs (SVC and tributaries, left SVC), cardiac (right atrium, coronary sinus) or umbilicovitelline (IVC, portal vein) veins (Brody 1942; Healey 1952; Neill 1956; Darling et al. 1957). According to some authors, bronchial veins could play a key role in the occurrence and course

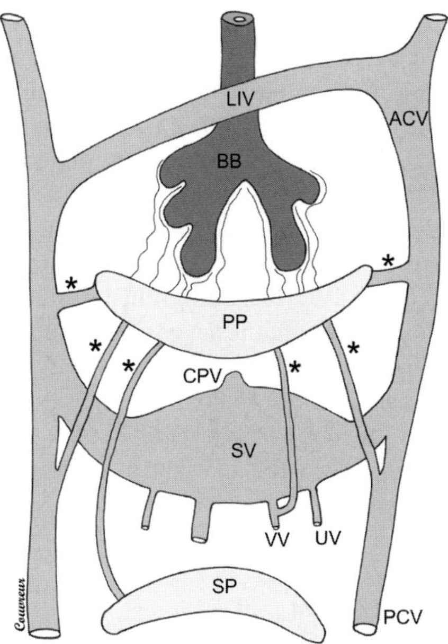

Fig. 21.1. Embryological anastomoses between the pulmonary plexus and the systemic veins (*stars*). *BB* bronchial buds, *ACV* anterior cardinal vein, *PCV* posterior cardinal vein, *PP* pulmonary plexus, *LIV* left innominate vein, *VV* vitelline vein, *UV* umbilical vein, *SV* sinus venosus, *CPV* common pulmonary vein, *SP* splanchnic plexus

of PAPVRs (Okamoto et al. 2004). Similarly, CT opacification of PVs through a reverse flow resulting in a R-to-L shunt have been described in patients with SVC syndrome (Grayet et al. 2001).

Second, any shift of the common PV with regard to the atrial septum during rotation of the sinus venosus to the right may result in part of the common PV being incorporated into the right side of the primitive atrium and may explain APVR into the right atrium or in the nearby located SVC, IVC and coronary sinus (Brody 1942; Healey 1952; Neill 1956). Depending on the degrees of shift and of incorporation of the common PV in the atrial wall, it may result in partial or total APVR in the right atrium or closely located structures (Snellen et al. 1968).

21.3 Normal Pattern of the Pulmonary Venous Return

Modal anatomy is found in around 70% of individuals and consists of four PVs, two superior and two inferior veins. Anatomical variations of number and branching patterns are related to under- or over-incorporation of the common PV into the left dorsal atrium, occurring during embryological development (Healey 1952; Ghaye et al. 2003). Under-incorporation, which can occur asymmetrically, may result into a confluence, either of both PVs on the same side, the most common variation found in 12–25% usually on the left side, or of both superior or inferior PVs (Healey 1952). The extreme situation is related to the rare persistence of the former common PV, eventually leading to cor triatriatum in case of narrowing of the common chamber opening into the left atrium (Grondin et al. 1964). On the other hand, over-incorporation beyond the first division is responsible for supernumerary or accessory PVs. An increase in number of PVs occurs more frequently on the right side (Budorick et al. 1989). Variations of the right middle lobe PV connection may also be frequently encountered, draining into the right superior PV in 53–69%, into the left atrium with an independent ostium in 17–23%, and into the right inferior PV in 3–8% (Tsao et al. 2001; Yazar et al. 2002). In the latter, pulmonary oedema or infarction of the middle lobe could result when ligation of right lower PV is performed during lower lobectomy (Remy-Jardin and Remy 1999). Similarly, the lingular vein has been reported to drain into the left inferior PV in 2.5% of cases (Sugimoto et al. 1998). More than three PVs and up to seven by side have been rarely reported, but one or more of these PVs usually present with an APVR in most cases (Healey 1952).

21.4 Global Anomalous Pulmonary Venous Return

In global or total APVR, no PV drains into the left atrium. PVs join directly behind the heart and drain into supracardiac veins (50%), cardiac structures (30%), infradiaphragmatic veins (15%), or mixed pattern (5%) (Healey 1952; Darling et al. 1957). ASD or patent ductus arteriosus is necessary for survival (Brody 1942; Healey 1952; Kalke et al. 1967). Cyanosis frequently occurs at birth or in early childhood. Blockage of APVR is a surgical emergency in the newborn. Other cardiovascular abnormalities are present in 36% of cases (Nakib et al. 1967). Mortality is around 40% during infancy, even after surgical correction (Fraser et al. 1999).

21.5 Partial Anomalous Pulmonary Venous Return

In PAPVRs, one or many PVs drain(s) into other structures than the left atrium. The number of anomalous PVs is variable. In two series of 28 and 43 patients, 53–71% had a single, 11–42% had two, 2–14% had three, 2% had four and 4% had six anomalous PVs (Ammash et al. 1997; Hijii et al. 1998). PAPVR usually drains into a reservoir located in the proximity, i.e., into (a) right-sided collector(s) for right lung PVs and into (a) left-sided for left lung PVs, but "cross-mediastinal" drainage may be occasionally seen. Similarly, upper PVs tend to drain into superiorly located reservoirs, while lower PVs drain in inferiorly located structures (Snellen et al. 1968). The left lower lobe shows the lower rate of PAPVR (Healey 1952).

Sixty to ninety percent of PAPVRs involve the right lung. Right-sided PAPVR usually drains into the SVC (18–59%), the azygos vein (1–3%), the right atrium (20–46%), or the supradiaphragmatic part of the IVC (1–5%). Left-sided PAPVR usually drains into the left innominate vein (LIV), either directly or via a vertical vein (15–21%), a persistent left SVC (LSVC) (8%), the coronary sinus (1–3%), a pericardiophrenic vein, or the hemiazygos vein. Exceptionally PAPVR can drain into the subclavian vein, left ventricle and thoracic duct. PAPVRs can drain into infradiaphragmatic structures (2–4%), including the IVC, hepatic veins and portal vein (Brody 1942; Healey 1952; Blake et al. 1965; Kalke et al. 1967; Ammash et al. 1997).

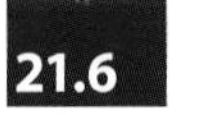

21.6 Types of PAPVR

21.6.1 Right Lung

21.6.1.1 PAPVR in the SVC or the Azygos Vein

PAPVR in the SVC or azygos vein concerns more frequently the right upper PV than the right lower PV (Fish et al. 1991). The most frequent is the connection of the right upper PV at the junction between the SVC and right atrium, directly above a sinus venosus type ASD (Blake et al. 1965). This type of PAPVR may be underdetected on CT, as findings are more subtle than for PAPVR in other locations, and as part of the corresponding PV may still be visible in the hilum (Haramati et al. 2003; Galetta et al. 2006). Similarly, differentiation between anomalous drainage into the azygos arch and the posterior aspect of the SVC may be difficult, particularly in the presence of streak artefacts due to dense contrast medium (CM) in the SVC (Fig. 21.2). When drainage occurs into the azygos vein, the azygos arch shadow is enlarged on frontal chest X-ray (Fig. 21.3) (Schatz et al. 1986; Thorsen et al. 1990; Posniak et al. 1993). Flow reversal in the SVC at the level of PAPVR and subsequent drainage via the LIV and a persistent LSVC has been reported (Fish et al. 1991).

21.6.1.2 PAPVR in the Right Atrium

PAPVR draining into the right atrium is usually a consequence of abnormal development of the septum secundum, which is shifted to the left. In consequence, one or both right-sided PVs drain into the right atrium (Hijii et al. 1998). PAPVR in right atrium is frequently associated with ASD (Kalke et al. 1967; Gustafson et al. 1989; Pucelikova et al. 2007).

21.6.1.3 PAPVR in the IVC

Anomalous drainage into the IVC represents 1–5% of all PAPVRs and concerns the whole right lung in 60–80% or one to two right lobe(s) in 20–40% (Mathey et al. 1968; Dupuis et al. 1992). Most cases are sporadic, but genetic factors have been suggested as familial cases are reported (Fraser et al. 1999). PAPVR in the IVC is also known as the Halasz syndrome or as the scimitar syndrome due to the demonstration of the "Turkish curved sword" aspect of the anomalous PV on frontal chest X-ray (Fig. 21.4) (Halasz et al. 1956). Nevertheless, the anomalous PV may be thin, straight or multiple (Godwin and Tarver 1986). Exceptional cases occur on the left side (D'Cruz and Arcilla 1964; Mardini et al. 1981). Drainage is either into the infra-diaphragmatic part of the IVC (76%) or at the junction between the IVC and right atrium (24%) (Dupuis et al. 1992). Accessory areas of drainage, including SVC, coronary sinus, right or left atrium, hepatic vein, portal vein and azygos vein have been reported in 37% (Mathey et al. 1968; Woodring et al. 1994; Schramel et al. 1995).

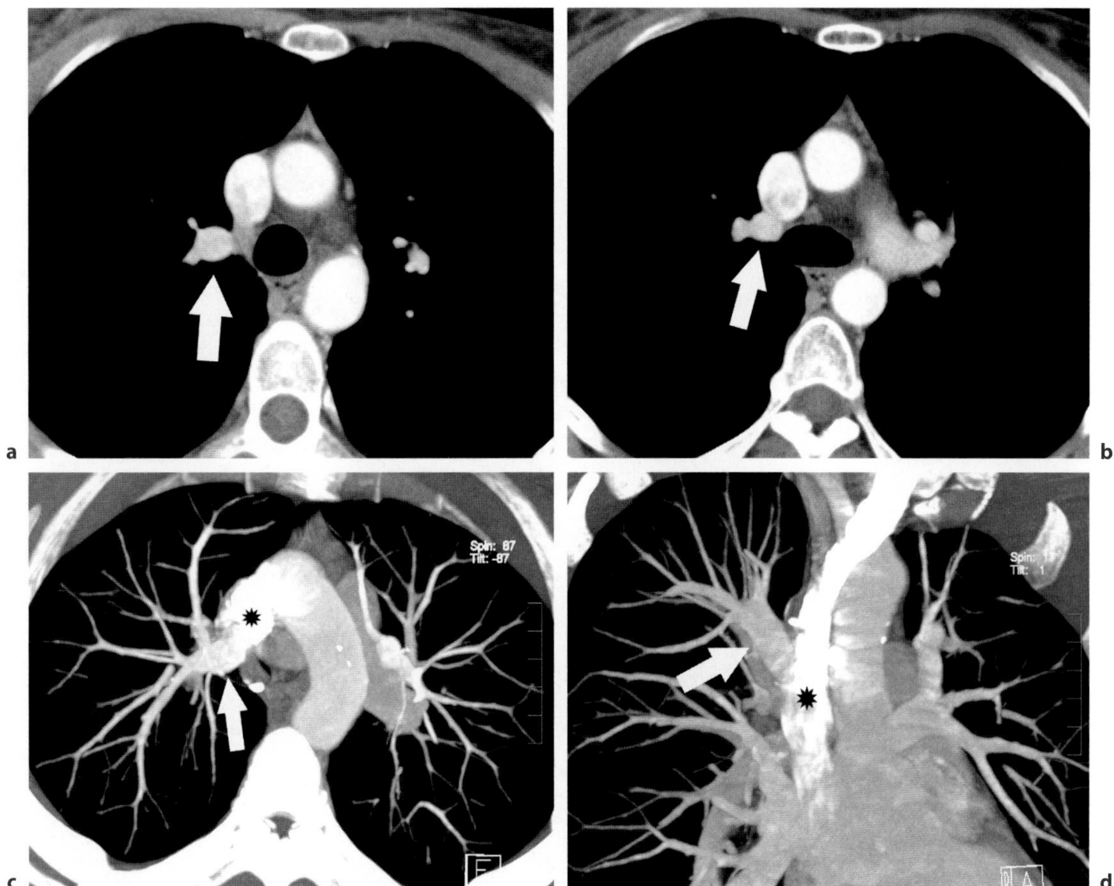

Fig. 21.2a–d. PAPVR at the junction between azygos vein and the SVC (*arrows*). The junction between PAPVR and systemic reservoir may be difficult to evidence due to high contrast in SVC (*stars*). Note dilatation of venous structures in the anomalous area compared to the other side on MIP reformatting (**c**,**d**). Three other right-sided PVs are draining into the left atrium (**d**)

The scimitar syndrome often, but not always, includes a spectrum of associated anomalies including (Halasz et al. 1956; Mathey et al. 1968; Dupuis et al. 1992):

- abnormal lobation of the right lung with mediastinal shift to the right, also called hypogenetic right lung syndrome
- "dextrocardia" – dextroposition – dextroversion of the heart
- pulmonary arterial anomalies (small ipsilateral pulmonary artery in half of patients)
- systemic arterial supply originating from the abdominal aorta and less frequently from thoracic descending aorta, which is responsible for further increase of the L-to-R shunt (48%)
- other tracheal or bronchial malformations (cysts or diverticula, bronchiectasis in up to 14%)
- accessory hemidiaphragm, diaphragmatic eventration
- horseshoe lung
- other cardiovascular anomalies in 25%, most frequently interatrial communication

The scimitar sign on chest X-ray may be absent or overlooked in more than 50% of the patients at initial presentation, particularly in children (Gazzaniga et al. 1969; Dupuis et al. 1992; Brown et al. 2003).

21.6.1.4 Others

Cases of right PAPVRs have been rarely reported in the subclavian vein, innominate vein, pericardiophrenic vein, hepatic vein, and portal vein or one of its tributaries (Brody 1942; Snellen et al. 1968; Mardini et al. 1981).

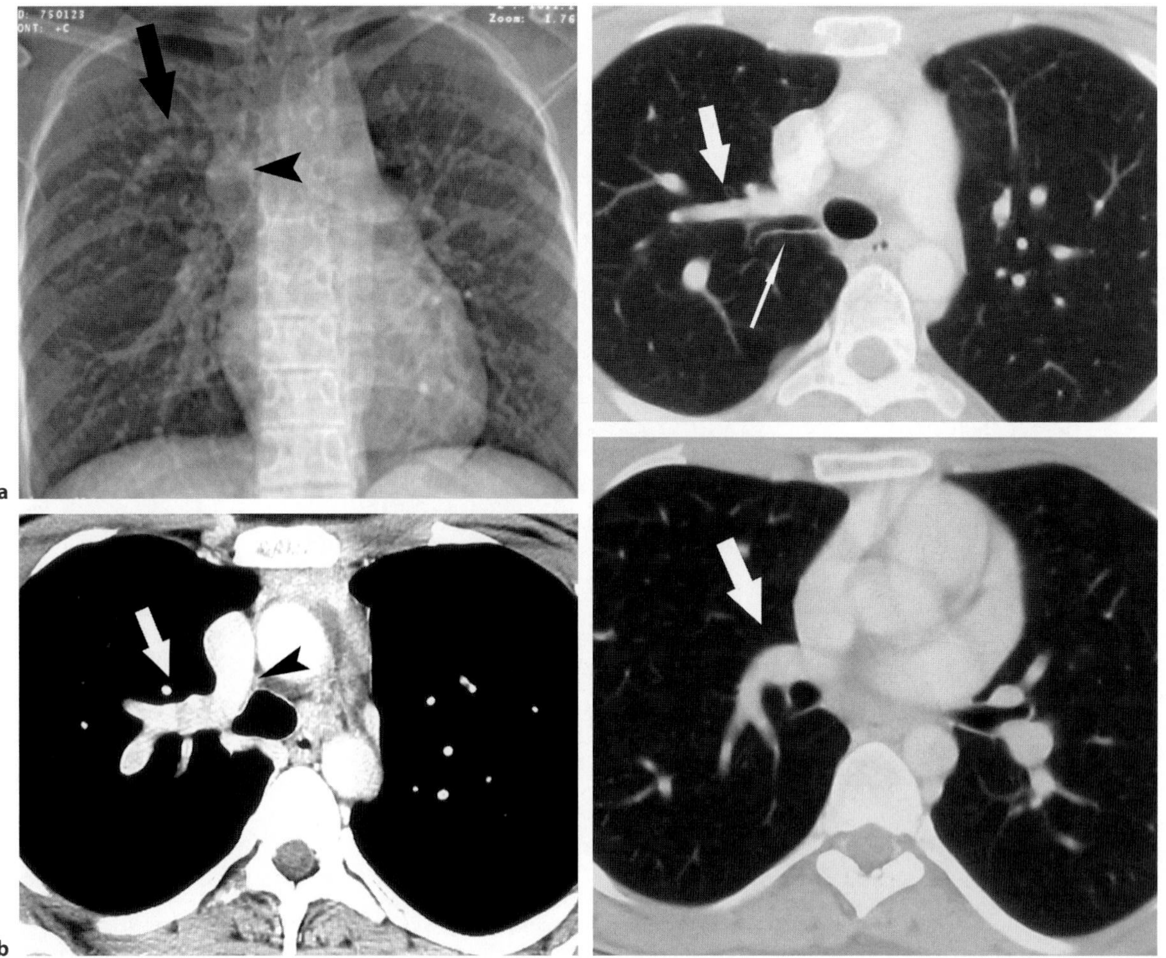

Fig. 21.3a–d. PAPVR of the right upper PV into the azygos vein. CT topogram and CT slices show a horizontal anomalous PV (*arrows*) draining into a dilated azygos arch (*arrowhead*). CT section shows associated tracheal bronchus ventilating the anomalous area (*thin arrow*). Note the absence of the right upper PV in the expected area in front of the right interlobar artery (*arrow* in **d**)

21.6.2 Left Lung

21.6.2.1 PAPVR in the Left Innominate Vein

PAPVR into the LIV directly or via a vertical vein is one of the most commonly recognized PAPVRs on CT (Fig. 21.5) (Pennes and Ellis 1986). The vertical vein is generally believed to represent the persistence of the embryonic left anterior CV. Usually it passes anteriorly to the aortic arch to terminate at the proximal part of the LIV. Sometimes the vertical vein courses more posteriorly, having a risk of compression between the left pulmonary artery and the left main bronchus (Nakib et al. 1967; Kastler et al. 2002). The expected part of the corresponding PV in the hilum is not found or is smaller. The anomalous drainage can concern the culminal vein (the lingular drainage being orthotopic), the left upper PV, or the whole left lung (Moes et al. 1967; Kissner and Sorkin 1986; Pennes and Ellis 1986; Van Meter et al. 1990).

21.6.2.2 PAPVR in a Persistent LSVC

Cases of PAPVR in a true persistent LSVC draining into the coronary sinus have been reported, usually from left lung PVs (Winter 1954; Peel et al.

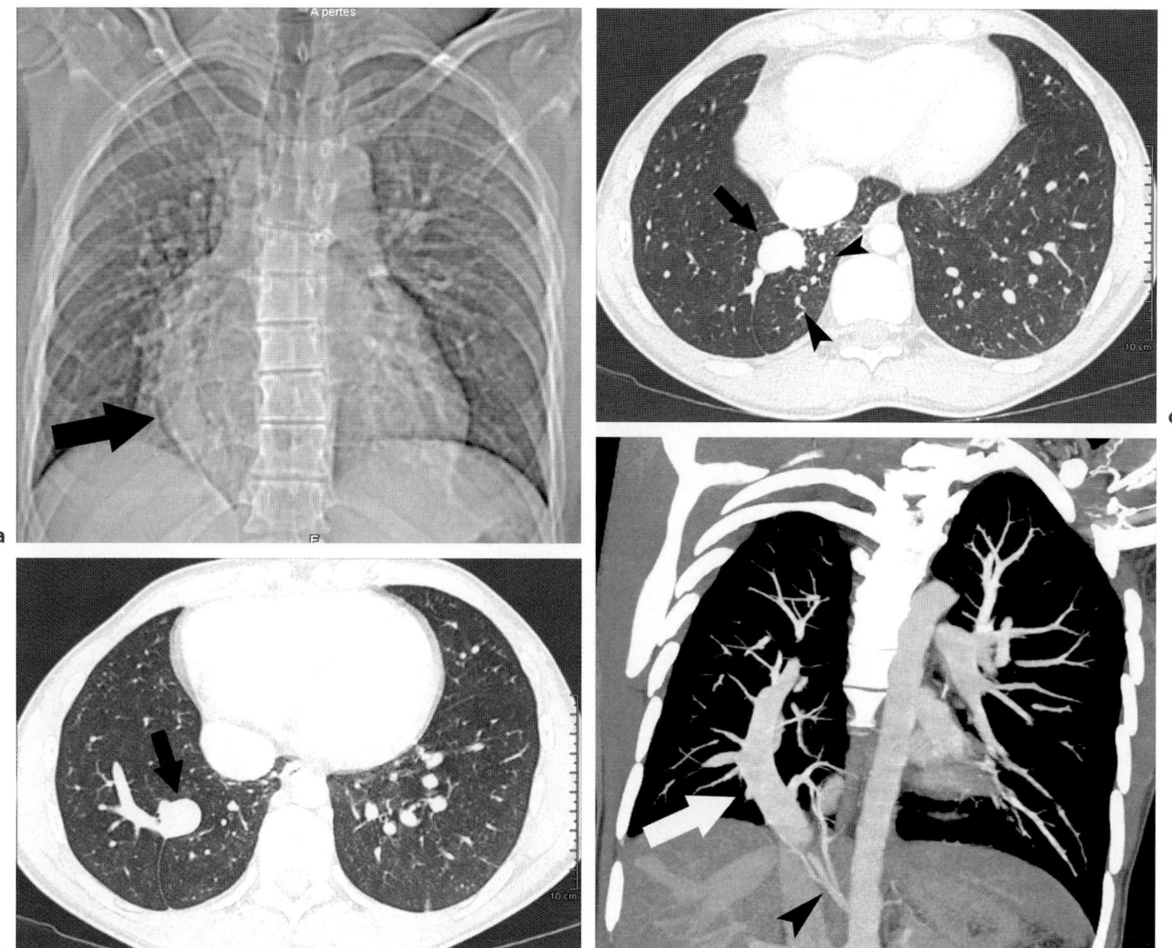

Fig. 21.4a–d. PAPVR draining into the IVC (*arrows*) (scimitar syndrome). Chest topogram shows the scimitar sign (*arrow* in **a**). Note a relative dextrocardia related to small right lung, accessory fissures (**b** and **c**), and systemic arteries arising from abdominal aorta (*arrowheads*). (Courtesy of Dr. A. Khalil, Hôpital Tenon, Paris)

1956; Snellen and Dekker 1963; Blake et al. 1965; Fish et al. 1991). PAPVRs in LSVC having simultaneous connections to the left atrium and LIV (most correctly called the levoatrio-cardinal vein in this condition) have been reported (Nakib et al. 1967; Snellen et al. 1968). Obstruction of venous return may be seen when the LSVC passes posteriorly instead of anteriorly to the left pulmonary artery as usually seen (Blake et al. 1965).

21.6.2.3
PAPVR in the Hemiazygos Vein

PAPVR in the hemiazygos vein is rare. A case of total anomalous drainage draining partially into the hemiazygos vein has been described (James et al. 1994).

21.6.2.4
PAPVR in the Coronary Sinus

PAPVR into the coronary sinus seems to occur more frequently from the left than the right lung (Blake et al. 1965; Snellen et al. 1968; Van Meter et al. 1990; Ammash et al. 1997). Infrequently the coronary sinus failed to drain into the right atrium. In atresia of the coronary sinus ostium, blood flow drains retrogradely into the left atrium through persistent Bochdalek foramen, or through LSVC into the right atrium (Blake et al. 1965).

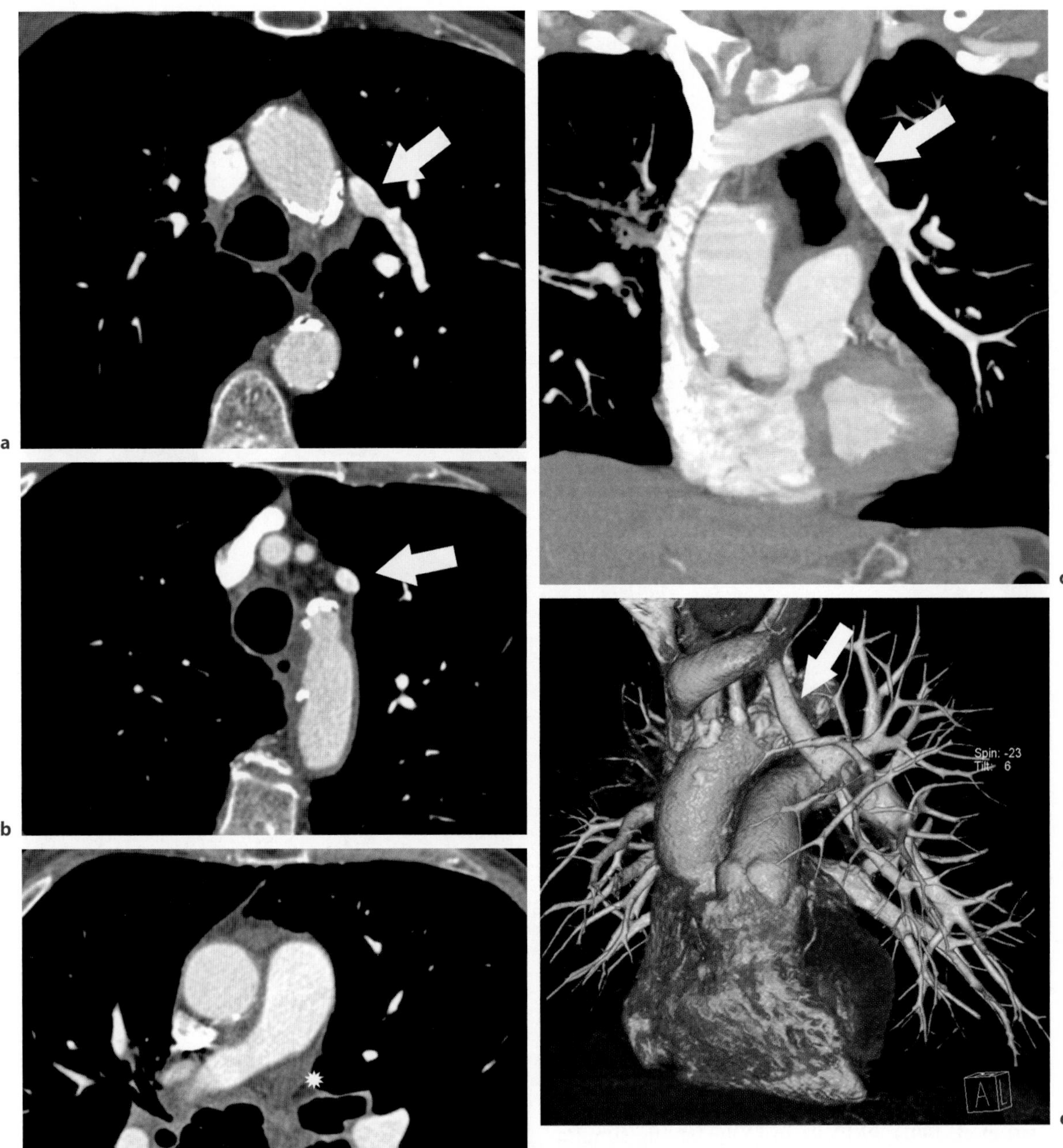

Fig. 21.5a–e. PAPVR of the left upper PV in the vertical vein. The left upper PV drains via a vertical vein (*arrows*) into a dilated LIV. Note that no vein is demonstrated in front of the left upper lobe and left main bronchi (*star*) (**c**)

21.6.2.5 Others

Left PAPVRs can drain into the IVC (D'Cruz and Arcilla 1964; Mardini et al. 1981), pericardiophrenic vein (Mardini et al. 1981), subclavian vein, portal vein, or gastric vein (Brody 1942; Kalke et al. 1967).

21.6.3 More Complex PAPVR

"Cross-mediastinal" drainages have also been reported, i.e., PAPVR of the left lung draining in the right atrium while the right PVs connect normally to the left atrium (Blake et al. 1965; Hijii et al.

1998), PAPVR of left lung PVs in the IVC (D'Cruz and Arcilla 1964; Mardini et al. 1981), or PAPVR of right lung into LSVC (Blake et al. 1965). Anomalous PVs can also originate from both lungs in a single patient in up to 7%, connecting together or separately to right or left systemic collectors of the mediastinum or to IVC (Fig. 21.6) (Blake et al. 1965; Nakib et al. 1967; Kalke et al. 1967; Snellen et al. 1968; Ammash et al. 1997; Hijii et al. 1998).

21.6.4 Connection of PV to Both Left Atrium and Right Atrium or Systemic Veins

In some cases a PV can join the left atrium normally, but in addition an anomalous connection exists between this PV or the left atrium and the right atrium or its systemic venous tributaries (Nakib et al. 1967). Such a connection is called a levoatriocardinal vein as it joins the left atrium to a derivate of the cardinal system, most frequently the LIV. Mitral atresia may be associated.

21.7 Differential Diagnosis of PAPVR

21.7.1 Abnormal Pathway of Segmental Pulmonary Vein

Segmental PVs can present with abnormal course that may simulate PAPVR. The most common ex-

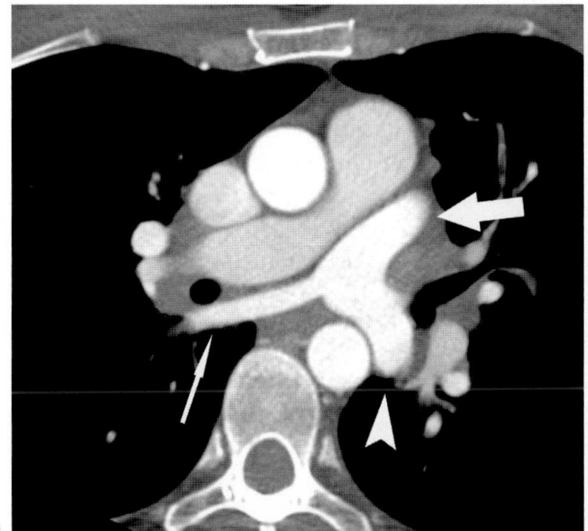
a

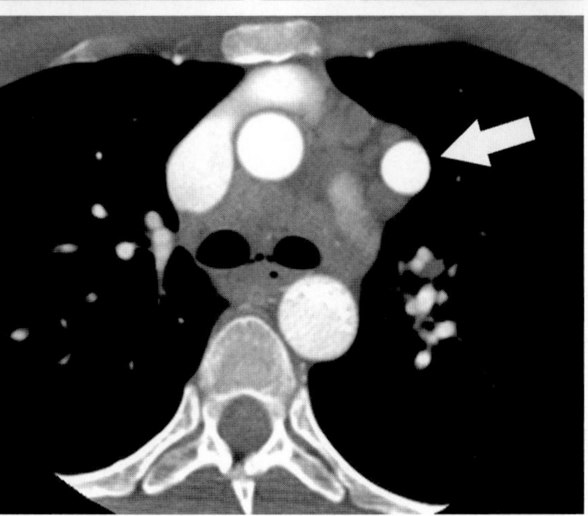
b

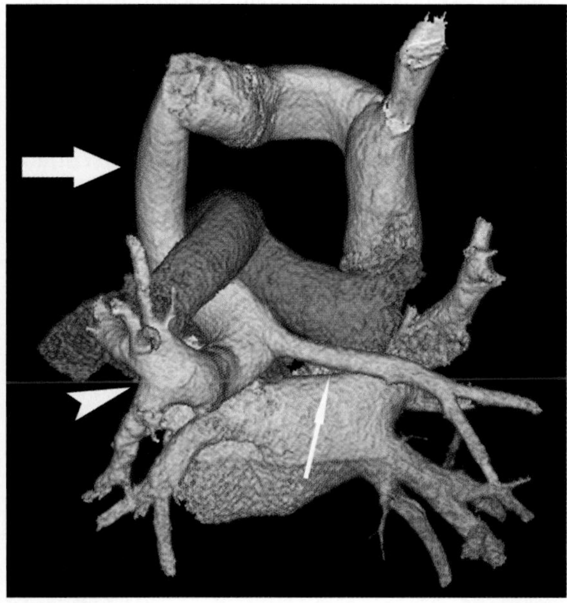
c

Fig. 21.6a–c. Complex PAPVR (acquired with ECG-gating). One right-sided PV (*thin arrow*) and two left-sided PVs (*arrowheads*) drain via a vertical vein (*arrow*) into a dilated LIV. Pulmonary arteries are coloured in blue in the posterior-view VRT reformat (**c**). (Courtesy of Dr. C. Deible and Dr. J. Lacomis, Pittsburg Medical Center, PA)

ample is the PV draining the posterior segment of the right upper lobe (right V3), passing posteriorly to the bronchus intermedius, and draining into the upper part of the right upper PV or directly into the left atrium (Fig. 21.7). The PV draining the superior segment of the right lower lobe (right V6) can also present a similar course.

21.7.2 Meandering Vein

Any dilated PV showing an anomalous course in the lung does not represent a PAPVR. In particular, any scimitar-shaped opacity located in the right paracardiac area is not pathognomonic of APVR in the IVC (Blake et al. 1965). The whole right pulmonary venous return may present as a varicose venous dilatation with anomalous scimitar-like course before entering the left atrium. Such abnormality results in a dilated vessel that may simulate vascular malformation or nodule on chest X-ray (Fig. 21.8). It has been called pseudo-scimitar syndrome, but should be better termed meandering vein to avoid confusion. Such anomaly may nevertheless be associated with other malformations, as also found in the scimitar syndrome (Goodman et al. 1972; Rey et al. 1986; Agarwal et al. 2004; Furuya et al. 2007). Therefore, scimitar syndrome and meandering vein cannot be differentiated by means of chest X-ray alone. The extreme situation is a PV presenting a scimitar course and connected both to the left atrium and the IVC (sometimes called pseudo-pseudo-scimitar syndrome) (Mohiuddin et al. 1966; Takeda et al. 1994; Tansel et al. 2006). Association with cor triatriatum has also been described (Becu et al. 1955; Grondin et al. 1964; Tansel et al. 2006).

Similarly, cases of meandering vein on the left side have been reported (Benfield et al. 1971; Tretheway et al. 1974). Cases of right-sided meandering vein crossing the mediastinum and draining into the left side of the left atrium have been reported (Goodman et al. 1972; Furuya et al. 2007). Possible embryologic explanation of meandering vein consists of atresia of a PV, the blood draining through intrapulmonary collaterals into another PV (Rey et al. 1986).

21.7.3 Left Superior Vena Cava

The vertical vein and the LSVC are generally believed to share a common embryonic origin, namely the persistence of a part of the left anterior CV. This accounts for radiographic and CT similarities between both entities. They should be easily differentiated. First, in LSVC two vessels are demonstrated immediately anterior to the left main bronchus (Chap. 20).

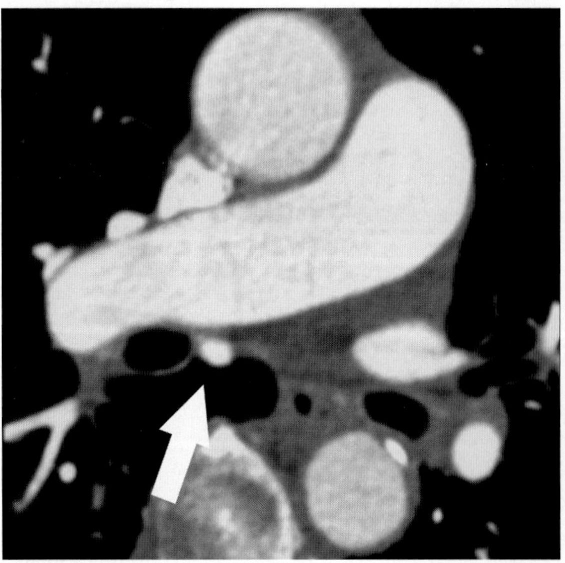
a

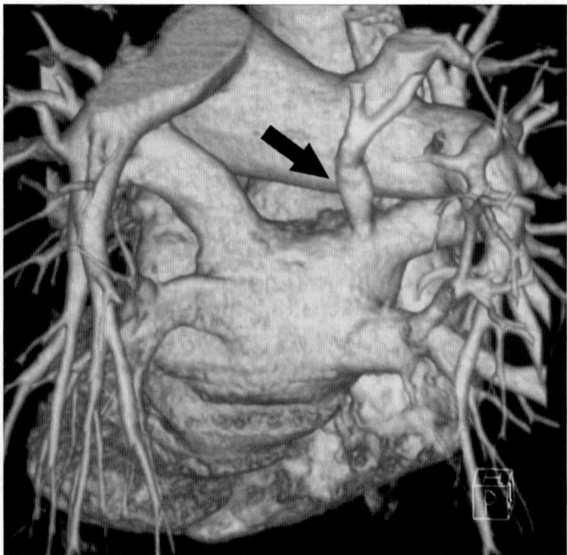
b

Fig. 21.7a,b. Variant of the course of RV3. Retrobronchial course of the PV draining the posterior segment of the right upper lobe (RV3) (*arrows*) into the roof of the junction of the right upper PV and left atrium. VRT reformat is a posterior view (**b**)

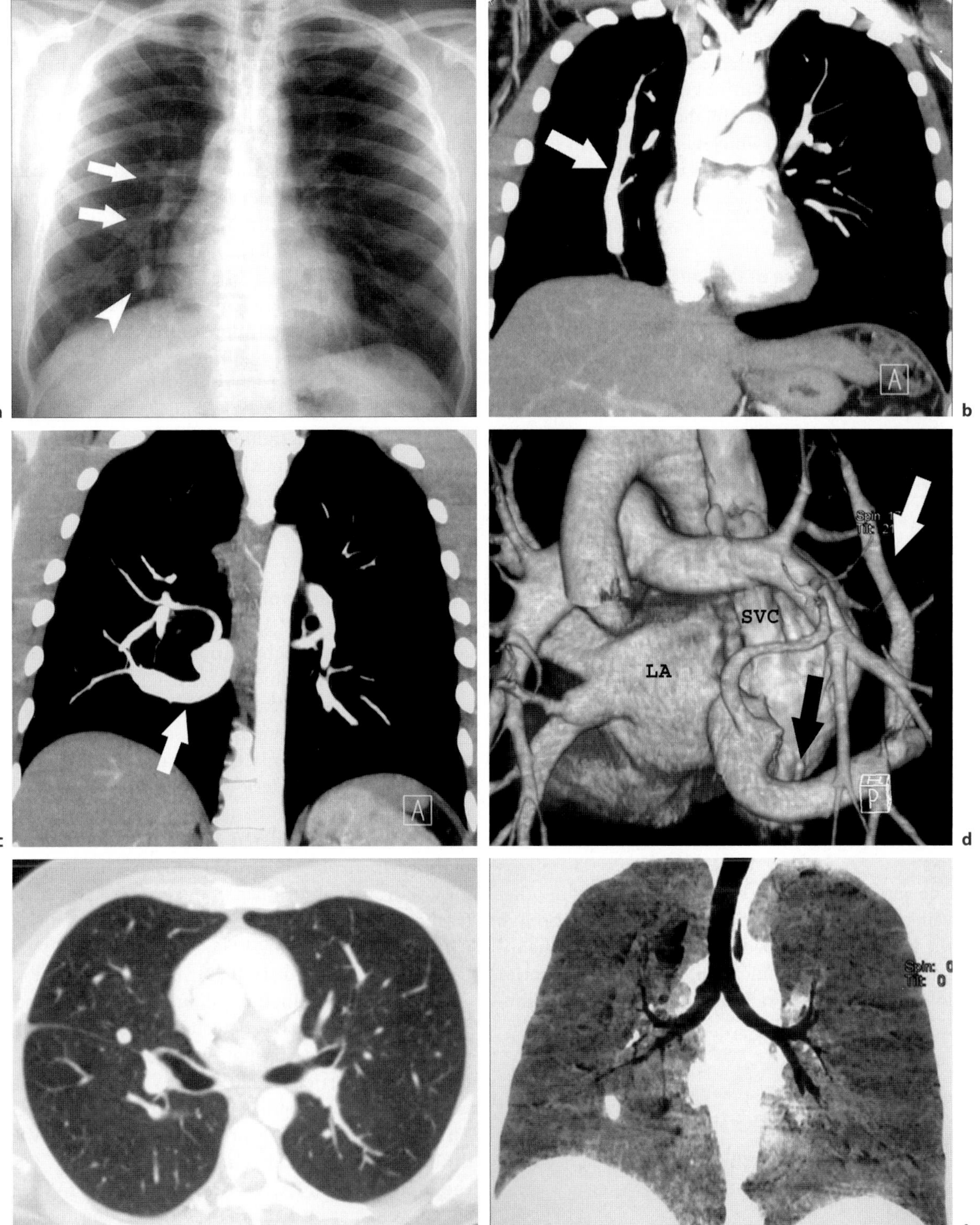

Fig. 21.8a–f. Meandering vein **a–f**. A scimitar vein (*arrows*) is seen in the right perihilar region and a rounded opacity in right paracardiac area (*arrowhead*) (**a**). The anomalous vein drains into the left atrium (**b,c,d**).The volume of the right lung is smaller than the left one (**a,e**) and shows a mirror left pattern of bronchial division in lungs (left isomerism) (**e,f**). Right lobar bronchi are slightly hypoplastic when compared to the left ones (**f**). *LA* left atrium, *SVC* superior vena cava

In PAPVR of the left upper PV, no or sometimes only one small vessel is seen in that location (Fig. 21.5). Second, blood flow is directed cranially in the vertical vein and caudally in LSVC. Third, when LSVC drains into the right atrium, the size of the coronary sinus will be dilated, which is not found in PAPVR of the left upper PV in the vertical vein.

21.7.4 Infra-Aortic Course of the Left Innominate Vein

In 0.015% of necropsies, the LIV can present with a vertical course paralleling the left border of the mediastinum, similar to the vertical vein and the LSVC (Chap. 20). The anomalous LIV, however, curves into the aorticopulmonary window, crosses the mediastinum to join the right innominate vein, and forms the SVC at the level of or caudal to azygos arch (Takada et al. 1992; Kim et al. 1994). Anomalous LIV can also be duplicated, one vein being in normal position and the other vein being infra-aortic (Takada et al. 1992). Infra-aortic LIV crossing the mediastinum below the pulmonary artery has also been described (Gerlis and Ho 1989). Infra-aortic LIV by itself has no clinical significance, but associated congenital heart diseases are reported in 33–85% (Gerlis and Ho 1989; Takada et al. 1992).

21.7.5 Others

The vertical vein must be distinguished from other veins that may present with a vertical course through the left side of the mediastinum, including the dilated pericardiophrenic vein, dilated left superior intercostal vein, or rare hemiazygo-caval continuation (Chap. 20).

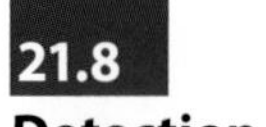

21.8 Detection of PAPVR

21.8.1 Chest X-Ray

Chest X-ray appearance will depend on the configuration of the APVR and degree of L-to-R shunt. In minor forms, chest X-ray may be normal or shows the uncommon course, often crescent-shaped, of the anomalous vein and the increased diameter of vessels in the anomalous area (Fig. 21.3) (Aldridge and Wigle 1965). Venous dilation may be explained by two factors. First, the abnormal vessels may drain a larger blood flow than usually. Second, PVs draining into the right atrium may have an increased blood flow, as they are subject to less resistance from atrial pressure and ventricular distensibilities than PV draining into the left atrium. In consequence, the arterial flow towards the anomaly is increased (Alpert et al. 1977; Saalouke et al. 1977). Abnormal mediastinal contour due to dilation of the vein collecting the PAPVR, i.e., the azygos arch or SVC, may be demonstrated (Pennes and Ellis 1986; Posniak et al. 1993; Haramati et al. 2003). Larger shunts may result in signs of right heart and pulmonary artery enlargement and pulmonary congestion (Kalke et al. 1967; Saalouke et al. 1977).

21.8.2 Computed Tomography

A more precise characterization of chest X-ray findings of PAPVR is achieved with CT (Thorsen et al. 1990; Haramati et al. 2003). In a series of 29 patients, cardiomegaly was seen in 48%, right atrial and right ventricle enlargement in 31%, enlarged central pulmonary arteries in 14%, and pulmonary venous congestion in 7% (Haramati et al. 2003). CT is currently considered as a first-line technique in the work-up of PAPVR, as it evidences the anomalous vein and its drainage, and shows associated tracheobronchial, lung or vascular abnormalities (Godwin and Tarver 1986; Dupuis et al. 1992; Remy-Jardin and Remy 1999).

Although examination should be performed with CM injection, the detectability of PAPVR is not greatly affected on non-enhanced CT acquisition (Haramati et al. 2003). PAPVR from the left lung is easier to recognize than from the right lung. This is due to the high proportion of left PAPVR draining via a vertical vein into a dilated LIV. On the contrary, right PAPVR draining into the SVC or azygos vein may be difficult to evidence, due to close anatomic relationships of vascular structures in this area, absence of intrapulmonary abnormal course of the anomalous PV, and frequent artefacts from dense contrast in the SVC and the right atrium.

Parameters of injection include high iodine concentration, i.e., 300–350 mg/ml and flow rate of

4–5 cc/s, with a bolus trigger placed in the ascending aorta or a fixed minimal start delay of 12–15 s. Saline flush helps reduce artefacts in the central PV from dense contrast in the SVC and the right atrium. Multiplanar and 3-D reformatting also helps in elucidating the course of abnormal vessels (Remy-Jardin and Remy 1999). In patients with complex malformation, an ECG-gated acquisition may be helpful (Fig. 21.6).

21.8.3 MRI

MR is able to provide the same morphological findings as CT (Thorsen et al. 1990). MR imaging may be helpful to assess direction of the flow inside vessels, severity of the shunt, and associated cardiac diseases (Fig. 21.9) (Masui et al. 1991; Vesely et al. 1991; White et al. 1997). Quantification of pulmonary to systemic flow ratio and L-to-R shunt can be assessed using flow-sensitive sequences (Marco de Lucas et al. 2003).

21.8.4 Digital Pulmonary Angiography

In the past, pulmonary angiography has frequently been required to confirm the diagnosis (Sider et al. 1984). Nevertheless, global pulmonary angiography may fail to demonstrate the number of anomalous PVs or their connections in up to 21%, and therefore selective injection should be obtained (Masui et al. 1991; Hijii et al. 1998).

21.8.5 Others

Endoesophageal and transthoracic echocardiography are complementary for the evaluation of PAPVR (Mehta et al. 1991; Ammash et al. 1997). Although it provides accurate assessment of right heart repercussions and detection of associated cardiac anomalies, it has been shown to have lower sensitivity in the detection of PAPVRs when compared to MR or angiography (Vesely et al. 1991,

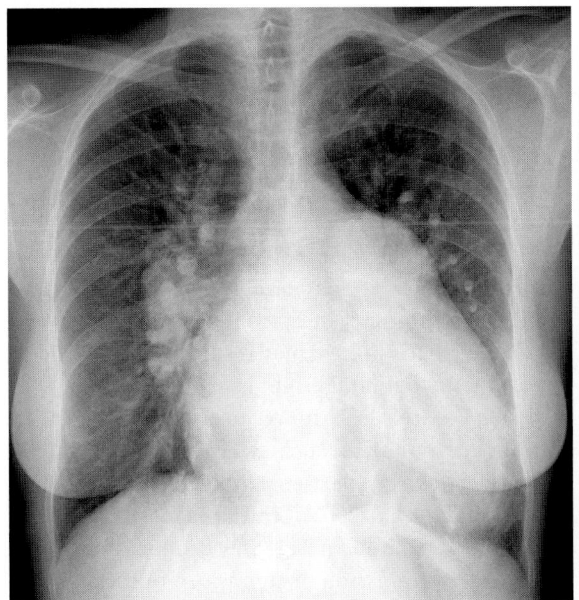

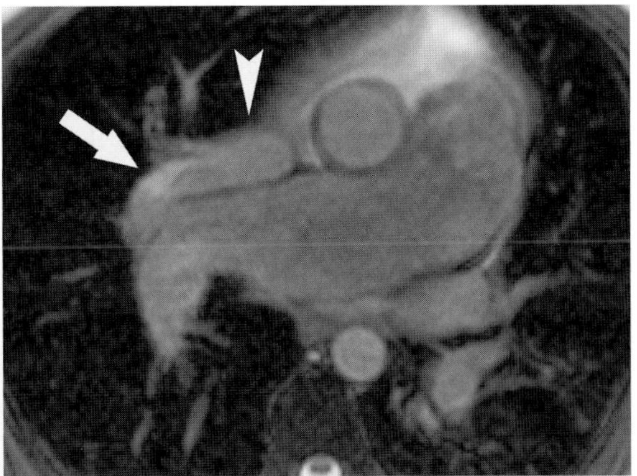

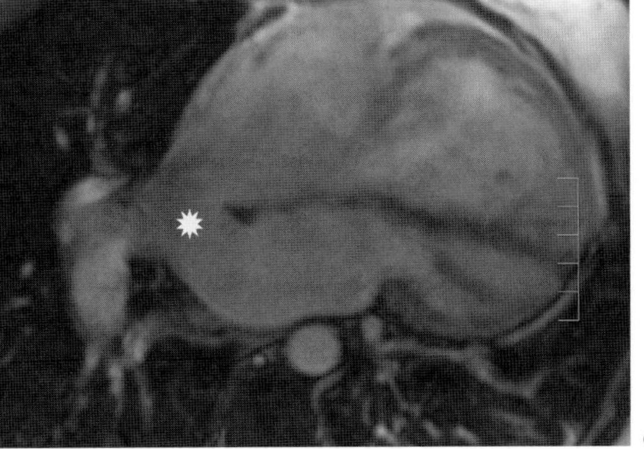

Fig. 21.9a–c. PAPVR and ASD. In a patient with PAPVR of the right upper lobe (*arrow*) into the lower part of SVC (*arrowhead*) and ASD (*star*), chest X-ray shows a severe cardiomegaly, increased pulmonary vasculature, signs of pulmonary hypertension, and decreased vascular pedicle related in part to a small-sized aortic arch. MR demonstrates a large sinus venosus-type ASD and, as a consequence, signs of severe cor pulmonale

Masui et al. 1991). Similar to MR, transoesophageal echocardiography estimates pulmonary to systemic flow ratio, but with a smaller field of view and often at the expense of general anaesthesia or heavy sedation (Marco de Lucas et al. 2003). In complex cases cardiac catheterization may still be useful before considering operative repair (Kalke et al. 1967; Saalouke et al. 1977; Fish et al. 1991; Brown et al. 2003). Oxygen saturation is always higher in collectors than in other systemic venous structures. Pulmonary artery pressures, resistances, and amplitude of the shunt can be measured.

21.9 Consequences of PAPVR

As demonstrated in some studies using the dilution method, abnormal connection of vessels does not necessarily mean abnormal drainage (Becu et al. 1955; Blake et al. 1965). Anomalous PVs can present with dual connections in the systemic vein and left atrium (Gazzaniga et al. 1969; Forbess et al. 1998; Peynircioglu et al. 2005). PAPVRs may be completely asymptomatic and incidentally discovered at CT. Most PAPVRs are similar to uncomplicated ASD, both resulting in L-to-R shunt (Kalke et al. 1967; Moes et al. 1967). PAPVRs result in elevated oxygen content in the collector and right heart cavities. Depending on their complexity, some PAPVRs may be symptomatic in children or adults.

Consequences of PAPVR will depend on many factors:

- presence of associated disease of the heart
- presence of associated broncho-pulmonary or vascular disease in the anomalous area
- number of anomalous PV
- site of connection of anomalous PV
- proportion of the cardiac output affected by the L-to-R shunt
- functional status of the normally draining pulmonary circulation
- associated disease of the normally draining lung
- surgical resection in the normally draining lung
- presence and degree of obstruction of PAPVR
- age of the patient

The most important factor is associated disease of the heart that is reported in 25–82% and should be systematically searched (Hijii et al. 1998). ASD, mainly of the sinus venosus type and inter-atrial communication, is found in up to 70% of patients, particularly in patients with PAPVR draining into the SVC or right atrium. Therefore, when present, symptoms, signs, and electrocardiogram findings are identical to those of ASD (Kalke et al. 1967; Van Meter et al. 1990; Ammash et al. 1997). The second sound is often widely split, and there are usually systolic and diastolic murmurs due to relative pulmonary and tricuspid stenoses (Fraser et al. 1999). Other cardiac anomalies, reported in up to 20% of patients, and associated lung and vascular anomalies are presented in Table 21.1.

Without associated cardiac anomalies, tolerance will depend on the proportion of the cardiac output affected by the L-to-R shunt. Most frequently, the abnormal PV drains around 25% of the cardiac output, which is generally asymptomatic (Black et al. 1992). In PAPVR of a whole lung, the abnormal drainage may represent 50% of the cardiac output and be associated with clinical symptoms (Brody 1942).

PAPVRs are also well-tolerated provided that there is no disease or surgical resection in the remaining lung (Kissner and Sorkin 1986). When not recognized before contralateral surgery, PAPVR of a single PV may result in life-threatening right heart failure in the early postoperative period (Black et al. 1992). In such circumstances, reimplantation of the abnormal PV should be simultaneously performed during or before major lung resection (Takei et al. 2002; Sakurai et al. 2005).

Whereas symptoms are generally absent in childhood, adults may develop fatigue and exertional dyspnoea. Depending on the severity of L-to-R shunt, pulmonary arterial hypertension, ranging from mild to occasionally severe, may rarely develop, particularly in adults with intact interatrial septum (Saalouke et al. 1977). This in turn may result in atrial arrhythmias and uncommonly right heart failure.

PAPVRs are also known to be associated with cardiac arrhythmias, such as atrial fibrillation and atrial tachycardia, particularly in PAPVR draining into SVC (Tse et al. 2003). Similar to total anomalous venous return, mild PAPVR may produce symptoms in case of compression or stenosis of the anomalous PV (Blake et al. 1965; Chanoine et al. 1988; Brown et al. 2003).

PAPVR may be responsible for asymmetric pulmonary oedema. In case of severe compression of the anomalous PV, pulmonary oedema may develop in the area with anomalous drainage. The same pattern can appear in right heart failure, due to direct transmission of elevated right venous pressure (Kissner and

Table 21.1. Malformations associated with PAPVRs

Heart malformations	Lung malformations
Atrial septal defect Cor triatriatum Common atrium Valves stenosis or atresia Ventricular septal defect Dextrocardia Truncus arteriosus Tetralogy of Fallot	Pulmonary sequestration Abnormal lung lobation Lung hypoplasia Bronchial stenosis Tracheal stenosis Bronchiectasis Horseshoe lung Cystic adenoid malformation
Vascular malformations	**Others**
SVC stenosis Left SVC Patent ductus arteriosus Peripheral pulmonary stenosis Aorta stenosis Meandering pulmonary vein Anomalies of aortic arch Anomalies of IVC Pulmonary artery atresia Transposition of great vessels Pulmonary arteriovenous fistula	Eventration of hemidiaphragm Hydrocephaly Vertebral malformations Bochdalek hernia Accessory diaphragm Hepatic herniation Situs inversus Spleen anomalies

Sorkin 1986). On the other hand, PAPVR may protect the area with anomalous drainage from pulmonary oedema in patients with left heart failure (Aldridge and Wigle 1965). Patients with scimitar syndrome may have additional symptoms, such as pulmonary infection or hemoptysis, due to the spectrum of associated anomalies (Mathey et al. 1968; Dupuis et al. 1992; Schramel et al. 1995; Brown et al. 2003).

21.10 Treatment

Medical treatment using vasodilators, digitalis and diuretics has limitations in PAPVRs, and surgical repair is the definite therapy (Kissner and Sorkin 1986; Brown et al. 2003). Surgical decision depends on two factors: the hemodynamic status and the associated cardiac malformations. In patients without associated anomalies, non-operative management is suitable, provided that clinical, echocardiographical and radiologic hemodynamic findings suggest a low-grade shunt (pulmonary to systemic flow ratio of less than 1.5) (Fish et al. 1991). A pulmonary to systemic flow ratio of more than 1.5:1 or 2:1 has been considered for surgical correction, regardless of associated cardiac defects (Saalouke et al. 1977; Van Meter et al. 1990; Hijii et al. 1998). Patients with scimitar syndrome and presenting with recurrent pulmonary infections may require surgical resection of the anomalous area (Schramel et al. 1995).

Some PAPVRs may be left uncorrected, when found as part of a complex cardiac malformation (Black et al. 1992). However, after correction of ASD, the residual shunt may worsen if the left heart is hypoplastic (Hijii et al. 1998). Therefore, surgical treatment is frequently designed to both exclude the L-to-R shunt and redirect the anomalous PV to the left atrium. Surgical treatment usually consists inredirecting pulmonary flow towards the left atrium trough patches, flaps or anatomical partitioning, or in end-to-side anastomosis of anomalous PV with left atrial appendage or left atrium (Gustafson et al. 1989; Van Meter et al. 1990; Brown et al. 2003). The main complication is thrombosis of the anomalous PV or systemic collecting vein that may be responsible for pulmonary infarction, pulmonary hypertension, or severe hemoptysis (Gustafson et al. 1989; Dupuis et al. 1992; Schramel et al. 1995; Hijii et al. 1998). Arrhythmias have also been reported as a complication (Kalke et al. 1967; Gustafson et al. 1989; Hijii et al. 1998). In rare conditions (dual drainage of the anomalous PV into both systemic veins and left atrium), percutaneous closure of an anomalous connection using coils or endograft has also been reported (Forbess et al. 1998; Peynircioglu et al. 2005).

References

Agarwal PP, Seely JM and Matzinger FR (2004) MDCT of anomalous unilateral single pulmonary vein. AJR Am J Roentgenol 183:1241–1243

Aldridge HE, Wigle ED (1965) Partial anomalous pulmonary venous drainage with intact interatrial septum associated with congenital mitral stenosis. Circulation 31:579–584

Alpert JS, Dexter L, Vieweg WV, Haynes FW, Dalen JE (1977) Anomalous pulmonary venous return with intact atrial septum: diagnosis and pathophysiology. Circulation 56:870–875

Ammash NM, Seward JB, Warnes CA, Connolly HM, O'Leary PW, Danielson GK (1997) Partial anomalous pulmonary venous connection: diagnosis by transesophageal echocardiography. J Am Coll Cardiol 29:1351–1358

Babb JD, McGlynn TJ, Pierce WS, Kirkman PM (1981) Isolated partial anomalous venous connection: a congenital defect with late and serious complications. Ann Thorac Surg 31:540–541

Becu LM, Tauxe WN, Dushane JW et al. (1955) Anomalous connection of pulmonary veins with normal pulmonary venous drainage; report of case associated with pulmonary venous stenosis and cor triatriatum. AMA Arch Pathol 59:463–470

Benfield JR, Gots RE and Mills D (1971) Anomalous single left pulmonary vein mimicking a parenchymal nodule. Chest 59:101–103

Black MD, Shamji FM, Goldstein W et al. (1992) Pulmonary resection and contralateral anomalous venous drainage: a lethal combination. Ann Thorac Surg 53:689–691

Blake HA, Hall RJ and Manion WC (1965) Anomalous pulmonary venous return. Circulation 32:406–414

Bliss DF 2nd, Hutchins GM (1995) The dorsal mesocardium and development of the pulmonary veins in human embryos. Am J Cardiovasc Pathol 5:55–67

Brody H (1942) Drainage of the pulmonary veins into the right side of the heart. Arch Pathol Lab Med 33:221–240

Brown JW, Ruzmetov M, Minnich DJ et al. (2003) Surgical management of scimitar syndrome: an alternative approach. J Thorac Cardiovasc Surg 125:238–245

Budorick NE, McDonald V, Flisak ME et al. (1989) The pulmonary veins. Semin Roentgenol 24:127–140

Chanoine JP, Viart P, Perlmutter N et al. (1988) Unusual ventilation-perfusion mismatch in partial anomalous venous return. Pediatr Radiol 18:497–498

Darling RC, Rothney WB and Craig JM (1957) Total pulmonary venous drainage into the right side of the heart; report of 17 autopsied cases not associated with other major cardiovascular anomalies. Lab Invest 6:44–64

D'Cruz IA, Arcilla RA (1964) Anomalous venous drainage of the left lung into the inferior vena cava. A case report. Am Heart J 67:539–544

Dupuis C, Charaf LA, Breviere GM et al. (1992) The "adult" form of the scimitar syndrome. Am J Cardiol 70:502–507

Fish FA, Davies J and Graham TP Jr (1991) Unique variant of partial anomalous pulmonary venous connection with intact atrial septum. Pediatr Cardiol 12:177–180

Forbess LW, O'Laughlin MP, Harrison JK (1998) Partially anomalous pulmonary venous connection: demonstration of dual drainage allowing nonsurgical correction. Cathet Cardiovasc Diagn 44:330–335

Fraser RS, Müller NL, Colman N et al. (1999) Developmental anomalies affecting the pulmonary vessels. In: Fraser RS, Müller NL, Colman N, Paré PD (eds) Fraser and Paré's diagnosis of diseases of the chest, 4th edn. Saunders, Philadelphia, pp 637–675

Furuya K, Kaku K, Yasumori K et al. (2007) Hypogenetic lung syndrome with anomalous venous return to the left inferior pulmonary vein: multidetector row CT findings. J Thor Imag 22:351–354

Galetta D, Veronesi G, Leo F et al. (2006) Anomalous right upper lobe venous drainage. Ann Thorac Surg 82:2272–2274

Gazzaniga AB, Matloff JM, Harken DE (1969) Anomalous right pulmonary venous drainage into the inferior vena cava and left atrium. J Thorac Cardiovasc Surg 57:251–154

Gerlis LM, Ho SY (1989) Anomalous subaortic position of the brachiocephalic (innominate) vein: a review of published reports and report of three new cases. Br Heart J 61:540–545

Ghaye B, Szapiro D, Dacher JN et al. (2003) Percutaneous ablation for atrial fibrillation: the role of cross-sectional imaging. Radiographics 23:S19–33

Godwin JD, Tarver RD (1986) Scimitar syndrome: four new cases examined with CT. Radiology 159:15–20

Goodman LR, Jamshidi A, Hipona FA (1972) Meandering right pulmonary vein simulating the Scimitar syndrome. Chest 62:510–512

Gotsman MS, Astley R, Parsons CG (1965) Partial anomalous pulmonary venous drainage in association with atrial septal defect. Br Heart J 27:566–571

Grayet D, Ghaye B, Szapiro D et al. (2001) Systemic-to-pulmonary venous shunt in superior vena cava obstruction revealed on dynamic helical CT. AJR Am J Roentgenol 176:211–213

Grondin C, Leonard AS, Anderson RC et al. (1964) Cor triatriatum: A diagnostic surgical enigma. J Thorac Cardiovasc Surg 48:527–539

Gustafson RA, Warden HE, Murray GF, Hill RC, Rozar GE (1989) Partial anomalous pulmonary venous connection to the right side of the heart. J Thorac Cardiovasc Surg 98:861–868

Halasz NA, Halloran KH, Liebow AA (1956) Bronchial and arterial anomalies with drainage of the right lung into the inferior vena cava. Circulation 14:826–846

Haramati LB, Moche IE, Rivera VT et al. (2003) Computed tomography of partial anomalous pulmonary venous connection in adults. J Comput Assist Tomogr 27:743–749

Healey JE Jr (1952) An anatomic survey of anomalous pulmonary veins: their clinical significance. J Thorac Surg 23:433–444

Hijii T, Fukushige J, Hara T (1998) Diagnosis and management of partial anomalous pulmonary venous connection. A review of 28 pediatric cases. Cardiology 89:148–151

James CL, Keeling JW, Smith NM et al. (1994) Total anomalous pulmonary venous drainage associated with fatal outcome in infancy and early childhood: an autopsy study of 52 cases. Pediatr Pathol 14:665–678

Kalke BR, Carlson RG, Ferlic RM et al. (1967) Partial anomalous pulmonary venous connections. Am J Cardiol 20:91–101

Kastler B, Clair C, Delabrousse E et al. (2002) Retours veineux systémiques et pulmonaires anormaux: aspects IRM et classification. Encycl Méd Chir (Elsevier, Paris) Radiodiagnostic-Coeur-Poumon 32-016-A-20:1–15

Kim HJ, Kim HS, Lee G (1994) Anomalous left brachiocephalic vein: spiral CT and angiographic findings. J Comput Assist Tomogr 18:872–875

Kissner DG, Sorkin RP (1986) Anomalous pulmonary venous connection. Medical therapy. Chest 89:752–754

Marco de Lucas E, Canga A, Sadaba P et al. (2003) Scimitar syndrome: complete anatomical and functional diagnosis with gadolinium-enhanced and velocity-encoded cine MRI. Pediatr Radiol 33:716–718

Mardini MK, Sakati NA, Nyhan WL (1981) Anomalous left pulmonary venous drainage to the inferior vena cava and through the pericardiophrenic vein to the innominate vein: left-sided scimitar syndrome. Am Heart J 101:860–863

Masui T, Seelos KC, Kersting-Sommerhoff BA et al. (1991) Abnormalities of the pulmonary veins: evaluation with MR imaging and comparison with cardiac angiography and echocardiography. Radiology 181:645–649

Mathey J, Galey JJ, Logeais Y et al. (1968) Anomalous pulmonary venous return into inferio vena cava and associated bronchovascular anomalies (the scimitar syndrome) Thorax 23:398–407

Mehta RH, Jain SP, Nanda NC et al. (1991) Isolated partial anomalous pulmonary venous connection: echocardiographic diagnosis and a new color Doppler method to assess shunt volume. Am Heart J 122:870–873

Moes CA, Goldman BS, Mustard WT (1967) Anomalous pulmonary venous drainage from the left lung into a left vertical vein. J Can Assoc Radiol 18:377–381

Mohiuddin SM, Levin HS, Runco V, Booth RW (1966) Anomalous pulmonary venous drainage. A common trunk emptying into the left atrium and inferior vena cava. Circulation 34:46–51

Nakib A, Moller JH, Kanjuh VI et al. (1967) Anomalies of the pulmonary veins. Am J Cardiol 20:77–90

Neill CA (1956) Development of the pulmonary veins; with reference to the embryology of anomalies of pulmonary venous return. Pediatrics 18:880–887

Okamoto K, Kodama K, Kawai K et al. (2004) An anatomical study of the partial anomalous pulmonary venous return with special references to the bronchial vein. Anat Sci Int 79:82–86

Peel AA, Blum K, Kelly JC et al. (1956) Anomalous pulmonary and systemic venous drainage. Thorax 11:119–134

Pennes DR, Ellis JH (1986) Anomalous pulmonary venous drainage of the left upper lobe shown by CT scans. Radiology 159:23–24

Peynircioglu B, Williams DM, Rubenfire M et al. (2005) Endograft repair of partially anomalous pulmonary venous connection with dual drainage. J Vasc Surg 42:1221–1225

Posniak HV, Dudiak CM, Olson MC (1993) Computed tomography diagnosis of partial anomalous pulmonary venous drainage. Cardiovasc Intervent Radiol 16:319–320

Pucelikova T, Kautznerova D, Vedlich D et al. (2007) A complex anomaly of systemic and pulmonary venous return associated with sinus venosus atrial septal defect. Int J Cardiol 115:e47–48.

Remy-Jardin M, Remy J (1999) Spiral CT angiography of the pulmonary circulation. Radiology 212:615–636

Rey C, Vaksmann G, Francart C (1986) Anomalous unilateral single pulmonary vein mimicking partial anomalous pulmonary venous return. Cathet Cardiovasc Diagn 12:330–333

Saalouke MG, Shapiro SR, Perry LW et al. (1977) Isolated partial anomalous pulmonary venous drainage associated with pulmonary vascular obstructive disease. Am J Cardiol 39:439–444

Sakurai H, Kondo H, Sekiguchi A et al. (2005) Left pneumonectomy for lung cancer after correction of contralateral partial anomalous pulmonary venous return. Ann Thorac Surg 79:1778–1780

Schatz SL, Ryvicker MJ, Deutsch AM et al. (1986) Partial anomalous pulmonary venous drainage of the right lower lobe shown by CT scans. Radiology 159:21–22

Schramel FM, Westermann CJ, Knaepen PJ et al. (1995) The scimitar syndrome: clinical spectrum and surgical treatment. Eur Respir J 8:196–201

Sider L, Fisher MR, Mintzer RA (1984) The evaluation of partial anomalous pulmonary venous return with the use of digital subtraction angiography. Chest 86:97–99

Snellen HA, Dekker A (1963) Anomalous pulmonary venous drainage in relation to left superior vena cava and coronary sinus. Am Heart J 66:184–196

Snellen HA, van Ingen HC, Hoefsmit EC (1968) Patterns of anomalous pulmonary venous drainage. Circulation 38:45–63

Sugimoto S, Izumiyama O, Yamashita A et al. (1998) Anatomy of inferior pulmonary vein should be clarified in lower lobectomy. Ann Thorac Surg 66:1799–1800

Takada Y, Narimatsu A, Kohno A et al. (1992) Anomalous left brachiocephalic vein: CT findings. J Comput Assist Tomogr 16:893–896

Takeda S, Imachi T, Arimitsu K et al. (1994) Two cases of scimitar variant. Chest 105:292–293

Takei H, Suzuki K, Asamura H et al. (2002) Successful pulmonary resection of lung cancer in a patient with partial anomalous pulmonary venous connection: report of a case. Surg Today 32:899–901

Tansel T, Harmandar B, Dayioglu E et al. (2006) Anomalous dual drainage of the right pulmonary veins in a patient with cor triatriatum: report of a case without scimitar sign. J Cardiovasc Surg (Torino) 47:75–78

Thorsen MK, Erickson SJ, Mewissen MW et al. (1990) CT and MR imaging of partial anomalous pulmonary venous return to the azygos vein. J Comput Assist Tomogr 14:1007–1009

Tretheway DG, Francis GS, MacNeil DJ et al. (1974) Single left pulmonary vein with normal pulmonary venous drainage: a roentgenographic curiosity. Am J Cardiol 34:237–239

Tsao HM, Wu MH, Yu WC et al. (2001) Role of right middle pulmonary vein in patients with paroxysmal atrial fibrillation. J Cardiovasc Electrophysiol 12:1353–1357

Tse HF, Lau CP, Lee KL et al. (2003) Atrial tachycardia arising from an epicardial site with venous connection between the left superior pulmonary vein and superior vena cava. J Cardiovasc Electrophysiol 14:540–543

Van Meter C, Jr., LeBlanc JG, Culpepper WS 3rd et al. (1990) Partial anomalous pulmonary venous return. Circulation 82(5 Suppl):IV195–198

Vesely TM, Julsrud PR, Brown JJ et al. (1991) MR imaging of partial anomalous pulmonary venous connections. J Comput Assist Tomogr 15:752–756

White CS, Baffa JM, Haney PJ et al. (1997) MR imaging of congenital anomalies of the thoracic veins. Radiographics 17:595–608

Winter FS (1954) Persistent left superior vena cava; survey of world literature and report of 30 additional cases. Angiology 5:90–132

Woodring JH, Howard TA, Kanga JF (1994) Congenital pulmonary venolobar syndrome revisited. Radiographics 14:349–369

Yazar F, Ozdogmus O, Tuccar E et al. (2002) Drainage patterns of middle lobe vein of right lung: an anatomical study. Eur J Cardiothorac Surg 22:717–720

Zylak CJ, Eyler WR, Spizarny DL et al. (2002) Developmental lung anomalies in the adult: radiologic-pathologic correlation. Radiographics 22:S25–43

Pulmonary Valvular Stenosis

22

Jacques Rémy and Kahimano Boroto

The three main causes of pulmonary valvular stenosis are (Amplatz and Moller 1993): commissural fusion of the pulmonary cusps causing a thickened, dome-like pulmonary valve, bicuspid pulmonary valve and valvular dysplasia. Previously known as trilogy of Fallot, two elements of this trilogy, hypertrophy of the right ventricle and right-to-left shunt through a patent foramen ovale, are the consequences of the pulmonary arterial stenosis (PVS). When the stenosis is limited to the pulmonary valves, and depending on the stenosis intensity, right ventricular systole causes a post-stenotic dilatation of the main pulmonary artery extending in the left main pulmonary artery (Fig. 22.1) due to their common leftward and backward orientation. Elevated pressure leads to muscular hypertrophy of the right ventricle, most marked in the outflow tract. Hypertrophy of the right ventricle leads to counterclockwise rotation of the heart. These changes in the orientation cause the post-stenotic jet to impact primarily on the left main pulmonary artery. PVS may be asymptomatic or associated with fatigue caused by decreased cardiac output. The stenosis can trigger a systolic murmur in the pulmonary outflow tract and electrocardiographic signs of right ventricular hypertrophy.

From a hemodynamic viewpoint, when the stenosis is minimal, there is neither post-stenotic dilatation nor right ventricular consequence. When the stenosis is narrow, there is no post-stenotic dilatation because the post-stenotic jet is poor, but the right ventricular hypertrophy is marked. When the stenosis is moderate, the post-stenotic jet dilates the pulmonary trunk far from the pulmonary annulus.

In cases of commissural fusion, the pulmonary valves appear moderately thickened and dome-shaped and can be identified even without ECG gating. The leaflets are more thickened in valvular dysplasia, which is usually not associated with post-stenotic dilatation. When performed with ECG gating, short axis views of the right ventricle show the thickened myocardium mainly in the right ventricular outflow tract during systole. Without ECG gating, the muscular wall of the right ventricular outflow tract can appear falsely thickened due to motion artifacts. Systolic reformations in the right ventricular short axis views allow for an analysis of the valves and of their dome-shaped appearance. Rarely, they may be calcified. The pulmonary annulus and the main pulmonary artery are moderately hypoplastic in case of valvular dysplasia.

Post-stenotic dilatation of the pulmonary artery contributes to the left hilum and may simulate a hilar or a mediastinal mass of non-vascular origin, such as thymic tumor, lymphadenopathy, mediastinal pleural mass or pericardial congenital defect (Cole et al. 1995).

Idiopathic aneurysm of the main PA with pulmonary valve regurgitation, important dilatation of the pulmonary trunk, up to 10 cm in diameter, dilatation of the annulus and normal pulmonary valves is one of the differential diagnoses of PVS (Shimokawa et al. 1997).

Watson syndrome is composed of mild mental retardation, short stature, PVS, café-au-lait spots and other signs of type I neurofibromatosis (Foster et al. 2006). Pulmonary hypertension is an important factor in the pathogenesis of pulmonary arterial aneurysm, dissection and rupture. Pulmonary valve agenesis or congenital or acquired insufficiency di-

J. Rémy, MD
Professor, Department of Radiology, C.H.R.U. de Lille, Hôpital Calmette, Boulevard du Prof. J. Leclercq, 59037 Lille Cédex, France
K. Boroto, MD
Department of Thoracic Imaging, University Center of Lille, Boulevard du Prof. J. Leclercq, 59037 Lille Cédex, France

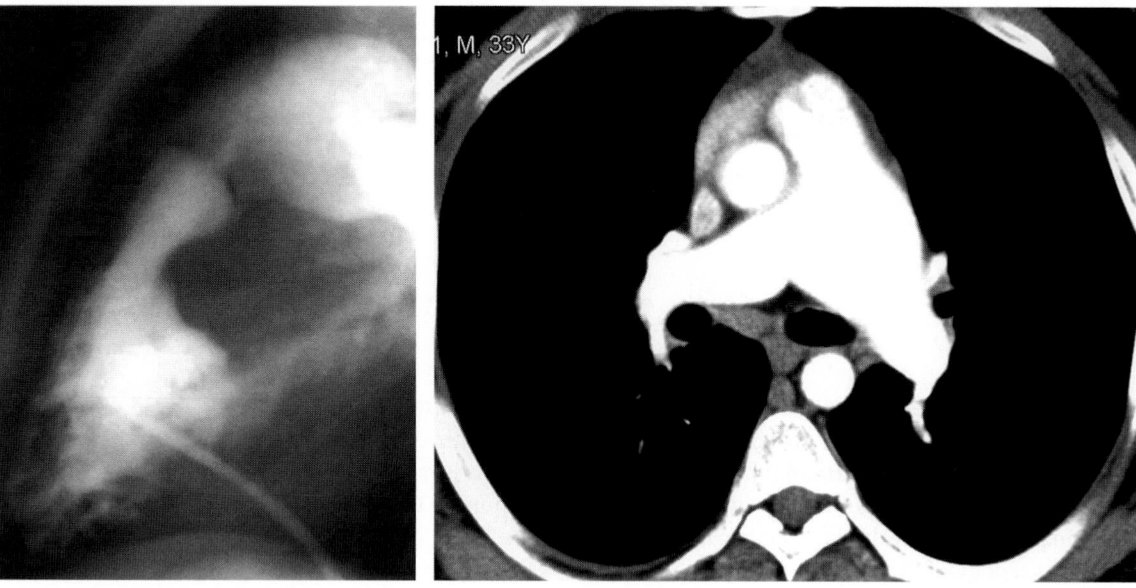

Fig. 22.1a,b. Typical right ventriculography of a pulmonary valvular stenosis (**a**). Moderate stenosis of the right ventricular outflow tract. Dome-shaped valvular stenosis with jet phenomenon responsible for the left pulmonary artery dilatation. In another patient, the selective dilatation of the left pulmonary artery is depicted, extending in the proximal part of the left descending PA (**b**). This acquisition should be performed with cardiac gating and systolic and diastolic short-axis reformations of the valvular apparatus

lates the pulmonary trunk. Structural arterial wall abnormalities either congenital (Marfan syndrome) or acquired (systemic lupus erythematosous) may be responsible for PA aneurysm. Massive embolus or left PA tumor can also massively dilate the hilar PA. The treatment of PA aneurysm implies the follow-up to detect a progressive increase in arterial diameter prior to its rupture or dissection, which represents an indication for surgery (Mastroroberto et al. 1997).

Reference

Amplatz K, Moller JH (1993) Radiology of congenital heart disease. Mosby Year Book Inc, St. Louis

ColeTJ, Henry DA, Jolles H, Proto AV (1995) Normal and abnormal vascular structures that simulate neoplasms on chest radiographs: Clues to the diagnosis. RadioGraphics 15:867–891

Foster JL, Bradley SM, Ikonomidis JS (2006) Pulmonary artery aneurysm and coronary artery disease in the clinical presentation of Watson syndrome. Ann Thorac Surg 82:740–742

Mastroroberto P, Chello M, Zofrea S et al. (1997) Pulmonary artery aneurysm. Ann Thorac Surg 64:585–586

Shimokawa S, Komokata T, Moriyama Y, Taira A (1997) Aneurysm of pulmonary trunk. Ann Thorac Surg 64:586–587

Right-to-Left Shunts

23

Loic Boussell, Philippe Douek, and Brett Elicker

CONTENTS

L. Boussel, MD
P. Douek, MD, Professor
Service de Radiologie, Hôpital Louis Pradel, 28 Avenue du Doyen Lépine, 69677 Bron Cédex, France
B. Elicker, MD, Assistant Professor
Department of Radiology, University of California, 505 Parnassus Avenue, San Francisco, CA 94122, USA

23.1 Introduction

A right-to-left shunt is defined as a cardiac shunt that allows deoxygenated blood to flow from the right heart to the left heart. The shunt may occur at different levels, and we will schematically distinguish among intra-cardiac, para-cardiac, related great vessel and intra-pulmonary shunts. They can be related to a congenital lesion (Higgins and Ross 2006; Baert et al. 2005) or post-surgical sequelae. CT scanners recently have made great progress in the evaluation of these shunts since cardiac imaging can now accurately be performed using cardiac gating. Indeed, even if the CT scanner does not allow quantifying the shunt, it can contribute to presurgical evaluation by providing some useful information about the location of the shunt and other cardiac- and vascular-associated lesions.

23.2 Intra-Cardiac Shunts

23.2.1 Direct Right-to-Left Shunts

23.2.1.1 Tetralogy of Fallot

Tetralogy of Fallot represents 10% of congenital heart disease (Hoffman and Kaplan 2002) and occurs in approximately 800 per 1,000,000 births. It is caused by an anterior misalignment of the conal septum, leading to the combination of a ventricular septal defect (VSD), a pulmonary stenosis and an aorta overriding the VSD. Right ventricular hypertrophy, which results from this combination, causes resistance to blood flow from the right ventricle to the narrowed pulmonary artery. The most frequently associated lesions are stenosis of the left pulmonary artery, bicuspid pulmonary valve, right-sided aortic arch, atrial septal defect (pentalogy of Fallot), partial or total anomalous pulmonary venous return and coronary artery anomalies. Tetralogy of Fallot can be part of other syndromes such as diGeorge syndrome (Lu et al. 2001).

Tetralogy of Fallot is easily diagnosed by CT scanner (Fig. 23.1). Indeed CT scanners allow visualizing the septal defect, measuring the size of the proximal aorta (which is larger than normal) and its position, and mostly estimating the narrowing of the pulmonary tract and the hypertrophy of the right ventricle. Surgical repair of tetralogy of Fallot consists of VSD closure associated with a complete release of infundibular stenosis and an enlargement of narrowed pulmonary artery. Careful preoperative assessment of coronary artery origin is required, in particular the search for a main coronary artery crossing anteriorly to the right ventricular outflow in the site of potential surgical repair. This mainly may happen in case of aberrant origin of the left main anterior interventricular coronary artery originating from the right coronary artery. The second important point is to provide detailed analysis of the pulmonary tract and pulmonary artery narrowing and look for additional stenosis on the pulmonary branches. Narrowing on the pulmonary arteries may indicate additional treatment, such as balloon angioplasty, and the presence of a coronary artery crossing the infundibulum may lead to changing the intervention into a Rastelli procedure.

After surgery, CT may be useful to assess early postoperative complications (pericarditis, remaining stenosis on the pulmonary arteries, etc.) and delayed complications such as aneurismal dilatation of the infundibular repaired area. Pulmonary valve regurgitation (PVR) and its long-term deleterious consequences on right ventricular function occur frequently and may impair long-term prognosis. Quantitative measurement of PVR cannot be performed with CT, but with MRI (phase-contrast imaging), which actually represents the current gold standard in this area.

23.2.1.2 Pulmonary Atresia

Pulmonary atresia is characterized by the absence of or a very narrow connection between the right ventricle and the pulmonary arteries. Pulmonary atresia can be separated into two groups depending on the presence or not of VSD.

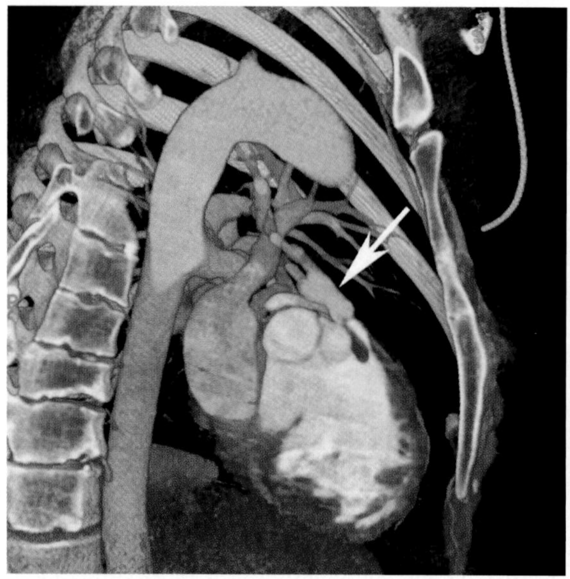

a

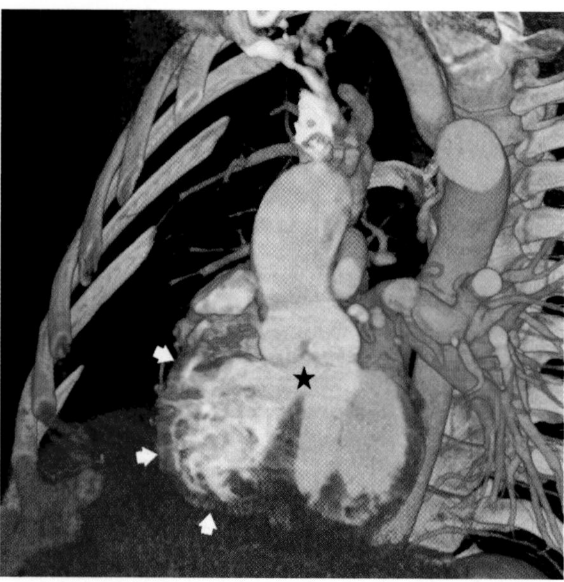

b

Fig. 23.1a,b. Tetralogy of Fallot. Three-dimensional reconstruction in sagittal (**a**) and oblique (**b**) views. The pulmonary stenosis (*long arrow*), the ventricular septal defect (*star*) with the overriding aorta and the right ventricular hypertrophy (*small arrows*) are well identified on the cardiac CT with EGC gating

23.2.1.2.1
Pulmonary Atresia with Ventricular Septum Defect

Pulmonary atresia with VSD is the extreme form of tetralogy of Fallot. It represents 2% of congenital heart defects. The atresia can be focal, located at the valve level or more extensive, involving the pulmonary artery and its proximal branches. The aorta is markedly large, overriding the VSD. Lung perfusion is provided by systemic-to-pulmonary collaterals (major aorto-pulmonary collateral arteries or MAPCAs) mainly originating from the descending aorta (through bronchial or intercostal arteries), internal thoracic arteries or even diaphragmatic and other abdominal branches (Norgaard et al. 2006). These MAPCAs generally present multiple stenoses and anastomoses between them and with the native pulmonary arteries.

CT scanners with 3D reconstruction are of particular interest to estimate the extension of the stenosis on the pulmonary tract, to measure the size of the native pulmonary arteries and to visualize the MAPCAs, their origin, size and position in the mediastinum. This information is required to make decisions about surgical strategies, as the complexity of the pulmonary tract and MAPCAs often leads to staged surgical procedures (staged focalization of MAPCAs to native pulmonary tract or complete one-stage unifocalization of the MAPCAs, establishment of a right ventricular outflow tract to pulmonary artery continuity with an homograft and repair of the VSD) and/or palliative systemic-to-pulmonary shunts (Blalock-Taussig anastomosis).

After surgery, CT can assess long-term complications, such as stenosis and calcification of the homograft. Whenever a new surgical procedure is planned, CT can assess the position of the homograft relative to the sternum (which can be injured during the sternotomy), the permeability of the previous palliative shunts and the anatomy of the coronary arteries. As in tetralogy of Fallot, pulmonary regurgitation and its long-term consequences cannot be properly assessed by CT.

23.2.1.2.2
Pulmonary Atresia with Intact Ventricular Septum

Pulmonary valve atresia with intact ventricular septum is a rare congenital lesion. Diagnosis always occurs early in life, either in newborns or at the fetal stage. It has a wide spectrum of anatomic heterogeneity and invokes a wide variety of treatment strategies. It is associated with a variable degree of right ventricular hypoplasia. The type of surgical repair depends on the size and shape of the right ventricle and goes from palliative shunts and total cavopulmonary derivation (Fontan operation) to a biventricular repair. As for pulmonary atresia with ventricular septum defect, a CT scanner can be used at the early diagnosis stage to study the systemic-to-pulmonary collaterals, but it often fails to properly estimate the size of the right ventricle. When a re-intervention is planned, the CT scanner provides reliable assessment of the palliative shunt permeability and of the mediastinum anatomy.

23.2.1.3
Double-Outlet Right Ventricle

Double-outlet right ventricle is a congenital heart defect with both great vessels arising for more than 50 percent of their orifice over the right ventricle. A VSD is associated in most of the cases. A CT scanner can help in the pre-surgical evaluation of the disease (Uehara et al. 2007) by showing:

- The relative position and the size of the great vessels, generally side by side, but sometimes the aorta is in the anterior position.
- The position of the VSD relative to the great vessels: a subaortic position is most common and is usually surgically corrected by the creation of a intraventricular tunnelization from the VSD to the aorta; a subpulmonary position ("Taussing-Bing heart"), an intermediate position close to the great vessel ("doubly committed") or one distant from it ("non committed") is less frequent and leads to more complex surgical repair.
- The potential associated anomalies, including coarctation of the aorta or pulmonary vein stenosis, or even abnormal origin of coronary arteries.

23.2.1.4
Complete Transposition of the Great Vessels

Complete transposition of the great vessels (TGV) is achieved when the aorta arises anteriorly from the right ventricle and the pulmonary artery posterior from the left ventricle. Its frequency is 800 per million of live births (Hoffman and Kaplan 2002). It results in a complete separation between systemic and pulmonary circulation, causing severe neonatal hypoxia. A VSD and/or an atrio-septal defect (ASD) are associated to allow blood oxygenation. According to the position of the aorta relative to the pulmonary artery, TGV is called D-TGV (the aorta is positioned anterior and on the right of pulmonary artery) or L-TGV (the aorta is positioned anterior and on the left of pulmonary artery). An abnormal origin of coronary arteries is associated in more than 50% of the cases. "Corrected TGV," currently called "double discordance," is a different cardiac disease, where the left atrium communicates with the right ventricle and with the aorta, whereas the right atrium communicates with the left ventricle and with the pulmonary artery. Despite its complex anatomy, it results in an absence of symptoms unless other lesions are associated (such as VSD or pulmonary stenosis).

Current repair of complete TGV consists in the arterial switch procedure: the roots of the great arteries are transected and reattached to the opposite ventricle (Fig. 23.2). VSDs and/or ASDs are closed concomitantly. In the presurgical evaluation, CT can confirm the transposition and its type. Careful analysis of the position and potential anomalies of coronary arteries is highly recommended preoperatively. Size and thickness of the left ventricle are important predictors of post-surgical outcome.

23.2.1.5 Truncus Arteriosus

The truncus arteriosus is thought to result from incomplete or failed septation of the embryonic truncus arteriosus. The anomaly is characterized by a single arterial trunk arising from the normally formed ventricles by means of a single semilunar valve (i.e., truncal valve). The common trunk typically straddles a ventricular defect in the outlet portion of the interventricular septum (i.e., conal septum). Four anatomical variants were described by Collette and Edwards (1949):

- Type I truncus in which the pulmonary trunk originates from the common trunk and gives rise to right and left pulmonary branches
- Type II truncus in which the pulmonary vessels arise independently from the posterior part of the ascending common trunk
- Type III truncus in which the pulmonary vessels arise farther laterally from the truncus
- Type IV truncus, which is now recognized to be a form of pulmonary atresia with VSD rather than truncus arteriosus.

Various abnormalities may be associated with and have an impact on management and outcome. Structural abnormalities of the truncal valve, including dysplastic and supernumerary leaflets, are frequently observed, with truncal valve regurgitation (moderate or severe) being present in at least 20% of patients. Similarly, proximal coronary artery abnormalities may be present, like a single coronary artery or an intramural course. The other major anomaly associated with truncus arteriosus is interruption of the aortic arch, which occurs between the left common carotid and subclavian arteries.

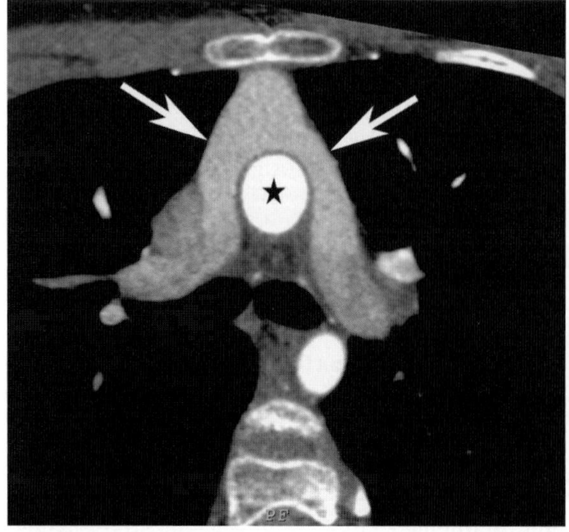

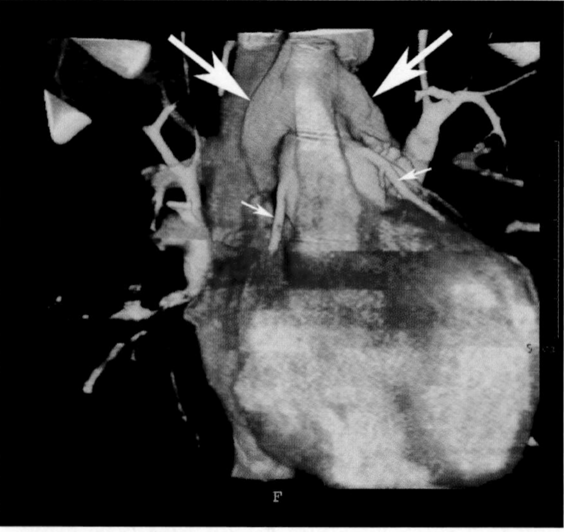

Fig. 23.2a,b. Correction of a transposition of the great vessels: the switch procedure. MPR reconstruction in axial view (**a**) and 3D reconstruction in coronal views (**b**). Aorta (*star*) is in posterior position relative to the pulmonary arteries (*large arrows*). The two pulmonary arteries are surrounding the aorta. Coronary arteries (*small arrows*) are well visualized

A CT scanner allows analyzing the relationship between aorta and pulmonary arteries and thus performing the Collette and Edwards' classification. It can also visualize the size of the pulmonary arteries, the origin of the coronary arteries and the associated anomalies. After surgery (which consists of the placement of a Rastelli tube between the right ventricle and the pulmonary arteries, previously separated from the truncus, and the closure of VSD), a CT scanner can assess focal stenosis of the pulmonary arteries or within the tube (due to thrombosis and/or endothelial proliferation).

23.2.1.6
Other Congenital Anomalies

Several other congenital disorders can lead to a situation similar to a right-to-left shunt. For example, in case of large ASD with a unique atrium aspect, blood coming from the pulmonary and the systemic circulation is mixed and leads to a cyanosis. A unique ventricle due a large VSD or to a mitral or tricuspid atresia can produce a similar situation. Similarly, a complete atrio-ventricular canal is also associated with a right-to-left shunt.

23.2.2
Inversion of Left-to-Right Shunts

Intra-cardiac left-to–right shunt can be reverted and become a right-to-left shunt when the pressure in the right cavities or in the arterial pulmonary system increases. In patients presenting with a large septal defect, with initial left-to-right shunting, Eisenmenger's syndrome (Benisty and Landzberg 1999) consists of an inversion of the shunt due to a secondary pulmonary hypertension. This hypertension results from the permanent overload of the pulmonary vascular bed, which causes a progressive elevation of the pulmonary blood pressure, leading to vascular injury and eventually irreversible elevation of pulmonary vascular resistances. It represents the final and dramatic evolution of untreated significant left-to-right shunts.

More frequently, an inversion of an ASD shunt occurs when arterial pulmonary pressure increases after a pulmonary embolism or during the evolution of chronic bronchitis. These shunts are often small and very difficult to assess by CT scanner (transesophageal echocardiography is a more reliable tool to address this issue).

Patency of the foramen ovale (PFO) is a particular type of ASD frequently occurring in the general population. Indeed, PFO can result in right-to-left shunt at the atrial level, even in the absence of elevated right heart pressure. In some situations, directional flow from the right atrium to the left atrium can cause paradoxal embolism and/or positional hypoxia. For example, the platypnea-ortodeoxia syndrome is characterized by severe hypoxia occurring in the supine position and due to PFO right-to-left shunt. Contrast transesophageal echocardiography, but not CT scanners, can evidence the shunt. Percutaneous closure of PFO is then performed in symptomatic patients.

23.3
Para-Cardiac Shunts

A right-to-left shunt can result form congenital or post-surgical anastomosis of either the systemic vein system or the pulmonary artery with the left atrium.

23.3.1
Congenital Abnormal Systemic Venous Connection

Persistent left superior vena cava is a common abnormality observed in 0.3% of the general population (Hoffman and Kaplan 2002). Generally, this left superior vena cava is connected to the coronary sinus, which is enlarged, and does not lead to a shunt. But in 10% of the cases, it is connected to the superior part of the left atrium (Fig. 23.3). The importance of the observed right-to-left shunt will then depend on the rest of the superior systemic venous system anatomy: it can go from a total superior systemic abnormal venous return if the right vena cava is absent to a less significant shunt if the left vena cava is small and the left innominate vein is patent.

Connection of the coronary sinus in the left atrium is rare and can be isolated or part of a more complex congenital heart anomaly. Abnormal connection of the inferior vena cava is very rare, but is more specifically associated with abnormal situs. In this situation, the inferior vena cava or some hepatic veins may directly connect to the left atrium.

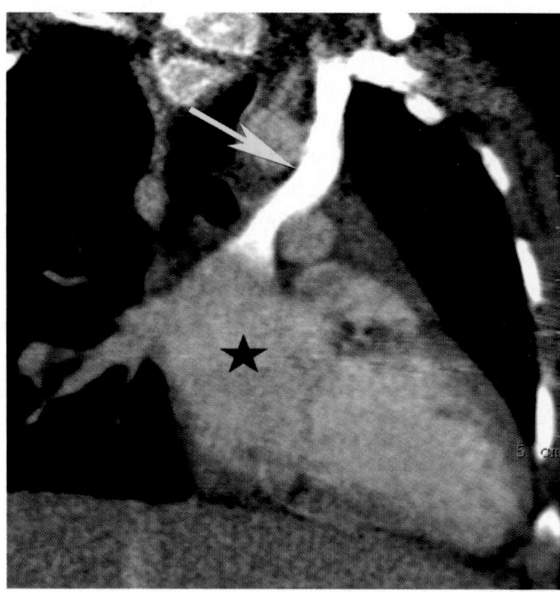

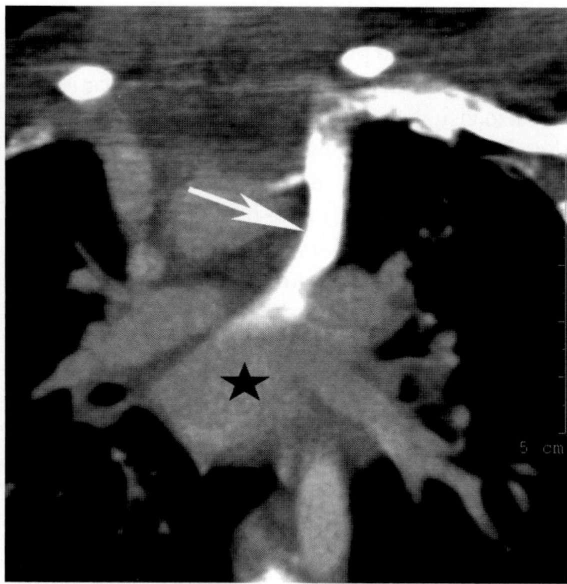

Fig. 23.3a,b. Abnormal connection between left superior vena cava and the left atrium. MPR reconstruction in sagittal (**a**) and coronal (**b**) views. The left superior vena cava (*arrow*) is directly connecting with the upper part of the left atrium, creating a direct right-to-left shunt

Finally, some embryological veins, like the levoatriocardinal vein between left pulmonary vein and the innominate vein (Jaecklin et al. 2003), may be patent, spontaneous or result from other major systemic vein obstruction (Ho et al. 1999) and create a right-to-left shunt.

CT scanners are of particularly high interest in the study of abnormal venous connections. The protocol may require a bi-brachial contrast injection, but it is best to perform a unilateral injection followed by two acquisitions: one at the end of the bolus injection and another 5 min later. In our experience this method allows to obtain some dynamic information since it visualizes the path of the high-contrast-filled vessel on the first pass and the rest of the venous anatomy on the second pass. We recommend using a 50 percent dilution of the contrast in order to limit blooming artifacts. The side of the injection depends on which structure has to be analyzed (the left arm to study a left superior vena cava, for example).

23.3.2 Post-Surgical Systemic to Pulmonary Connection

Surgically created right-to-left shunts can be necessary in some particular situations and lead to a de facto right-to-left shunt. For example, the univentricular correction of an obstruction on the left outflow tract (Damus procedure) leads to a complete mixing of blood from the right and left circulation.

23.4 Vascular Pulmonary Shunts

23.4.1 Introduction

Extra-cardiac vascular shunts result in an abnormal connection between arterial and venous pulmonary vessels. Congenital arteriovenous fistulas are much more common than acquired; however, all arteriovenous fistulas (AVFs) demonstrate direct connections between pulmonary arteries and veins. Since blood bypasses the pulmonary capillaries, microbubble contrast echocardiography is an important modality used for detection. Agitated saline is injected intravenously. As the microbubbles are absorbed within the lung, they should not be visualized in the left-sided cardiac chambers in a normal patient. If an intracardiac shunt is present, contrast is typically seen in the left heart soon after injection.

If an intrapulmonary shunt is present, contrast is seen in the left heart, but after a short delay. CT is a complimentary modality for identification of the cause of a shunt.

23.4.2
Congenital Pulmonary Arteriovenous Malformations (PAVMs)

Approximately 40–60% of patients with PAVMs have Osler-Weber-Rendu (Dines et al. 1983), otherwise known as hereditary hemorrhagic telangiectasia (HHT). The classic trio of HHT includes telangiectasia, epistaxis and family history. However, the defining abnormality is multi-organ involvement by arteriovenous malformations. Of all patients with HHT, 5–15% have PAVMs. The majority of PAVMs are simple, with one feeding artery and one draining vein. PAVMs usually present as a round or lobulated subpleural nodule demonstrating a feeding artery and draining vein (Fig. 23.4). Complications include pulmonary hemorrhage, pleural hemorrhage, systemic arterial embolization and abscess formation. PAVMs are typically treated with coil embolization when they are symptomatic or when the feeding artery is >3 mm, regardless of symptoms.

23.4.3
Acquired Vascular Pulmonary Shunts

23.4.3.1
Hepatopulmonary Syndrome

Hepatopulmonary syndrome (HPS) is characterized by vasodilatation of the pulmonary arteriolar bed in association with cirrhosis or any other cause of portal hypertension (e.g., Budd-Chiari). The liver dysfunction results in a cascade whose end result is the over-production of vasoactive substances, particularly nitrous oxide. As many as 20% of patients presenting for orthotopic liver transplant will meet criteria for this syndrome. Hypoxemia may result because of V/Q mismatching and intrapulmonary shunting. This shunting is exacerbated by the presence of intrapulmonary vascular malformations in some patients, also associated with HPS. The CT

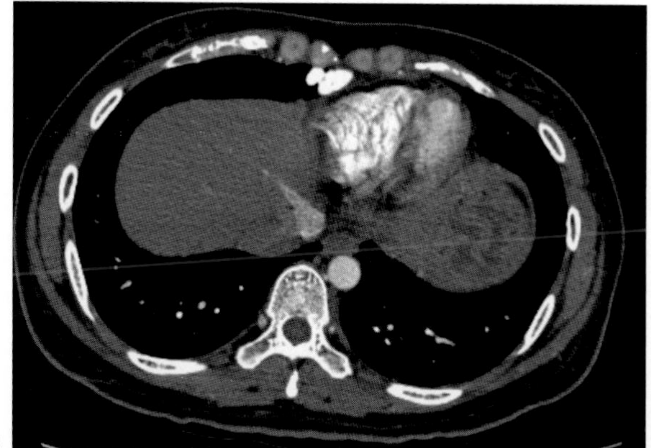
a

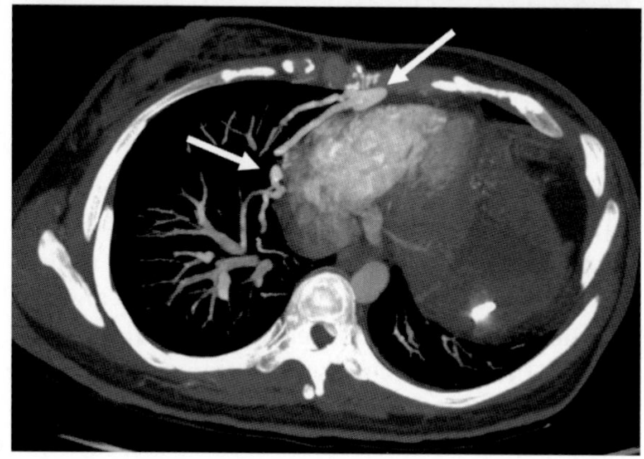
b

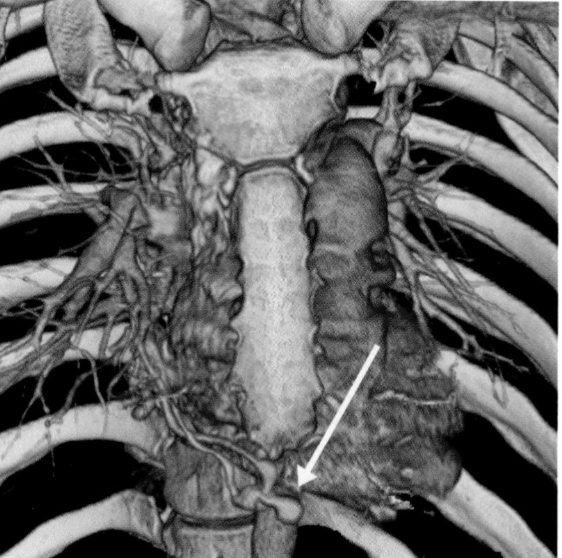
c

Fig. 23.4a–c. A 30-year-old female with hereditary hemorrhagic telangiectasia with multiple AVMs. Axial CT through the lung base (**a**) shows a large saccular AVM in the medial right middle lobe. Oblique MIP (**b**) in the same region demonstrates two AVMs (*arrows*). Both are simple with one feeding artery and one draining vein. Volume-rendered image (**c**) nicely demonstrates the morphology and vascular supply to the AVM in the right middle lobe

findings of HPS are vascular dilatation of small distal arteries in the periphery of the lung extending near to the pleural surface (McAdams et al. 1996) (Fig. 23.5).

23.4.3.2
Vascular Metastases

Highly vascular metastases may be associated with shunting, primarily because of small arteriovenous fistulas. These are rarely symptomatic; however, large arteriovenous fistulas may occasionally be associated with significant shunting and subsequent hypoxemia. The most common tumors to demonstrate pulmonary arteriovenous fistulas include renal cell carcinomas, thyroid carcinomas, sarcomas and choriocarcinoma. The rare triton tumor, a malignant neurogenic tumor with rhabdomyoblastic differentiation, has been described as a cause of intrapulmonary shunting. Extra-pulmonary arteriovenous fistulas, as seen with osseous metastases from renal cell carcinoma, are more common and may result in high-output cardiac failure.

23.4.3.3
Rasmussen Aneurysms

One of the rare complications of pulmonary tuberculosis is the Rasmussen aneurysm. In one review of autopsy findings, the prevalence of this complication was approximately 4–5% in patients with chronic cavitary disease. Cavitary tuberculosis adjacent to a pulmonary artery branch may cause weakening of the arterial wall from deposition of granulation tissue and fibrosis. This may eventually rupture with the typical clinical presentation being hemoptysis. Rarely, an arteriovenous communication may form from direct extension to a pulmonary vein.

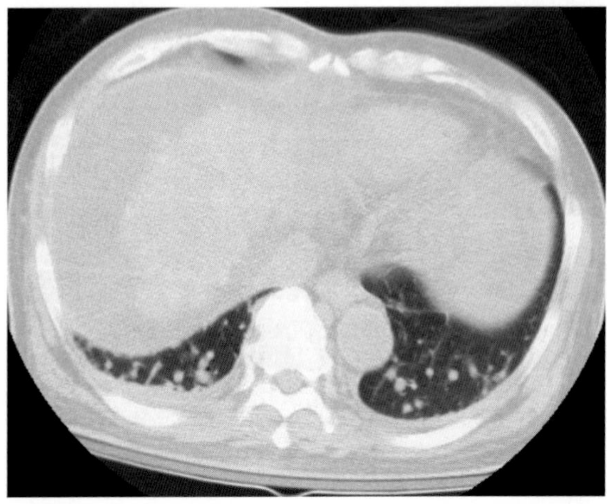

Fig. 23.5. A 56-year-old male with cirrhosis and hepatopulmonary syndrome. CT through the lung bases demonstrates very dilated arteries extending to the immediate supleural lung regions

23.4.3.4
Traumatic Arteriovenous Fistula

Direct arteriovenous communications in the setting of penetrating trauma are very rare, with only approximately ten reported cases in the literature (Dairywala et al. 2005). The most common associated injuries are gunshot wounds. Patients may present with acute hypoxemia, but a delayed presentation remote from the traumatic injury is not uncommon.

23.4.3.5
Septic Emboli

Septic embolization to the lung is a rare cause of an acquired arteriovenous fistula. This is most frequently seen in intravenous drug users with right-sided endocarditis (Stagaman et al. 1990). Embolization to a pulmonary arterial branch results in weakening of the wall and pseudoaneurysm formation. This may eventually erode into a pulmonary vein producing a direct connection. As with other direct arteriovenous communications, this complication may result in systemic arterial embolization, particularly in the setting of recurrent or untreated endocarditis.

23.5
Parenchymal Shunts

23.5.1
Introduction

Intrapulmonary shunting is a common cause of impaired blood oxygenation. To understand the impact of intrapulmonary shunts, knowledge of lung physiology is essential. In an ideal situation, alveolar ventilation (Va) and lung perfusion (Q) are matched (1:1) so that there is maximum transfer of oxygen and carbon dioxide between the alveolar airspace and pulmonary capillary. In the normal upright patient, there is proportionally more ventilation than perfusion in the upper lungs (Va/Q >1) and less ventilation than perfusion in the lower lungs (Va/Q <1). This results in a baseline ventilation/perfusion mismatch and a small physiologic shunt, as not all blood is able to fully participate in gas exchange.

Reductions in alveolar ventilation will result in an increase in this shunt. This may occur because of either airway obstruction or an alveolar filling process. Both serve to decrease the amount of oxygen and increase the amount of carbon dioxide within alveoli. The normal response to hypoxia is vasoconstriction in an attempt to redirect blood flow away from diseased regions; however, this mechanism can only incompletely compensate.

Clinically shunting may present with dyspnea and respiratory failure in addition to an elevated systemic arterial pCO_2 and decreased pO_2. If the shunt is severe enough, increasing the inspired oxygen content will not result in an increase in arterial pO_2 because there is little to no gas exchange at the alveolar level.

23.5.2 Atelectasis

Atelectasis is the most common cause of an intrapulmonary shunt. As the alveoli are airless, there is no gas exchange between the alveoli and pulmonary capillaries. The degree of shunt will be proportional to the extent of collapse (Hedenstierna et al. 1986). Shunting may occur with any of the types of atelectasis (obstructive, passive, adhesive and cicatricial); however, passive atelectasis is the most commonly encountered form in clinical practice. Some of the most frequent clinical scenarios include anesthesia during surgery and patients who are supine for long periods of time.

On both chest X-rays and CTs, it is easy to underestimate the amount of lung affected by atelectasis because of volume loss. The radiographic findings of atelectasis are segmental regions of opacity with displacement of fissures and other signs of volume loss. With obstructive atelectasis, the lung typically appears airless as bronchial obstruction eventually results in complete resorption of air in both alveoli and bronchi. Air bronchograms are frequently seen on CT in patients with passive atelectasis as the airways are not obstructed.

23.5.3 Rounded Atelectasis

Significant shunting related to rounded atelectasis is very rare. Since it is a focal process associated with an adjacent pleural abnormality, the degree of lung affected is typically relatively small. This is evidenced by the fact that rounded atelectasis is rarely symptomatic and is typically discovered as an incidental finding in the evaluation of a patient with significant asbestos exposure.

23.5.4 Pneumonia

Pneumonia is a very common cause of intrapulmonary shunting. There are two main elements that may contribute to this shunt. First, inflammatory infiltrates replace normal air within the alveoli, preventing gas exchange between the alveolar spaces and pulmonary capillaries. Second, certain infections, particularly viruses, may produce airway inflammation and narrowing. This can result in decreased alveolar ventilation even when alveoli distal to the obstructed bronchi are normally aerated. As with atelectasis, the degree of shunting is proportional to the volume of lung affected.

23.5.5 Bronchioloalveolar Cell Carcinoma

Bronchioloalveolar cell carcinoma (BAC) spreads via lepidic growth, disseminating via the surfaces of alveolar septa and bronchial walls. The mucinous subtype of BAC often is associated with extensive mucin production that fills the alveolar spaces and further prevents normal gas exchange. Despite this alveolar filling process, perfusion to regions involved by tumor is typically normal, creating a significant shunt in larger tumors (Fishman et al. 1974). This is in contrast to other lung tumors and inflammatory processes in which perfusion tends to decrease because of reflex vasoconstriction. Bronchioloalveolar cell carcinomas that produce large shunts present with large regions of consolidation that are often multi-focal. Centrilobular nodules may also be seen, reflecting endobronchial spread of the tumor (Fig. 23.6).

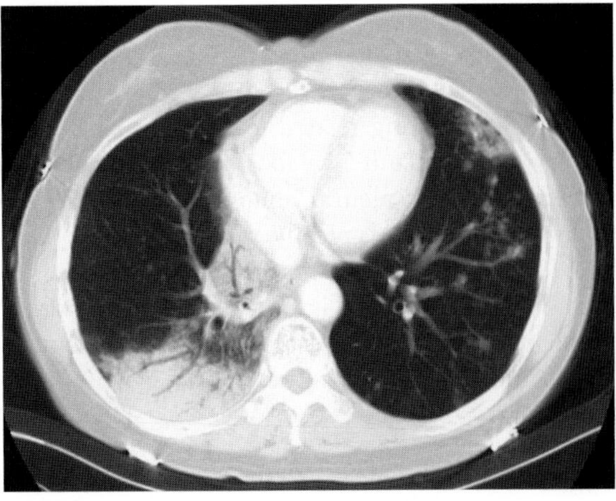

Fig. 23.6. A 56-year-old female with bronchioloalveolar cell carcinoma. CT shows multi-focal regions of consolidation and centrilobular nodules. This reflects both alveolar and airway spread of tumor

23.5.6 Tracheal or Bronchial Obstruction

Any cause of decreased alveolar ventilation may cause a ventilation/perfusion mismatch. The processes already described prevent gas exchange through alveolar filling or complete airway obstruction with alveolar collapse. However, incomplete obstruction of airways may also produce decreased ventilation and an associated V/Q mismatch. The end result is a lower oxygen level and higher carbon dioxide level within the alveolar spaces and thus within the blood. As opposed to the processes above, patients with incomplete airway obstruction have some residual ventilation, albeit decreased. Because of this, increasing the inspired oxygen tends to improve the patient's hypoxemia except in severe cases. Radiographically incomplete airway obstruction may present with varying degrees of segmental opacity or lucency depending upon the severity of obstruction and whether air trapping is present.

23.6 Conclusion

Although it cannot directly quantify the shunt, the CT scanner provides useful information about the origin of a right-to-left shunt and the anatomy of the involved structure to properly guide surgical options. However, MRI is often preferred to CT scanners for its ability to quantify flows and measure ventricular function, and because of the absence of irradiation. Nevertheless, CT has several advantages. First, its excellent spatial resolution allows analysis of small arterial structures, such as MAPCAs and coronary arteries. Then, the examination time is much shorter in CT (a few seconds) than in MRI (20 to 30 min). This last element is particularly important in young children in whom prolonged anesthesia time can hardly be achieved. Finally, MRI fails to identify intra-pulmonary shunts and to evaluate the impact of the underlying pathology (tetralogy of Fallot, for example) on lung perfusion and development. Therefore, cardiac CT should not be considered concurrently with MRI or other techniques in right-to-left shunt imaging, but as an alternative method with specific indications.

References

Baert A, Dymarkowski S, Sartor K (2005) Clinical cardiac MRI. Springer, Berlin Heidelberg New York

Benisty JI, Landzberg MJ (1999) Eisenmenger's syndrome. Curr Treat Options Cardiovasc Med 1:355–362

Collett RW, Edwards JE (1949) Persistent truncus arteriosus; a classification according to anatomic types. Surg Clin North Am 29:1245–1270

Dairywala IT, Lokhandwala J, Patrick H, Talucci R, Jain D (2005) Severe refractory hypoxemia following a gunshot injury. Chest 127:398–401

Dines DE, Seward JB, Bernatz PE (1983) Pulmonary arteriovenous fistulas. Mayo Clin Proc 58:176–181

Fishman HC, Danon J, Koopot N, Langston HT, Sharp JT (1974) Massive intrapulmonary venoarterial shunting in alveolar cell carcinoma. A case report. Am Rev Respir Dis 109:124–128

Hedenstierna G, Tokics L, Strandberg A, Lundquist H, Brismar B (1986) Correlation of gas exchange impairment to development of atelectasis during anaesthesia and muscle paralysis. Acta Anaesthesiol Scand 30:183–191

Higgins C, Roos AD (2006) MRI and CT of the cardiovascular system, 2nd edn). Lippincott Williams & Wilkins, Philadelphia

Ho HT, Horowitz AL, Ho AC (1999) Systemic to pulmonary venous communication (right-to-left shunt) in superior vena cava obstruction demonstrated by spiral CT. Br J Radiol 72:712–713

Hoffman JI, Kaplan S (2002) The incidence of congenital heart disease. J Am Coll Cardiol 39:1890–1900

Jaecklin T, Beghetti M, Didier D (2003) Levoatriocardinal vein without cardiac malformation and normal pulmonary venous return. Heart 89:1444

Lu JH, Chung MY, Betau H, Chien HP, Lu JK (2001) Molecular characterization of tetralogy of fallot within Digeorge critical region of the chromosome 22. Pediatr Cardiol 22:279–284

McAdams HP, Erasmus J, Crockett R, Mitchell J, Godwin JD, McDermott VG (1996) The hepatopulmonary syndrome: radiologic findings in ten patients. AJR Am J Roentgenol 166:1379–1385

Norgaard MA, Alphonso N, Cochrane AD, Menahem S, Brizard CP, d'Udekem Y (2006) Major aorto-pulmonary collateral arteries of patients with pulmonary atresia and ventricular septal defect are dilated bronchial arteries. Eur J Cardiothorac Surg 29:653–658

Stagaman DJ, Presti C, Rees C, Miller DD (1990) Septic pulmonary arteriovenous fistula. An unusual conduit for systemic embolization in right-sided valvular endocarditis. Chest 97:1484–1486

Uehara M, Funabashi N, Ogawa Y, Minamino T, Komuro I (2007) Double outlet right ventricle demonstrated by multislice computed tomography. Int J Cardiol 121:218–220

Medical Applications of Integrated Cardiothoracic Imaging

Diseases of the Pericardium

MDCT: Evaluation of Congenital and Acquired Diseases of the Pericardium

24

Paul Stolzmann, Borut Marincek, and Hatem Alkadhi

CONTENTS

P. Stolzmann, MD
B. Marincek, MD, Professor
H. Alkadhi, MD, PD
Institute of Diagnostic Radiology, University Hospital Zurich, Raemistrasse 100, 8091 Zurich, Switzerland

24.1 Introduction

The clinical mainstay of diagnostic imaging of the pericardium is transthoracic or transesophageal echocardiography. However, when imaging of the pericardium with echocardiography is hampered by a restricted acoustic window or when there is discrepancy between the clinical and the echocardiographic findings, magnetic resonance imaging (MRI) is considered as a second-line imaging modality. MRI has the advantage of providing superior soft tissue contrast as compared to all other imaging modalities. In addition, MRI is not operator-dependent and relies less on the patients' constitution than echocardiography.

The advent of multi-detector row computed tomography (CT) with increased temporal and spatial resolution has considerably improved the imaging capabilities of this technique. Because the isotropic data enable images in any arbitrary plane and orientation, even complex anatomic structures can be visualized. Traditionally, CT has not been used as a primary imaging modality of pericardial disease, but as an alternative to echocardiography when MRI was contraindicated. The strengths of CT derive from its capability to image the entire mediastinum, including the pericardium in a short time period with a high spatial resolution. As compared to echocardiography, CT provides a larger field of view, allowing the examination of the entire chest and the detection of associated abnormalities in the mediastinum and lungs. With multi-detector CT technology, the anatomy of the pericardium is routinely clearly displayed even when images are acquired without electrocardiography (ECG) gating. In recent years, images of the pericardium have been acquired as an adjunct to the increasingly performed cardiac CT examination. This requires that the radiologist is familiar with the normal anatomy and with the most common imaging features of pericardial disease. This chapter describes the normal anatomy of the pericardium along with its appearance in CT and lists the imaging features of the most relevant pericardial diseases, such as pericarditis, effusion, neoplasms, as well as congenital anomalies.

24.2 CT Anatomy

24.2.1 General Anatomy and Physiology of the Pericardium

The pericardium is composed of the visceral and the parietal layer. The visceral pericardium is a serous membrane consisting of a single layer of mesothelial cells that are adherent to the epicardial surface. The parietal pericardium is composed of a largely acellular, fibrous layer about 2 mm in thickness. The parietal pericardium forms a flask-shaped outer sac that surrounds most parts of the heart. Much of the ascending aorta, pulmonary trunk, short segments of pulmonary veins and the caval veins are located intra-pericardially. The phrenic nerves are the only non-cardiac macrostructures that are enveloped by the parietal pericardium.

As the visceral pericardium reflects near the origins of the great vessels, it forms the inner layer of the parietal pericardium (Fig. 24.1). The pericardial cavity lies in between and contains up to 50 ml of serous fluid, which provides lubrication between the layers. The exact amount may vary among different individuals.

The parietal pericardium has attachments to the diaphragm, sternum, costal cartilage and dorsal spine. Ventral insertions to the sternum are present, while only some patients show attachments to the dorsal spine. These attachments ensure a relatively fixed position of the heart regardless of respiration phase and body position.

Another important function of the parietal pericardium is provided by bundles of collagen and elastic fibres that are stretched during each single cardiac cycle. Thereby, the pericardium yields a higher stiffness at end-diastole, which has a restraining effect on cardiac volume (Hamilton et al. 1994). Furthermore, the pericardium functions as a barrier to infection. Although the pericardium serves these many important functions, it is not essential for life.

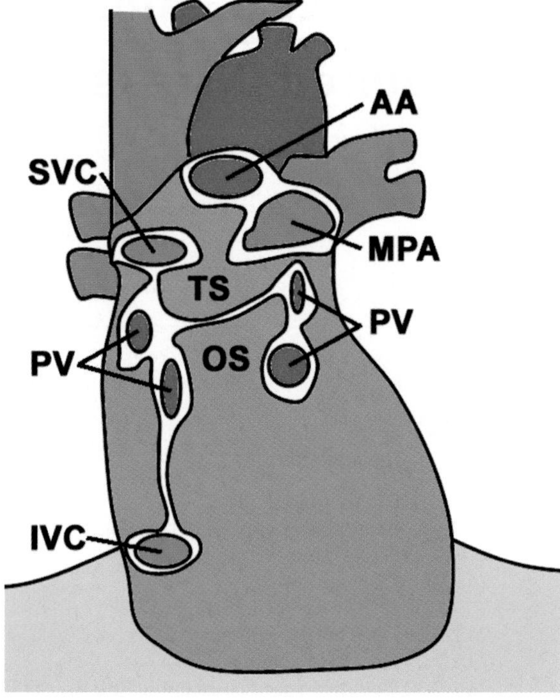

Fig. 24.1. Pericardial cavity and reflections of serosal layers (*scheme*, view from anterior). The pericardium encloses the ascending aorta (*AA*), the main pulmonary artery (*MPA*), the superior (*SVC*) and the inferior vena cava (*IVC*), and the pulmonary veins (*PV*). The transverse sinus (*TS*) is posterior to the left atrium, the oblique sinus (*OS*) inferiorly

24.2.2 CT Anatomy of Pericardial Structures

The pericardial cavity lies between variable amounts of epicardial and pericardial adipose tissue, which provides a natural tissue contrast. On CT, the ventral and caudal portions of the pericardium are generally visualized best (Fig. 24.2). The normal parietal pericardial is seen as a pencil-thin curvilinear line of 1 to 2 mm of thickness, but can focally appear thicker at the sites of its major attachments.

The ventral parts of the fibrous parietal pericardium are regularly visualized, while the dorsal aspects of the parietal pericardium are primarily seen at the caudal insertions and occasionally at the level of the left atrium and ventricle. The cephalad portion is usually not visualized because of lacking fat in this area. It can be identified with abnormal thickening or when a pericardial effusion displaces it ventrally (Vesely et al. 1986).

As described above, the inner serosal layer reflects at the great vessels and forms the pericardial

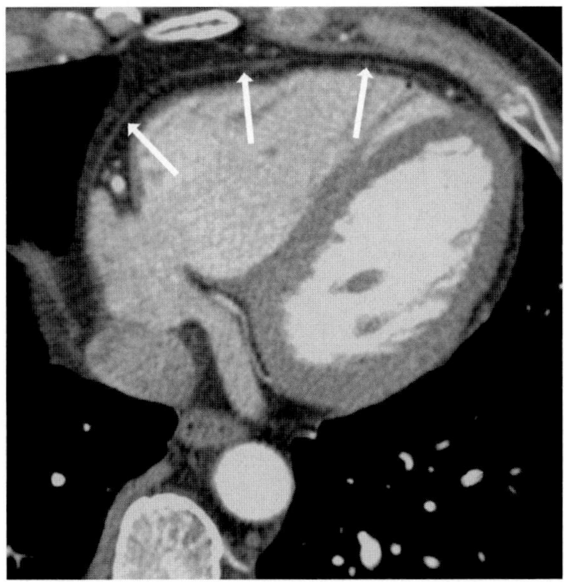

Fig. 24.2. Normal anterior pericardium. The pericardium appears as a *thin line* in the anterior mediastinum (*white arrows*)

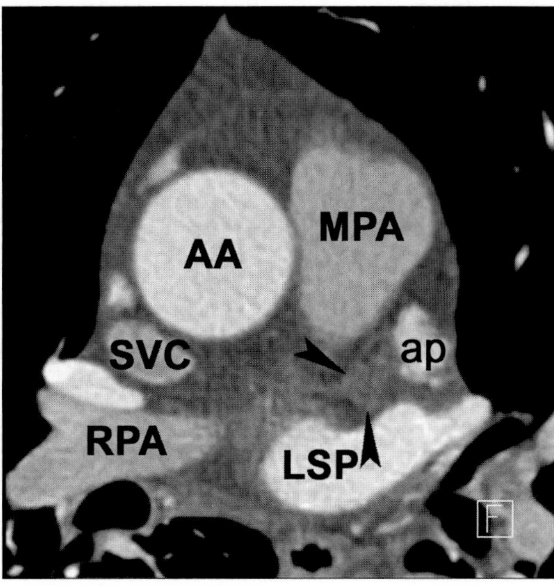

Fig 24.3. Transverse sinus of the pericardium (*arrowheads*). CT inferior to the RPA at the level of the left atrial appendage (*ap*). Ascending aorta (*AA*), main pulmonary artery (*MPA*), the superior vena cava (*SVC*), left superior pulmonary vein (*LSP*), right pulmonary artery (*RPA*)

recesses (Fig. 24.1). These serosal reflections surround two complex tubes. The first tube encloses the aorta and pulmonary trunk. The second encloses both the superior and the inferior vena cava, and additionally contains the four pulmonary veins. The transverse sinus is located above and posterior to the left atrium and represents the transition zone of the two tubes. It is divided into the superior aortic recess (anterior and posterior portion), the inferior aortic recess, the right pulmonic recess and the left pulmonic recess (Vesely et al. 1986). Finally, the oblique sinus proper includes the postcaval recess and the left and right pulmonary venous recesses. Misinterpretation of these pericardial recesses as mediastinal abnormalities may have an important clinical impact (Vesely et al. 1986, Batra et al. 2000) (see Sect. 2.2.3).

24.2.2.1 The Transverse Sinus

Superior Aortic Recess

The transverse sinus is situated above the left atrium and behind the aorta and the pulmonary trunk (Fig. 24.3). The superior division of the transverse sinus represents the superior aortic recess, which normally is divided into two parts, the anterior and the posterior portion. The anterior superior aortic recess lies in front of the ascending aorta, whereas the posterior superior aortic recess lies behind (Fig. 24.4a,b). Both are connected. The anterior superior aortic recess passes anteriorly to the aorta and the pulmonary trunk and forms a fissure between these vessels. Fluid in this pericardial recess has a well-circumscribed contour with a snout-shaped extension. It may drape in front of the aorta and pulmonary artery.

The posterior portion of the superior aortic recess is seen on CT as a half-moon-shaped fluid collection adjacent to the posterior wall of the ascending aorta, usually at the level of the right pulmonary artery.

Inferior Aortic Recess

The inferior aortic recess of the transverse sinus extends between the aortic root and the right atrium (Fig. 24.5). This recess is subdivided into a right and a left pulmonic recess. The left pulmonic recess lies laterally to the left pulmonary artery and extends posteriorly to the proximal right pulmonary artery. The right pulmonic recess extends posteriorly below the right pulmonary artery (Groell et al. 1999).

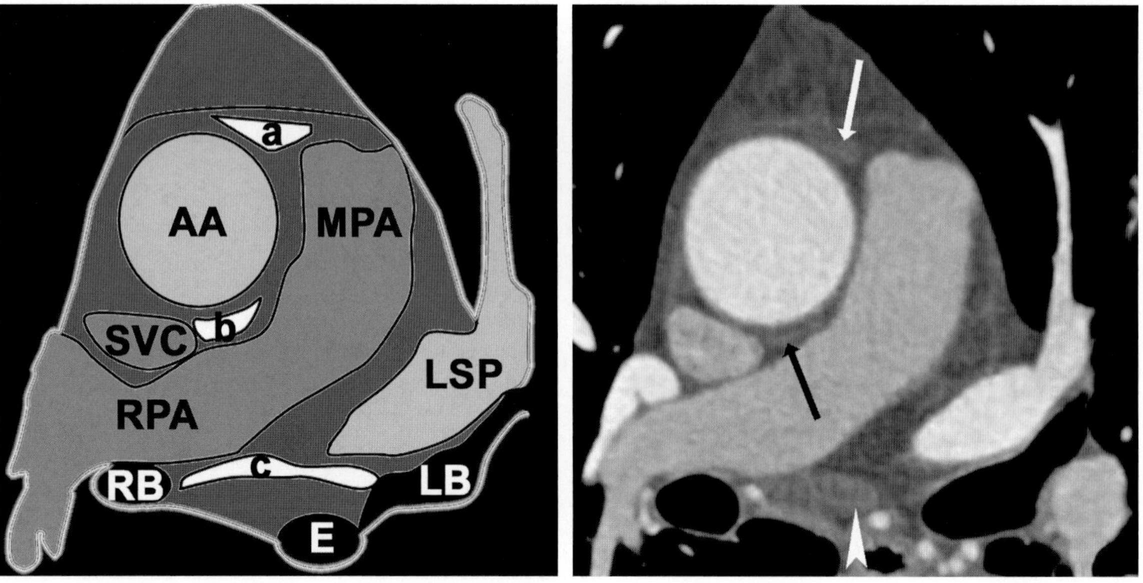

Fig. 24.4a,b. Pericardial sinuses and recesses. (**a**) *Cross-sectional drawing* of the ascending aorta (*AA*), right bronchus (*RB*), left bronchus (*LB*), esophagus (*E*), left superior pulmonary vein (*LSP*), main pulmonary artery (*MPA*), right pulmonary artery (*RPA*), anterior superior aortic recess (*a*), posterior superior aortic recess (*b*), posterior pericardial recess of oblique sinus (*c*). (**b**) Corresponding CT. The anterior portion of the superior aortic recess is ventrally (*white arrow*) and the posterior portion dorsally of the ascending aorta (*black arrow*). The posterior recess of the oblique sinus is posterior to the RPA and between the RB and LB (*white arrowhead*)

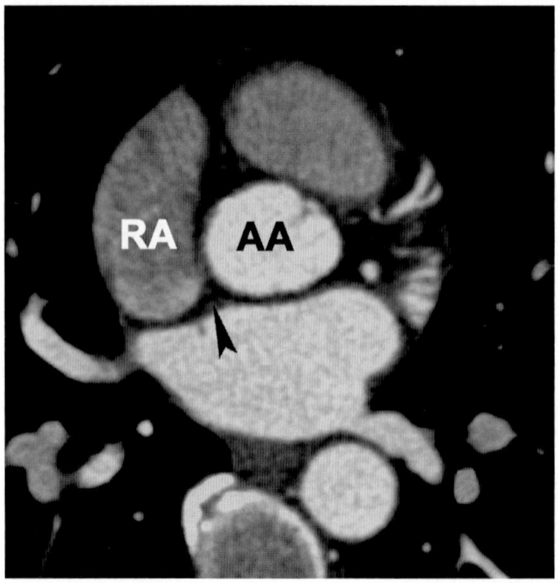

Fig. 24.5. Inferior aortic recess. The inferior aortic recess (*black arrowhead*) extends behind the ascending aorta (*AA*) and the right atrium (*RA*)

24.2.2.2
The Oblique Sinus

The oblique sinus lies posterior to the left atrium and to the left pulmonary artery (Groell et al. 1999). The superior portion of this sinus is called the posterior pericardial recess. This pericardial cavity is separated from the transverse sinus by a double reflection of serous pericardium and includes the post-caval recess as well as the left and right pulmonary venous recesses. These extensions may reach the subcarinal region.

Pulmonary Venous Recess

The left and right pulmonary vein recesses are between the superior and inferior pulmonary veins on each side (Fig. 24.6).

Postcaval Recess

The postcaval recess is posterior and lateral to the superior caval vein and between the inferior vena cava and the coronary sinus. The postcaval recess is bounded by the superior caval vein and the right superior pulmonary vein.

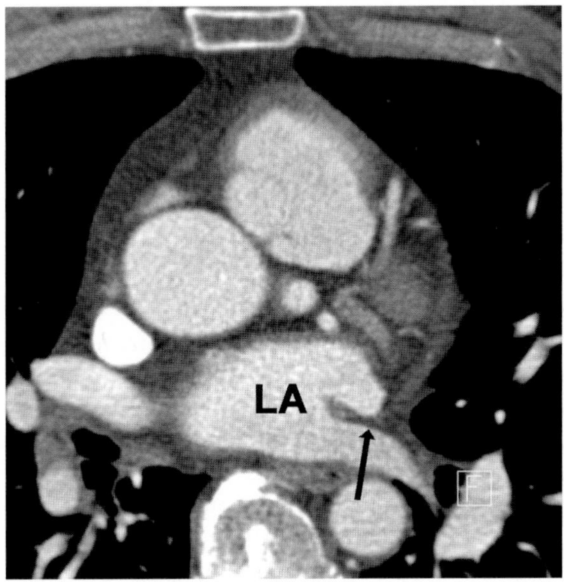

Fig. 24.6. Pulmonary vein recess. The pulmonary vein recess (*black arrow*) is between the superior and inferior pulmonary veins. Left atrium (*LA*)

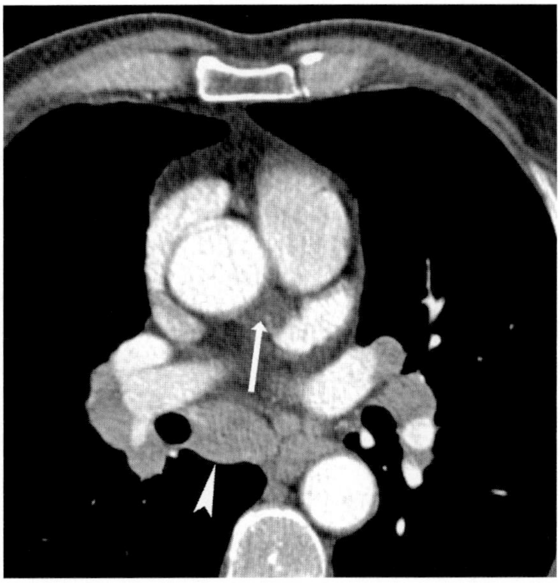

Fig. 24.7. Transverse CT of a patient with infracarinal adenopathy (*white arrowhead*). The small fluid collection in the transverse sinus (white *arrow*) could be mistaken for another lymphadenopathy

24.2.2.3 Modality-Specific Anatomic Pitfalls

Pericardial fluid can collect in the various above-described sinuses of the pericardial reflections. As these collections may mimic dissection flaps, bronchogenic cysts or adenopathy, they can be mistaken as pathologies (Choi et al., 2000). Especially in oncologic imaging, misinterpretation of pericardial fluid as adenopathy can lead to inaccurate clinical staging and inappropriate patient management and therapy (Fig. 24.7).

Rarely, the extensions of the superior recess may lie more cranially in a right paratracheal location (Aronberg et al. 1984). This ectopic location has been defined as a high-riding pericardial recess (Choi et al. 2000). Knowledge of this anatomic variant prevents mistaking it for a right para-tracheal lymph node (Truong et al. 2003). The prevalence of a high-riding superior pericardial recess is 2%. Differentiation of this recess from aorto-pulmonary window adenopathy is possible based on the typical location and appearance: since fluid in the sleeve can be seen anterior and posterior to the vein, adenopathy typically occurs only on one side of the vein, with possible concomitant narrowing of the vein (Batra et al. 2000).

On the other hand, fluid in the oblique sinus can imitate abnormalities in the posterior mediastinum, such as pathologies of the esophagus or descending thoracic aorta. Fluid in the oblique sinus may also be mistaken for subcarinal or bronchopulmonary lymph nodes. Also, at the level of the inferior pulmonary vein recess, pericardial fluid in this sleeve can be misinterpreted as adenopathy.

In order to differentiate between these fluid collections, the radiologist has to determine carefully the allocation. Fluid in the sleeves can be seen anterior and posterior to the vein, whereas adenopathy typically occurs only on one side of the vein. The reverse, narrowing of the vein, is most frequently caused by lymph nodes.

24.3 CT Techniques for Diagnosis of Pericardial Disease

During early stages of CT application, cardiac CT interpretation was limited by the effects of motion artifacts. With the introduction of ECG gating, image reconstruction may be synchronized to the movements of the heart. Newer scanners provide a high temporal resolution of up to 83 ms allowing the accurate depiction of coronary arteries without motion artifacts. On the other hand, the pericardium can be visualized consistently with high accuracy without ECG gating. This is facilitated by the isotropic spatial resolution allowing multiplanar reformations in any arbitrary plane.

CT scanning of the pericardium should cover the full range from the tracheal bifurcation to the diaphragm. In the routine clinical setting, patients are examined in the supine position. Views in the lateral decubitus position may be of additional value when encapsulated effusions are suspected. When examining the pericardial recesses, it may be of value to reconstruct thin-section CT images that permit reformatted images in coronal, sagittal or oblique planes (Kodama et al. 2003).

The use of contrast media is recommended in patients with suspected pericarditis, encapsulated pericardial effusions and cardiac or intra-pericardial masses (Gross et al. 1983).

Although echocardiography is the most widely used technique for pericardial imaging, MRI and more recently CT allow for the detection of practically all diseases of the pericardium. Consequently, three-dimensional studies are of high value in the accurate determination for percutanous puncture sites. Information about the adjacent lung anatomy in order to avoid a pneumothorax and measurements of distances (i.e., between the skin and the pericardial sac) may routinely be obtained.

24.4 Classifications and Detection of Pericardial Disease in CT

24.4.1 Congenital Diseases of the Pericardium

Congenital anomalies of the pericardium are rare. They are classified as congenital absence or defects of the pericardium, pericardial cysts and developmental tumors of the pericardium.

24.4.1.1 Congenital Absence or Defects of the Pericardium

A compromise of the vascular supply to the pleuropericardial membrane during embryologic development is associated with congenital absence or defects in the pericardium. Congenital absences of the pericardium can be classified into three groups (Moore et al. 1953):

- Left-sided absence, meaning the left heart and lung are in the same cavity with preservation on the right (60%).
- A foramen-like defect, mostly on the left side (20%).
- Total absence or rudimentary development (20%).

Absence or defects occur with a frequency of 1:10,000 in autopsies and are three times more often in males (male to female ratio 3:1) (Maisch et al. 2004). The variation in size is wide. Defects of the pericardium are frequently associated with large defects in the parietal pleura through which the lung can herniate (Hipona et al. 1964) or other congenital anomalies of the heart. Patients may present with a patent ductus arteriosus, a defect of the interventricular septum, a tetra- or pentalogy of Fallot, as well as with a lung sequestration in around 30% (Maisch et al. 2004, Rao et al. 1981).

Absence or defects of the left pericardium usually cause no symptoms. Vague chest pain may occur and increase in the left lateral position due to volume loading of the cardiac chambers. Several studies described a herniation of the atrium (Robin et al. 1975) or of the ventricle through a congenital pericardial defect. A herniation of the atrium or of the ventricle may also be found in postoperative patients (Fig. 24.8) (Dober et al. 2006). Acute symptoms occasionally occur during exercise when the appendage or the apical ventricle herniates. However, absence or defects of the pericardium are commonly an incidental finding. Contrast-enhanced CT and MRI are the modalities of choice for the diagnosis. The evidence of an interruption of the pericardial continuity may be directly seen or may be denoted by the recognition of a direct contact between the heart and the lungs.

24.4.1.2 Pericardial Cysts

Pericardial cysts are a benign congenital anomaly in the middle mediastinum. They may also be acquired after cardiothoracic surgery. Pericardial cysts are caused by an incomplete coalescence of fetal lacunae forming the pericardium and result when a portion of the pericardium is isolated during embryonic development. Histological examinations have shown pericardial cysts and diverticula

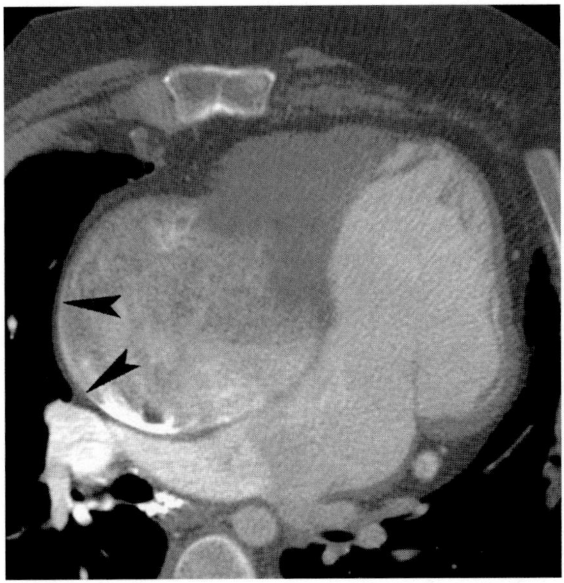

Fig. 24.8. Partial herniation of the right atrium (*black arrowheads*) bulging dorsolaterally (transverse oblique multiplanar CT reconstruction). This 22-year-old previously underwent a Fontan procedure for tetralogy of Fallot repair

to be fluid-filled outpouchings of the parietal pericardium (Feigin et al. 1977). Therefore, they are thought to emerge from persistent blind-ending ventral pericardial recesses. Pericardial cysts occur at a rate of 1 per 100,000 persons. They represent 6% of mediastinal masses and 33% of mediastinal cysts (Wang et al. 2003). Fifty-one to 71% percent of congenital cysts are located at the right cardiophrenic angle, 28–38% at the left and 8–11% in the superior mediastinum (Patel et al. 2004). Seventy-five percent of the cysts cause no associated clinical symptoms. Most commonly they are depicted incidentally during routine chest X-ray or echocardiography. The size of pericardial cysts varies from 1 to 5 cm. It is unknown whether a particular size or position of the cyst is associated with a higher complication rate. Symptomatic patients most commonly complain about chest pain, persistent cough and dyspnea, which are usually due to compression of adjacent organs (Feigin et al. 1977). Cardiac tamponade, obstruction of right main stem bronchus and sudden death represent life-threatening emergencies. Cardiac tamponade is secondary to an intra-pericardial rupture of the cyst or spontaneous hemorrhage into the cyst. Other complications include obstruction of the right ventricular outflow tract, inflammation and infection, pulmonary stenosis, partial erosion into adjacent structures, atrial fibrillation and congestive heart failure. A few pericardial cysts resolve spontaneously, likely from rupture into the pleural space. The rates of spontaneous resolution or complications have not been reported so far (Feigin et al. 1977).

Contours of these cysts are usually well defined and round. On CT, they present as unilocular or multilocular low-attenuation and thin-walled space-occupying lesions (Maisch et al. 2004). Their attenuation is slightly higher than water density and does not enhance after intravenous contrast administration (Fig. 24.9a,b).

Since cysts may also be located in the superior mediastinum, the differential diagnoses should include intrapericardial, bronchogenic cysts and cystic teratomas. The management of pericardial cysts includes follow-up, percutaneous drainage or resection. Follow-up is performed with repeated CT scans, MRI or echocardiography.

24.4.2 Acquired Diseases of the Pericardium

24.4.2.1 Pericarditis

Pericarditis is defined as a state of inflammation of the pericardium that is secondary to infection (viral, fungal or bacterial), myocardial infarction, radiotherapy, uremia, systemic autoimmune diseases or drug-related (Maisch et al. 2004).

Viral pericarditis is the most common infection and results from a direct viral attack and antiviral immune response. The entero-, echo-, adeno-, Epstein-Barr, herpes simplex, influenza, parvo B19 or hepatitis C virus may be causative. The cytomegalovirus is most often seen in immunocompromised hosts (Campbell et al. 1995). The treatment consists of resolving the symptoms and preventing recurrences.

Fungal pericarditis mainly occurs in immunocompromised patients or in the course of endemic-acquired fungal infections. *Histoplasma* and *Coccidioides* are mainly causative in endemic areas, whereas *Candida*, *Aspergillus* and *Norcardia* are non-endemic. The clinical picture varies and includes the full spectrum of pericardial diseases. Antifungal medication represents the treatment of choice.

Bacterial pericarditis is a rare entity and usually manifests as a purulent effusion or empyema. Again,

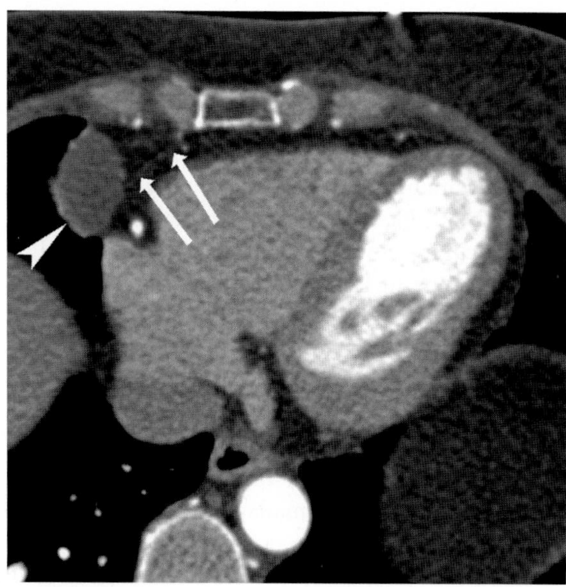

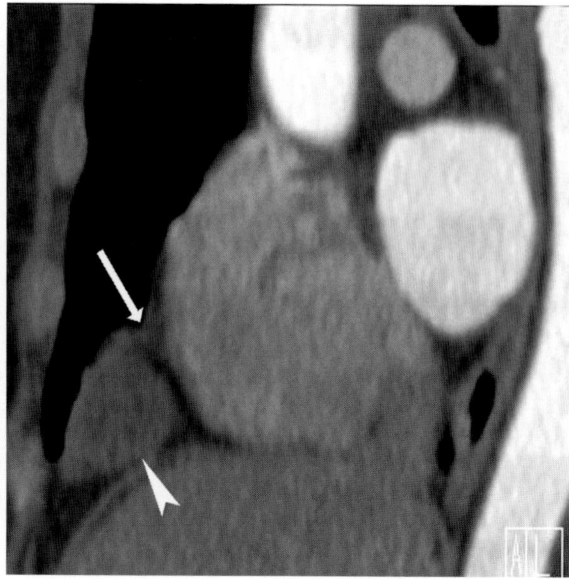

Fig. 24.9a,b. Pericardial cyst. Transverse CT (**a**) and sagittal oblique multiplanar CT reconstruction (**b**). Pericardial cyst (*white arrowhead*) at right cardiophrenic angle with adherence to the pericardium (*white arrows*)

a wide variety of organisms, such as staphylococcus, pneumococcus and streptococcus, can be causative (Sagrista-Sauleda et al. 1993). In patients with proven tuberculosis, tuberculous pericarditis is likely. Often, purulent pericarditis is fatal if untreated. Open surgical drainage and pericardectomy are required in patients with dense adhesions, loculated and thick purulent effusion, or progression to constriction (Maisch et al. 2004).

Postinfarction pericarditis may occur as an early (pericarditis epistenocardica) or as a delayed form (Dressler's syndrome). Dressler's syndrome manifests within weeks to several months after myocardial infarction. Postsurgical pericarditis usually develops within days after cardiac/pericardial injury (Maisch et al. 2004).

Radiation-induced pericarditis is seen in 3–20% of patients who have received mediastinal radiotherapy. This complication most often occurs months or years after treatment (Adams et al. 2003).

Uremia is a common cause of pericarditis, producing large pericardial effusions. Six to ten percent of patients with acute or chronic renal failure are affected. Pericarditis results from inflammation of the visceral and parietal pericardium and correlates with the degree of azotemia. Dialysis-associated pericarditis is present in 13% of patients who undergo dialysis and is due to inadequate dialysis and/or fluid overload (Maisch et al. 2004).

Autoreactive pericarditis can be a sequela of a variety of systemic autoimmune diseases, e.g., rheumatoid arthritis, systemic lupus erythematosus, progressive systemic sclerosis, dermatomyositis, mixed connective tissue disease and vasculitides, and sarcoidosis. It manifests with a high number of lymphocytes and mononuclear cells, the presence of antibodies against heart muscle tissue and inflammation of the epi- or endomyocardium. The exclusion of an infective pericarditis is needed for the diagnosis. The management consists of intensifying the treatment of the underlying disease.

Drug-related pericarditis is rare. Management is based on the discontinuation of the causative agent and symptomatic treatment. Pericarditis can remain clinically silent or present with a sudden onset of typical signs and symptoms, including chest pain, dyspnea, fever, friction rub, ST-segment and T-wave changes, and decreased QRS voltage. A prodrome of fever, myalgia and malaise is common. Acute pericarditis can be dry, fribrinous, but most commonly manifests with effusion, and pericardial thickening may be seen in chronic states (>3 months) (Maisch et al. 2004).

Acute Pericarditis

Acute pericarditis may be a self-resolving benign disease. The associated fluid can be a transudate or an exsudate depending on the underlying cause. Transudates are most frequently found in post-surgical pericarditis, uremia, connective tissue disorders or after myocardial infarction, whereas exudates mainly occur in infective pericarditis (Maisch et al. 2004). On plain films of the chest, a sudden increase of the cardiac silhouette suggests the presence of a pericardial effusion. Echocardiography is the most often used technique in this clinical setting, while CT and MRI similarly show a smoothly thickened pericardium (Table 24.1). CT acquisition in the venous phase after contrast-administration better visualizes the hyper-attenuating pericardium than an acquisition during the arterio-venous phase that is usually performed in standard thoracic CT studies (Fig. 24.10a,b). However, there is so far no literature analyzing the best contrast enhancement phase for diagnosing acute pericarditis.

Chronic Pericarditis

An irregular pericardial thickening is the hallmark of chronic pericarditis. The normal thickness of the pericardium is less than 2 mm and a thickness of more than 4 mm is considered abnormal. Chronic pericarditis may be associated with calcifications (Table 24.1) (Fig. 24.11). CT will show pericardial enhancement after intravenous contrast administration. Occasionally, the differentiation on CT between a small effusion from pericardial thickening may be difficult. A pericardial thickening accompanied by clinical findings of heart failure is highly suggestive of constrictive pericarditis (Wang et al. 2003).

Constrictive Pericarditis

Constrictive pericarditis is a clinical syndrome characterized by a hampered expansion of the heart because of a rigid, chronically inflamed and thickened pericardium that limits diastolic filling of the ventricles. The most frequent causes are idiopathic conditions, cardiac surgery, tuberculosis and other infectious diseases, neoplasms, radiation therapy, renal failure and connective tissue diseases.

The clinical symptoms resemble congestive states that are caused by myocardial or chronic liver diseases. Decompensation may lead to venous congestion, hepatomegaly, pleural effusions and ascites. Patients complain about fatigue, peripheral edema, breathlessness, weight gain, abdominal discomfort, nausea, edema and abdominal swelling (Hoit 2007).

The CT demonstration of an irregularly thickened pericardium without or with calcifications in the proper clinical setting is essentially diagnostic (Table 24.1) (Fig. 24.12). A thickened pericardium without an impaired diastolic filling is indicative of acute or chronic pericarditis, but not necessarily of constrictive pericarditis. Although absence of a thickened pericardium argues against the diagnosis of constriction, it does not rule out constrictive pericarditis. In these patients microstructural changes predominantly cause chronic constriction. However, the presence of any pericardial calcification in a patient suspected of constriction should be considered as significant (Wang et al. 2003).

Additional imaging findings in constrictive pericarditis include distorted contours of the ventricles and tubular-shaped ventricles. Dilatation of the atria, the coronary sinus, the inferior caval vein and the hepatic veins may also be present (Table 24.1) (Wang et al. 2003).

Pericardiectomy is the definitive treatment in constrictive pericarditis, but is unwarranted in any state of disease when the risk of surgery is increased (30% to 40% mortality) (Seifert et al. 1985). The definition of the location of the focal pericardial thickening facilitates the surgical approach.

Table 24.1. CT features in pericarditis

	Pericardium	Enhancement of pericardium	Additional findings
Acute pericarditis	Smoothly th ickened	+++	Effusion
Chronic pericarditis	Irregularly thickened, ev. calcifications	+++	Effusion
Constrictive pericarditis	Irregularly thickened, ev. calcifications	+/–	Distorted contours and tubular-shaped ventricles, dilatation of atria, coronary sinus, inferior vena cava and hepatic veins

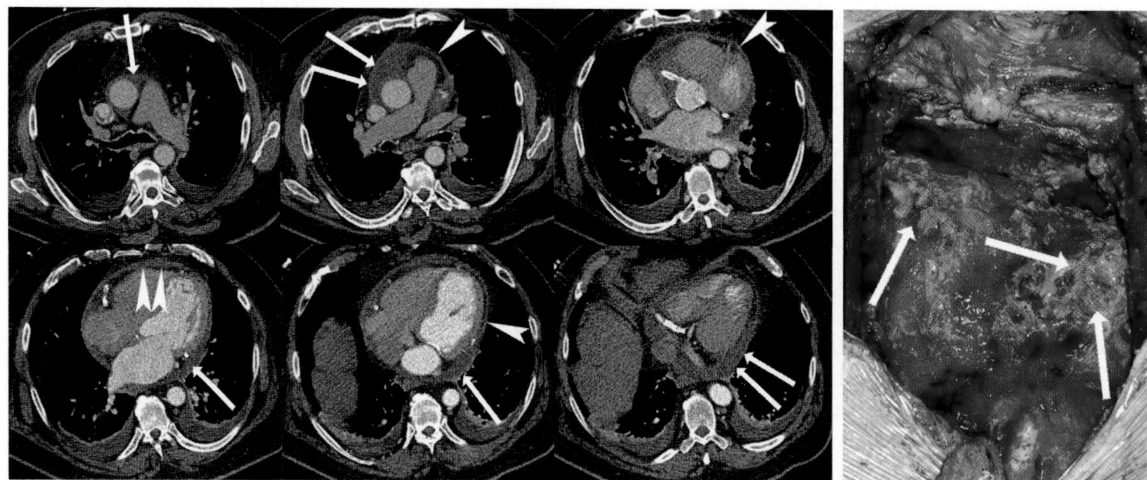

Fig. 24.10a,b. Acute bacterial pericarditis. Cranio-caudal CT images show a circular pericardial effusion (*white arrows*) with contrast enhancement of smoothly thickened pericardium (*white arrowheads*) (**a**). A localized, purulent infection (*arrows*) of the anterior pericardium was seen intraoperativly (**b**)

24.4.2.2 Pericardial Effusion

The pericardial cavity normally contains 50 ml of serous fluid. Pericardial effusion defines the presence of an abnormal amount and/or composition of fluid. It can be caused by a variety of local and systemic disorders and may appear as a transudate (hydropericardium), exudate or pyopericardium. Large effusions are common with neoplastic, tuberculous, cholesterol (chylous) and uremic pericarditis, as well as in myxoedema and parasitosis. After heart transplantations, pericardial effusions are seen as a result of a small donor heart in a large pericardial cavity or after immunotherapy with cyclosporine (Maisch et al. 2004). Loculated effusions are more common after surgery, trauma or in purulent pericarditis.

Slowly accumulating effusions cause the pericardium to stretch. They can exceed a liter in volume. When the fluid is rapidly filling the pericardial cavity, the presence of a normal pericardium can be detrimental by showing a limited ability to distend quickly (Breen 2001). For these reasons, slowly developing large effusions can be remarkably asymptomatic, whereas rapidly accumulating small effusions can create a tamponade, i.e., a compressive disorder due to an increased intrapericardial pressure (Maisch et al. 2004). In large pericardial effusion, the heart may move freely within the pericardial cavity, which is called a "swinging heart."

Although CT can accurately detect a pericardial effusion, echocardiography is considered the primary diagnostic tool. The volume of effusion is usually graded by echocardiography as small (echo-free space in diastole <10 mm), moderate (echo-free space 10–20 mm) or large (echo-free space >20 mm). CT measurements of the attenuation of the fluid may be useful for the determination of the etiology.

Hemopericardium

Blood within the pericardial cavity is considered as a specific entity of pericardial effusion. The blood may be secondary to trauma, aortic dissection (Fig. 24.13a,b), malignancy, infection, uremia or coagulopathy. Furthermore, a hemopericardium may be due to anticoagulation agents that are required after valve replacement or following open heart surgery.

A hemopericardium may become hemodynamically significant, leading to cardiac tamponade (see Sect. 4.2.4). Thoracotomy and immediate surgical repair will be necessary to stabilize the hemodynamics.

24.4.2.3 Pneumopericardium

A pneumopericardium is a rare finding and defined as the presence of air within the pericardial cavity. It

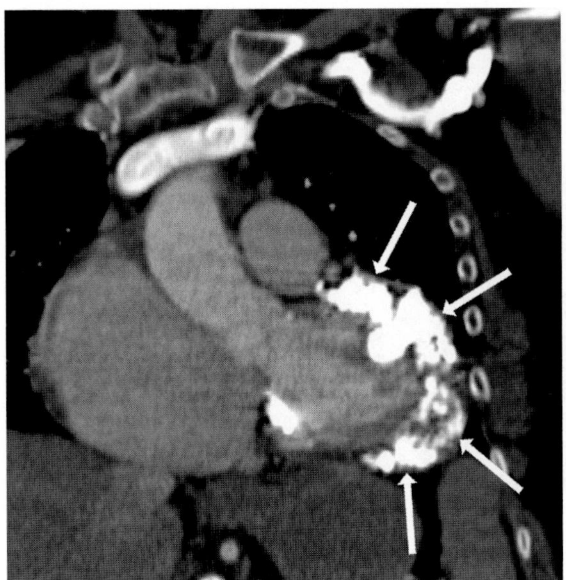

Fig. 24.11. Chronic pericarditis with extensive pericardial calcifications (*white arrows*) (coronal CT reconstruction)

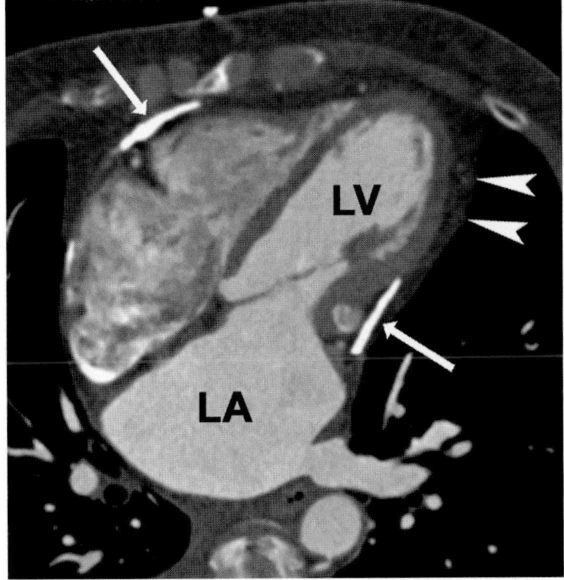

Fig. 24.12. Constrictive pericarditis (transverse end-diastolic CT). Irregularly thickened (*arrowheads*), calcified (*arrows*) pericardium. The left ventricle (*LV*) is tubular-shaped; the left atrium (*LA*) is dilated

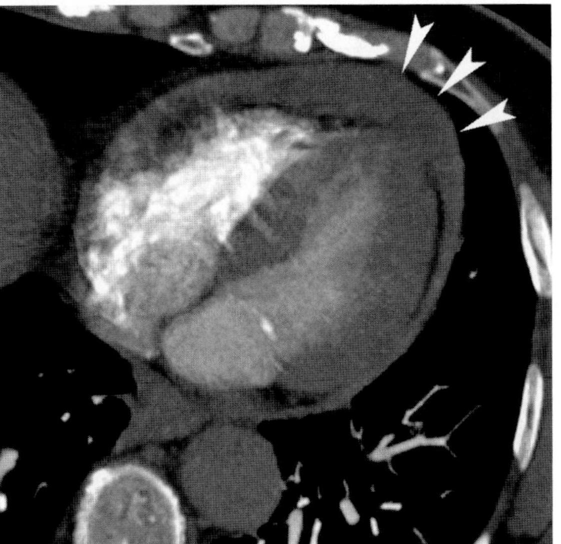

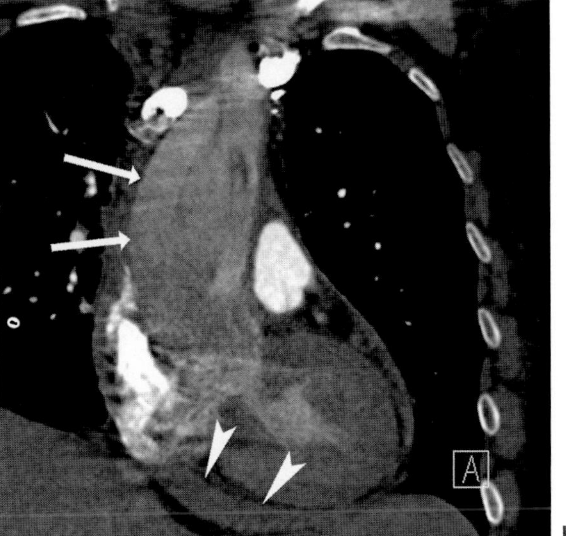

Fig. 24.13a,b. Hemopericardium secondary to dissection of ascending aorta. Transverse CT shows a large amount of blood within pericardial cavity (*arrowheads*) (**a**). Coronal multiplanar CT reconstruction visualizes the dissecting aneurysm (*arrows*) and the concomitant hemopericardium (*arrowheads*) (**b**)

occurs when air is trapped as a one-way valve. When the amount of air is increasing, it may become hemodynamically significant. A pneumopericardium may be traumatic or non-traumatic. High-speed blunt deceleration injuries represent the most frequent traumatic causes (Fig. 24.14a–c).

Less common causes are thoracic procedures, endoscopy, or positive pressure ventilation. Non-traumatic causes are acute asthma and esophageal lesions, such as peptic ulceration, carcinoma and spontaneous rupture (Sharma et al. 2007). Infrequent causes are intrapericardial perforation of a lung abscess or a tuberculous cavity and pericarditis secondary to gas-forming organisms (Grandhi et al. 2004).

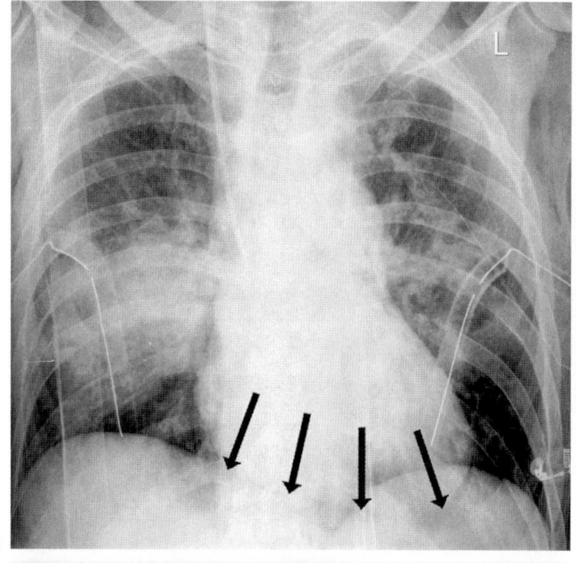

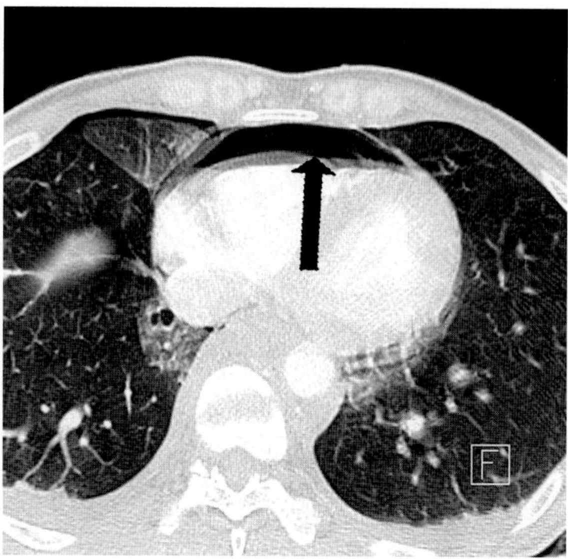

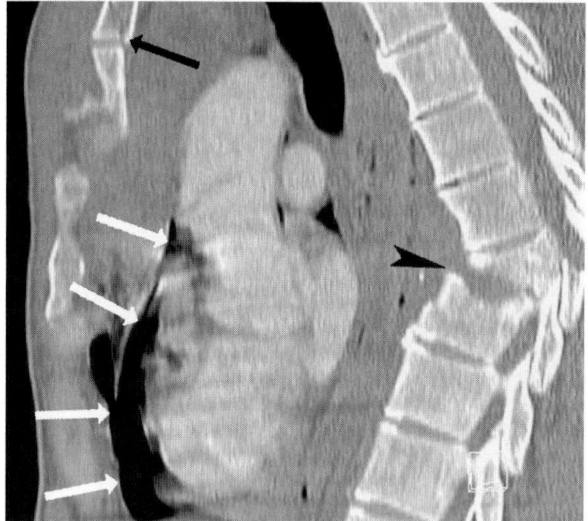

Fig. 24.14a–c. Pneumopericardium after deceleration trauma. Chest radiography demonstrates a rim of air (*black arrows*) below the cardiac silhouette (**a**). Transverse CT in lung window setting depicts the pneumopericardium (*black arrow*) (**b**). Sagittal CT reconstruction shows pneumopericardium (*white arrows*) and collateral sternal (*black arrow*) and vertebral fractures Th 7/8 (*black arrowhead*) (**c**)

The diagnosis is usually made on plain chest films. Chest radiography will show air surrounding the heart and a fine white line representing the pericardium. The cranial contour of the diaphragm may be visualized by air, which is referred to as the "continuous diaphragm sign" (Sharma et al. 2007). CT is valuable in confirming the diagnosis and may detect concomitant injuries to neighboring structures.

Since a pneumopericardium is usually self-limited and does not require a specific therapy, the placement of a chest tube is sufficient in patients with a concomitant pneumothorax. Immediate surgery is necessary when the patient suffers from a tear of the tracheobronchial tree or the esophagus (Sharma et al. 2007). Endoscopy must be performed with caution as insufflation of air may exacerbate cardiac tamponade. Early detection of a hemodynamically significant pneumopericardium is essential for an effective management.

24.4.2.4
Tamponade

Cardiac tamponade is defined as a hemodynamic condition that is characterized by equal elevation of atrial and pericardial pressures, a pulsus paradoxus and a reduced systemic pressure.

The importance of pericardial restraint of ventricular filling at physiologic cardiac volumes remains controversial, but there is an agreement on the size of the pericardial reserve volume. Hence, pericardial effects become significant when the reserve volume is rapidly exceeded. This may occur when there is a rapid increase of the blood volume or the heart size (e.g., acute mitral and tricuspid regurgitation, pulmonary embolism, RV infarction). In contrast, chronic stretching of the pericardium results in "stress relaxation," which explains why large, but slowly developing effusions do not produce a tamponade (Hoit 2007).

Cardiac tamponade may be acute or chronic. Acute tamponade may occur as a complication of cardiac surgery, myocardial infarction or a dissecting hematoma of the ascending aorta. Occasionally, it represents an uncommon complication of percutaneous biopsy. Acute cardiac tamponade is a potentially life-threatening condition resulting from a rapid fluid or air accumulation within the pericardial cavity.

Chronic cardiac tamponade is regarded as a continuum ranging from mild (pericardial pressure of <10 mmHg) to severe states (pericardial pressure of >15 to 20 mmHg). Mild chronic tamponade is frequently asymptomatic, whereas patients with moderate chronic tamponade and especially severe chronic tamponade suffer from precordial discomfort and progressive dyspnea (Hoit 2007).

The removal of small amounts of pericardial fluid yields a considerable improvement of the clinical condition. Prompt pericardiocentesis is reasonable if cardiac tamponade is severe.

24.4.2.5
Neoplasms of the Pericardium

Primary benign and malignant neoplasms of the pericardium are infrequent. Teratomas and mesotheliomas are the leading primary solid masses. Secondary malignancies are far more common.

CT features that may elucidate the etiology of a mass include location, extent, cystic or solid tissue composition, effect on cardiac chambers and enhancement pattern. An accurate assessment is of paramount importance with regard to surgical resection. Therefore, echocardiography, CT and MRI may all be employed.

Benign Neoplasms

Teratomas

Pericardial teratomas are benign germ cell neoplasms that typically affect infants and children. They are similar to extrapericardial teratomas and contain derivatives of all three germ layers, i.e., mature endodermal, mesodermal and ectodermal elements. Tissues discovered in intrapericardial teratomas are diverse and include neuroglia, cartilage, skeletal muscle, liver, intestine, pancreas and glandular tissue. Pericardial teratomas are usually right-sided masses, which typically have contact to one of the great vessels via a pedicle (Grebenc et al. 2000).

On chest radiography, teratomas present with an enlarged cardiomediastinal silhouette. On CT, they frequently exhibit a multicystic appearance, with the cysts showing a high variability in size. The complex multilocular cystic mass may compress the heart and the great vessels. Formed calcified teeth may also be present within the lesion (Grebenc et al. 2000).

Although teratomas are benign lesions, intrapericardial teratoma is life-threatening due to tamponade and requires urgent surgical intervention with pericardiocentesis in nearly all cases. Excision brings immediate relief of symptoms. The prognosis of surgically treated patients is good. In the fetus, tamponade due to an intrapericardial teratoma is a common cause of death (Aldousany et al. 1987).

Lipomas

Percardial lipomas account for approximately 10% of all primary cardiac tumors (Grande et al. 1998). Most frequently, they are found incidentally during imaging or at autopsy. Cardiac lipomas of the heart can arise from the endocardium, myocardium or pericardium. They are typically found in adults, although patients of all ages may be affected.

The circumscribed, spherical or elliptical masses of homogeneous yellow fat are composed of mature adipocytes usually entrapped in a capsule. They are reported as single lesions; however, multiple lipomas have occurred with congenital heart defects and tuberous sclerosis. The patients are usually asymptomatic, although symptoms of heart disease due to a mass effect may occur (Grebenc et al. 2000).

Both CT and MRI are useful for the diagnosis. Pericardial lipomas are diagnosed on CT based on their low attenuation (below -70 HU) and on MRI on the basis of signal intensities of fatty tissue. They appear as predominantly homogeneous masses, but may display internal soft-tissue septa or scattered strands of higher attenuation tissue. After intravenous contrast administration, lipomas demonstrate poor contrast enhancement. Information regarding the relationship of the mass to the coronary arteries is valuable for preoperative planning and in determining resectability. Symptomatic cardiac lipomas are treated with surgical resection, and patients generally have a good outcome.

Hemangiomas

Cardiac hemangiomas account for approximately 5%–10% of all benign cardiac neoplasms (Zeina et al. 2007). They may involve the endocardium, myocardium or pericardium. At the time of diagnosis, the majority of patients are older than 50 years with an age range from 18 days to 76 years (Brodwater et al. 1996). Most patients are asymptomatic; in a few cases, however, atypical chest pain or symptoms of a hemopericardium and cardiac tamponade may be present.

Hemangiomas are of endothelial cell origin with a remaining uncertainty whether hemangiomas are true neoplasms or developmental vascular anomalies. In general, endothelial cells form large, interconnecting vascular spaces divided by varying amounts of connective tissue. With regard to their morphology and size, they are classified as capillary, cavernous or venous hemangiomas (McAllister 1979).

Pericardial hemangiomas typically arise from the visceral pericardium, and most of them are of the cavernous entity. They are usually solitary and well circumscribed. A true capsule is rare, and microscopic extension into the epicardium or myocardium is not uncommon (McAdams et al. 1994). On CT, pericardial hemangiomas present as unilateral masses between 1 and 13 cm in size and with sharply marginated, smooth borders. They normally appear heterogeneous on native CT scans and show an intense centripetal enhancement after intravenous contrast administration. This suggest the diagnosis and can assist in preoperative surgical planning (Brodwater et al. 1996).

Fibromas

The incidence of pericardial fibromas is 2–3% of all primary cardiac tumors (Burke et al. 1994). Patients may present with non-specific symptoms, such as heart failure, arrhythmias, cyanosis and chest pain. Pericardial fibromas may be stable in size for years, and sometimes even tumor regression has been observed.

Fibromas are cellular, fibroblast-rich tumors with little collagen in infants, whereas tumors in adults are composed predominantly of collagen. In approximately 50% of the cases, spots of calcification and less commonly ossification may be found. Examinations of resected cardiac fibromas reveal firm or rubbery masses. Cysts, hemorrhage or necrosis is not present.

On chest radiography, an enlargement of the cardiac silhouette is the most frequent finding. On CT, pericardial fibromas present as large, solid masses with scattered calcifications and well-circumscribed margins. They show a heterogeneous enhancement pattern after intravenous contrast administration (Tilling et al. 2006). Accurate assessment of the extent is necessary prior to surgical excision. Post-surgical tumor recurrence is very rare (Burke et al. 1994).

Primary Malignant Neoplasms

Mesotheliomas

Pericardial mesotheliomas are primary malignant neoplasms that arise from the mesothelial cells of the pericardium. The term is used to describe tumors localized to the pericardium and does not apply to primary pleural tumors that secondarily invade the pericardium. Although pericardial mesotheliomas represent less than 1% of all malignant mesotheliomas, they account for 50% of all primary pericardial tumors (Kaul et al. 1994). There appears to be some causal effect of asbestos exposure, but a definite association has not been established yet due to the rarity of this lesion. Patients with pericardial mesotheliomas show an age peak in the mid-40s, with males predominantly affected. Clinical symptoms include chest pain, cough, dyspnea and palpitations. A diffuse pericardial involvement may present with symptoms and signs that mimic pericarditis or cardiac tamponade. Advanced tumors may show widespread metastases.

Malignant mesotheliomas are firm and homogenous in macroscopic appearance. Histology demonstrates a biphasic tumor composed of epithelial areas, which resemble a carcinoma, and spindled areas similar to a sarcoma. Malignant pericardial mesotheliomas typically form multiple coalescing pericardial masses that obliterate the pericardial cavity and constrict the heart. Although there may be slight infiltration of the outer epicardium, significant myocardial invasion is rare (Kaul et al. 1994).

Conventional X-ray of a pericardial mesothelioma typically visualizes an enlargement of the cardiac silhouette and an irregular cardiac contour. CT readily demonstrates enhancement of a pericardial soft-tissue mass as well as irregular, diffuse pericardial thickening and pericardial effusion (Fig. 24.15) (Grebenc et al. 2000).

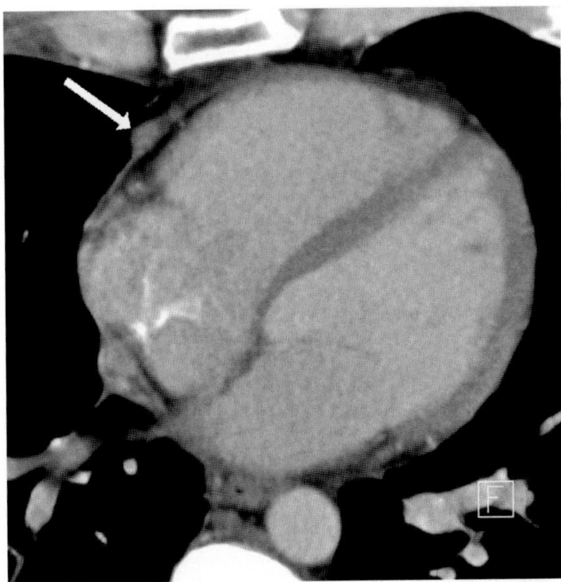

Fig. 24.15. Pericardial mesothelioma. Contrast enhancement of right-sided soft-tissue mass (*white arrow*) with irregular, diffuse pericardial thickening

Surgery combined with radiation therapy may be palliative, but the prognosis of all patients is extremely poor, even of those who are treated, with survivals of 6 months to 1 year after diagnosis (Kaul et al. 1994).

Lymphomas

Primary cardiac lymphomas involve the heart or the pericardium at the time of diagnosis, with no evidence of extracardiac manifestation. Although primary cardiac lymphomas are rare, they can be observed with higher frequencies in immunocompromised patients, e.g., in association with the acquired immunodeficiency syndrome. This is important since 16%–28% of patients with primary extracardial lymphomas present with cardiac involvement (Grebenc et al. 2000). The mean age of the patients is approximately 60 years, with a reported age range of 13 to 90 years and a slight male predominance. Symptoms include unresponsive, rapidly progressive heart failure, arrhythmias, chest pain, cardiac tamponade and superior vena cava syndrome.

The pathology of pericardial lymphomas is typically that of the non-Hodgkin's type and shows multiple solid, white nodular masses with a fish-flesh, homogeneous appearance. Sometimes foci of necrosis occur. In most of the cases, more than one cardiac chamber is involved. Also, the coronary arteries may be affected. Pericardial effusion is usually massive. Cytologic characteristics of this pericardial fluid are diagnostic in two thirds of the cases. However, exploratory thoracotomy and biopsy are often required for a definitive diagnosis (Nand et al. 1991).

Chest radiographs of patients with primary cardiac lymphoma usually demonstrate an enlarged cardiac silhouette and signs of heart failure. On CT, cardiac lymphomas have a nodular appearance (Fig. 24.16). They are iso-attenuating relative to the myocardium, after intravenous contrast administration, a heterogeneous enhancement pattern is seen (Dorsay et al. 1993). Pericardial lymphoma is less likely to demonstrate necrosis or extend into the heart chambers when compared with sarcomas. Differential diagnoses include thymomas, germ-cell tumors, atypical teratomas and metastases.

The prognosis for patients with pericardial lymphoma is very poor. Surgery has not proven to improve prognosis, although operative reduction of the tumor may be an effective palliation. However, early diagnosis and chemotherapy may result in remission and therefore may result in longer survivals (Nand et al. 1991).

Sarcomas

Pericardial sarcomas are rare malignant mesenchymal neoplasms. They are by definition confined to the heart or pericardium at the time of diagnosis with no evidence of extracardiac primary neoplasm. Various types of sarcomas may affect the heart.

Angiosarcomas

Cardiac angiosarcomas are the most common malignant primary cardiac neoplasms with a frequency of 37% in surgical studies and a slight predominance in males. Usually, clinical signs of right-sided heart failure or tamponade are seen. Systemic signs, such as fever and weight loss, may also be present in the clinical history.

Angiosarcomas consist of endothelial cells that form ill-defined anastomotic vascular spaces, although there may also be large avascular areas of spindle cells. Two types of angiosarcomas can be differentiated:

- A loculated, often polypoid tumor mass most often occurs in the right atrium and shows involvement of the pericardium
- The second morphologic type is a diffusely infiltrative mass extending along the pericardium.

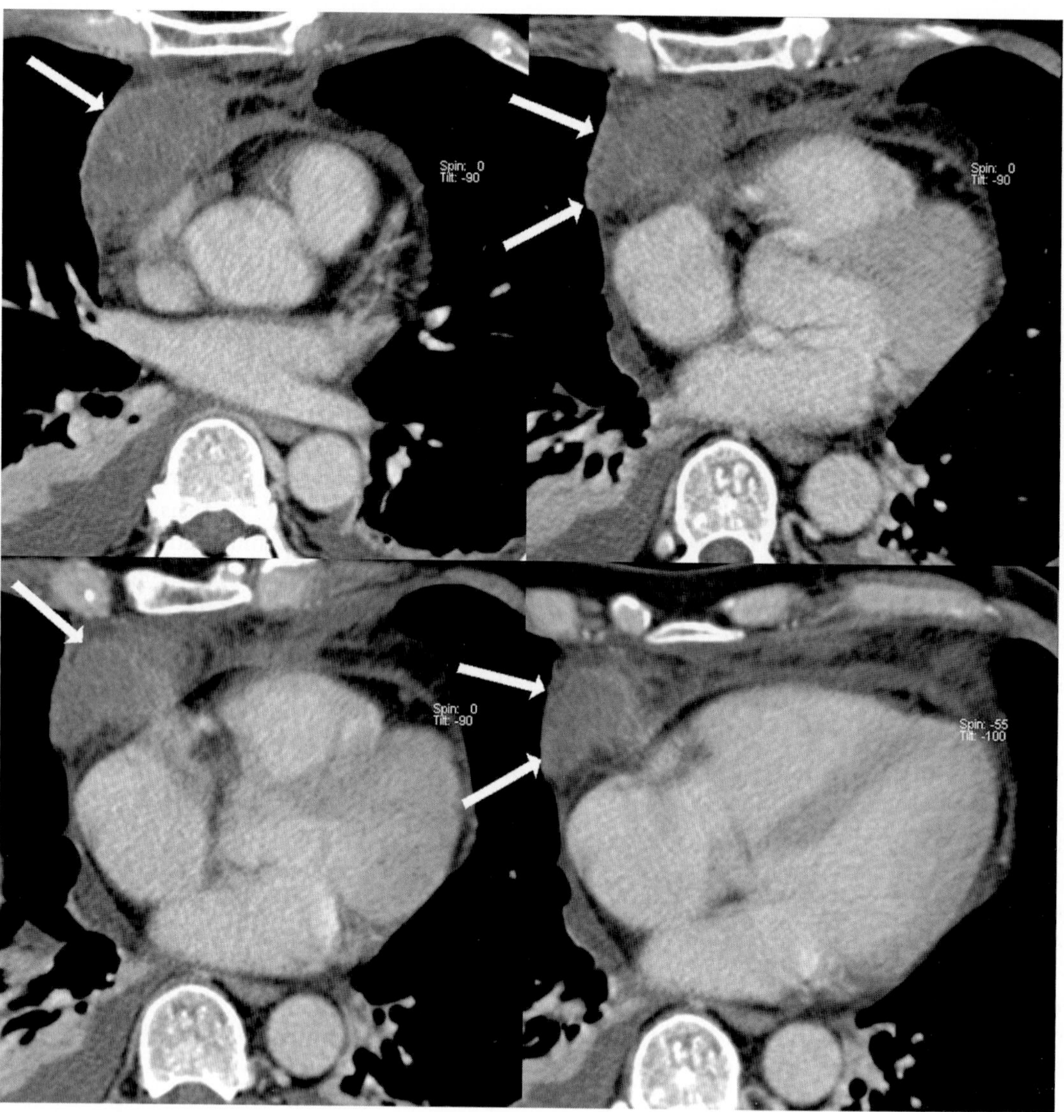

Fig. 24.16. Pericardial B-cell lymphoma (cranio-caudal CT images). Broad-based, nodular and contrast-enhancing neoplasm (*white arrows*) with irregular ill-defined borders extending from ascending aorta to right cardio-phrenic angle

Both types may show infiltration of the pericardium, compression of cardiac chambers and involvement of the great vessels. On CT, the pericardial cavity is obliterated with hemorrhagic, necrotic tumor debris in almost all cases. CT shows a mass of low-attenuation with a heterogeneous enhancement pattern after intravenous contrast administration.

Chemotherapy, surgery, radiation therapy, as well as heart transplantation are considered to be therapeutic options. However, prognosis is poor with survivals ranging from 12 to 30 months due to the frequently delayed diagnosis (Araoz et al. 1999).

Undifferentiated Sarcomas

Undifferentiated sarcomas represent the second most frequent cardiac sarcoma (Fig. 24.17a,b). These neoplasms lack specific histological or immunohistochemical features.

CT is helpful in the evaluation as it demonstrates the broad-based tumor attachment, potential myocardial and mediastinal invasion, as well as extension into the great vessels and pulmonary metastases, when present. Pericardial undifferentiated sarcomas are characterized by pericardial thickening, nodularity and heterogeneous enhancement pattern after

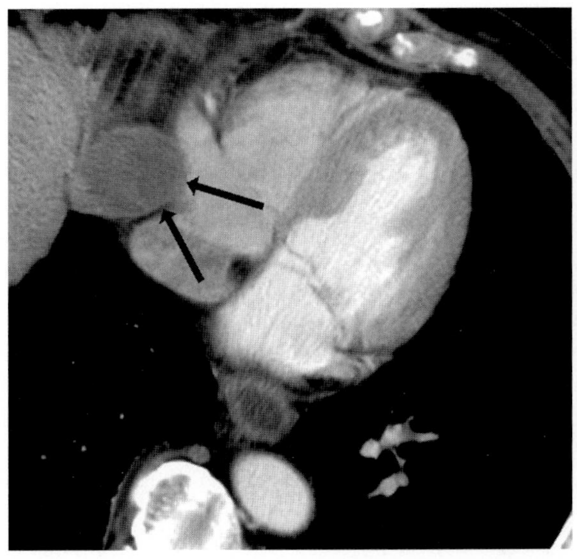

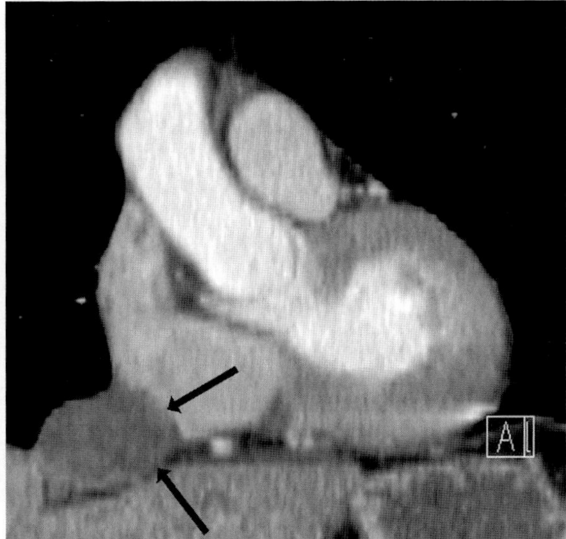

Fig. 24.17a,b. Undifferentiated high-grade sarcoma of pericardium. Transverse CT (**a**) and coronal oblique multiplanar reconstruction (**b**) show a low-attenuating inhomogeneous neoplasm (*black arrows*) in the anterior mediastinum

intravenous contrast administration. Non-enhancing areas typically correspond to necrosis.

These highly aggressive lesions are uniformly fatal. The mean survivals of affected patients range from 3 months to 1 year. Surgery offers palliation of symptoms secondary to obstruction and improves survival (Grebenc et al. 2000).

Liposarcomas

Primary cardiac liposarcomas arise from the atria or the ventricles and invade the pericardium. Affected patients most often present with shortness of breath or arrhythmia; fever and weight loss may also occur (Rafajlovski et al. 2001).

At macroscopic examinations, tumors are usually large in size and multilobulated with areas of necrosis and hemorrhage. Despite the name, liposarcomas show no or only little macroscopic fat. Pericardial involvement may present with thickening, tumor nodules, or effusion. Since primary cardiac liposarcomas only have little macroscopic fat, this entity can be excluded in the differential diagnosis of fatty cardiac tumors. Even well-differentiated liposarcomas have a higher CT number than normal fat (Puvaneswary et al. 2000).

Fibrosarcomas

The predilection site of pericardial fibrosarcomas is the left atrium. Patients most often present with congestive heart failure. Macroscopically, the neoplasm presents as a lobulated and soft mass lesion with a gelatinous appearance and necrotic areas. Microscopic examination will demonstrate fibroblasts. On CT, pericardial fibrosarcomas show low-attenuation values with possible areas of necrosis and may mimic mesotheliomas. Prognosis is very poor (Lionarons et al. 1990).

Secondary Malignant Neoplasms

Secondary malignant neoplasms of the pericardium are more common than primary. About two thirds of all cardiac metastases involve the pericardium. Malignancies metastasizing to the pericardium are, in order of decreasing frequency: mesotheliomas of the pleura, carcinomas of the lung, ovarian tumors, cancer of the stomach and of the prostate (Bussani et al. 2007). The pericardium can be involved by hematogeneous or lymphatic spread or by contiguous invasion. Clinical presentations of pericardial metastases are highly variable. Pericardial effusion is common and may be the sole symptom of an unrecognized metastasizing cancer.

Nearly all cardiac metastases manifest in patients with a known advanced extra-cardiac primary neoplasm (Fig. 24.18a,b). Hence, the distinction between primary and secondary cardiac neoplasms can be made only on the basis of the clinical history.

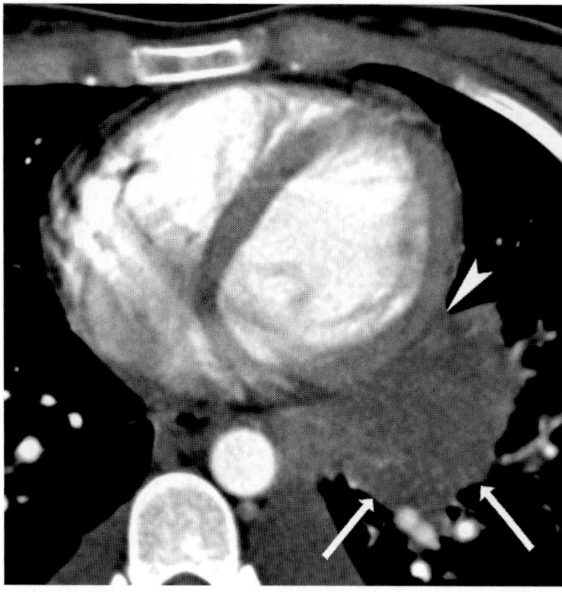
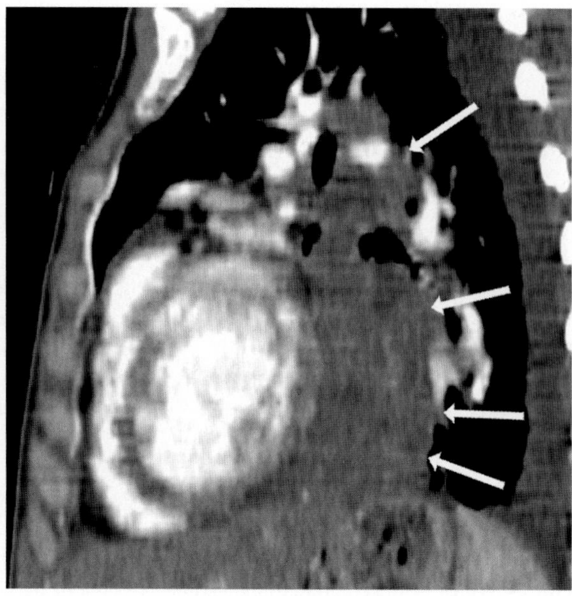

Fig. 24.18a,b. Pericardial metastasis of an occipital melanoma. Transverse CT image (**a**) and sagittal reconstruction (**b**). Large irregular tumor mass (*white arrows*) with inhomogeneous enhancement after intravenous contrast administration and direct contact to the pericardium (*white arrowhead*). Prior abdominal staging showed additional metastases in liver, ovaries and spleen

24.5 Conclusions

- Since the pericardium is well displayed in a large number of routine CT examinations, knowledge of its normal anatomy as well as of the most relevant pericardial diseases, such as pericarditis, effusion, neoplasms and congenital anomalies, is important for their correct interpretation.
- Although echocardiography is the reference imaging modality regularly used to examine the pericardium, CT allows for the detection of practically all diseases of the pericardium because of high soft tissue contrast and demonstration of pericardial calcifications.
- CT imaging should be used when findings at echocardiography are non-conclusive or in conflict with clinical findings, and when MRI is contraindicated. Intravenous contrast administration is recommended in patients with suspected pericarditis, encapsulated pericardial effusion and neoplasms.
- CT and MRI provide a larger field of view than echocardiography and clearly depict adjacent structures. Therefore, three-dimensional studies are of high value in the surgical planning and for the accurate determination for percutanous puncture sites.

References

Adams MJ, Lipshultz SE, Schwartz C, Fajardo LF, Coen V, Constine LS (2003) Radiation-associated cardiovascular disease: manifestations and management. Semin Radiat Oncol 13:346–356

Aldousany AW, Joyner JC, Price RA et al. (1987) Diagnosis and treatment of intrapericardial teratoma. Pediatr Cardiol 8:51–53

Araoz PA, Eklund HE, Welch TJ, Breen JF (1999) CT and MR imaging of primary cardiac malignancies. Radiographics 19:1421–1434

Aronberg DJ, Peterson RR, Glazer HS, Sagel SS (1984) The superior sinus of the pericardium: CT appearance. Radiology 153:489–492

Batra P, Bigoni B, Manning J et al. (2000) Pitfalls in the diagnosis of thoracic aortic dissection at CT angiography. Radiographics 20:309–320

Breen JF (2001) Imaging of the pericardium. J Thorac Imaging 16:47–54

Brodwater B, Erasmus J, McAdams HP, Dodd L (1996) Case report. Pericardial hemangioma. J Comput Assist Tomogr 20:954–956

Burke AP, Rosado-de-Christenson M, Templeton PA, Virmani R (1994) Cardiac fibroma: clinicopathologic correlates and surgical treatment. J Thorac Cardiovasc Surg 108:862–870

Bussani R, De-Giorgio F, Abbate A, Silvestri F (2007) Cardiac metastases. J Clin Pathol 60:27–34

Campbell PT, Li JS, Wall TC et al. (1995) Cytomegalovirus pericarditis: a case series and review of the literature. Am J Med Sci 309:229–234

Choi YW, McAdams HP, Jeon SC et al. (2000) The "high-riding" superior pericardial recess: CT findings. AJR Am J Roentgenol 175:1025–1028

Dober I, Alkadhi H (2006) [Herniation of the heart after pneumonectomy-rare, but life threatening]. Rofo 178:229–231

Dorsay TA, Ho VB, Rovira MJ et al. (1993) Primary cardiac lymphoma: CT and MR findings. J Comput Assist Tomogr 17:978–981

Feigin DS, Fenoglio JJ, McAllister HA, Madewell JE (1977) Pericardial cysts. A radiologic-pathologic correlation and review. Radiology 125:15–20

Grande AM, Minzioni G, Pederzolli C et al. (1998) Cardiac lipomas. Description of three cases. J Cardiovasc Surg (Torino) 39:813–815

Grandhi TM, Rawlings D, Morran CG (2004) Gastropericardial fistula: a case report and review of literature. Emerg Med J 21:644–645

Grebenc ML, Rosado de Christenson ML, Burke AP et al. (2000) Primary cardiac and pericardial neoplasms: radiologic-pathologic correlation. Radiographics 20:1073-1103; quiz 1110–1071, 1112

Groell R, Schaffler GJ, Rienmueller R (1999) Pericardial sinuses and recesses: findings at electrocardiographically triggered electron-beam CT. Radiology 212:69–73

Gross BH, Glazer GM, Francis IR (1983) CT of intracardiac and intrapericardial masses. AJR Am J Roentgenol 140:903–907

Hamilton DR, Dani RS, Semlacher RA et al. (1994) Right atrial and right ventricular transmural pressures in dogs and humans. Effects of the pericardium. Circulation 90:2492–2500

Hoit BD (2007) Pericardial disease and pericardial tamponade. Crit Care Med 35:S355–364

Hipona FA, Crummy AB Jr (1964) Congenital pericardial defect associated with tetralogy of Fallot. Herniation of normal lung into the pericardial cavity. Circulation 29:132–135

Kaul TK, Fields BL, Kahn DR (1994) Primary malignant pericardial mesothelioma: a case report and review. J Cardiovasc Surg (Torino) 35:261–267

Kodama F, Fultz PJ, Wandtke JC (2003) Comparing thin-section and thick-section CT of pericardial sinuses and recesses. AJR Am J Roentgenol 181:1101–1108

Lionarons RJ, van Baarlen J, Hitchcock JF (1990) Constrictive pericarditis caused by primary liposarcoma. Thorax 45:566–567

Maisch B, Seferovic PM, Ristic AD et al. (2004b) Guidelines on the diagnosis and management of pericardial diseases executive summary; The Task Force on the Diagnosis and Management of Pericardial Diseases of the European Society of Cardiology. Eur Heart J 25:587–610

McAdams HP, Rosado-de-Christenson ML, Moran CA (1994) Mediastinal hemangioma: radiographic and CT features in 14 patients. Radiology 193:399–402

McAllister HA Jr (1979) Primary tumors of the heart and pericardium. Pathol Ann 14 Pt 2:325–355

Moore TC, Shumacker HB Jr (1953) Congenital and experimentally produced pericardial defects. Angiology 4:1–11

Nand S, Mullen GM, Lonchyna VA, Moncada R (1991) Primary lymphoma of the heart. Prolonged survival with early systemic therapy in a patient. Cancer 68:2289–2292

Patel J, Park C, Michaels J et al. (2004) Pericardial cyst: case reports and a literature review. Echocardiography 21:269–272

Puvaneswary M, Edwards JR, Bastian BC, Khatri SK (2000) Pericardial lipoma: ultrasound, computed tomography and magnetic resonance imaging findings. Australas Radiol 44:321–324

Rafajlovski S, Tatic V, Stepic V (2001) Primary liposarcoma of the pericardium. Vojnosanit Pregl 58:205–207

Rao KS, Gupta BK, Roa VH, Sankaran K (1981) Congenital pericardial defect with persistent left superior vena cava associated with tetralogy of Fallot. Indian J Chest Dis Allied Sci 23:201–204

Robin E, Ganguly SN, Fowler MS (1975) Strangulation of the left atrial appendage through a congenital partial pericardial defect. Chest 67:354–355

Sagrista-Sauleda J, Barrabes JA, Permanyer-Miralda G, Soler-Soler J (1993) Purulent pericarditis: review of a 20-year experience in a general hospital. J Am Coll Cardiol 22:1661–1665

Seifert FC, Miller DC, Oesterle SN et al. (1985) Surgical treatment of constrictive pericarditis: analysis of outcome and diagnostic error. Circulation 72:II264–273

Sharma A, Agrawal S, Gupta M (2007) Evolving pneumopericardium. Heart 93:738

Tilling L, Hudsmith L, Goldman J, Becher H (2006) Imaging of pericardial tumours: a case report. Cardiovasc Ultrasound 4:29

Truong MT, Erasmus JJ, Gladish GW et al. (2003) Anatomy of pericardial recesses on multidetector CT: implications for oncologic imaging. AJR Am J Roentgenol 181:1109–1113

Vesely TM, Cahill DR (1986) Cross-sectional anatomy of the pericardial sinuses, recesses, and adjacent structures. Surg Radiol Anat 8:221–227

Wang ZJ, Reddy GP, Gotway MB et al. (2003) CT and MR imaging of pericardial disease. Radiographics 23 Spec no:S167–180

Zeina AR, Zaid G, Sharif D et al. (2007) Images in cardiovascular medicine. Huge pericardial hemangioma imaging. Circulation 115:e315–317

Medical Applications of Integrated Cardiothoracic Imaging

Functional Imaging of the Chest

Lung Perfusion

25

Ernst Klotz, Jacques Rémy, François Pontana, Jean-Baptiste Faivre, Vittorio Pansini, and Martine Rémy-Jardin

CONTENTS

25.1 Part I: Technical Introduction

In this section we will discuss the use of contrast-enhanced CT techniques to assess pathological changes of pulmonary parenchymal perfusion. Perfusion strictly defined is "blood flow per unit volume or mass" of tissue. We will see that this quantity is not easy to measure directly for the lung. In a looser sense the term perfusion is often used as a synonym for any parameter (quantitative or qualitative) related to tissue hemodynamics such as relative blood volume or simply regional level of tracer enhancement.

Perfusion measurements usually are based on injecting a tracer into the blood circulation and following its dilution and distribution in vessels and tissues. Perfusion scintigraphy and SPECT, for instance, use radiolabeled macroaggregated albumin as tracer. These tracer particles are large enough to eventually get stuck in the pulmonary parenchymal capillaries after intra-venous injection. As their distribution rate is approximately proportional to blood flow, measuring the number of particles regionally retained in the capillaries by one static measurement is a measure of gross perfusion, i.e., flow per unit of aerated lung tissue. The small tracer particles of the typical iodine contrast media used for CT, contrastingly, quickly traverse lung parenchyma with a typical transit time of not much more than 5 s. Calculating quantitative perfusion values based on indicator dilution theory therefore requires multiple dynamic acquisitions with a temporal resolution in the order of 1 s. The feasibility of this approach has been shown in a pioneering EBT study (Schoepf et al. 2000), but has not made it into wider clinical use. This might be due to the limited availability of EBT, the only partial lung coverage, and the relatively high radiation exposure due to multiple expositions. If this will change with the recent availability of whole lung dynamic acquisitions by 4D spiral techniques remains to be seen.

In the meantime relatively simple techniques that rely on a semi-quantitative analysis of parenchymal iodine distribution and can often be performed as an easy adjunct to standard CTA-type examinations have emerged. Their methodological basis and their clinical value will be the topic of this chapter.

E. Klotz, Dipl. Phys.
Computed Tomograpy Division, Siemens Healthcare Sector, Siemensstrasse 1, 91301 Forchheim, Germany
J. Rémy, MD, Professor
F. Pontana, MD
J-B. Faivre, MD
V. Pansini, MD
M. Rémy-Jardin, MD, PhD, Professor
Department of Thoracic Imaging, C.H.R.U. de Lille, Hospital Calmette, Boulevard du Prof. J. Leclercq, 59037 Lille Cédex, France

25.1.1 Analysis of Iodine Enhancement

In the following we will try to describe with relatively simple mathematics which effects influence the quantification of enhancement after the injection of iodine contrast media and how enhancement can alternatively be determined with dual-energy CT. We will only describe a static analysis. This corresponds to scans taken at an approximately constant level of enhancement in the pulmonary vasculature. Such relative plateau states are reached in the later phase of injection protocols.

CT values describe X-ray attenuation relative to that of water. The historic definition of Hounsfield units (HU) scales this ratio by 1,000 and defines the origin of the scale (i.e., no attenuation or air) as -1,000. By this convention water has a CT number of zero, and all structures attenuating less than water have negative values. This is a simple convention, but occasionally appears to create slight confusion in the medical literature when percent "signal" changes are sometimes reported as relative to the CT value. The "signal" that CT measures is attenuation, however; and in order to avoid any confusion, we will use "Hounsfield attenuation" ρ instead of the CT value in the mathematical analysis:

$$\rho = 1000 + CT_{value} \tag{25.1}$$

Note that differences of ρ and CT value, i.e., enhancement and noise, are identical.

25.1.2 Single-Energy Analysis

If one assumes a voxel of normal lung parenchyma contains tissue, blood, and air, its attenuation ρ_0 will be

$$\rho_0 = (1-\nu)[(1-f_b)\rho_t + f_b\rho_b] \tag{25.2}$$

ρ_t and ρ_b are the attenuation of tissue and blood, respectively. f_b is the fraction of perfused tissue without air that is filled with blood; ν is the fraction of the voxel filled with air (passive ventilation). f_b an be interpreted as the fractional blood volume of the actual lung tissue (without air), and being able to determine its regional distribution would be close to a valuable perfusion measure. Including other non-perfused components such as edema is straightforward, but as they do not change the general principle, they are omitted for simplicity reasons.

Equation 25.2 directly shows why there is an anterior-posterior gradient of CT numbers in the supine position. As the normal pressure in the pulmonary circulation is only equivalent to a water column of about 15 cm, gravity leads to a downward fluid shift increasing f_b and reducing ν when tissue components move closer together. Both effects increase attenuation ρ_0. Screaton et al. (2003) had noted a reduction of the CT number by about 100 HU after total balloon occlusion of one pulmonary artery in an animal experiment. If one assumes that absence of perfusion pressure after an occlusion leads to a significant collapse of the vessels, Equation 25.2 predicts at least the order of magnitude correctly: If a cardiac output of 5 l/min traverses the lung with a mean transit time of 6 s and is distributed over a total lung volume of 5 l, an approximate gross blood volume of 10% results. Removing this changes CT numbers by about 100 HU. Figure 25.1a shows that this effect, although faint, is also present for regional occlusions.

What happens if we add contrast media to the right circulation by intra-venous injection? The iodine mixes with the blood plasma in the right ventricle and when entering the pulmonary circulation can be assumed to be well distributed and diluted by at least a factor of 20. Therefore, volume change can be neglected. The attenuation of a voxel will then be

$$\rho_{CM} = (1-\nu)[(1-f_b)\rho_t + f_b\rho_b + f_b\rho_{iod}] \tag{25.3}$$

ρ_{iod} is the attenuation of the iodine diluted in the plasma component of blood. It is a constant for each patient, but its absolute value depends on kV, injection protocol, and cardiac output. Figure 25.1b shows that while missing iodine in areas after an occlusion can be seen when looking closely, they are mostly obscured by the strong variation of the underlying lung structures. They become prominent if we subtract the pre-contrast from the post-contrast scan (Fig. 25.1c). This is equivalent to subtracting Equation 25.2 from Equation 25.3, which yields

$$\Delta\rho_{SE} = \rho_{CM} - \rho_0 = (1-\nu) f_b \rho_{iod} \tag{25.4}$$

If necessary, ρ_{iod} could be determined from an ROI in the pulmonary artery, but even when doing so, we never get f_b alone; iodine maps are always

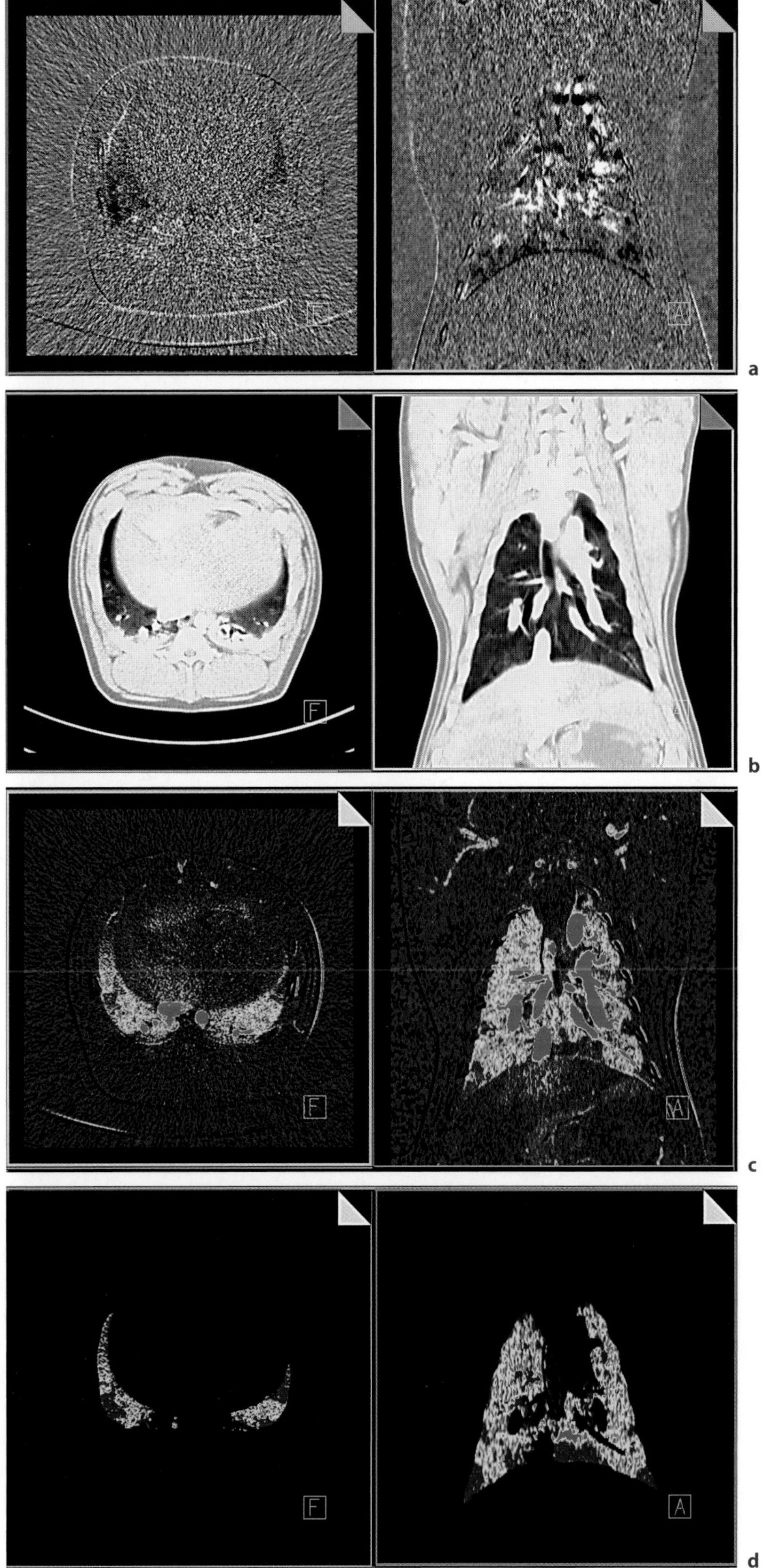

Fig. 25.1a–d. Experimental PE study (provided by Joachim Wildberger, MD, Aachen, Germany). A healthy pig was injected with fresh blood clots. Plain CT scans were performed before and after the injection of the clot material. A dual-energy CT scan was performed after injection of iodine contrast. **a** Registered subtraction of plain CT before and after clot injection. Despite artifacts around vessels and small differences, some perfusion defects are already visible, probably caused by at least partially collapsed vessels. **b** Mean energy images after contrast media injection. Although hypodensities are visible, they are difficult to delineate against the heterogeneous background. **c** Color-coded subtraction of the plain CT from the post-contrast CT scan shows typical subsegmental enhancement defects. **d** Dual-energy perfused blood volume images including lung isolation and vessel removal show equivalent information

"ventilation weighted." This is not a problem per se and in particular does not impede the analysis of the effect of vascular occlusions, such as in PE. It should simply be kept in mind when interpreting enhancement images.

Color-mapped subtraction of pre- and post contrast scans based on Equation 25.4, such as the one depicted in Figure 25.1c, has been used with very good results in experimental PE studies on animals using elastic registration techniques (Wildberger et al. 2001, 2005). Transferring the technique into clinical routine, however, was not very successful. It turned out it is not robust enough. This can be explained by its sensitivity to slight ventilation mismatches that can be avoided in rigorous experimental setups, but not in clinical practice.

The magnitude of the error caused by a small breath-hold mismatch can be estimated by calculating the attenuation change, which falsely mimics or obscures enhancement. If one assumes blood and tissue to have CT numbers close to water, then a change Δv causes a change in attenuation of

$$\Delta\rho_v = \Delta v[(1-f_b)\rho_t + f_b\rho_b] \approx \Delta v\rho_t \tag{25.5}$$

v varies roughly between 0.5 and 0.8 (expiration to inspiration). A mere 5% change of breath-hold level causes a Δv of about 0.015, which in turn results in a CT number change of 15 HU. This is already 50% of a typical normal parenchymal enhancement (Groell et al. 1999). An additional error source is low-frequency variation of the CT numbers due to the presence of large contrast-media-filled cavities in the thorax that are not present in the pre-contrast scan and on subtraction again mimic or obscure pathological enhancement patterns. Both problems can be avoided by using an alternate approach based on the simultaneous acquisition of post-contrast data with dual-energy.

25.1.3 Dual-Energy Analysis

Dual-energy scanning exploits the fact that the attenuation of materials significantly different in their chemical composition from water-like soft tissues strongly depends on the spectral quality of the X-rays used. This is particularly true for materials or mixtures containing elements with higher atomic numbers, such as calcium (in bone) or iodine (in contrast media). The photo-electric effect is more prominent for these materials and causes them to attenuate lower energy photons much more than higher energy ones in comparison to soft tissue. While the CT number of water is by definition the same for an X-ray spectrum of, e.g., 80 kV and 140 kV, adding a certain amount of iodine to water increases the CT number about twice as much at 80 kV than at 140 kV. This effect allows extracting the relative amount of iodine without performing a non-contrast scan. For a simplified mathematical analysis, we can neglect the small spectral dependence of soft tissue and blood versus the twofold change caused by iodine. The attenuation measured with two different spectral qualities, kV_{Hi} and kV_{Lo}, after iodine contrast injection will then be

$$\rho_{CM,kVHi} = (1-v)[(1-f_b)\rho_t + f_b\rho_b + f_b\rho_{iod,kVHi}] \tag{25.6a}$$

$$\rho_{CM,kVLo} = (1-v)[(1-f_b)\rho_t + f_b\rho_b + f_b\rho_{iod,kVLo}] \tag{25.6b}$$

Simple subtraction yields an expression similar to Equation 25.4.

$$\Delta\rho_{DE} = (1-v) f_b(\rho_{iod,kVLo} - \rho_{iod,kVHi}) \tag{25.7}$$

Like in the single-energy subtraction analysis, $(\rho_{iod,kVLo} - \rho_{iod,kVHi})$ is a constant for every patient and could be determined from an ROI in the pulmonary artery. As the regional variation is sufficient for a diagnosis most of the time, this is usually omitted. If the two acquisitions are performed simultaneously as they are in a dual-source scanner, there will be no ventilation mismatch, and as both scans are influenced in a similar fashion by large contrast-filled cavities, the influence of artifacts will be smaller as in single-energy subtraction.

Similar color-coded maps can be calculated from Equation 25.7 as from Equation 25.4, both depicting ventilation-weighted blood volume. Figure 25.1d shows an example that is additionally enhanced by segmenting the lungs and by removing major vessels. Comparing Figures 25.1d and 25.1c shows that the parenchymal enhancement information is equivalent. Post-processed maps such as in Figure 25.1d can be fused with the contrast images providing a blending of morphological and functional information. The clinical examples shown in the rest of this chapter were all generated using this technique.

25.2 Part II: Clinical Applications

25.2.1 General Considerations

Lung perfusion leads pulmonary blood into the gas-exchanging parenchyma, an area characterized by a very close distance between the inhaled air and blood. The air-blood barrier itself is composed at least of an endothelial and an epithelial cell sharing a fused basement membrane (MURRAY 1986). Consequently, the lung derives its function from the interaction of ventilation and perfusion, the latter having been shown to be spatially heterogeneous (GLENNY 1998). Until now, the evaluation of lung microcirculation has not been accessible to standard CT, whereas there are numerous clinical situations in which a combined approach of structural and functional analysis of the pulmonary circulation would be clinically relevant. Focusing on the diagnosis of acute pulmonary embolism, there are several justifications for a combined approach of morphology and function. The dogma according to which normal ventilation and perfusion scintigrams exclude acute pulmonary embolism is often contradicted by CT angiographic findings. Moreover, perfusion defects are not always seen with the concurrent presence of morphological alterations of pulmonary arteries. Lastly, the quantitative assessment of the effect of pulmonary embolism on tissue perfusion may bear more important information for patients' management than the direct visualization of emboli by CT angiography alone. Enlarging this concept to respiratory disorders as a whole, we can anticipate the superiority of a CT examination enabling the radiologist to provide both structural and functional information from the same data set.

Perfusion imaging is based on quantification of the enhancement in tissue and blood at certain time points following intravenous administration of contrast medium (Table 25.1) (MILES 2006). These enhancement data are used to calculate blood flow, blood volume, and blood-vessel permeability for each voxel. Enhancement of lung microcirculation depends on the volume and flow within the capillary bed. It also depends on the site of administration of contrast medium, namely, via a peripheral vein, a central venous catheter with its extremity positioned at the level of the superior vena cava or a right-sided cardiac cavity. Within normal lung parenchyma, the iodine content of the capillary bed can be assimilated to the "parenchymographic" phase of a conventional or digital angiogram. Using single-slice CT scans, the mean enhancement of the lung parenchyma was 29.8 HU in the normally perfused lung and was calculated as 12.3 HU in lung segments with reduced perfusion (WILDBERGER et al. 2005a). CT perfusion based on dual energy, as further described, does not provide analysis of blood flow per time unit, namely actual perfusion, but reflects the iodine content within the lung parenchyma at the time of surveying a given anatomical region. The time at which the iodine content is measured will vary according to the table position. If actual perfusion were to be evaluated with dual energy, this would require to focus on a limited volume of acquisition and to evaluate the iodine concentration of this anatomical volume over time with an improved analysis of iodine with dual energy by mean of its absorptiometric characteristics. Limited to the assessment of the iodine content, dual-energy perfusion imaging enables recognition of normal, hyper- or hypoperfused lung areas. From a clinical standpoint, this can be assimilated to perfusion imaging.

Table 25.1. True perfusion imaging is obtained when the circulating blood is analyzed in time points of the same acquisition volume following intravenous injection of a marker (i.e., dynamic acquisition after contrast medium injection)

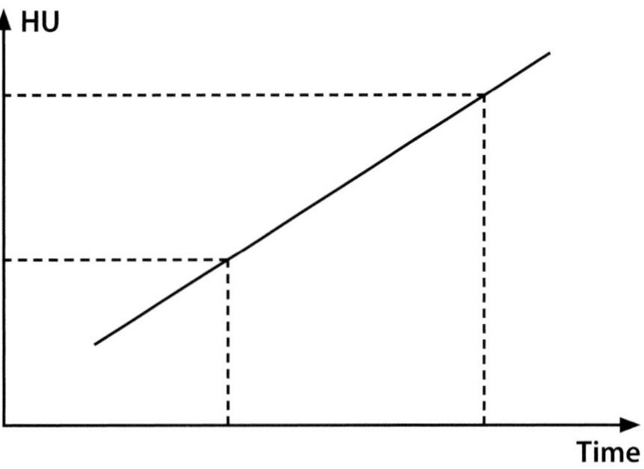

Our knowledge on the transit time of an iodinated bolus through lung microcirculation suffers from some uncertainties (GIL and CIUREA 1996). Because of the continuous nature of data acquisition over the entire thorax, it is likely that the "capillary" phase differs from top to bottom of the volume scanned, especially in case of long scan times. The duration of the iodine transit through the microcirculation

Table 25.2. Parameters potentially influencing the transit time of an iodinated bolus within the capillary bed (Caplin 1996)

Systemic venous return
Right heart: right atrium, right ventricle, tricuspid annulus
Pulmonary vascular resistance
Left heart: left atrium, left ventricle, mitral annulus
Aorta and peripheral systemic arteries

Table 25.3. Variations of physiological parameters between steady state and exercise

	Steady state	Physical exercise
Systolic PA pressure (mmHg)	20	30
Diastolic PA pressure	10	11
Mean PA pressure	10	20
Pulmonary blood flow (l/min)	6.5	16.2
Heart rate	70	>100
Cardiac output (l/min)	6.3	16.2
Right atrial pressure (mmHg)	3 à 5	1
Left atrial pressure (mmHg)	5	10
Wedge pressure*	5	10
Capillary volume	75 ml	>200 ml
Pulm vascular resistance (mmHg /l/min)	1.45	6.9

* Wedge pressure refers to the retrograde pressure coming from pulmonary capillaries and small-sized pulmonary veins. Post-capillary pulmonary hypertension secondary to obstructive lesions at the level of pulmonary veins is characterized by an elevated pulmonary wedge pressure. However, a postcapillary obstacle at the level of small-sized veins may be responsible for a hemodynamic profile of precapillary hypertension

is also influenced by the patient's age, the level of pulmonary vascular resistance, the degree of lung inflation as well as numerous additional parameters summarized in Table 25.2. The arterial stiffness of the aorta and peripheral systemic arteries have an impact on left ventricular function, which in turn also influences the pulmonary circulation. After the age of 60 years, the volume and density of pulmonary capillaries is known to be reduced by 50% to 60% compared to younger subjects (Rouatbi et al. 2006). From conventional angiographic experience, one can quote the systolic-diastolic variability of the pulmonary blood flow, easily observed when small amounts of contrast medium were administered. Similar findings can be observed on pulmonary CT angiograms obtained during the early phase of contrast medium injection, leading to an inhomogeneous attenuation within proximal pulmonary arteries.

25.2.2 Physiological Basis of Lung Perfusion Imaging

The pulmonary blood circulates into conducting vessels before reaching the capillary bed, which occupies 85 to 95% of the overall alveolar surface, i.e., 130 m^2. For an adult of average size, the capillary bed of each lung contains approximately 250 ml of blood, with great variations in the physiological parameters with the patient's age and physical exercise (Table 25.3). Several characteristics of the pulmonary circulation are worth emphasizing. The pulmonary blood flow varies between 5 to 8 l/min in an adult at rest, reaching 20 to 30 l/min during exercise for a trained individual (Murray 1986). The pulmonary vascular bed is thus able to cope with a four- to five-fold increase in blood flow without noticeable elevation of pulmonary artery pressure. The level of pulmonary artery pressure is only one-fifth of systemic pressure. Pulmonary vascular resistances are low.

There are two types of peripheral pulmonary vessels, namely extraalveolar and the alveolar vessels (Gil and Ciurea 1996). Extra-alveolar vessels, composed of small-sized arterioles and venules, are surrounded by a connective tissue sheath at the level of which the pressure is negative. Because the interstitial pressure becomes more negative during inflation, the extra-alveolar vessels become enlarged (wider and longer) during inspiration; they become smaller (narrower and shorter) during expiration. The alveolar vessels, located within the alveolar walls and assimilated to the "capillary vessels," become compressed during lung inflation and even collapse when the alveolar pressure is abnormally increased. The highest pulmonary vascular resistances are found at this anatomical level (Naeije 1996). Changes in left atrial pressure have considerable influence on pulmonary vascular resistance. Pulmonary blood flow varies during the cardiac cycle. Seventy percent of right ventricular ejection fraction is retained within pulmonary arteries during systole. It is distributed to the capillaries during diastole. If the blood volume within pulmonary vessels varies with the cardiac cycle, it remains constant over several cycles. There is a systolic distension of pulmonary arteries following the ventricular systolic contraction, leading to variations in the arterial diameter between systole and diastole. The gravitational stratification of lung perfusion into four zones described by West et al. (1964) and Hughes et al. (1968) is also present in supine position, albeit less marked. The greatest anteroposterior differences in pulmonary blood flow are found in the lower third of the thorax where the highest lung volume is observed. These gravitational differences have also been demonstrated in experimental studies (Reed and Wood 1970; Hakim et al. 1987, 1988). However, the influence of gravity is less pronounced in the supine position compared to the upright position owing to the smaller anteroposterior diameter of the chest, i.e., 20 cm, compared to the height of the chest in the upright position, i.e., 30 cm. The gravity-dependent gradient in lung attenuation after administration of iodinated contrast medium can be analyzed with dynamic CT (Wolfkiel and Rich 1992). In the supine position, the anteroposterior gradient in lung attenuation is more pronounced at low lung volumes owing to the combined effect of low alveolar volumes, alveolar collapse, and redistribution of blood flow in the dependent portions of the lung. Gurney (1991) has summarized the physiological modifications of lung ventilation and perfusion detectable with morphologic CT. The closing volume corresponds to the lung volume at which small airways, mainly composed of bronchioles, are collapsed. It is primarily reached in the dependent portions of the lung because of the self-compression of the lung. The complex relationships between ventilation and perfusion within consolidated lung parenchyma areas can be approached by CT. Lung perfusion can be reduced or suppressed in cases of pulmonary vascular occlusion or hypoxic vasoconstriction. However, lung perfusion can be maintained in areas of airspace consolidation, and thus is responsible for a parenchymal right-to-left shunt. CT also has the potential to help define the level of pulmonary arterial obstruction beyond which pulmonary infarction occurs, currently only hypothetical. CT is also expected to help investigate the reversibility of hypoxic vasoconstriction according to its pathophysiology and its potential treatments (Tsai et al. 2004).

25.2.3 Lung Perfusion Imaging

Blood perfusion of tissues refers to the delivery of oxygen and nutrients to cells through capillaries. Conventional perfusion measurements based on the uptake or washout radionuclide tracers have led to the identification of "perfusion" with "blood flow" in the tissue (Le Bihan 1992). To measure perfusion, several conventional approaches have been used. Microspheres are particles that are trapped before they enter the capillaries. Their deposition in the tissue reflects the blood flow. Diffusible tracers are exchanged with the tissue. By monitoring tracers' concentration time course in the tissue, one can evaluate their rate of delivery to the tissue and thus perfusion. Pure intravascular tracers do not cross the capillary wall. By visualizing the passage of tracers through the tissue capillaries, one may directly determine the blood flow rate.

Dynamic imaging methods have been used to estimate arterial, venous, and capillary transit times, as well as capillary flow distributions (Schoepf et al. 2004). These methods involve two types of image data collection regimes (Hoffman et al. 1995, 2004). *Inlet-outlet detection* is typically used for conducting vessels and whole organ analysis; this analysis is achievable with CT. The other data collection regime is referred to as *residue detection*. Residue detection is typically used for analysis of microvasculature, wherein the individual vessels are below the resolution of the imaging system. The normal transit time of an iodinated bolus within lung microcirculation varies between 5 to 7 s. On the basis of single-source CT, two approaches have been investigated for the detection of perfusion abnormalities, one using color-coded maps of lung density in humans (Wildberger et al. 2001; Herzog et al. 2003; Coulden et al. 2000), while other authors have investigated a substraction technique using precontrast and postcontrast conventional CT images in experimental animal studies (Screaton et al. 2003; Wildberger et al. 2005b). Although both approaches demonstrated the detectability of perfusion defects by CT, the feasibility of this approach in clinical practice has substantial limitations pertaining to scanning times and levels of radiation exposure to the patient.

The recent availability of dual-source CT and the subsequent possibility to scan patients with dual energy offers another alternative for lung functional imaging. Preliminary experiences have shown that this technique could be applied to the analysis of lung perfusion, with radiation doses below the legally required levels (Johnson et al. 2007). This technique is based on basis material decomposition into three elements, i.e., air, soft tissues, and iodine (Kalender 1986). It allows characterization of the iodine content within microcirculation at a specific time and within a given volume, arbitrarily chosen during the contrast medium transit time. Iodine is a non-diffusible tracer that does not enter the tissue (Le Bihan 1992). Its concentration within the surveyed volume reflects regional blood, which is not, stricto sensu, perfusion imaging. The iodine map provided with dual-energy CT could be described as CT microangiography.

25.2.3.1 Protocol for Dual-Energy CT Angiography

CT examinations can be obtained using a scanning protocol similar to that obtained in routine clinical practice, as recently reported by Pontana et al. (2008a) in the clinical setting of acute pulmonary embolism. The tube voltages are set at 140 and 80 kV, with the tube current adjusted to six-fold for the 80 kV over the 140-kV tube, i.e., 50 and 330 mAs to compensate for the lower photon input at the lower voltage. Collimation is 32×0.6 mm with z-flying spot, enabling reconstruction of 64 slices per rotation; the gantry rotation time is 0.33 s with a pitch of 0.5. In this study, the acquisitions were acquired from top to bottom of the chest. The injection protocol was similar to that of a standard CT angiogram obtained with single energy on a similar 64-slice CT scanner (120 ml of a 35% contrast agent; flow rate: 4 ml/s). The scan was initiated by bolus tracking within the ascending aorta with a threshold of 100 HU to trigger data acquisition. These examinations were systematically obtained with an automatic angular (x, y) modulation of the milliamperage. The average scanning time of the entire thorax was 13 s. The mean DLP value for dual-energy CT angiography was 275 ± 37 mGy.cm.

25.2.3.2 Image Reconstruction

From each data set, two categories of images can be reconstructed, i.e., the "diagnostic scans" and the "lung perfusion scans." The diagnostic scans correspond to contiguous 1-mm-thick transverse CT scans of the chest, generated from the raw spiral projection data of tube A and tube B. The averaged images of both tubes (60% from the acquisition with tube A; 40% from the acquisition with tube B), used for diagnostic reading by the radiologists, consist of lung and mediastinal images, reconstructed with standard reconstruction kernels with a field of view adapted to the patient's size.

Lung perfusion scans are generated after determination of the iodine content of every voxel of the lung parenchyma on the separate 80- and 140-kVp images. Three series of images can be created: (1) native perfusion scans; (2) MIPs of lung perfusion; (3) fused images of native perfusion scans and mediastinal diagnostic scans (Fig. 25.2). Native perfusion scans and MIP images of lung perfusion can be generated as grayscale or color-coded images (Fig. 25.3). All generated images can be displayed as transverse scans, completed, whenever necessary, by coronal and sagittal reformations. Figure 25.4 illustrates the three categories of axial perfusion scans that can be generated from dual-energy CT angiography. It is noticeable that each data set can also be used to generate virtual noncontrast images, useful to extract iodine when intramural or endoluminal calcifications of pulmonary arteries are searched for.

25.2.3.3 Clinical Applications

25.2.3.3.1 Acute Pulmonary Embolism

Dual-energy CT angiography offers the unique advantage of a precise morphological analysis of the pulmonary vessels, airways, and lung parenchyma, combined with an insight into the distribution of iodine within peripheral lung circulation. With regard to the diagnosis of acute pulmonary embolism, it has recently been shown that dual-energy CT can detect endoluminal clots on averaged images of tubes A and B as efficiently as single-source CT angiography (Pontana et al. 2008a). In this study, the authors have also validated the detectability of perfusion defects beyond obstructive clots. Perfusion defects in the adjacent lung parenchyma have the typical territorial triangular shape well known from pulmonary angiographic, scintigraphic, and MRI perfusion studies (Fig. 25.5). Dual-energy CT angiography can lead to the depiction of perfusion defects without direct identification of peripheral endoluminal clots, located within subsegmental or more distal

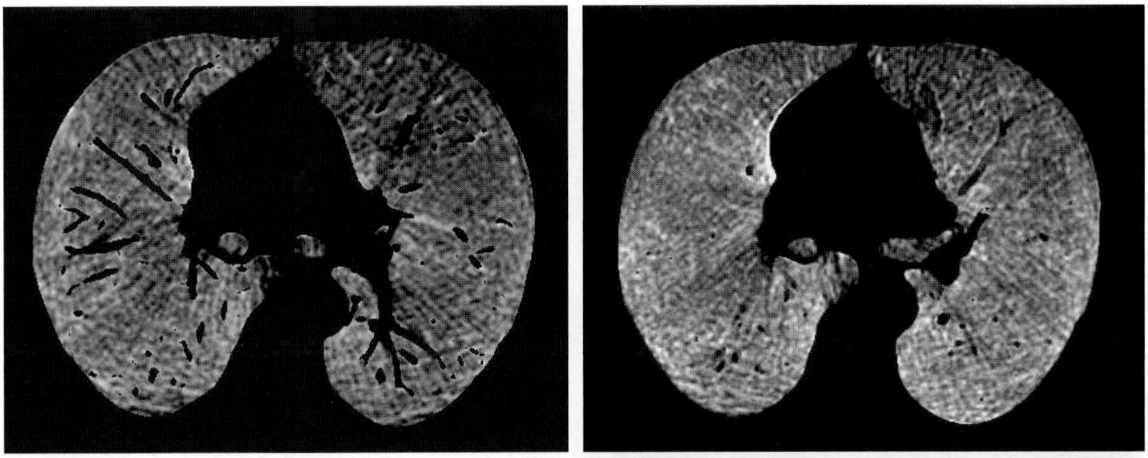

Fig. 25.2a–c. A 58-year-old male with a normal CT angiogram and normal perfusion scans. This example illustrates the three series of lung perfusion scans generated from each data set (from Pontana et al. 2008a). **a** Native perfusion scan, 2-mm thick, obtained at the level of the upper lung zones. **b** Maximum intensity projection, 4-mm thick, obtained at the same level as that of **a**. Note the more homogeneous appearance of lung perfusion compared to **a**. **c** Fusion of the native perfusion scan and the mediastinal diagnostic scan, both reconstructed with the same section thickness (2-mm thick) at the same anatomical level. The fused image allows simultaneous depiction of lung perfusion and surrounding anatomical structures

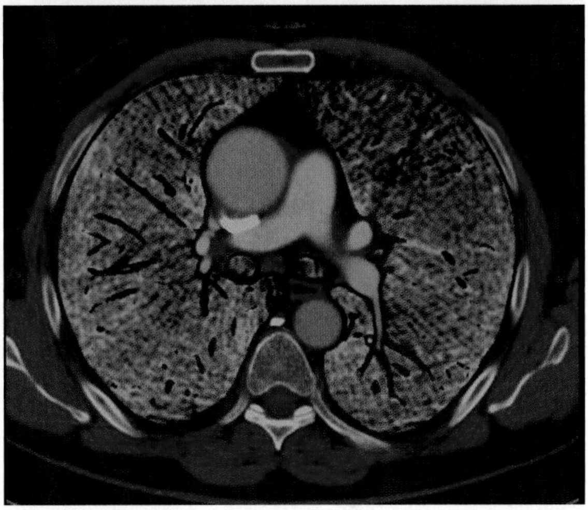

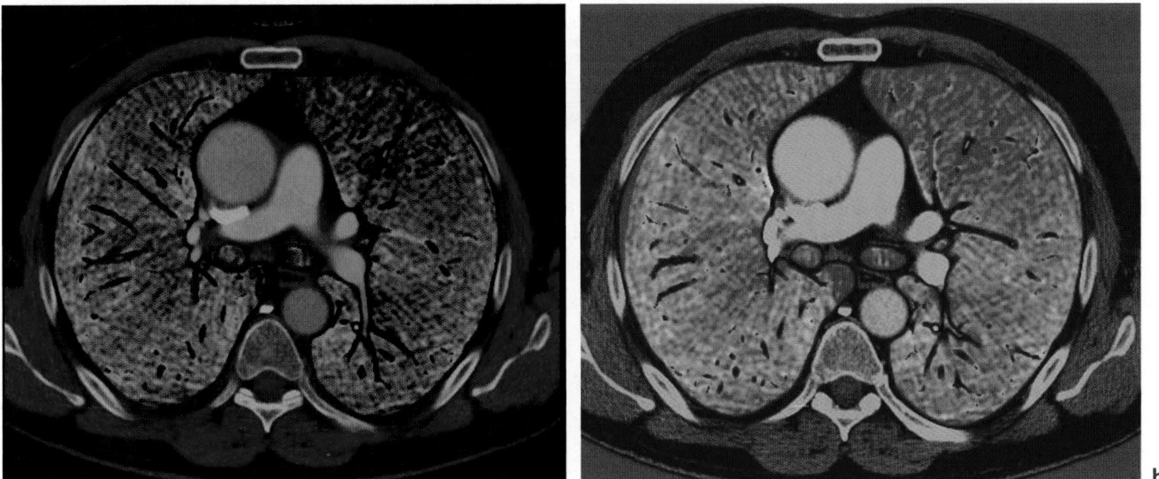

Fig. 25.3a,b. Same patient as that of Figure 25.2. This example illustrates the two variants of perfusion scans. **a** Perfusion scan, 2-mm thick, obtained at the level of the pulmonary trunk bifurcation. This image is generated as a grayscale image. **b** Same image as that shown on **a**, generated as a color-coded image

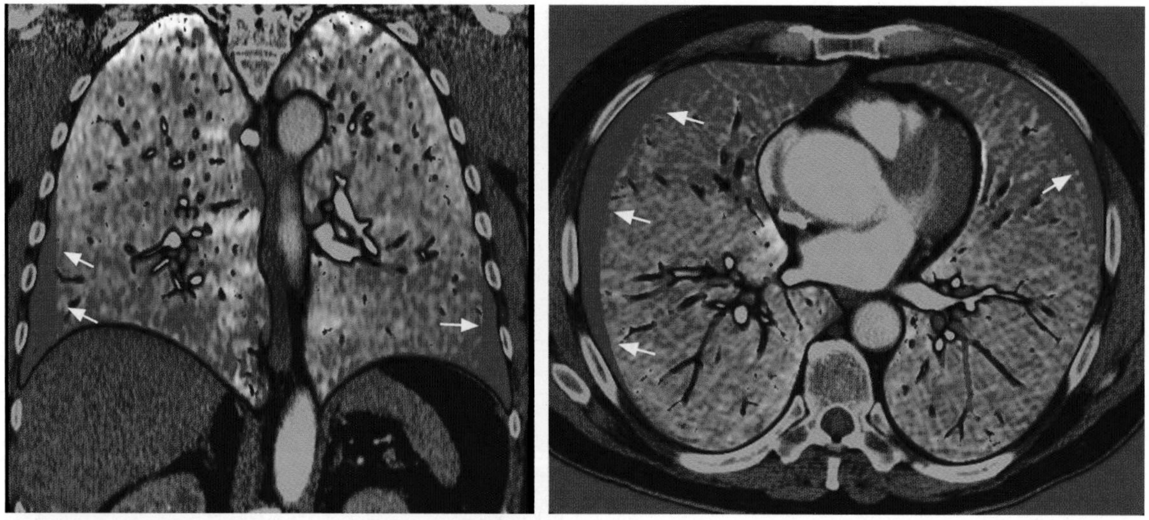

Fig. 25.4a,b. Same patient as that of Figure 25.2. Normal lung perfusion scans displayed in coronal (**a**) and sagittal (**b**) planes. Note the presence of an asymmetric peripheral rim (*arrows*), devoid of perfusion information, due to the smaller size of the tube B

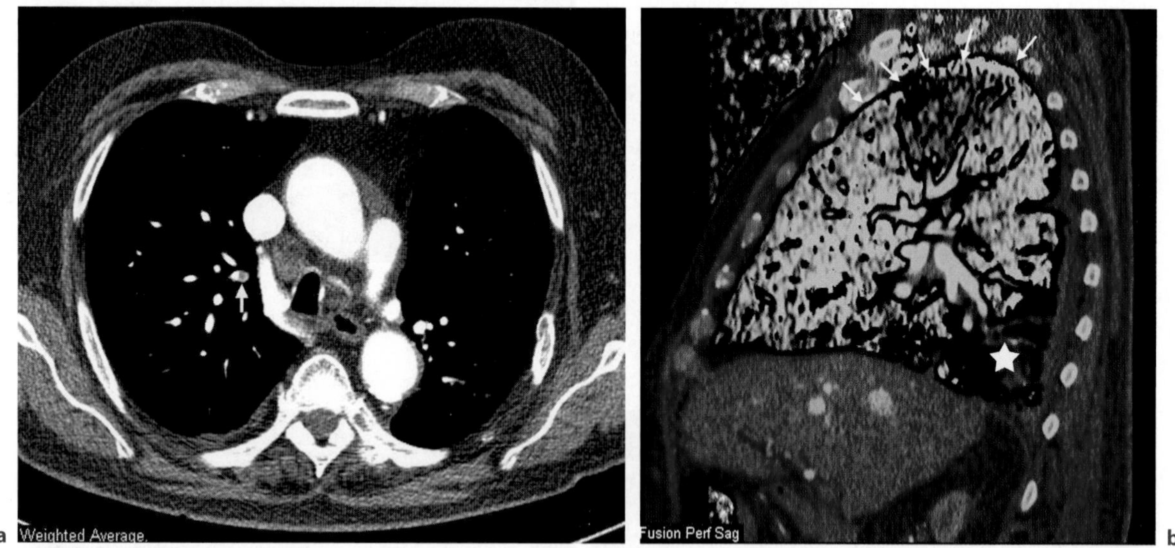

Fig. 25.5a,b. Patient referred for a clinical suspicion of acute pulmonary embolism. **a** Transverse CT scan obtained from dual-energy CT angiography (averaged image from tube A and tube B), showing an endoluminal clot within the apical segmental artery of the right upper lobe (*arrow*). **b** Perfusion scan, 2-mm thick. This sagittal plane allows depiction of a perfusion defect (*arrows*), triangular in shape, in the lung segment supplied by the occluded artery. The *stars* points to a right lower lobe consolidation

branches. Dual-energy CT can also help differentiate lung infarction from nonspecific peripheral lung consolidation, sometimes mimicking a Hampton's bump. Another advantage of dual-energy CT is the ability to use the diagnostic information available from tube B, set at 80 kV. As this tube voltage optimizes the contrast-to-noise ratio within pulmonary vessels, it can help detect peripheral endoluminal clots, known to be better visualized than on images acquired at 120 or 140 kV (Gorgos et al. 2008). The iodine map can also be used as an additional parameter in the assessment of pulmonary artery obstruction score in the clinical context of acute pulmonary embolism.

25.2.3.3.2
Chronic Pulmonary Embolism (PE)

Similar to that achievable for acute pulmonary embolism, dual-energy CT angiography can allow the depiction of perfusion defects beyond chronic clots (Fig. 25.6). Three vascular characteristics of chronic pulmonary embolism can benefit from dual-energy CT. First, chronic PE is responsible for a mosaic pattern of lung attenuation, characterized by areas of ground-glass attenuation with enlarged vascular sections, intermingled with areas of normal lung attenuation and smaller vascular sections. When present, these findings are highly suggestive of redistribution of blood flow, but they are not systematically observed in chronic pulmonary embolism. In such circumstances, dual-energy CT has the potential to recognize ground-glass attenuation of vascular origin by means of the high iodine content within the areas of ground glass attenuation, thus enabling to distinguish them from ground-glass attenuation secondary to bronchiolalveolar diseases (Pontana et al. 2008b). Second, chronic PE can lead to the development of calcifications within partially or completely occlusive chronic clots as well as within pulmonary artery walls when chronic PE is complicated by longstanding and/or severe pulmonary hypertension. Such calcifications can be detected by means of virtual non-contrast imaging, always accessible from dual-energy CT. Third, the images generated at 80 kV can be used to improve the visualization of the systemic collateral supply present in chronic PE, originating from bronchial, but also nonbronchial systemic arteries. Lastly, it should be underlined that dual-energy CT angiography can allow depiction of lipiodol embolization of the pulmonary arteries after endovascular treatment of esophageal gastric varices, liver chemoembolization or percutaneous vertebroplasty.

25.2.3.3.3
Small Airway Diseases

Asthma

Bronchoconstriction in asthma leads to heterogeneous regional ventilation, itself responsible for changes in regional perfusion. Some uncertainty persists over the extent of regional perfusion alterations and their spatial correlation with altered regional ventilation. In a recent study, Harris et al. (2006) have demonstrated that the heterogeneous and patchy regional distribution of ventilation during bronchoconstriction was accompanied by physiologically relevant shifts in perfusion, which tended

a
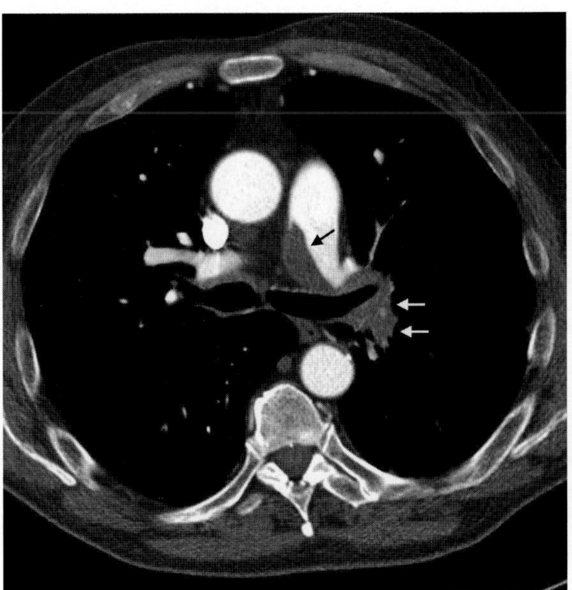

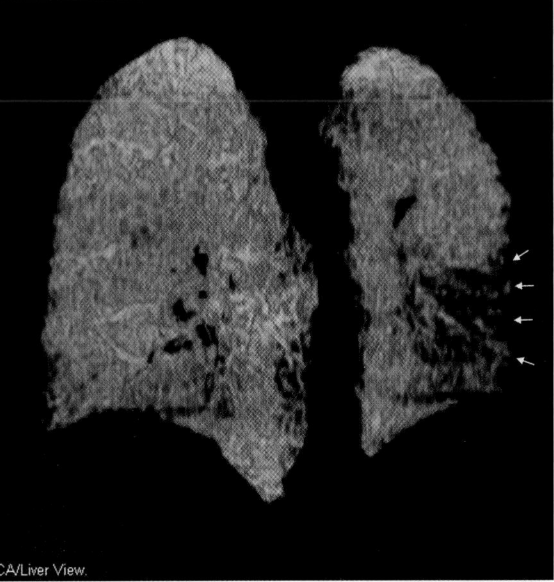

b

Fig. 25.6a,b. Dual-energy CT angiography in a 64-year-old patient referred for worsening of dyspnea related to chronic pulmonary embolism. **a** Transverse CT scan obtained at the level of the left pulmonary artery (averaged image from tube A and tube B), showing an endoluminal filing defect, extending from the pulmonary trunk (*black arrow*), partially obstructed, to the left interlobar pulmonary artery (*white arrows*), which is completely obstructed. **b** Coronal perfusion scan, 2-mm thick, obtained in the posterior part of the thorax, showing a large perfusion defect within the left lower lobe (*arrows*)

to reduce the regional mismatch between ventilation and perfusion. This is the first quantitative evaluation of regional redistribution of perfusion in asthmatics before and after bronchoconstriction induced by metacholin, investigated with positron emission tomography. In asthmatics, perfusion CT imaging can demonstrate multiple regional perfusion defects, closely correlated with areas of altered ventilation identified as areas of air trapping on expiratory scans. A potential explanation for these alterations of ventilation and perfusion could be the hypoxic vasoconstriction within severely hypoventilated areas. The reversibility of perfusion defects can be demonstrated after inhaled corticosteroid treatment.

Chronic Obstructive Pulmonary Disease (COPD)

Alterations in pulmonary perfusion are present in numerous stages of smoking-related respiratory diseases. Figure 25.7 illustrates the alterations of lung perfusion in a patient with a severe form of emphysema. It has long been established that COPD can lead to pulmonary hypertension, generally limited to an increase in the mean pulmonary artery pressure to 25–35 mmHg (Chaouat et al. 2005; Naeije 2005; Barberà et al. 2003). However, mean pulmonary artery pressures higher than 40 mmHg are not uncommon in advanced COPD. In healthy smokers, lung scintigraphy has already demonstrated the presence of perfusion defects, which can also be depicted in normal non-smoking subjects (Fedullo et al. 1989; Wallace et al. 1981, 1982). Investigating endothelial dysfunction in pulmonary arteries of patients with mild COPD, Peinado et al. (1998) have shown that endothelial dysfunction of pulmonary arteries is already present in patients with mild COPD. In these patients as well as in smokers with normal lung function, some arteries show thickened intimas, suggesting that tobacco consumption may play a critical role in the pathogenesis of pulmonary vascular abnormalities in COPD. Several structural changes in early stages of COPD have been described in experimental models, including proliferation of smooth muscle fibers within peribronchiolar arterioles and deposition of collagen and elastin in the thickened intima (Yamato et al. 1997; Santos et al. 2002). In preliminary studies, Hoffman et al. (2006) have demonstrated an increased heterogeneity of local mean transit times of the contrast agent within pulmonary microvasculature of smokers with normal pulmonary function tests. The increased coefficient of variation showed up only when sampling of regional blood flow occurred in regions no larger than

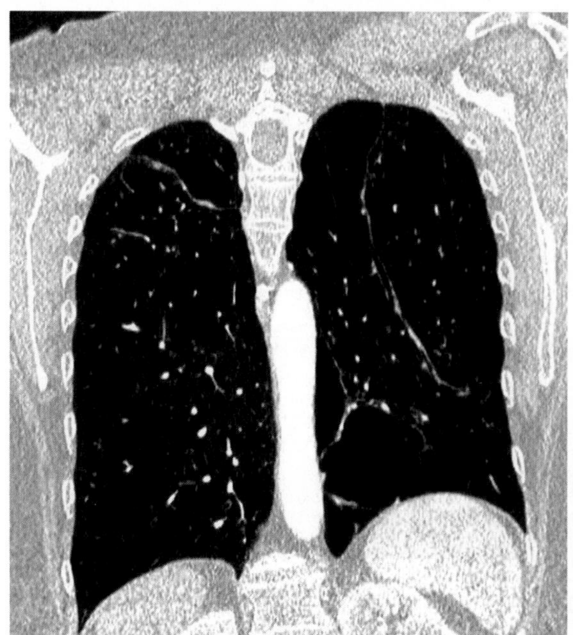

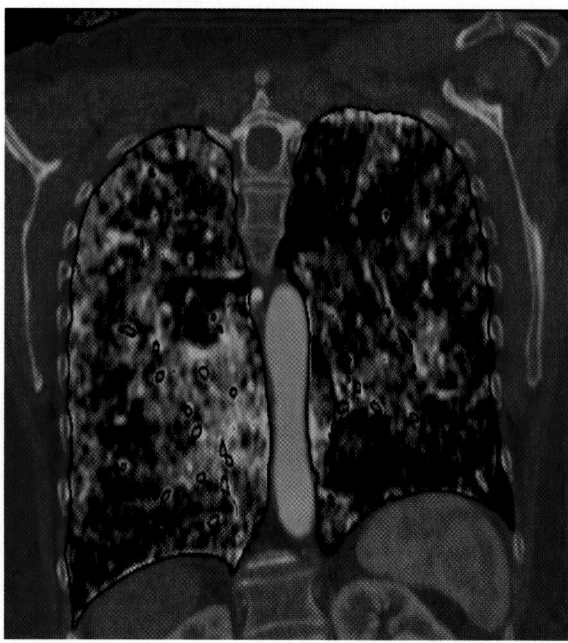

Fig. 25.7a,b. Heavy smoker with a severe form of emphysema, investigated with dual-energy CT angiography. Note the heterogeneity of lung perfusion (**b**) within lung areas devoid of major structural changes (**a**)

3×3 voxels, i.e., 1.2 mm, which correspond to $\frac{1}{5}$ to $\frac{1}{10}$ of an acinus.

These structural alterations are worth considering for dual-energy CT when keeping in mind the epidemiologic burden represented by COPD, a disease expected to become the third leading cause of morbidity worldwide. Dual-energy CT has the potential to allow precise evaluation of this large category of patients. First, dual-source CT used with single- or dual-energy and without ECG gating allows significant dose reduction for CT angiographic examinations of the chest. This advantage is clinically relevant for smokers in whom there is an almost multiplicative risk for lung carcinoma derived from tobacco smoke and radiation dose. Second, dual source, single energy with ECG gating is particularly well adapted for the screening and evaluation of associated cardiovascular co-morbidities. Third, acquisitions based on dual source, single energy and high pitch, i.e., ultrahigh temporal resolution imaging, are well adapted for the management of patients with acute exacerbation of COPD. In this subset of clinical situations, one should underline the high prevalence of acute PE (Tillie-Leblond et al. 2006). Lastly, dual-source, dual-energy CT has the potential to depict perfusion defects in smokers that can be observed prior to the development of structural alterations within the lung parenchyma.

25.2.3.3.4 Diseases of the Pulmonary Circulation

Pulmonary Hypertension

When a patient is referred for pulmonary hypertension of unknown origin, CT plays an important role owing to its ability to evaluate noninvasively central and peripheral pulmonary arteries. Four conditions share a heterogeneous spatial distribution of the underlying vascular lesions. They include chronic pulmonary embolism, primitive pulmonary hypertension, pulmonary veno-occlusive disease, and pulmonary capillary hemangiomatosis. With regard to these entities, pathologic reports indicate dilated alveolar capillaries in pulmonary veno-occlusive disease and proliferation of capillaries within alveolar walls in pulmonary capillary hemangiomatosis. Such capillary proliferation can lead to ground-glass opacity in diffuse, geographic, mosaic, perihilar, patchy, or centrilobular patterns (Itoh et al. 2003). Reports from pulmonary arteriographic findings and perfusion scintigraphic findings have already documented these peripheral vascular lesions (Frazier et al. 2007; Lippert et al. 1998) that are likely to be detectable using dual-energy CT angiography.

Follow-up of Pulmonary Arteriovenous Malformations Treated by Embolotherapy

In approximately 10% of cases, embolotherapy of pulmonary arteriovenous malformations is complicated by clinical and/or radiological symptoms suggestive of pulmonary infarction. This situation can be observed after occlusion of proximal or distal portions of the pulmonary arterial bed. It has been reported after an asymptomatic period extending from a few hours to several months after the embolization procedure. It could be reasonably envisaged to perform the follow-up of occluded pulmonary arteriovenous malformations with dual-energy CT to analyze the regional alterations induced by the endovascular procedure.

25.2.3.3.5 Preoperative Assessment of Postoperative Pulmonary Function

Recent postprocessing developments have allowed the lobar quantification of lung perfusion using dual-energy CT (Pansini et al. 2008). The clinical indications for perfusion quantification can be found among patients requiring prediction of lung function prior to endoscopic or surgical procedures. One indication could be the evaluation of patients with severe emphysema prior to surgical or endoscopic lung volume reduction. Another category could be patients with non-small cell lung cancer in whom surgery is considered only in cases of adequate respiratory reserve.

Different techniques have been used to predict postoperative lung function. One technique is called the simple lung segment-counting technique, based on the counting of the number of functioning segments that will be preserved and the number of those that will be resected. It requires preoperative FEV1 (forced expiratory volume in 1 s) and provides an accurate prediction provided that the segments have normal ventilation and perfusion function. This is far from being the case of numerous patients undergoing lung surgery for tumoral indications, either because of the patient's previous history of respiratory disease or because of the concurrent presence of lung carcinoma and COPD. Scintigraphic techniques, sometimes coupled to CT, can evaluate the postoperative predicted residual forced expiratory volume in 1 s by measuring the radioactivity counts of the affected lobe or segments with breath-hold single-photon emission tomography (Sudoh et al. 2006). Quantitative lung perfusion scan with tomographic imaging can also be obtained with single-photon emission computed tomography (Piai et al. 2004). Quantitative ventilation-perfusion traditional scintigraphy does not seem to be superior to the simple segment counting technique to predict postoperative lung function in lobectomy patients (Win et al. 2004). It is likely that the iodine map achievable with dual-energy CT angiography could also provide quantitative information on the lobar perfusion that could be then coupled to the morphological information on the corresponding anatomical regions.

25.2.3.3.6 Additional Potential Indications

Several additional indications for dual-energy CT angiography are worth considering in clinical practice. Following lung transplantation, postoperative complications can occur at the level of the arterial and venous anastomoses, as well as graft-versus-host rejections at the level of small airways, both situations in which depiction of lung perfusion abnormalities could complement the usual morphological analysis. In patients with a previous history of occupational exposure to asbestos fibers, it may be sometimes difficult to assess the diagnosis of round atelectasis with a high degree of certainty. In such circumstances of indeterminate lung consolidation where the main differential diagnosis remains lung carcinoma, it could be clinically relevant to add information on the perfusion pattern within the consolidated area. The expected pattern is that of a highly perfused zone in case of round atelectasis, whereas tumoral perfusion will be more variable. Dual-energy CT angiography could also lead to the noninvasive diagnosis of right-to-left shunt through a highly perfused round atelectasis.

25.2.3.4 Advantages and Limitations of Perfusion Imaging

In the current status of investigation of dual energy, four main advantages of perfusion imaging can be found. First, the functional information provided with dual-energy CT is obtained in addition to precise morphological information at the level of the pulmonary and systemic circulations, but also at the level of the airways and lung parenchyma. Precise analysis of all these compartments provides more precise investigation of chest disorders than previously achievable with single-source CT angiography. Second, dual-energy CT can help understand isolated perfusion defects. Despite the current absence of direct information on lung ventilation with CT, one can use air trapping on expiratory scans to investigate perfusion defects in the context of normal lung parenchyma and airways. In the presence of air trapping, perfusion abnormalities can be the consequence of hypoxic vasoconstriction observed with small-airway disease; in the absence of air trapping, one should consider a link with a pulmonary vascular disease. The radiation dose of dual-energy CT angiography is lower than that of lung scintigraphy. Owing to the above-mentioned list of information that can be obtained with dual-energy CT, it is likely that this technique will be considered in the management of numerous chest disorders. If perfusion scintigraphy is sufficient for the diagnosis of acute pulmonary embolism (Pistolesi), one should reasonably envisage replacing it by dual-energy CT angiography, which combines morphological and functional approaches. Lastly, dual energy can take advantage of spectral optimization, directly applicable to the analysis of peripheral pulmonary and systemic arteries.

Some limitations of dual energy need to be underlined. First, as previously pointed out, it is neither a true perfusion imaging nor a blood flow imaging. It should not be separated from ventilation imaging. The current limitation should be overcome by the possibilities of spectral resolution of inhaled xenon and krypton. The bolus tracking, with a ROI positioned within the pulmonary trunk or ascending aorta, is not adapted to the physiology or pathophysiology of pulmonary circulation. The time needed to survey the entire thorax far exceeds the transit time within lung microcirculation. The current temporal limitations of dual-energy CT may lead to masking pulmonary perfusion alterations as increased systemic arterial supply may mimic regular pulmonary arterial blood supply on monophasic, contrast-enhanced pulmonary CT imaging (Boll et al. 2005). Consequently, one should integrate the presence of hypertrophied systemic arteries on the averaged scans and consider them as an indirect indicator of mixed pulmonary and systemic perfusion patterns.

Conclusion

The potential physiologic markers for the assessment of COPD (Malher and Criner 2007) require imaging techniques such as CT and MR to evaluate bronchial reactivity, hyperpolarized gas for investigating lung ventilation with MR, quantification of bronchial lumina, and airway walls. A one-step structure-function imaging with CT becomes possible in the assessment of lung vascular disorders. Dual-energy ventilation studies with xenon and krypton have been published, and the radiologist should also be aware of the opportunities and challenges of developing new functional imaging biomarkers (Schuster 2007).

References

Barberà JA, Peinado VI, Santos S (2003) Pulmonary hypertension in chronic obstructive pulmonary disease. Eur Respir J 21:892–905

Boll DT, Lewin JS, Young P et al. (2005) Perfusion abnormalities in congenital and neoplastic pulmonary disease: comparison of MR perfusion and multislice CT imaging. Eur Radiol 15:1978–1986

Caplin JL (1996) Radionuclide studies of the pulmonary circulation. In: Peacock AJ (ed) Pulmonary circulation. Chapman and Hall Medical, London

Chaouat A, Bugnet AS, Kadaoui N et al. (2005) Severe pulmonary hypertension and chronic obstructive pulmonary disease. Am J Respir Crit Care Med 172:189–194

Coulden RA, Brown SJ, Clements L et al. (2000) Mosaic perfusion in pulmonary hypertension: how does multislice CT compare with perfusion scintigraphy. Radiology 217:S384–S385

Fedullo PF, Kapitan KS, Brewer NS et al. (1989) Patterns of pulmonary perfusion scans in normal subjects. Smokers 30 to 49 years of age. Am Rev Respir Dis 139:1155–1157

Frazier AA, Franks TJ, Mohammed TLH et al. (2007) Pulmonary veno-occlusive disease and pulmonary capillary hemangiomatosis. RadioGraphics 27:867–882

Gil J, Ciurea D (1996) Functional structure of the pulmonary circulation. In: Peacock AJ (ed) Pulmonary circulation. Chapman and Hall Medical, London

Glenny RB (1998) Blood flow distribution in the lung. Chest 114:8S–16S

Gorgos A, Remy-Jardin M, Tacelli N, Boroto A, Duhamel A, Remy J (2008) Evaluation of peripheral pulmonary arteries at 80 kV and at 140 kV: Dual-energy CT assessment in 40 patients. (abstract) (accepted, RSNA)

Groell R, Peichel KH, Uggowitzer MM, Schmid F, Hartwagner K (1999) Computed tomography densitometry of the lung: a method to assess perfusion defects in acute pulmonary embolism. Eur J Radiol 32:192–196

Gurney JW (1991) Cross-sectional physiology of the lung. Radiology 178:1–10

Hakim TS, Dean GW, Lisbona R (1988) Effect of body posture on spatial distribution of pulmonary blood flow. J Appl Physiol 64:1160–1170

Hakim TS, R Lisbona R, Dean GW (1987) Gravity-independent inequality in pulmonary blood flow in humans. J Appl Physiol 63:1114–1121

Harris RS, Winkler T, Tgavalekos N (2006) Regional pulmonary perfusion, inflation, and ventilation defects in bronchoconstricted patients with asthma. Am J Respir Crit Care Med 174:245–253

Herzog P, Wildberger JE, Niethammer MU et al. (2003) CT perfusion imaging of the lung in pulmonary embolism. Acad Radiol 10:1132–1146

Hoffman EA, Clough AV, Christensen GE (2004) The comprehensive imaging-based analysis of the lung: a forum for team science. Acad Radiol 11:1370–1380

Hoffman EA, Simon BA, McLennan G (2006) A structural and functional assessment of the lung via multidetector-row computed tomography. Proc Am Thorac Soc 3:519–534

Hoffman EA, Tajik JK, Kugelmass SD (1995) Matching pulmonary structure and perfusion via combined dynamic multislice CT and thin-slice high-resolution CT. Comput Med Imaging Graphics 19:101–112

Hughes JMB, JB Glazier JB, Maloney JE et al. (1968) Effect of extra-alveolar vessels on distribution of blood flow in the dog lung. J Appl Physiol 25:701–712

Ito K, Ichiki T, Ohi K et al. (2003) Pulmonary capillary hemangiomatosis with severe pulmonary hypertension. Circ J 67:793–795

Johnson TRC, Kraub B, Sedlmair M, Grasruck M, Bruder H, Morhard D et al. (2007) Material differentiation by dual energy CT: Initial experience. Eur Radiol 17:1510–1517

Kalender WA, Perman WH, Vetter JR et al. (1986) Evaluation of a prototype dual-energy computed tomographic apparatus. I. Phantom studies. Med Phys 13:334–339

Le Bihan D (1992) Theoretical principles of perfusion imaging. Application to magnetic resonance imaging. Invest Radiol 27:S6–S11

Lippert JL, White CS, Cameron EW et al. (1998) Pulmonary capillary hemangiomatosis: radiographic appearance. J Thorac Imaging 13:49–51

Mahler DA, Criner GJ (2004) Assessment tools for chronic obstructive pulmonary disease. Proc Am Thorac Soc 4:507–511

Miles KA (2006) Perfusion imaging with computed tomography: brain and beyond. Eur Radiol 16(S7):M37–M43

Murray JF (1986) The normal lung. The basis for diagnosis and treatment of pulmonary disease, 2nd edn. WB Saunders, Philadelphia

Naeije R (1996) Pulmonary vascular function. In: Peacock AJ (ed) Pulmonary circulation. Chapman and Hall Medical, London

Naeije R (2005) Pulmonary hypertension and right heart failure in chronic obstructive pulmonary disease. Proc Am Thorac Soc 2:20–22

Pansini V, Remy-Jardin M, Faivre JB, Perez T, Duhamel A, Remy J (2008) Assessment of lobar pulmonary perfusion in COPD patients: preliminary experience with dual-energy CT angiography (abstract). Accepted, RSNA 2008

Peinado VI, Barberà JA, Ramirez J et al. (1988) Endothelial dysfunction in pulmonary arteries of patients with mild COPD. Am J Physiol 274:L908–L913

Piai DB, Quagliatto Jr R, Toro I et al. (2004) The use of SPECT in preoperative assessment of patients with lung cancer. Eur Respir J 24:258–262

Pontana F, Faivre JB, Remy-Jardin M, Flohr T, Schmidt B, Tacelli N, Pansini V, Remy J (2008a) Lung perfusion with dual-energy multidetector-row CT (MDCT): Feasibility for the evaluation of acute pulmonary embolism in 117 consecutive patients. Acad Radiol (accepted for publication)

Pontana F, Faivre JB, Remy-Jardin M, Pansini V, Duhamel A, Remy J (2008b) Lung perfusion with dual-energy multidetector-row CT (MDCT): Can it help recognize ground glass opacities (GGO) of vascular origin? (abstract). Accepted, RSNA

Reed JH, Wood EH (1970) Effect of body position on vertical distribution of pulmonary blood flow. J Appl Physiol 28:303–311

Rouatbi S, Ouahchi YF, Ben Salah C et al. (2006) Facteurs physiologiques influençant le volume capillaire pulmonaire et la diffusion membranaire. Rev Mal Respir 23:211–218

Santos S, Peinado VI, Ramirez J et al. (2002) Characterization of pulmonary vascular remodelling in smokers and patients with mild COPD. Eur Respir J 19:632–638

Schoepf UJ, Bruening R, Konschitzky H, Becker CR, Knez A, Weber J, Muehling O, Herzog P, Huber A, Haberl R, Reiser MF (2000) Pulmonary embolism: comprehensive diagnosis by using electron-beam CT for detection of emboli and assessment of pulmonary blood flow. Radiology 217:693–700

Schoepf UJ, Wildberger JE, Niethammer M et al. (2004) Pulmonary perfusion. In: Functional imaging of the chest. Kauczor HU (ed).Springer, Berlin-Heidelberg-New York 175–190

Schuster DP (2007) The opportunities and challenges of developing imaging biomarkers to study lung function and disease. Am J Respir Crit Care Med 176:224–230

Screaton NJ, Coxson HO, Kalloger SE, Baile EM, Nakano Y, Hiorns M, Mayo JR (2003) Detection of lung perfusion abnormalities using computed tomography in a porcine model of pulmonary embolism. J Thorac Imaging 18:14–20

Sudoh M, Ueda K, Kaneda Y et al. (2006) Breath-hold single-photon emission tomography and computed tomography for predicting residual pulmonary function in patients with lung cancer. J Thorac Cardiovasc Surg 131:994–1001

Tillie-Leblond I, Marquette CH, Perez T et al. (2006) Pulmonary embolism in patients with unexplained exacerbation of chronic obstructive pulmonary disease: prevalence and risk factors. Ann Intern Med 144:390–396

Tsai BM, M Wang M, MW Turrentine MW et al. (2004) Hypoxic pulmonary vasoconstriction in cardiothoracic surgery: basic mechanisms to potential therapies. Ann Thorac Surg 78:360–368

Wallace JM, Moser KM, Hartman MT et al. (1981) Patterns of pulmonary perfusion scans in normal subjects. Am Rev Respir Dis 124:480–483

Wallace JM, Moser KM, Hartman MT et al. (1982) Patterns of pulmonary perfusion scans in normal subjects. The prevalence of abnormal scans in young smokers. Am Rev Respir Dis 125:465–467

West JV, Dollery CT, Naimark A (1964) Distribution of blood flow in isolated lung; relation to vascular and alveolar pressures. J Appl Physiol 19:713–724

Wildberger JE, Klotz E, Ditt H, Spüntrup E, Mahnken AH, Günther RW (2005) Multislice computed tomography perfusion imaging for visualization of acute pulmonary embolism: animal experience. Eur Radiol 15:1378–1386

Wildberger JE, Niethammer MU, Klotz E, Schaller S, Wein BB, Günther RW (2001) Multi-slice CT for visualization of pulmonary embolism using perfusion weighted color maps. Rofo 173:289–294

Wildberger JE, Schoepf UJ, Mahnken AH et al. (2005a) Approaches to CT perfusion imaging in pulmonary embolism. Semin Roentgenol 40:64–73

Win W, Laroche CM, Groves AM et al. (2004) Use of quantitative lung scintigraphy to predict postoperative pulmonary function in lung cancer patients undergoing lobectomy. Ann Thorac Surg 78:1215–1218

Wolfkiel CJ, Rich S (1992) Analysis of regional pulmonary enhancement in dogs by ultrafast computed tomography. Invest Radiol 27:211–216

Yamato Y, Sun JP, Churg A et al. (1997) Guinea pig pulmonary hypertension caused by cigarette smoke cannot be explained by capillary bed destruction. J Appl Physiol 82:1644–1653

Medical Applications of Integrated Cardiothoracic Imaging

Miscellaneous

Pulmonary Embolism from Cardiac Origin

26

Lorenzo Bonomo, Anna Rita Larici, Fabio Maggi, Laura Menchini, Andrea Caulo, and Maria Luigia Storto

CONTENTS

26.1 Introduction and Classification

Pulmonary embolism (PE) is a pathologic condition in which a blood clot as well as some neoplastic or infectious material migrates from any part of the body through the right heart and stops in the pulmonary arterial circulation. It is a life-threatening condition either when presenting as an acute or massive disease or when presenting as a chronic condition followed by repeated episodes.

The different types of pulmonary embolism can be classified on the basis of the embolic material:

1. Thromboembolism (embolism of thrombus or blood clot)
2. Fat embolism (embolism of fat droplets)
3. Air embolism (embolism of air bubbles)
4. Gas embolism (embolism of blood gas, such as oxygen, nitrogen and helium)
5. Septic embolism (embolism of pus containing bacteria)
6. Tissue embolism (embolism of small fragments of tissue)
7. Foreign body embolism (embolism of foreign materials, such as talc and other tiny objects).

Three different pathways can be recognized for PE: anterograde pathway, in which the embolus follows the direction of blood flow; retrograde pathway, typical of high-weighted emboli that may oppose the blood flow; paradoxical or crossed embolism, in which the embolus crosses from the venous to the arterial blood system. This latter condition can be observed in association with congenital heart diseases such as atrial or ventricle septal defects.

26.2 Etiology, Symptoms, and Clinical Findings

The vast majority of pulmonary emboli implicate embolization of thrombotic material arising from the lower extremity or pelvic veins (Tapson 2008). There is also a less conspicuous part of emboli originating from the right heart chambers or from catheter tips and intracardiac devices (Torbicki et al. 2003).

The most frequent cardiac diseases and conditions that may lead to clot formation and pulmonary artery embolization are:

- right-sided endocarditis from intracardiac catheter tips, after cardiac surgery with septic complication, in intravenous drug abusers, in patients with pacemaker or venous central catheters, in

L. Bonomo, MD, Professor
A. R. Larici, MD
F. Maggi, MD
L. Menchini, MD
A. Caulo, MD
Department of Bioimaging and Radiological Sciences, Catholic University, Largo Agostino Gemelli 8, 00168 Rome, Italy
M. L. Storto, MD, Professor
Department of Radiology, University of Chieti, Via dei Vestini, 66100 Chieti, Italy

congenital heart diseases and in long-term hemodialyzed patients with prosthetic vascular access devices;
- valvular diseases, in association or not with atrial fibrillation;
- atrial fibrillation alone (primary or secondary to atrial dilatation and aneurysms, a very rare entity in the right heart);
- ventricular dysfunction secondary to myocardial infarction;
- cardiac neoplasms, either primary, originating from the right heart, or of metastatic origin;
- cardiac surgery; in this conditions PE is usually attributed to embolization from thrombus within the deep venous system, but in a few cases it truly originates from the heart. Cases of PE after cardiac surgery due to late onset heparin-induced thrombocytopenia have also been reported (Badmanaban et al. 2003);
- coagulation disorders like the anti-phospholipids syndrome, essential thrombocitosis, protein C or S deficiency and Behçet disease;
- "paradoxical embolism", emboli originating from left heart chambers associated with some form of cross-circulation allowing the embolic mass to pass from the left to the right side of the heart.

A rare cause of pulmonary embolism of cardiac origin reported in the literature is the presence of a hydatic cyst of the right heart chambers that may break off and embolize in the pulmonary arterial bed (Lahdhili et al. 2002).

PE of septic origin may be found in *right-sided endocarditis*, which occurs predominantly in intravenous drug users (Carrel et al. 1993; Weisse et al. 1993), in intensive care patients with peripheral or central venous catheters (Fig. 26.1), or following surgery, most often involving the tricuspid valve (Robbins et al. 1986b), in patients with pacemakers (Fig. 26.2) and in patients with congenital heart diseases. Right-sided endocarditis accounts for only 5–10% of cases of infective endocarditis (Chan et al. 1989). It has been estimated that up to 76% of cases of endocarditis among intravenous drug abusers involve the right heart, compared with only 9% in non-addict patients. In the typical case of infective endocarditis, the offending organism is bacterial and affects valves on the left side (mitral or aortic) previously abnormal because of rheumatic disease or congenital defects. Fungal endocarditis, by contrast, is usually right-sided and causes larger vegetations with a greater likelihood of embolization. After reviewing 270 published cases of fungal endocarditis (*C. Albicans* 24%, *non-Albicans Candida* spp. 24%, *Aspergillus* spp. 24%), Ellis et al. (2001) found that the major risk factors were non-cardiac surgery, vascular lines, immunocompromised patients, and injection drug abuse. The majority of cases involve the tricuspid valve. Pulmonary valve endocarditis is mostly associated with tricuspid valve endocarditis, whereas isolated pulmonary valve endocarditis is extremely rare (Cremieux et al. 1985). Eustachian valve endocarditis remains a distinctly rare identity with less than 20 reported cases (Sawhney et al. 2001; San Roman et al. 2001). There have been isolated cases of infective endocarditis involving the interventricular septum or right ventricular free wall of individuals diagnosed with ventricular septal defect (Zijlstra et al. 1986). Cases of isolated right ventricular outflow tract vegetation have been recently reported (Uppal et al. 2000; Cosson et al. 2003). In some studies a significant correlation between vegetation size and incidence of complication, including PE, has been demonstrated (Robbins et al. 1986a; Davila et al. 2005).

In all these conditions of infective endocarditis involving the right heart chambers or valves, patients often present with septic pulmonary emboli, which may be life threatening, especially in HIV-positive intravenous drug users. Clinical symptoms include cough, fever, pleuritic chest pain, hemoptysis, and dyspnea.

Infective endocarditis must be suspected, according to Duke's criteria, in presence of fever of unknown origin, often spiking, continuous presence of microorganisms in the bloodstream determined by serial collection of blood cultures, vegetation on valves on echocardiography and murmurs suggestive of valvular regurgitation (Nucifora et al. 2007).

Atrial dysrhythmia is well accepted as a predisposing factor to pulmonary embolism (Johnson et al. 1971) because of the known association of atrial fibrillation with right atrial thrombosis (Carmicheal and Martin 1991). Alteration in the kinetic of atrial contraction, in the absence of valvular or congenital heart disease, is in fact associated with a significant increase of right atrial thrombi (Aberg 1969) resulting from blood stasis and turbulence of blood flow, which predispose to thrombus formation (Goldhaber 1998). In a large study population, a rate of 1.8% of embolic complications from atrial fibrillation has been reported (Levy et al. 1999).

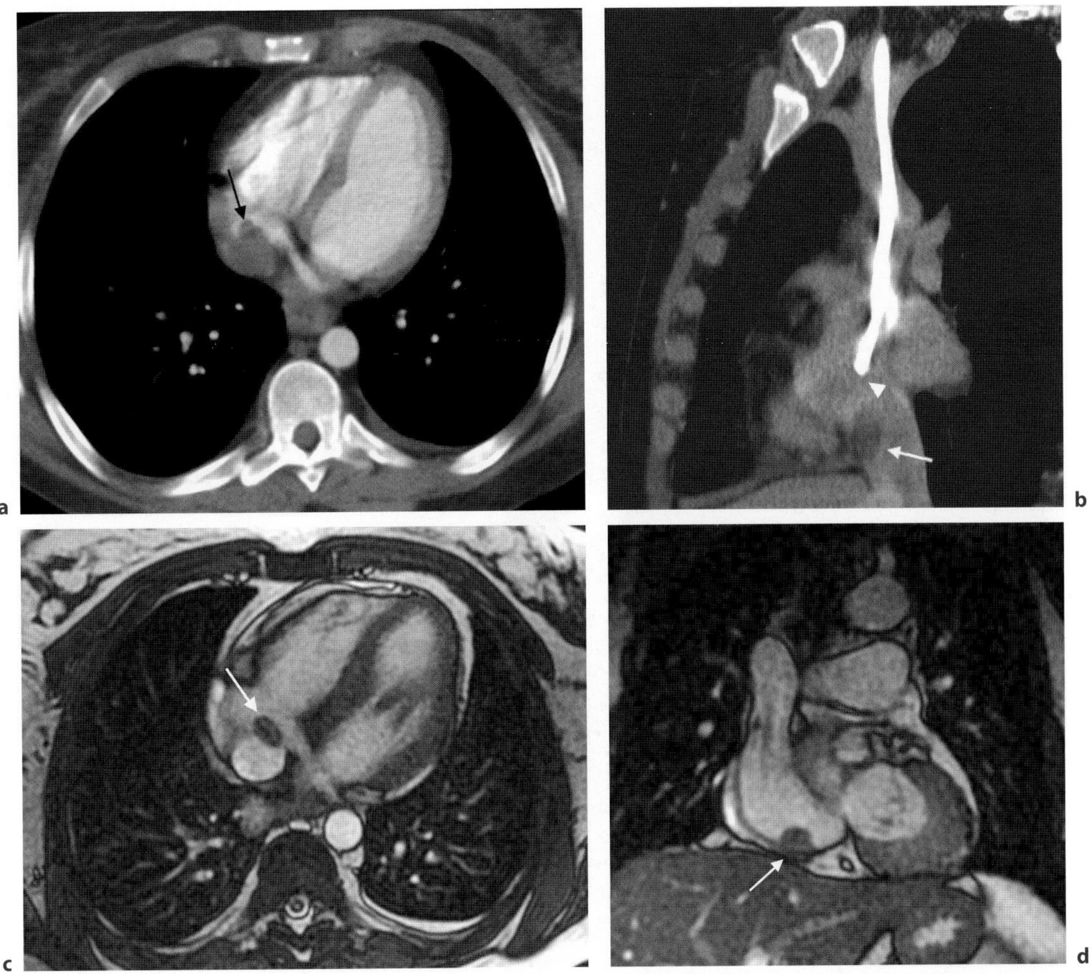

Fig. 26.1a–d. Right atrial thrombus in a patient with central venous catheter. Contrast-enhanced CT images in the axial (**a**) and sagittal (**b**) plane show a small filling defect in the right atrium, adjacent to the inferior vena cava (*arrows*). The tip of a central venous catheter in the right atrium is seen on the sagittal image (*arrowhead*). T2-weighted MR images (**c**,**d**) better depict the right atrial thrombus (*arrows*) proximal to the end of venous catheter

Among conditions of the heart that may determine pulmonary embolism, *benign or malignant heart tumors* have to be included and taken into account. Right-sided cardiac tumors are rare and most commonly found in the right atrium (McAllister and Fenoglio 1978).

Among primary benign or malignant cardiac tumors for which embolization in the pulmonary artery circulation has been reported, cardiac myxomas, papillary fibroelastomas, lymphomas, rhabdomyosarcomas, liposarcomas and angiosarcomas must be mentioned; however, other cardiac neoplasms, for which a direct embolizing potential is not documented, may account for pulmonary embolism in reason of their disturbance on cardiac conduction that generate arrhythmogenic events.

Myxoma is the most common type of primary cardiac tumor in adults (50% approximately of all primary cardiac tumors) and occurs in about 75% of cases in the left atrium, from 5 to 20% in the right atrium and in only 3–4% of cases in the right ventricle. Most myxomas arise in the region of the fossa ovale (90%) (Reynen 1995). Embolism in case of a right heart myxoma from tumor fragmentation and embolization into the pulmonary arteries occurs in 10% of the cases, often leading to massive pulmonary artery obstruction (Parsons and Detterbeck 2003). *Papillary fibroelastomas* are rare benign cardiac tu-

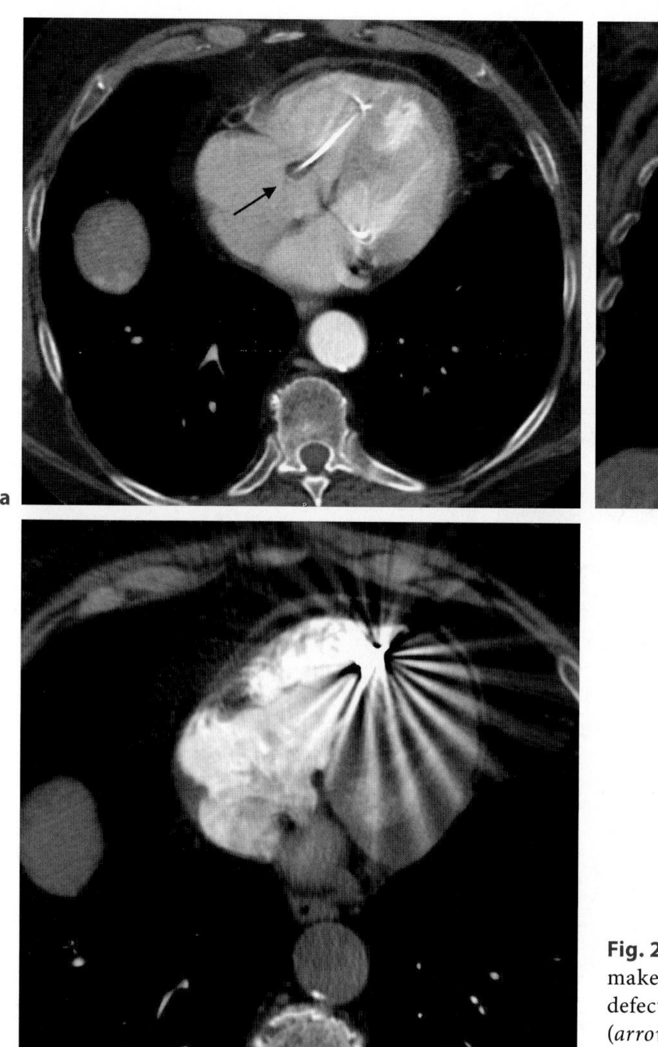

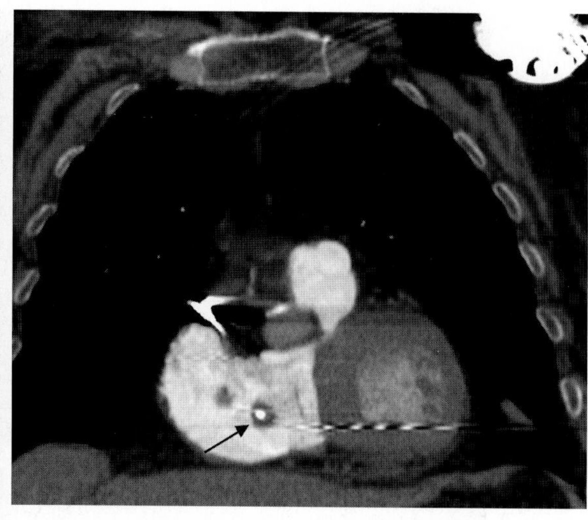

Fig. 26.2a–c. Right atrial thrombus in a patient with pacemaker. Contrast-enhanced CT scans (**a**,**b**) show a filling defect in the right atrium, around the pacemaker electrode (*arrows*), close to the tricuspid valve. Streak artifacts from the metallic tip of the pacemaker electrode are also shown (**c**)

mors typically attached to left-sided valves. Papillary fibroelastomas are friable tumors that are likely to form surface thrombus and have the potential to embolize (Sun et al. 2001; Neerukonda et al. 1991). *Lymphomas* account for 5% of primary malignant cardiac tumors. However, they are extremely rare and represent only 1% of all (benign and malignant) primary cardiac tumors (Daus et al. 1998). Lymphomatous involvement of the heart and/or pericardium usually occurs by dissemination, whereas cardiac involvement as the initial presenting manifestation of malignant non-Hodgkin's lymphoma is extremely rare. Cardiac lymphoma, as well, has been reported to cause pulmonary embolism (Skalidis 1999).

Fig. 26.3a–g. A 26-year-old woman with right atrial angiosarcoma. On the unenhanced CT image (**a**), a slightly hypodense, oval lesion showing peripheral nodular hyperdensity can be seen in the right atrium (*arrows*). Contrast-enhanced CT images (**b**,**c**) demonstrate a solid lesion arising from the free wall of the right atrium (*arrows*) and showing inhomogeneous enhancement with peripheral nodular hemorrhage. The right ventricle is displaced to the left. Right pleural effusion and bilateral lower lobe compression collapse are also present. The CT scan performed 3 months after heart transplant (**d**) shows a nodular pericardial recurrence along the right cardiac border (*arrow*). On the subsequent follow-up CT scan performed 2 months later (**e**), the nodular recurrence is increased in size, despite chemotherapy. A lytic lesion involving the vertebral body of T10 is also present (**f**,**g**) (*arrows*) ▷

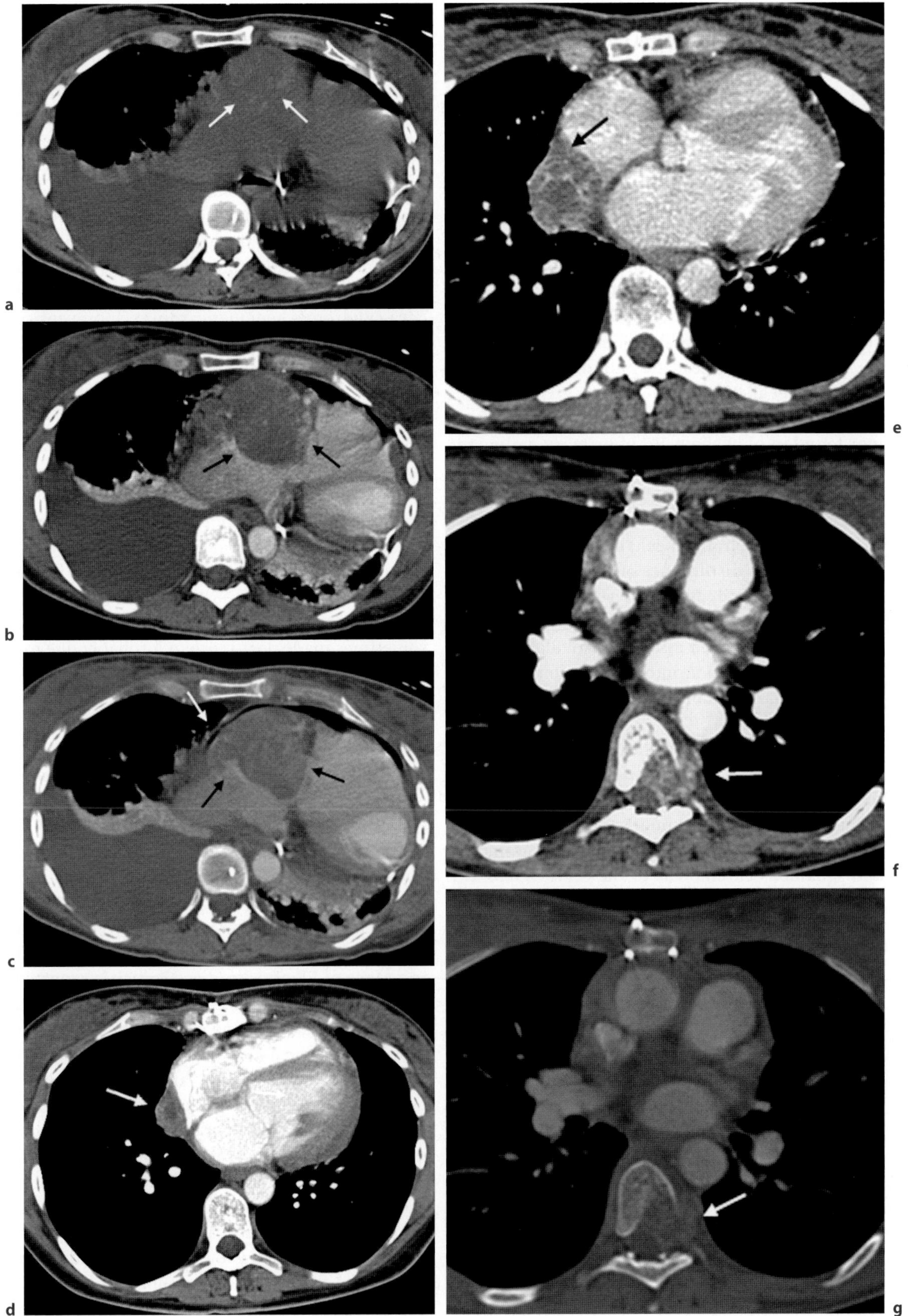
a
b
c
d
e
f
g

Among malignant primary cardiac tumors (Araoz 1999) that may have a potential to embolize (Pinto et al. 2005), sarcomas are the most common. *Angiosarcoma*, a very aggressive histological entity, is the most frequent one, accounting for about 30% of primary cardiac sarcomas. Most often it arises in the right atrium near the atrioventricular groove (80%) (Burke 2008) (Fig. 26.3).

Embryonal *rhabdomyosarcomas* account for 10% of all primary cardiac sarcomas and represent the most common cardiac malignancy in infants and children. They usually arise from the ventricular walls and frequently interfere with valvular motion because of their intracavitary bulk (Castorino et al. 2000); they may lead to pulmonary embolism (Tsutsumi et al. 2005).

Primary cardiac *liposarcoma* is a rare cardiac tumor found in only about 1% of primary malignant tumors of the heart. Cardiac liposarcomas are usually bulky tumors (Butany et al. 2005) that can be associated with functional complications, the most common of which are mechanical obstruction of blood flow, with disturbance of venous return, cardiac tamponade and compression of the right atrium. In a recently published case report, a cardiac liposarcoma was associated also with valvular regurgitation, direct extension into the pulmonary artery with pulmonary embolism and atrial arrhythmias (Uemura et al. 2004).

Intracavitary *cardiac metastasis*, although rare, may occur in patients with widespread metastatic disease. Tumors that have a potential to metastasize to the heart are ovarian tumors, uterine leiomyosarcoma, chorioncarcinoma, endometrial carcinoma and squamous carcinomas of the cervix (Senzaki et al. 1999). These may present as intracardiac obstruction and occasionally cause pulmonary emboli (Borsaru et al. 2007).

There is also a small part of all cardiac tumors that do not directly determine pulmonary embolism, but may participate in clot formation in the pulmonary arteries, since they may lead to conduction disturbances. These cardiac neoplasms that may be involved in alterations of cardiac function and conductance are cardiac fibromas, paragangliomas, lymphangiomas, lipomas and rhabdomyomas.

Symptoms of cardiac tumors are often misleading although severe and catastrophic complications, such as embolization, coronary occlusion, syncope, loss of consciousness, infection and sudden death, may occur. Clinical manifestations vary depending upon the size and location of the tumors rather than the histology per se. Atrial locations present with mitral or tricuspid inflow obstruction, superior or inferior vena cava obstruction, systemic or pulmonary emboli, supraventricular arrhythmia, embolic events, or tamponade. Patients with cardiac neoplasm may have conduction abnormalities, malignant ventricular arrhythmias from myocardial infiltration, and low voltage complex from pericardial infiltration and may present with sudden death. Unexplained chest pain, hemoptysis, systolic or diastolic murmurs, cough, syncope, progressive respiratory failure, right-sided heart failure, superior vena cava syndrome, hemopericardium, supraventicular arrhythmias, ventricular tachycardia and sudden cardiac death or recurrent unexplained pericardial effusion, clubbing, anemia, cardiomegaly, signs of cor pulmonale or metastatic manifestations may be the first presentation signs and symptoms in case of cardiac tumors. Tumor emboli, if present, typically appear with progressive dyspnea over days to weeks, are sometimes accompanied by hemoptysis and may cause increased pulmonary arterial pressure leading to right ventricular failure. The tumors may also lead to hemodynamic obstruction. Right atrial tumors may mimic tricuspid stenosis. The diagnosis is sometimes made post-mortem, probably due to the rarity of certain tumors and the non-specificity of the presenting symptoms.

Cardiac metastases should be suspected in oncology patients if they develop inexplicable heart failure, neurological deficits, or recurrent pulmonary emboli, particularly when no peripheral source of emboli can be identified.

PE as a consequence of *cardiac surgery* is well documented in the literature and is usually attributed to embolization from a thrombus within the deep venous system; however, in many patients deep vein thrombosis (DVT) cannot be identified. The incidence of PE after cardiac surgery is reported to be very low, partly because systemic anticoagulation with heparin during cardiopulmonary bypass prevents the formation of DVT (Josa et al. 1993; Gillinov et al. 1992). In a large study of adult patients undergoing cardiac surgery, the incidence of pulmonary emboli was 0.6%, and was more frequent in patients with coronary artery disease (Lahtinen et al. 2006). Of course, in postoperative patients it could be difficult to assess the real cause of PE, but when a diagnosis of DVT is excluded, the real incidence of PE is very low (McGiven and Bunton 2000). The formation of thrombi within the right atrium has been reported after surgical repair of an atrial septal defect (Hawe 1969); moreover, right atrial thrombi arising in situ after coronary artery bypass surgery have been reported in very few premortem cases (Hyman et al. 1997). Formolo et al. (1981) reported a case of fatal PE after coronary bypass surgery. The mechanism of right atrial thrombus formation in this case is likely due to cannulation of the right atrium during cardiopulmonary bypass. Presumably, suture material used to close the atriotomy site or endocardial damage from the tip of the cannulation catheter creates a nidus for thrombus formation. Atrial fibrillation in the postoperative period causes stasis of blood within the right atrium, further increasing the risk of thrombus formation.

Heparin-induced thrombocytopenia (*HIT*) is an immune-mediated adverse drug reaction that may be associated with limb- or life-threatening thrombosis, which is successfully treated by cessation of heparin administration and by using alternative anticoagulant therapy (Walls et al. 1990).

As already said, PE of cardiac origin has a right-sided location; however, in a few cases, left-sided sources have been described (Ishihara et al. 2002). PE of left-sided origin, the so-called "*paradoxical embolism*," may be the result of a left-sided thrombus embolization in the pulmonary arterial circulation via an interatrial septal defect (Fig. 26.4). The most frequent sources of PE are left atrial thrombi, often the result of mitral valve stenosis or atrial fibrillation, and left-sided neoplasms (Seagle et al. 1985).

Cardiac hydatidosis cyst is a rare parasitic disease, caused by the development of the embryonic form of *Echinococcus granulosus* in humans, and is seen in 0.2–3% of patients with echinococcal disease (Tejada et al. 2001). Cardiac hydatidosis is often primitive and unique; however, it may also develop after the rupture of a pericardial hydatid cyst. The right ventricle localization is exceptional and may be revealed by cystic rupture. Hydatid pulmonary embolism generally occurs after an intracardial rupture of the right ventricle hydatid cyst (Bayezid et al. 1991).

PE may present with various symptoms, and its clinical presentation is proteiform depending on the extent of pulmonary vascular occlusion and pre-existing cardio-pulmonary function. The most

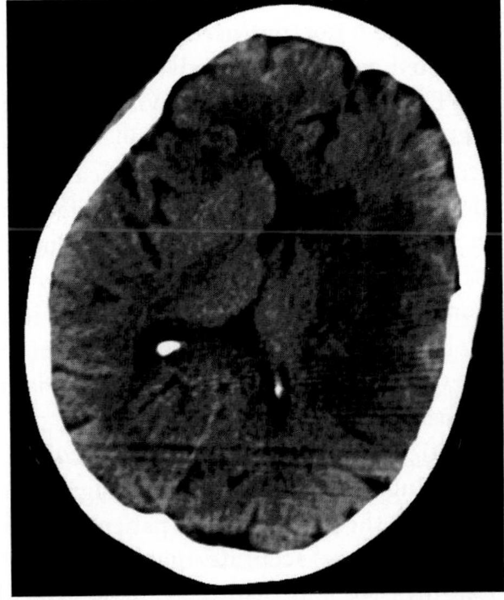

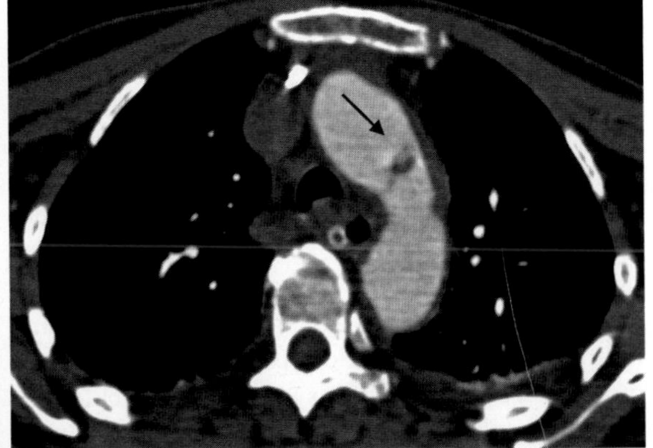

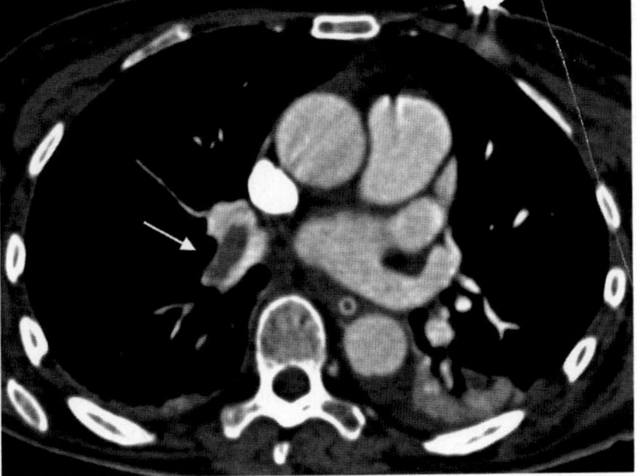

Fig. 26.4a–c. Paradoxical pulmonary embolism in a patient with atrial septal defect. Axial non-enhanced CT image of the head (**a**) shows a large hypodense area due to acute ischemia on the left hemisphere. Axial contrast-enhanced CT images demonstrate filling defects in the lumen of the aortic arch (**b**) (*black arrow*) and in the right inferior lobar pulmonary artery (**c**) (*white arrow*). The atrial septal defect, not evident on CT scans, was confirmed at echocardiography

frequent symptom associated with the disease is dyspnea; less frequently it is associated with cough, hemoptysis, sweating and pleuritic chest pain. Its clinical presentation may demonstrate tachycardia and tachypnea. Fever can occur; DVT and PE are often overlooked causes of fever. When present, pulmonary infarction is typically characterized by pleuritic chest pain, fever and occasionally hemoptysis (Shiber and Santana 2006).

Chronic thromboembolic pulmonary hypertension causes symptoms and signs of right heart failure, including exertional dyspnea, easy fatigue and peripheral edema that develops over months or years.

At blood analysis PE may present with hypoxia, hypocapnia with increased pH for compensatory tachypnea, or hypercapnia with decreased pH for global respiratory failure, and with increased LDH and liver enzymes (Masotti et al. 2000).

26.3 Diagnosis and Imaging Findings

Diagnosis of PE is challenging because symptoms and signs are nonspecific and diagnosing tests are either imperfect or invasive. Diagnosis starts by including PE in the differential diagnosis of nonspecific symptoms, such as dyspnea, pleuritic chest pain, fever, hemoptysis and cough (Shiber and Santana 2006). Thus, PE should be considered in the differential diagnosis of patients suspected of having such conditions as cardiac ischemia, heart failure, COPD exacerbation, pneumothorax, pneumonia, sepsis, acute chest syndrome (in sickle cell patients) and acute anxiety with hyperventilation (Wang et al. 2005).

Initial evaluation of PE should include pulse oxymetry and chest radiography. Radiographic findings are often nonspecific and include atelectasis, focal infiltrates, elevated hemidiaphragm, or pleural effusion. The classic findings of focal loss of vascular markings (Westermark sign), a peripheral wedge-shaped opacity (Hampton hump), or enlargement of the right descending pulmonary artery (Palla sign) are suggestive of PE with a respective specificity of 92%, 82%, and 80%, but quite uncommon (Worsley et al. 1993). The chest radiograph can also help to exclude pneumonia and pneumothorax that may mimic PE clinically.

Pulse oxymetry provides a quick way to assess oxygenation; hypoxemia is one sign of PE and requires further evaluation. ABG (arterial blood gas) measurement may show an increased alveolar to arterial oxygen (A–a) gradient or hypocapnia; the presence of one or both of these parameters is moderately sensitive for PE, although it is nonspecific (Tapson 2008).

ECG most often shows tachycardia and various ST-T wave abnormalities, which are non-specific for PE.

In case of thrombotic pulmonary embolism, useful tests for diagnosing or ruling out PE are *D-dimer* (Harrison and Amundson 2005), V/Q scanning, Doppler ultrasonography, CT angiography and echocardiography. There is no universally accepted algorithm for the best choice and sequence of tests; however, one common approach is to screen patients with D-dimer, obtain lower extremity ultrasonography when D-dimer is positive and progress to CT angiography (or V/Q scanning) if sonography is negative. Positive D-dimer, ECG, ABG measurements, chest X-ray and echocardiograms are adjunctive tests that lack sufficient specificity to be diagnostic alone.

Until recently, V/Q scan has represented the main imaging modality in the diagnosis of PE. In patients with PE, *V/Q scans* detect areas of lung that are ventilated, but not perfused (mismatch); results are reported as low, intermediate, or high probability of PE, based on patterns of V/Q mismatch. A completely normal scan excludes PE with nearly 100% accuracy, but a low probability scan still carries a 15% likelihood of PE. Perfusion defects may occur in other abnormal conditions, including pleural effusion, pulmonary mass, pulmonary hypertension, pneumonia and COPD. With an intermediate probability scan, there is 30 to 40% probability of PE; with a high probability scan, there is an 80–90% probability of PE (Pioped 1990).

Introduced in the late 1980s, *helical CT* is rapidly replacing scintigraphy as the imaging modality of choice in the assessment of patients with suspected PE. It is more accurate than scintigraphy, rapid, non-invasive and readily available. Helical CT directly demonstrates intraluminal clots as filling defects (Gurney 1993). Moreover, the most important advantage of CT over other imaging modalities is that both mediastinal and pleuro-parenchymal structures are evaluated so that, in the absence of PE, CT often provides an alternative diagnosis including aortic dissection, pneumonia, lung cancer, and pneumothorax (Remy-Jardin et al. 2003). Most of these diagnoses are amenable to CT visualization, so that in many cases a specific etiology for the patients' symptoms and important additional diagnoses can be established.

The main impediment for the unanimous acceptance of computed tomography as the new modality of choice for the diagnosis of acute PE has been the limitation of accurate detection of small peripheral emboli. Early studies comparing single-slice CT to selective pulmonary angiography demonstrated high accuracy of CT in detecting PE to the segmental arterial level (Remy-Jardin et al. 1992), but suggested that subsegmental pulmonary emboli could be overlooked by CT scanning (Goodman et al. 1995). With the advent of multi-detector row helical CT scanners, even the subsegmental pulmonary arteries can now be evaluated, allowing a more accurate identification of PE even at the subsegmental level. The current generation of multidetector CT (MDCT) scanners now allows acquisition of the entire chest with 1-mm or sub-millimeter resolution within a short single breath-hold. Shorter breath-hold times benefit patients with underlying lung disease and reduce the percentage of non-diagnostic CT scans. Probably the most important advantage of MDCT is improved diagnosis of small peripheral emboli. The high spatial resolution of MDCT data sets now allows evaluation of pulmonary vessels down to sixth order branches and significantly increases the detection rate of segmental and subsegmental pulmonary emboli (Schoepf et al. 2002; Patel et al. 2003). CT also appears to be the most cost-effective modality in the diagnostic algorithm of PE compared to algorithms that do not include CT, but are based on other imaging modalities (ultrasound, scintigraphy, pulmonary angiography) (Van Erkel et al. 1996).

In comparison with CT, the clinical relevance of *magnetic resonance* (*MR*) for the assessment of PE is low. Nevertheless, since there are some potential advantages of MR over CT (e.g., radiation-free method, better safety profile of MR contrast media, capability of functional imaging), MR might be considered as a valuable alternative in the assessment of suspected PE in patients who cannot tolerate contrast media and in young patients. Gadolinium-enhanced MR angiography (MRA) is an excellent non-invasive diagnostic technique for pulmonary embolism because its sensitivity and specificity are high, as confirmed by a recent review article (Stein et al. 2003). An advantage of MRA over multidetector CT angiography is that images of ventilation can be obtained if noble gases, such as helium 3 or xenon 129, are used (Altes et al. 2005).

Echocardiography as a diagnostic test for PE is controversial. It is a useful test, with a sensitivity of about 80%, for detecting right ventricular dysfunction that occurs when pulmonary artery pressure exceeds 40 mmHg. Estimation of pulmonary artery systolic pressure using Doppler flow signals gives additional useful information about the severity of acute PE. Even if the absence of right ventricular dysfunction or pulmonary hypertension makes the diagnosis of a large PE unlikely, this does not exclude the diagnosis of a smaller one.

Cardiac marker testing is evolving as a useful mean of stratifying mortality risk in patients with acute PE. Elevated troponin levels can signify right ventricular strain. Elevated brain natriuretic peptide (BNP) and pro-BNP levels are not helpful, but low levels appear to signify good prognosis. The clinical role of these tests remains to be determined, because they are not specific either for right ventricular strain or for PE.

Pulmonary angiography (*PA*) has traditionally been considered the standard of reference for the diagnosis of PE; however, it is an invasive technique and is seldom performed, even in major academic centers. Due to technical advances, in 2007 MDCT pulmonary angiography fulfilled the conditions to replace PA as the reference standard for diagnosis of acute PE (Remy-Jardin et al. 2007).

When a *cardiac origin for PE* is suspected, MDCT angiography is recommended for a combined assessment of lungs, heart, and cardiac structures and pulmonary vessels. With the advent of ECG-gating during CT acquisition, a free motion artifact imaging of the heart and chest in a single breath-hold can be obtained.

In the presence of valve *endocarditis* ECG-gated MDCT of the chest allows combined diagnosis of valve endocarditis and septic pulmonary embolism on the same imaging modality. Characteristic CT findings in septic pulmonary embolism consist of discrete nodules with varying degrees of cavitation and subpleural, wedge-shaped, heterogeneous areas of increased attenuation with rim-like peripheral enhancement. In many cases a vessel can be seen leading directly to the nodules ("feeding vessel" sign). In a study by Coche et al. (2006), a retrospective ECG-gated 16-slice CT of the entire chest was performed with 16 × 1.5-mm collimation. The entire chest was imaged in one breath-hold during 20 s, after injection of contrast medium. Multiple nodules of various sizes, some with necrotic centers and feeding vessels in the peripheral areas, suggestive of septic emboli, were identified. CT images reconstructed retrospectively at systolic and diastolic phase revealed an elongated hypodense mass, implanted on the tricuspid valve and confirmed by transesophageal echocardiography (TEE). TEE is particularly useful in diagnosing pulmonary valve endocarditis because, in the adult, the pulmonary valve is the most difficult valve to visualize with transthoracic echocardiography (TTE) (Shively et al. 1991).

In case of PE secondary to *cardiac echinococcosis*, the source of emboli may be the rupture of a cystic lesion in the right cardiac chamber. Both CT and MR angiography have been reported to demonstrate occlusion of the pulmonary arteries and their branches by cystic lesions (Dursun et al. 2008).

Acute atrial fibrillation can be associated with PE (Fig. 26.5). To treat patients with atrial fibrillation, radio-frequency catheter ablation (RFCA) of the distal pulmonary veins and posterior left atrium is increasingly used by cardiac interventional electrophysiologists. MDCT provides detailed anatomic information by 3D visualization of the pulmonary veins and the left atrium, allowing accurate placement of intracardiac ablation catheters (Lacomis et al. 2003). In this clinical setting, MDCT could also assess right heart chambers and pulmonary arteries, identifying possible cardiac thrombi and PE.

Primary or secondary cardiac neoplasms, before the advent of cross-sectional imaging, were frequently diagnosed only at autopsy. Nowadays they can be detected in living patients and are usually treated successfully. The plain chest radiograph is abnormal in about 80% of cases, but the findings are nonspecific and may include an abnormal or enlarged cardiac contour, pulmonary edema, or an enlarged azygous vein (Bogren et al. 1980). Echocardiography remains the most efficient method for the initial diagnosis and provides high resolution real-time images whose quality has further improved with the introduction of new ultrasonographic imaging techniques, such as tissue harmonics (Thomas and Rubin 1998). Echocardiography is an optimal modality for imaging small masses (<1 cm) or masses arising from valves and can also image velocities with Doppler, which allows for assessment of presence, degree, and location of obstructions to blood flow or valve regurgitation (Engberding et al. 1993).

Cardiac tumors at echocardiography may appear as an echogenic, nodular, or lobulated mass in the right heart chambers, with or without pericardial effusion or direct pericardial extension, in case of malignant neoplasm.

All patients with PE of unknown origin should undergo early echocardiography to exclude intracardiac masses or thrombi. TTE may demonstrate dilatation of the right heart chambers and the presence of mass located in the right atrium or ventricle, which can show a low or high degree of motion and eventually a free-floating movement suggestive of a mobile thrombus. It may as well demonstrate prolapse through the leaflets of the tricuspid valve during diastole and evaluate left and right ventricular function. Nevertheless, TEE is a well-accepted superior technique in comparison with TTE in the evaluation of right atrial tumors, providing better visualization of the atria and the great vessels. Therefore, TEE should be considered in patients with right atrial masses, even when these tumors have been demonstrated with TTE (Leibowitz et al. 1995).

However, as image acquisition with MDCT and magnetic resonance imaging has steadily become faster, these modalities are playing an increasingly important role in the evaluation of cardiac neoplasms. Soft tissue contrast of both CT and MR imaging is superior to that of echocardiography, and both modalities allow imaging of the entire mediastinum and evaluation of extracardiac extent of disease. They add useful information regarding tumor location, its morphological features, extent, and the presence of local invasion and associated mediastinal and/or pulmonary involvement. They can also offer some degree of histological characterization of the tumor by the identification of fat, calcifications, fibrous tissue, melanin, hemorrhage, or cystic changes (Araoz et al. 1999) (Fig. 26.3). Although MDCT is faster, easier to perform, and has more reliable image quality, MR has higher soft tissue contrast, helpful in detection of tumor infiltration, and greater flexibility in the selection of imaging planes and technical parameters (Siripornpitak and Higgins 1997). Administration of contrast material in MR may also be of help in the differential diagnosis between tumor and bland thrombus, as tumors usually enhance, and can characterize tumor vascularity, differentiating between benign tumors and angiosarcoma with a "sunray appearance" (Bruna and Lockwood 1998). In addition, the pathophysiological effect of the tumor on the myocardial hemodynamics can be assessed by using dynamic imaging techniques in MR that allow characterization of ventricular function, inflow or outflow obstruction, and valve regurgitation.

MDCT with cardiac gating also gives helpful information in patients with cardiac neoplasms, for

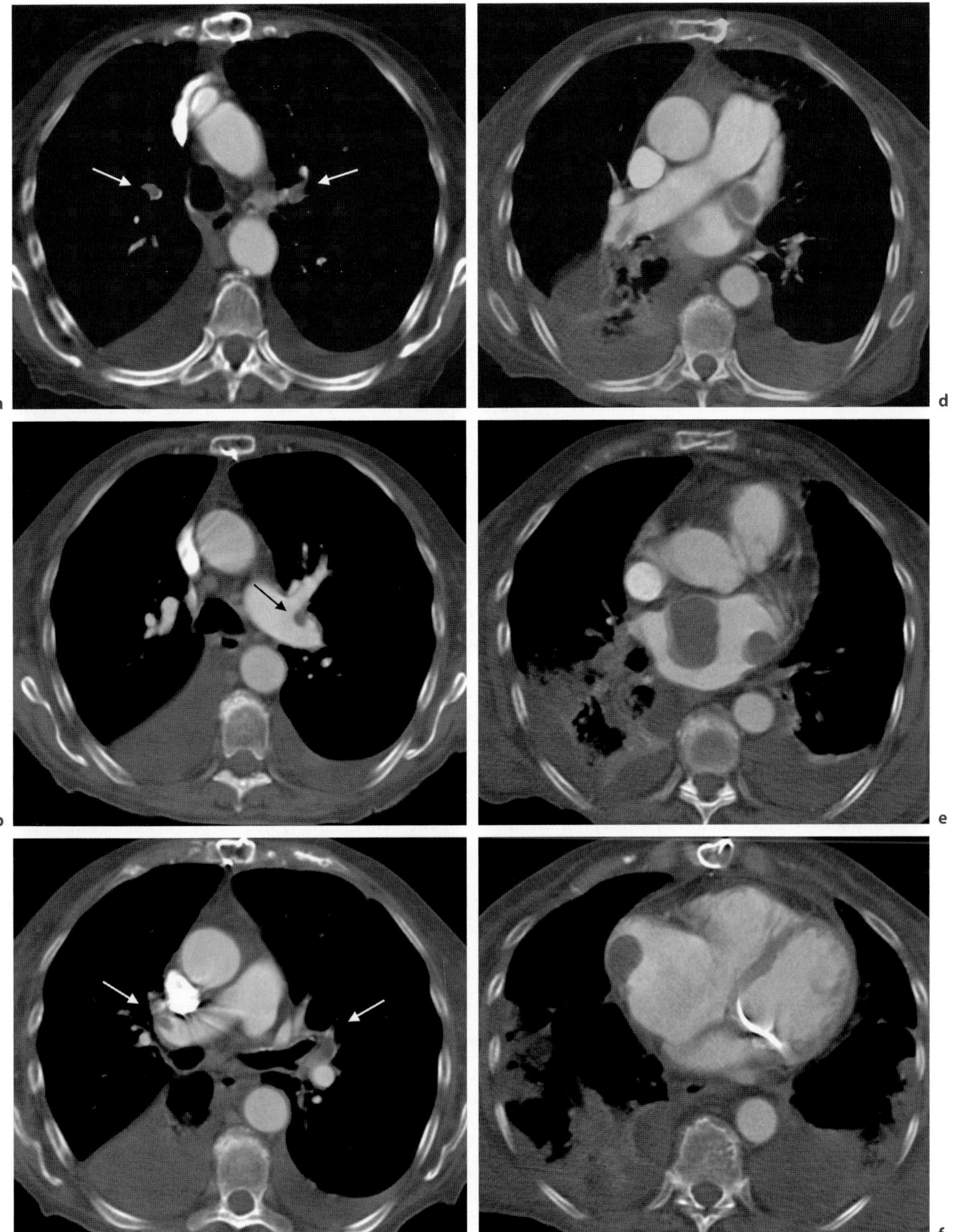

Fig. 26.5a–f. Pulmonary embolism in a patient with acute atrial fibrillation and mitral valve replacement. Contrast-enhanced CT scans (**a–c**) (*arrows*) show multiple and bilateral emboli within lobar and segmental pulmonary arteries. More caudal images through the atria (**d–f**) demonstrate multiple filling defects in both left and right atrium and within the left atrial appendage. Enlargement of the main pulmonary arteries is also seen

staging purpose and/or to rule out PE, not provided by other techniques, specifically echocardiography and MR (Tatli and Lipton 2005). MDCT angiography also helps to assess the anatomy of the coronary arteries and the great vessels in relation to the tumor, as well as to define the tumor vascular supply, an important issue when surgery is planned.

For what concerns *myxoma*, the most common cardiac neoplasm, at echocardiography, the characteristic narrow stalk is the most important distinguishing feature, followed by tumor mobility and distensibility (Obeid et al. 1989). When these characteristics are seen, myxoma can be diagnosed with a high degree of confidence, especially if the tumor is also attached to the interatrial septum. Myxomas demonstrate variable internal echocardiographic features. They may be homogeneous or have central areas of hyperlucency representing hemorrhage and necrosis (Rahilly and Nanda 1981). Echogenic foci of calcification may also be detected. Broad-based, nonmobile myxomas may also occur, but they are indeterminate at echocardiography. The thin, delicate stalk of myxomas usually cannot be defined at CT or MR imaging, although a generally narrow base of attachment is suggestive of, but probably not definitive for, a diagnosis of myxoma; because tumor mobility and distensibility also cannot be depicted, tumor location is the other important distinguishing feature. A mass that arises from the interatrial septum from a narrow base of attachment may be identified as a cardiac myxoma with a high degree of confidence. Other CT and MR imaging findings are variable and reflect gross pathologic features. Because of their gelatinous nature, myxomas usually have heterogeneous low attenuation at CT. Calcification is frequently seen (Tsuchiya et al. 1984). CT may occasionally show myxomas prolapsing through cardiac valves, which is a common finding at echocardiography. Myxomas tend to have markedly increased signal intensity in T2-weighted images. However, they may have areas of decreased signal intensity due to the presence of calcification or to magnetic susceptibility artifacts caused by hemosiderin (Masui et al. 1995). Contrast enhancement in myxomas is usually heterogeneous, which also likely reflects the presence of necrotic areas within the tumor, but intense enhancement may be seen.

Cardiac surgical procedures may have a not elevated, but considerable intrinsic risk of pulmonary embolism. In the post-surgical period, MDCT scans may evaluate both the good outcome of cardiac surgery and the pulmonary parenchyma and mediastinum and therefore identify the presence of PE, when suspected. In the late year a new diagnostic scanning technique, dual-source computed tomography (DSCT), has been developed; it shows great diagnostic potential in patients before or after cardiac surgery, providing a high diagnostic accuracy in the detection of coronary artery stenosis and in the assessment of patients who received aortic valve replacement (Nikolau et al. 2007). DSCT, due to its better temporal and spatial resolution, also allows the depiction of PE at a subsegmental level with high accuracy. Therefore, this new modality could become the best non-invasive imaging technique in this clinical setting.

Paradoxical embolism, a left-sided origin of an acute pulmonary embolism, should be suspected when an atrial septal defect is present. In these cases, TEE can confirm this finding and often identifies the embolic source in the left atrium.

26.4 Treatment

In case of infective endocarditis and pulmonary embolism, the treatment consists of a high dose of antibiotics administered by the intravenous route to maximize the diffusion of antibiotic molecules into vegetations from the blood filling the cambers of the heart. This is necessary because neither the heart valves nor the vegetations adherent to them are supplied by blood vessels. Antibiotics are continued for a long time (2–6 weeks); specific drug regimens differ depending on the classification of the endocarditis as subacute or acute. Fungal endocarditis requires specific anti-fungal treatment. Surgical removal of the valve is necessary in patients who fail to clear micro-organism from their blood in response to antibiotic therapy or in patients who develop cardiac failure resulting from destruction of a valve by infection. A removed valve is usually replaced with an artificial valve that may either be mechanical (metallic) or obtained from animals, generally pig (bioprosthetic valves). In cases without extensive valve destruction, a conservative surgical treatment is possible, with removal of vegetations sparing the valve and extraction of pulmonary emboli (Tanaka et al. 1989).

The treatment reserved for cardiac tumors is surgical, with TEE during surgery providing useful information about secondary valve damage caused by the tumor or detecting rare biatrial or multilocular myxomas. The use of TEE is then recommended as an intraoperative routine during resection of cardiac masses; bicaval cannulation is also recommended to avoid tumor fragmentation. Hypotermic circulatory arrest is the method of choice and provides good view for embolectomy (Allard et al. 1995). Repetitive recurrences are rare (1.3%), while asymptomatic recurrences are observed in young patients who have a familiar history of tumor or multifocal myxomas. Embolectomy of the pulmonary artery is performed in a way similar to that of chronic pulmonary thromboembolectomy (Ando et al. 1999).

Malignant cardiac tumors have a poor prognosis, because they typically present with metastasis, most frequently to the lung and the liver. Treatment is a combination of surgery and radiation with or without sarcoma-type chemotherapy. Heart transplantation is a consideration if metastatic disease is not identified (Gowdamarajan and Michler 2000).

When metastatic disease of the heart is diagnosed, the treatment is generally palliative, aimed at reducing the obstruction to blood flow by the tumor and providing symptomatic relief. The options remain very limited and depend on the type of primary tumor and its response to chemotherapy or radiotherapy, the extent of intracardiac and extracardiac involvement and the general status of the patient. Irrespective of the treatment, the prognosis remains very poor.

Pulmonary embolism after cardiac surgery is a complication reported in the literature, most of which occur when a DVT is diagnosed (Frizzelli et al. 2008), and the mortality is very high (34%). Early diagnosis and appropriate treatment are essential. Standard therapy for pulmonary embolism includes systemic anticoagulation with heparin and warfarin. In patients not candidates for systemic anticoagulation, caval interruption is only indicated to prevent recurrent pulmonary embolism when a DVT coexists.

26.5 Summary

Cardiac diseases or devices that may cause pulmonary embolism are not a common situation in the daily clinical practice. There are arrhythmogenic diseases, neoplasms, cardiac surgery and valve infective diseases that may account for an increased risk of PE. Diagnosis in all these conditions is based on clinical and anamnestic data and on various diagnostic procedures. CT, especially new generation scanners such as MDCT, is a useful diagnostic tool for better visualization of both pulmonary arterial circulation and cardiac anatomy assessment. Moreover, with the newest 64-slice scanners it is possible to obtain optimal visualization of cardiac structures almost without any of the motion artifacts that were documented with the older CT scanners, allowing cardiac and pulmonary imaging in only one breath-hold, also in patients with pulmonary disease and dyspnea as well as in subjects with cardiac arrhythmias. DSCT is a promising, new scanning technique for the evaluation of such patients, allowing volume-rendered images for almost the entire cardiac cycle with no motion artifacts.

References

Aberg H (1969) Atrial fibrillation. I. A study of atrial thrombosis and systemic embolism in a necropsy material. Acta Med Scand 185:373–379

Allard MF, Taylor GP, Wilson JE et al. (1995) Primary cardiac tumors. In: Goldhaber SZ, Braunwald E (eds) Cardiopulmonary diseases and cardiac tumors. Atlas of heart disease. Current Medicine, Philadelphia, pp 3:15.1–15.22

Altes TA, Mai VM, Munger TM et al. (2005) Pulmonary embolism: comprehensive evaluation with MR ventilation and perfusion scanning with hyperpolarized helium-3, arterial spin tagging, and contrast-enhanced MRA. J Vasc Interv Radiol 16:999–1005

Ando M, Okita Y, Tagusari O et al. (1999) Surgical treatment for chronic thromboembolic pulmonary hypertension under profound hypothermia and circulatory arrest in 24 patients. J Card Surg 14:377–385

Araoz PA, Eklund HE, Welch TJ et al. (1999) CT and MR imaging of primary cardiac malignancies. Radiographics 19:1421–1434

Badmanaban B, Sachithanandan A, Hunter I et al. (2003) Massive pulmonary embolism due to late onset heparin-induced thrombocytopenia following coronary bypass graft surgery: successful treatment with lepidurin. J Card Surg 18:316–318

Bayezid O, Ocal A, Isiko O et al. (1991) A case of cardiac hydatid cyst localised on the interventricular septum and causing pulmonary emboli. J Cardiovasc Surg 32:324–326

Bogren HG, De Maria AN, Mason DT (1980) Imaging procedures in the detection of cardiac tumors, with emphasis on echocardiography: a review. Cardiovasc Intervent Radiol 3:107–125

Borsaru AD, Lau KKK, Solin P (2007) Cardiac metastasis: a cause of recurrent pulmonary emboli. Br J Radiol 80:50–53

Bruna J, Lockwood M (1998) Primary heart angiosarcoma detected by computed tomography and magnetic resonance imaging. Eur Radiol 8:66–68

Burke A, Jeudy J, Virmani R (2008) Cardiac tumors: an update. Heart 94:117–123

Butany J, Nair V, Naseemuddin A et al. (2005) Cardiac tumors: diagnosis and management. Lancet Oncol 6:219–228

Carmichael AJ, Martin AM (1991) Pulmonary embolism: a complication of right atrial thrombi due to atrial fibrillation. J R Soc Med 84:313

Carrel T, Schaffner A, Vogt P et al. (1993) Endocarditis in intravenous drug addicts and HIV infected patients. Possibilities and limitations of surgical treatment. Heart Valve Dis 2:140–147

Castorino F, Masiello P, Quattrocchi E et al. (2000) Primary cardiac rhabdomyosarcoma of the left atrium: an unusual presentation. Tex Heart Inst J 27:206–208

Chan P, Ogilby JD, Segal B (1989) Tricuspid valve endocarditis. Am Heart J 117:1140–1146

Coche E, Mauel E, Beauloye C et al. (2006) Tricuspid valve endocarditis and septic pulmonary emboli illustrated by ECG-gated multi-slice CT of the chest. Eur Heart J27:20

Cosson S, Kevorkian JP, Milliez P et al. (2003) A rare localization in right-sided endocarditis diagnosed by echocardiolgraphy: a case report. Cardiovasc Ultrasound 1:10

Cremieux AC, Witchitz S, Malergue MC et al. (1985) Clinical and echocardiographic observations in pulmonary valve endocarditis. Am J Cardiol 56:610–613

Daus H, Bay W, Harig S et al. (1998) Primary lymphoma of the heart: report of a case with histological diagnosis of the transvenously biopsied intracardiac tumor. Ann Hematol 77:139–141

Dàvila PM, Navas E, Fortùn J et al. (2005) Analysis of mortality and risk factors associated with native valve endocarditis in drug users: The importance of vegetation size. Am Heart J 11:1099–1106

Dursun M, Terzibasioglu E, Yilmaz R et al. (2008) Cardiac hydatid disease: CT and MRI findings. Am J Roentgenol 190:226–232

Ellis M, El-Abdely H, Sandridge A et al. (2001) Fungal endocarditis: evidence in the world literature, 1965–1995. Clin Infect Dis 32:50–62

Engberding R, Daniel WG, Erbel R et al. (1993) Diagnosis of heart tumors by transoesophageal echocardiography; a multicenter study in 154 patients. Eur Heart J 14:1223–1228

Formolo JM, Giraldo A, Shors CM (1981) Fatal pulmonary embolism from massive right atrial thrombus post coronary artery bypass surgery. Am Heart J 101:510

Frizzelli R, Tortelli O, Di Comite V et al. (2008) Deep venous thrombosis of the neck and pulmonary embolism in patients with a central venous catheter admitted to cardiac rehabilitation after cardiac surgery: a prospective study of 815 patients. Intern Emerg Med Epub: 21 Mar

Gillinov AM, Davis EA, Alberg AJ et al. (1992) Pulmonary embolism in the cardiac surgical patient. Ann Thorac Surg 53:988–991

Goldhaber SZ (1988) Optimal strategy for diagnosis and treatment of pulmonary embolism due to right atrial thrombus. Mayo Clin Proc 63:1261–1264

Goodman LR, Curtin JJ, Mewissen MW et al. (1995) Detection of pulmonary embolism in patients with unresolved clinical and scintigraphic diagnosis: helical CT versus angiography. Am J Roentgenol 164:1369–1374

Gowdamarajan A, Michler RE (2000) Therapy for primary cardiac tumors: Is there a role for heart transplantation? Curr Opin Cardiol 15:121–126

Gurney JW (1993) No fooling around: Direct visualization of pulmonary embolism. Radiology 188:618–619

Harrison A, Amundson S (2005) Evaluation and management of the acutely dyspneic patient: the role of biomarkers. Am J Emerg Med 23:371–378

Hawe A, Rastelli GC, Brandenburg RO et al. (1969) Embolic complications following repair of atrial septal defects. Circulation 39:185–191

Hyman R, Kralis DG, Ross JJ et al. (1997) Pulmonary embolism from in situ right atrial thrombus after coronary artery bypass surgery. J Am Soc Echocardiogr 10:760–762

Ishihara Y, Hara H, Saijo T et al. (2002) Left atrial thrombus causing pulmonary embolism by passing through an atrial septal defect. Circ J 66:109–110

Johnson JC, Flowers NC, Horan LG (1971) Unexplained atrial flutter: a frequent herald of pulmonary embolism. Chest 60:29–34

Josa M, Siouffi SY, Silverma AB et al. (1993) Pulmonary embolism after cardiac surgery. J Am Coll Cardiol 22:1553–1554

Lacomis JM, Wigginton W, Fuhrman C et al. (2003) Multidetector row CT of the left atrium and pulmonary veins before radio-frequency catheter ablation for atrial fibrillation. Radiographics 23:S35–S48

Lahdhili H, Hachicha S, Ziadi M, Thameur H (2002) Acute pulmonary embolism due to the rupture of a right ventricle hydatid cyst. Eur J Cardiothorac Surg 22:462–464

Lahtinen J, Ahvenjarvi L, Biancari F et al. (2006) Pulmonary embolism after off-pump coronary artery bypass surgery as detected by computed tomography. Am J Surg 192:396–398

Leibowitz G, Keller NM, Daniel WG et al. (1995) Transoesophageal versus transthoracic ecocardiography in the evaluation of right atrial tumor. Am Heart J 10:1224–1227

Lévy S, Maarek M, Coumel P et al. (1999) Characterization of different subsets of atrial fibrillation in general practice in France: The ALFA study. Circulation 99:3028–3035

Masotti L, Ceccarelli E, Cappelli R et al. (2000) Pulmonary embolism in the elderly: clinical, instrumental and laboratory aspects. Gerontology 46:205–211

Masui T, Takahashi M, Miura K et al. (1995) Cardiac myxomas: identification of tumoral haemorrhage and calcification on MR images. Am J Roentgenol 164:850–852

McAllister HA, Fenoglio JJ (1978) Tumors of the cardiovascular system. In: Hartman WH, Cowan WR. Atlas of tumor pathology. Second series, fascicle 15.Armed Forces Institute of Pathology, Washington, DC , pp 20–25

McGiven J, Bunton R (2000) Pulmonary embolism after cardiac surgery. Heart Lung Circ 9:A179

Neerukonda SK, Janntz RD, Vijay NK et al. (1991) Pulmonary embolisation of papillary fibroelastomas. Arising from the tricuspid valve. Heart Inst J 18:132–135

Nikolaou K, Saam T, Rist C et al. (2007) Pre- and postsurgical diagnostics with dual-source computed tomography in cardiac surgery. Radiologe 47:310–318

Nucifora G, Badano L, Hysko F et al. (2007) Pulmonary embolism and fever. Clinical update. Circulation 115:e–73–e176

Obeid AI, Marvast M, Parker F et al. (1989) Comparison of transthoracic and transoesophageal echocardiography in diagnosis of left atrial myxoma. Am J Cardiol 63:1006–1008

Parsons AM, Detterbeck FC (2003) Multifocal right atrial myxoma and pulmonary embolism. Ann Thorac Surg 75:1323–1324

Patel S, Kazerooni EA, Cascade PN (2003) Pulmonary embolism: optimization of small pulmonary artery visualization at multi-detector row CT. Radiology 227:455–460

Pinto DS, Blair BM, Schwartzstein RM et al. (2005) A sailor's heartbreak. N Engl J Med 353:934–939

PIOPED Investigators (1990) Value of the ventilation/perfusion scan in acute pulmonary embolism. Results of the prospective investigation of pulmonary embolism diagnosis (PIOPED). JAMA 263:2753–2759

Rahilly GT, Nanda NC (1981) Two-dimensional echocardiographic identification of haemorrhages in atrial myxomas. Am Heart J 101:237–239

Remy-Jardin M, Remy J, Wattinne L et al. (1992) Central pulmonary thromboembolism: diagnosis with spiral volumetric CT with the single-breath-hold technique–comparison with pulmonary angiography. Radiology 185:381–387

Remy-Jardin M, Mastora I, Remy J (2003) Pulmonary embolus imaging with multislice CT. Radiol Clin North Am 41:507–519

Remy-Jardin M, Pistolesi M, Goodman LR et al. (2007) Management of suspected acute pulmonary embolism in the era of ct angiography: A statement from the Fleischner Society. Radiology 245:315–329

Reynen K (1995) Cardiac myxomas. N Engl J Med 333:1610–1617

Robbins MJ, Frater RW, Soeiro R et al. (1986a) Influence of vegetation size on clinical outcome of right-sided infective endocarditis. Am J Med 80:165–171

Robbins MJ, Soeiro R, Frishman WH et al. (1986b) Right-sided valvular endocarditis: aetiology, diagnosis, and an approach to therapy. Am Heart J 111:128–135

San Roman JA, Vilacosta I, Sarria C et al. (2001) Eustachian valve endocarditis: is it worth searching for? Am Heart J 142:1037–1040

Sawhney N, Palakodeti V, Raisinghani A et al. (2001) Eustachian valve endocarditis: a case series and analysis of the literature. J Am Soc Echocardiogr 14:1139–1142

Schoepf U, Holzknecht N, Helmberger TK et al. (2002) Subsegmental pulmonary emboli: Improved detection with thin-collimation multidetector-row spiral CT. Radiology 222:483–490

Seagle RL, Nomeir AM, Watts LE et al. (1985) Left atrial myxoma and atrial septal defect with recurrent pulmonary emboli. South Med J 78:992–994

Senzaki H, Uemura Y, Yamamoto D et al. (1999) Right intraventricular metastais of squamous cell carcinoma of the uterine cervix: an autopsy case and literature review. Pathol Int 49:447–452

Shiber JR, Santana J (2006) Dyspnea. Med Clin North Am 90:453–4579

Shively B, Gurule F, Roldan C et al. (1991) Diagnostic value of transoesophageal compared with transthoracic echocardiography in infective endocarditis. J Am Coll Cardiol 18:391–397

Siripornpitak S, Higgins CB (1997) MRI of primary malignant cardiovascular tumors. J Comput Assist Tomogr 21:462–466

Skalidis EI, Parthenakis FI, Zacharis EA et al. (1999) Pulmonary tumor embolism from primary cardiac B-cell lymphoma. Chest 116:1489–1490

Stein PD, Woodard PK, Hull RD et al. (2003) Gadolinium-enhanced magnetic resonance angiography for detection of acute pulmonary embolism. Chest 124:2324–2328

Sun JP, Asher CR, Yang XS et al. (2001) Clinical and echocardiographic characteristics of papillary fibroelastomas: a retrospective and prospective study in 162 patients. Circulation 103:2687–2693

Tanaka M, Abe T, Hosokawa S et al. (1989) Tricuspid valve *Candida endocarditis* cured by valve-sparing debridement. Ann Thorac Surg 48:857–858

Tapson VF (2008) Acute pulmonary embolism. N Engl J Med 358:1037–1052

Tatli S, Lipton MJ (2005) CT for intracardiac thrombi and tumors. Int J Cardiovasc Imaging 21:115–131

Tejada JC, Saavedra J, Molina L et al. (2001) Hydatid disease of the interventricular septum causing pericardial effusion. Ann Thorac Surg 71:2034–2036

Thomas JD, Rubin DN (1998) Tissue harmonic imaging: why does it work? J Am Soc Echocardiogr 11:803–808

Torbicki A, Galié N, Covezzoli A et al. (2003) Right heart thrombi in pulmonary embolism. Results from the International Cooperative Pulmonary Embolism Registry. J Am Coll Cardiol 41:2245–2251

Tsuchiya F, Kohno A, Saitoh R et al. (1984) CT findings of atrial myxoma. Radiology 151:139–143

Tsutsumi K, Aida Y, Ohno T et al. (2005) Primary cardiac rhabdomyosarcoma following a uterine leiomysarcoma. Jpn J Thorac Cardiovasc Surg 53:458–462

Uemura S, Watanabe H, Iwama H et al. (2004) Extensive primary cardiac liposarcoma with multiple functional complications. Heart 90:e48

Uppal KM, Nuno IN, Schwartz DS et al. (2000) Isolated right ventricular outflow tract mass presenting as hemoptysis. Ann Thorac Surg 70:2158–2159

Van Erkel AR, van Rossum AB, Bloem JL et al. (1996) Spiral CT angiography for suspected pulmonary embolism: a cost-effectiveness analysis. Radiology 201:29–36

Walls JT, Curtios JJ, Silver D et al. (1990) Heparin-induced thrombocytopenia in patients who undergo open heart surgery. Surgery 108:686–692

Wang CS, FitzGerald JM, Schulzer M et al. (2005) Does this dyspneic patient in the emergency department have congestive heart failure? JAMA 294:1944–1956

Weisse AB, Heller DR, Schimenti RJ et al. (1993) The febrile parenteral drug user: a prospective study in 121 patients. Am J Med 94:274–280

Worsley DF, Alavi A, Aronchick JM et al. (1993) Chest radiographic findings in patients with acute pulmonary embolism: observations from the PIOPED Study. Radiology 189:133–136

Zijlstra F, Fioretti P, Roelandt JR (1986) Echocardiographic demonstration of free wall vegetative endocarditis complicated by a pulmonary embolism in a patient with a ventricular septal defect. Br Heart J 55:497–499

Pectus Excavatum and the Heart

27

Lorenzo Bonomo, Giuseppe Macis, and Andrea Caulo

CONTENTS

L. Bonomo, MD, Professor
G. Macis, MD
A. Caulo, MD
Department of Bioimaging and Radiological Sciences, Catholic University, Largo Agostino Gemelli 8, Rome 00168, Italy

27.1 General Considerations

Pectus excavatum (PE) is a congenital malformation characterized by a depression of the sternum and of the adjacent rib cartilage that modifies the conformation of the chest with the appearance of a concavity of the anterior wall. This deformity, characterized by a sternal depression and known by various names (pectus excavatum, funnel chest, and cobbler's chest) represents the most common deformity of the chest wall (90%) and affects 1 in 1,000 live births (Mansour et al. 2003; Fonkalsrud 2003) with a prevalence in male subjects of 5:1 (M/F 5:1) (Fonkalsrud 2003). It is also the most frequently surgically treated malformation. The modality of hereditary transmission has not yet been established, but it is commonly accepted that patients with PE report other relatives affected by thoracic malformations.

PE has been found in twins and, in many cases, in various generations of the same family, many of whose members were carriers of altered connective tissue, suggesting that a defective connective tissue gene (i.e., fibrillin, collagen and B growth factor) (Creswick et al. 2006) could be at the base of the pathogenic process.

PE is, in fact, associated with congenital diseases of the connective tissue, such as Marfan syndrome, Elher-Danlos syndrome, osteogenesis imperfecta, Poland syndrome, Klippel-Fiel syndrome (Williams and Crabbe 2003) and, more rarely, with congenital heart disease (Shamberger et al. 1988). The malformation, barely evident at birth, becomes apparent around the first year of life when the child begins to stand and is even more visible after 4 or 5 years, becoming more serious during puberty. The defect stabilizes at around 18–20 years with the complete ossification of the rib cage. The sternal depression is created by the posterior angulation of two components: the body of the sternum starting from the second cartilage and the costal cartilage itself.

27.2 Physiopathology

Several hypotheses have been suggested to explain the deformity. Importance has been attributed to a fibrous ligament that could connect the sternum to the diaphragm or to the insufficient development of the anterior fibers of this muscle; such alterations would condition the depression of the sternum through an abnormal mechanism of traction (Brodkin 1953). More realistic is the current recognition of the importance of the genesis of PE as an anomalous costal cartilage growth pushing the sternum in a backwards direction (Ravitch 1961).

It is a complex and often asymmetric defect, complicated by the fact that the affected person tends to somehow curve himself around the deformity, arching his shoulders towards the malformation while pushing out the abdomen. Such changes in posture become permanent and, in time, impossible to modify.

In patients with PE, a paradoxical inspiratory reentry of the sternum is observed, particularly evident in very young children and in deep breathing in all carriers. PE presents with different clinical forms and levels of gravity: from mild malformations that require only corrective physical exercises to much more severe forms for which surgery is the only solution.

PE is asymptomatic in the majority of cases and manifests with a visible alteration of the thoracic conformation. However, although it is generally agreed that PE is a condition that has great psychological implications for the carrier, who is conscious of his potentially disfiguring condition, the clinical idea that the mechanical compression of the heart caused by moderate-severe PE determines organic cardiac and pulmonary alterations is becoming more diffuse. Alterations include compression of the right cardiac chambers (Mocchegiani et al. 1995), compression of the pulmonary infundibulum, prolapse of the mitral valve (Shamberger et al. 1987), tricuspid stenosis (Hoeffel 2000), compression of the inferior vena cava (Yalamanchili et al. 2005), alteration of the conduction and restrictive pulmonary syndrome (Lawson et al. 2005).

Patients complain of greater fatigability, evident in infants when eating and in older patients when engaging in intense physical activity. Subjectively, these patients complain of effort dyspnea, reduced tolerance to physical activity compared to their peers, chest pain and palpitations. In this condition, the anteroposterior diameter of the thorax is clearly reduced with the heart compressed and displaced to the left. The extent of previous fatigability is often only realized after the deformity has been surgically repaired. In recent years efforts have been made to use appropriate tests in order to measure limitations in individuals; generally, however, such tests measure tolerance to physical activity only indirectly.

Malek et al. (2003) recently reported that the maximum amount of oxygen that can be transported and consumed at the muscular level (VO2 max) during exercise of progressive intensity was 75% in patients with PE compared to healthy controls. This suggests a certain level of compromise at the cardiac level as consumption of oxygen depends largely on the proportional increase of output with effort.

The capacity for physical exercise is further conditioned by the body position as the degree of sternal compression varies with posture. The right atrium and ventricle are, in fact, compressed by the pectus, particularly when the patient is in a standing position. The physiopathologic mechanism of compression and the reduced ventricular filling have been well documented by Zhao et al. (2000). They carried out exercise tests using an ergometer bicycle on patients with PE and on controls, both in supine and sitting positions, acquiring, contemporaneously, an echocardiogram and measurement of stroke volume. In patients with PE both maximum oxygen consumption (VO2 max) and stroke volume were significantly inferior to those of controls during the exercise test in sitting position. Stroke volume did not, however, differ in either group during exercise in the supine position. From the above, we can deduce that patients present a real limitation on physical exercise of cardiac origin.

The natural history of PE has been modified over the years as progressive surgical procedures have been proposed to correct the most debilitating cases. The type of intervention performed has evolved in time from a highly invasive technique often with serious complications to a less-invasive technique, more suitable to physiological modifications and a growing organism.

From the 1950s until the early 1990s, surgical correction of the more serious forms of PE consisted of a series of long, complex procedures that entailed incision and resection of costal cartilage and a sternal ostoetomy associated with various forms of internal fixation. Following such invasive procedures, several postoperative complications could arise, sometimes with fatal consequences. For this reason, bearing in mind that many pediatric surgeons were sure that this defect was purely cosmetic surgery of PE, it was progressively abandoned and reserved for single sporadic cases.

Subsequently, a minimally invasive surgical technique was introduced by DONALD NUSS (NUSS et al. 1998a, 1998b, 2002): a metal bar is inserted through two small lateral incisions made in the chest wall, the PE indentation is pushed outwards, the bones are repositioned and the malformation is thus corrected. This operation does not interfere with the development of the thorax or induce respiratory insufficiency due to a non-expandable chest.

27.3 Indications for Surgery and Evaluation with Diagnostic Imaging

In PE the indication for surgery remains extremely limited in spite of the simplicity of the Nuss technique. The condition is classified as mild, moderate, or serious based on objective radiological parameters that can be assessed both on chest radiography and CT imaging. Only patients with moderate-severe malformations are candidates for surgical correction.

The radiogram of the thorax is the first examination to be performed on patients with PE and is followed by CT. In some institutions (DERVEAUX et al. 1989; OHNO et al. 2001; BARAUSKAS 2003), the severity of the deformity is, however, still assessed using only chest X-ray based on the criterion of lowest possible radiation exposure in those children with a "benign"-type pathology. The authors would like to point out that axial CT exposes children to an amount of radiation that exceeds the benefit it produces and sometimes requires the sedation of very young patients. The radiographic examination of the chest in children with PE should be performed in the two projections, in orthostatism, in deep inspiration phase and at a film-focal distance of 180 cm. The radiographic picture of PE is characterized by different findings.

In the lateral view, a depression in the lower third of the sternum is easily diagnosed: also evident is any direct contact between the heart and the anteriorly depressed sternum and between the heart and the thoracic spine posteriorly. Sometimes, in cases of sternal rotation, the sign of a double border that simulates the presence of a space-occupying process in the anterior mediastinum can be observed (SOTEROPOULOS et al. 1979). In the posteroanterior view the heart appears rotated and moved to the left: these anatomical modifications can produce multiple signs such as (GULLER and HABLE 1974):

- Disappearance of the second right cardiac arch following the dislocation of the right cardiac margin inside the right paraspinal line, or, in more serious cases, over the midline of the thoracic spine: this demonstrates the extent of the leftward shift of the heart.
- The aspect of the "mitral" heart produced by the rectilinearity of the left cardiac profile and of the prominence of the second arch caused by the rotation of the heart to the left.
- Enlargement of the right hilum following the rotation-dislocation of the heart that projects the vessels of the right hilum, rendering them more evident and simulating a middle lobe pathology: this sign indicates the lack of projected superimposition between the heart and vessels of the middle and right inferior lobes. The increase in density of the right paracardiac parenchyma can also be created by the compression produced by the depressed ribs pressing on the pulmonary parenchyma and thus simulating a pulmonary infiltrating process.
- Dislocation of the aorta towards the left: this is one of the mort frequent signs resulting as a consequence of the cardiac shift.
- Obliteration of the middle-inferior segment of the descending aortic interface (TAKAHASHI et al. 1992) as a result of the cardiac rotation, which causes contact between the junction of the inferior pulmonary vein and/or the surface of the left atrium with the wall of the descending aorta.
- Curved acute angle appearance of the anterior arches of the ribs due to the congenital deformity.

The evaluation of PE in order to determine the need for surgical repair is traditionally based on the indications of severity derived from the chest radiograph. The fundamental indices are the vertebral index (VI) and the fronto-sagittal index (FSI). The vertebral index (VI) is the percentage ratio between the minimum sagittal diameter measured from the ventral surface of the sternum at the point of deepest depression and the sagittal diameter of the vertebral body at the same level. The fronto-sagittal index is the percentage ratio between the maximum internal transverse diameter of the thorax and the minimum sagittal diameter. Ohno suggests that patients with values of VI > 27 and FSI < 29 be submitted for surgical repair (Ohno et al. 2001).

Kilda et al. (2007), in order to evaluate the severity of PE, utilized both the indices measured on the thorax and Haller's index measured using one axial CT scan at the point of deepest depression: this author also adds to the preoperative evaluation the indices of thoracic flattening and of asymmetry, measured using one CT scan. Values of VI > 30, FSI < 30 and HI > 3.3 are considered by the author as being severe and an indication for surgical repair. Values of VI < 30, FSI > 30 and HI < 3.3 are low and therefore preclude surgery. The alteration of only one of the indices classifies the condition as moderately serious and should therefore be surgically repaired.

The index of thoracic flattening is derived from the ratio between the transverse diameter doubled and divided by the sum of the right and left sagittal diameters by chest radiograph; with a result of < 2, the chest is considered 'flat', > 2 means that the chest is of normal conformation. The asymmetry index is derived from the inverse ratio between the right and the left sagittal diameters. The thoracic wall is considered asymmetric and the left hemithorax more convex if the index is < 0.05, the right side is more convex, and prominent if the index has a value > 0.05. The indices described are always utilized in the postoperative evaluation in order to measure the amount of improvement of the thoracic conformation.

Following a preliminary surgical, pulmonary and cardiological examination, proposed surgical candidates, following the Nuss technique, undergo CT scan (Lawson et al. 2006; Sidden et al. 2001). The complete extension of the chest is studied with spiral CT or MDCT. MDCT must be performed using the protocol established for chest CTA. The study extends in a cranio-caudal direction, 80 kVp per patient weighing less than 45 kg and > 80 kVp in those weighing more, with milliamps as low as possible according to the patient's weight (Paterson and Frush 2007). CTA is performed with thin thickness (< 1 mm), detector collimation of 0.75 or 0.6 and pitch from 1.0 to 1.5. The delay in acquisition of the scan is determined using a "bolus tracking" system connected to a ROI on the aorta. If the delay is to be calculated using the empirical method, one criterion could be to start the scan at 12–13 s in children weighing less than 15 kg and at 20–25 s in those weighing more. Scans are performed in a cranio-caudal direction during one breath in cooperating patients and at normal breathing in those unable to hold their breath. In order to examine cardiac alterations and large vessels with this protocol, ECG gating is not necessary. Volumetric data can be reconstructed at 3–5 mm for a routine examination or at 1–2 mm for multiplanar and three-dimensional reconstructions. Radiological evaluation must take the following into account.

27.3.1 Haller's Index

In 1987 Haller and co-workers formulated a pectus index based on the measurements of axial CT of several thoracic diameters as objective parameters of the gravity of PE representing an advance on the indices calculated on a standard radiogram (Haller et al. 1987; Nakahara et al. 1987; Clausner et al. 1991). Haller's index is defined as the maximum transverse diameter of the chest (T) measured from the internal margin of the rib on one side to the internal margin of the controlateral rib, divided by the minimum anteroposterior diameter (A), positioned on the same plane but perpendicular to T, from the ventral surface of the depressed sternum or from the most inward costal cartilage as far as the anterior surface of the vertebral body or its horizontal tangent (T/A) obtained at the point of greatest sternal depression (Fig. 27.1). In patients with symmetrical sternal deformity, Haller's index is calculated from the internal surface of the depressed sternum to the anterior surface of the corresponding vertebral body.

In asymmetrical deformities, however, the deepest point of the sternal depression is not located on the same sagittal plane as the dorsal vertebra and, to obtain the index, it is necessary to trace a tangent tranversal line to the anterior surface of the spine and another tangent to the internal surface of the most sunken cartilage and then measure the distance between these two lines, which corresponds to the smallest anteroposterior diameter.

Normal children and teenagers have a Hiller's index of between 1.9 and 2.2 from 0 to 6 years and from 2.3 to 2.7 from 6 to 14 years: all values are less

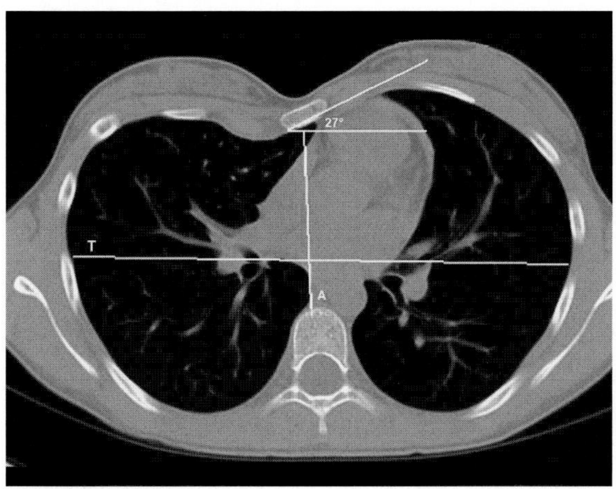

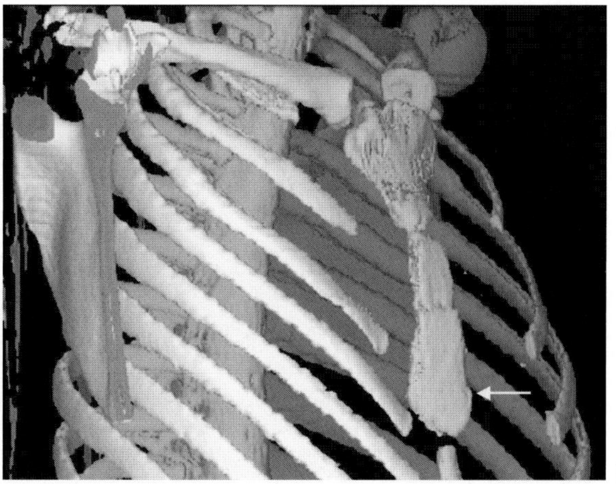

Fig. 27.1a,b. The severity of malformation is evaluated using Haller's index (*HI*) obtained by the ratio between the internal transverse diameter (*T*) of the chest divided by the A-P diameter (*A*). In this case (**a**), the diameters are 22.7 and 7.9 cm respectively, and the HI is 2.87. The malformation is therefore mild, and the surface of contact between the heart and the thoracic wall is reduced. In the same image the sternal torsion angle was calculated (27°), also classified as mild. Oblique 3D reconstruction (**b**) clearly shows the sternal torsion to the right (*arrow*). The slight "cup"-shaped sternal depression is located at the lower third of the sternum

than 3 (Daunt et al. 2004). In subjects with mild PE, the value is less than 3.2, moderate when the index is between 3.2 and 3.5 and severe when the value is over 3.5. Values over 3.25 are considered serious and an indication for surgical intervention.

27.3.2 Morphological Traits of PE

We can distinguish two morphological types of concavity based on the shape of the depression viewed in the axial section or on a middle-sagittal plane (Cartoski et al. 2006). "Cup" PE is when the depression is deep and circumscribed, delimited by steep walls that affect a limited portion of the sternum without alterations of the adjacent anatomical structures, particularly of the ribs. Widespread or so-called "saucer" PE (Fig. 27.2) is when the depression affects the entire sternum and sometimes the manubrium and extends to the ribs as far as the mammillary lines. The depression is therefore widened and determines a more or less relevant decrease of the anteroposterior diameters of the thorax.

Three-dimensional, multiplanar and 3D volume-rendering reconstructions permit the depiction of cup or saucer morphological-type characteristics (when viewed laterally, in oblique projection or in sagittal reconstruction). In the cup type, there is a funnel-shape and a short caudo-cranial diameter. In the saucer type, a valley-like depression can be observed that extends to the ribs adjacent to the sternum.

27.3.3 Length of Sternal Involvement on Cranio-Caudal Axis

In cup PE, the circumscribed depression is contained to one part of the sternum, prevalently the lower third. In saucer PE, the depression is much more extensive (Fig. 27.3); it should also be noted that those depressions classified as cups during the preliminary surgical examination or with photographic documentation are sometimes found to be saucers when studied by CT.

These notably long pectus excavatums can have a compressing effect on the upper part of the thorax, affecting both the trachea and the esophagus. This distinction, easily detected and measured by CT, is fundamental to surgical planning in order to decide on both the number of steel bars to be used and their position. Short PE has a lesser impact on the internal thoracic organs and surgery can be performed using one metal arch only. Extensive saucer PE must be corrected surgically with the positioning of two metal arches as a condition affecting such a large part of the chest and sternum cannot be corrected with one single bar.

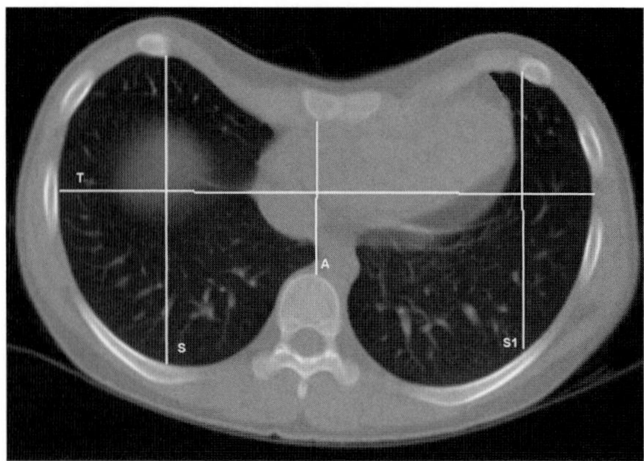

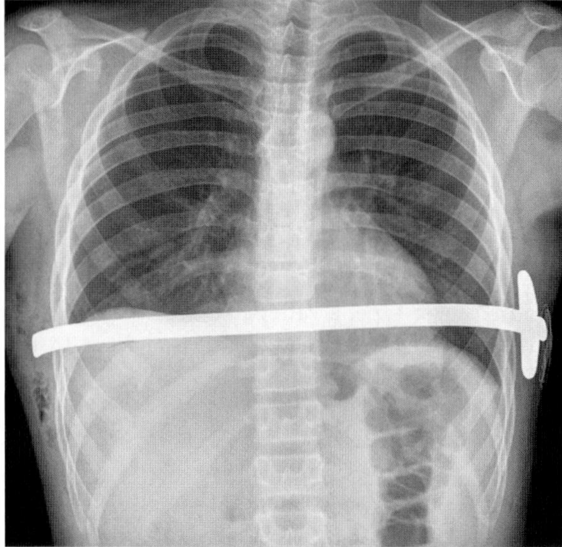

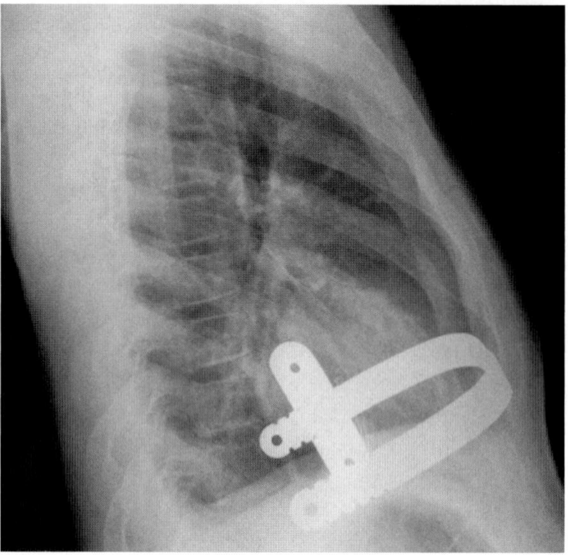

Fig. 27.2a–c. CT scan (**a**) shows a severe pectus whose indentation extends to the adjacent ribs and is classified as "saucer" PE. The transverse diameter (*T*) (25.8 cm), the A-P diameter (*A*) at the level of the sternal depression (7 cm) and the sagittal diameters (*S*, *S1*) of both hemithoraces (*right*: 14.3 cm; *left*: 12.8 cm) were measured. Consequently, the severe Haller's index (3.68) and the index of chest flattening (the ratio between the double transverse diameter divided by the sum of right and left diameters: 1.9; NV 1.49±0.12) can be calculated and is shown to be severe. Chest radiographs (**b**,**c**) show the metal bar in position and tethered by the vertical stabilizer. In the lateral projection, the correct position of the bar is shown; its anterior surface is pushing forward the depressed sternum

27.3.4 Symmetry

Another fundamental criterion that must be diagnosed with imaging is the degree of symmetry. The symmetry of the hemithoraxes is easily evaluated using CT, both through axial images that permit visualization of the thorax 'from inside' with a perception superior to that seen externally during the preliminary surgical examination and through three-dimensional reconstructions if images are acquired using MDCT. In seriously asymmetrical deformities, the left hemithorax is pushed outwards, while the heart is completely enclosed. In this condition, the sternum turns towards the right, towards the point of greatest depression and asymmetry. The symmetry of the hemithoraxes is defined by the relationship between the internal sagittal diameters (DX/SIN X100), thus indicating the prominence of one of the two hemithoraxes.

27.3.5 Sternal Torsion

A further essential morphological criterion that should be addressed in the report of the CT examination is sternal torsion. Sternal torsion corresponds to the angle of rotation of the sternum on its longitudinal axis: this is easily measured using a specific function on the work station or by placing a transparency, with the angle already traced, onto the printed image. Torsion is considered mild if the angle described is less than 30°and severe if more than 30° (Fig. 27.4).

Rotation in extreme cases can reach 90°, so that which should be the ventral surface of the sternum forms the left side of the more depressed part of the concavity. It is important to define precisely the degree of rotation as this also conditions the shaping of the metal arch that must be adapted for each individual patient. A sternum markedly rotated does not

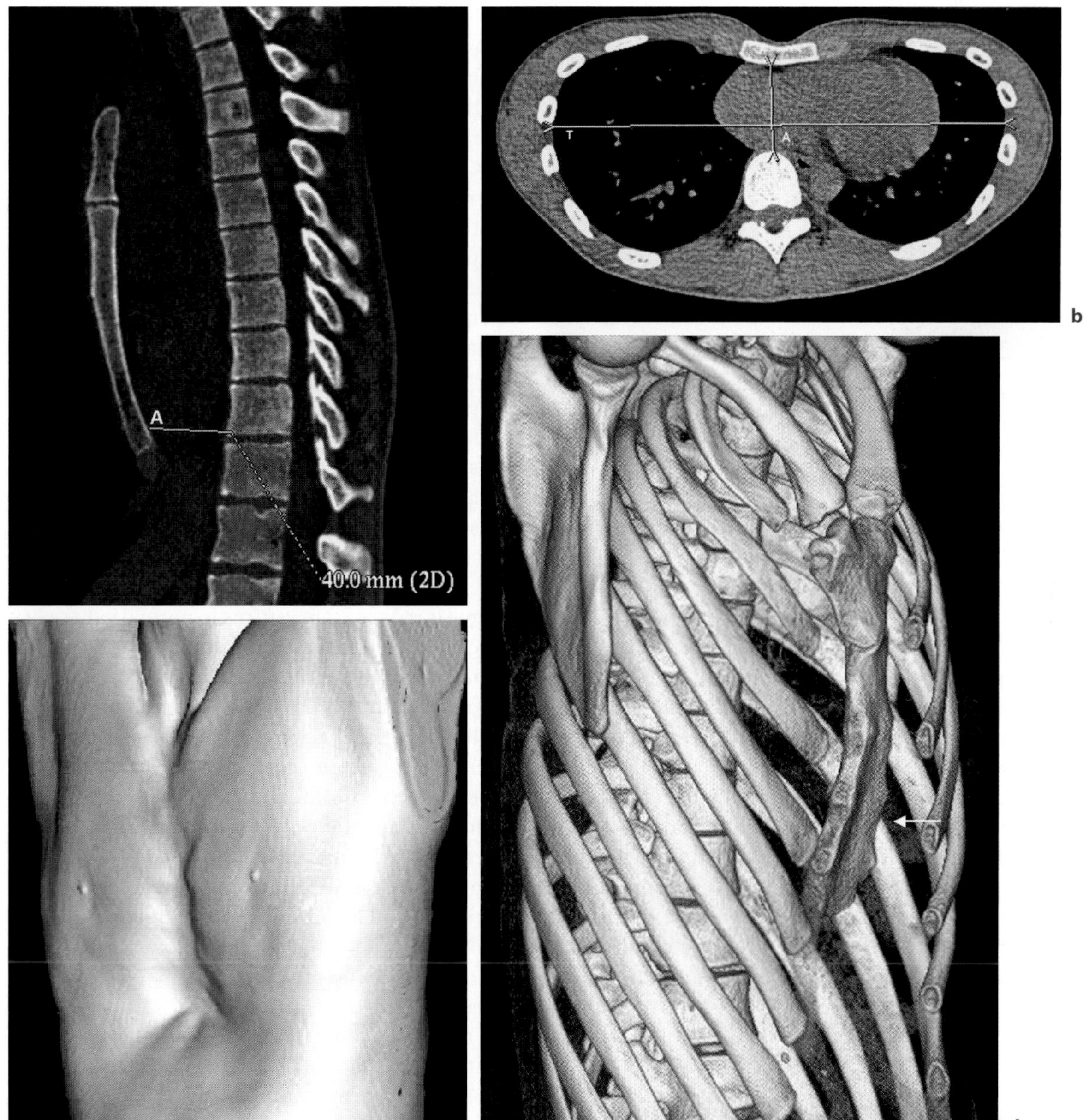

Fig. 27.3a–d. Patient studied with multi-detector CT multiplanar sagittal reconstruction (**a**) shows a pectus excavatum with an extremely reduced (4 cm) anteroposterior diameter and a long craniocaudal extension of the sternal depression. In the axial scan (**b**), Haller's index (6.5) is measured: it defines a severe PE. The degree of thoracic flattening defined by the flattening index is 2.3 (NV 1.49±0.12). In this scan the wide surface of contact and the slight compression exerted by the depressed sternum on the free wall of right cardiac chambers is evidenced. The 3D rendering display for soft tissues (**c**) provides a "photographic" representation of the outer surface of the pectus: consequently, based on morphology, it is classified as "saucer" type, that is, a wide PE involving almost the entire sternum below the manubrium and extending to the ribs as far as the mammilary line. The 3D rendering display for bones (**d**) provides an extremely good representation of the thoracic cage and the markedly depressed sternum (*arrow*) with a minimal torsion to the right. (Courtesy of Prof. Paolo Tomà)

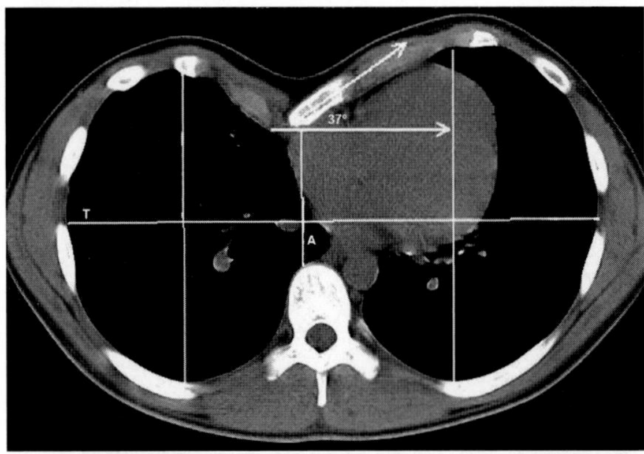

Fig. 27.4. Axial CT scan of a patient with pectus excavatum. The image shows a severe sternal torsion to the right (torsion angle: 37°). Haller's index (transverse diameter: 27.4 cm; A-P diameter: 6.8 cm) is 3.68, indicating a severe condition requiring surgical correction. A large surface of contact between the heart and the anterior thoracic wall is observed

always return to the correct morphology after surgical repair; sometimes a slight bump remains on the dorsal surface. For this reason there is a clear difference in the cosmetic result of corrective surgery in those with and without previous sternal torsion. Sternal torsion can be better evaluated in the reconstruction 3D filter for the bone in the cranio-caudal projection; the sternum rotates on its longitudinal axis, generally towards the right. The prominent indentation of the right costal cartilage that shortens the distance between the inferior costochondral junction and the midline of the sternum can also be well seen.

27.4 Cardiac Compression

In PE the heart must be evaluated for its possible compression, dislocation in the left side of mediastinum and distortion of its entire conformation (Hoeffel et al. 2000; Howard 1959). The position of the heart and its relationship with the markedly rotated sternum should be well documented. The compression can be either fixed or dependent on the postural position of the patient (Bevegard et al. 1960; Beiser et al. 1972). In the first case it is present in clino- and orthostatism and in the latter the cardiac compression occurs in orthostatism only. The deformity of the anterior thoracic wall can sometimes completely dislocate the heart from the left hemithorax, which then becomes a protective mechanism against the compression.

In the morphological assessment of severity of PE, CT images document that the sternum depression reduces the cardiac dimensions, distorts and alters the morphology of some cardiac chambers. The compression of the heart against the thoracic spine can cause volumetric constriction of the left atrium but, more commonly, also of the right cardiac chambers and in particular of the ventricular components: free-wall, tricuspid valve, inflow and outflow tracts and pulmonary valve. The extent of the compression is related to the severity of PE (Hoeffel et al. 2000; Crossland et al. 2006; Kowalewski et al. 1999).

The physiopathological consequence of the compression in PE is the limited filling of the right cardiac chambers causing an increase in filling pressure. During exercise in the upright position, stroke volume is reduced, but returns to normal value when exercise is performed in the supine position. This is confirmed by the fact that surgical intervention completely removes the signs and symptoms.

Clinically, PE is perceived as serious functional disturbances such as premature fatigability, dyspnea even during mild physical activity and low resistance and tolerance to prolonged effort. The indexes of severity measured on the axial CT images quantify, as described previously, the depth of the depression and a particularly high value of Haller's index, which nevertheless has a low sensitivity to identify those cases of postural cardiac compression in orthostatism only.

A more precise assessment of the right ventricular function in PE should be carried out using methods that study the heart more closely, such as echocardiography or MRI. Coln et al. (2006) recently reported a case study of 123 patients with PE studied preoperatively by CT for morphological evaluation and with color Doppler echocardiography for the assessment of cardiac function. In 117 cases the presence of cardiac compression was confirmed, showing a pattern similar to that of constrictive pericarditis, characterized by the reduction of right stroke volume during exercise stress test. This compression also caused distortion of the fibrous skeleton of the heart and consequently a high incidence of associated mitral valvular disease. All cardiac alterations regressed after the removal of cardiac compression by correction of the thoracic deformity using a Nuss metal bar.

In conclusion, the results of this study show that the main functional cardiac alteration in patients with PE is due to cardiac compression, which can be completely resolved by surgical repair.

27.5 Pectus Excavatum and Mitral Valve Prolapse

Patients with PE present a higher incidence of mitral valve prolapse (MVP) compared to the general population. The MVP valve should be considered a clinical syndrome, resulting from various pathogenetic mechanisms that affect one or more parts of the valvular apparatus: the leaflets, tendinous cords, papillary muscles and the valvular annulus. It is the most common form of valvular cardiac disease and is present in 0.6–2.4% of the general population. Patients with deformities of the thoracic cage, such as pectus excavatum, show an incidence of MVP between 30 and 65% according to case studies (Saint-Mézard et al. 1986; Udoshi et al. 1979). Subjects are generally symptomatic.

In patients with thoracic anomalies (pectus excavatum, scoliosis, straight back syndrome, flat thorax) and MVP, a reduction of the anteroposterior diameter of the thoracic cage has been observed, suggesting a pathogenetic role of thoracic deformities in the genesis of MVP in this particular group of subjects. Therefore, a functional MVP would be considered. In these cases the valvular prolapse is secondary to the compression of the heart against the thoracic spine, followed by distortion of the mitral valve annulus.

Raggi was the first author to study mitral valve prolapse in thoracic deformities using electron beam CT (EBCT) (Raggi et al. 2000). In the normal subject, the global aspect of the heart seen by CT is rounded and the contact with the thoracic wall is either minimal or completely absent. By studying a large number of patients with MVP and thoracic deformity, Raggi et al. found, in 82% of cases, the presence of a greater surface area contact between the heart and thoracic wall, thus determining a real "trap" or compression of the heart, able to cause distortion of the mitral valvular apparatus and consequent prolapse. Specifically, morphological and quantitative CT data reported by the authors supporting the theory of cardiac "entrapment" are summarized as follows:

1. Reduction of the anteroposterior diameter of the thorax measured from the internal surface of the thoracic wall to the anterior face of the corresponding vertebral body.
2. Increase of the area of contact between the heart and the internal surface of the thoracic wall, expressed by the product between the sagittal and axial extensions as observed in CT reconstructions.
3. Increase of the angle formed between the mitral valvular plane and that which passes through the atrial septum, which goes from rectangle to obtuse angle and which, when widened, provides a quantitative index of the progression of distortion of the mitral annulus.

The same author has described two morphological types of thorax that can cause cardiac distortion and consequent MVP:

1. Eight-shaped thorax in the horizontal position such as in pectus excavatum: sternum depression associated with approaching of the thoracic spine to the sternal axis.
2. Backward C-shape thorax characterized by a reduced anteroposterior diameter, as observed in straight back syndrome.

In these conditions the heart is trapped in a thoracic cavity too small for its size, causing the distortion of cardiac conformation in an attempt to adapt to the inadequate dimensions. The compression of the cardiac chamber inside a small space therefore causes a ventricular-valvular distortion with subsequent enlarging of the mitral valve annulus and the onset of MVP. An acquired condition of functional-type MVP thus occurs, secondary to a skeletal anomaly, and must therefore be corrected surgically.

In a recent study, the high frequency of mitral valve disease has been reported in 123 patients with pectus excavatum who subsequently underwent surgical repair (Coln et al. 2006). All patients underwent chest CT and cardiological evaluation using color Doppler echocardiography and treadmill exercise stress test. The results showed that 106 patients (86.1%) were symptomatic during the exercise test and 36 of them (34%) referred to pre-syncopal episodes on moving from the supine to orthostatic position. It should be noted that Haller's morphological index (HI) did not identify all symptomatic patients as some demonstrated a HI between 2.4 and 3 and others < 3.25. Therefore, in these patients, morphological study of the heart was carried out by basic color Doppler echocardiography in the supine position and then in orthostatism during the exercise stress test in order to identify those subjects with pectus excavatum and compromised cardiac function not identified by Haller's index when measured using CT.

From the results reported by the authors, at echocardiography 117 subjects (95%) presented compression of the cardiac chambers, a picture similar to that of constrictive pericarditis. Specifically, 46% of these showed anomalies of the mitral valve apparatus; 29 patients (54%) presented mitral insufficiency in the absence of prolapse and 25 (46%) had a MVP not associated with valvular regurgitation; in 3 patients, mitral regurgitation was associated with tricuspid regurgitation and in 1 with aortic regurgitation. Among the six subjects (5%) in whom no cardiac compression was demonstrated, two presented a MVP and four reported a symptomatic cardiac arrhythmia. All patients underwent Nuss' minimally invasive correction, obtaining a marked improvement of symptoms. At 2-month and 2-year follow-up after surgical repair, patients were reassessed by color Doppler echocardiography at rest and during exercise stress test: 93% (100 patients) presented morphologically and functionally normal cardiac chambers with valvular apparatus normally functioning; 7% still presented an MVP. Postoperative results confirm, therefore, both an acquired and functional origin of this form of MVP, which can regress after corrective surgery with an excellent prognosis. In this group of patients there were, in fact, no noted cases of complications, which sometimes form part of the natural history of MVP, such as:

27.5.1 Infective Endocarditis

Transitory ischemic cerebral attacks (TIA) and transitory changes of the visus, secondary to fibrinous embolism, involve the ophthalmic artery or posterior cerebral vessel of circle of Willis.

27.5.2 Rupture of Tendinous Cords

These include arrhythmias (atrial fibrillation, arrhythmias, ventricular tachycardia), sudden death (long QT, bradyrythmias and asystolia by abnormal vagal hypertonus secondary to autonomic dysfunction) and progressive worsening of mitral insufficiency with evolution to cardiac failure. In conclusion, color Doppler echocardiography can be considered the gold standard method for studying MVP when pectus excavatum is present.

The study of mitral valve prolapse (MVP) by color Doppler echocardiography permits a diagnosis of certainty through identification of the systolic movement (billowing) of one or both valve leaflets in the left atrium with or without mitral regurgitation. Using mono-dimensional echocardiography (M-Mode), sudden movement of one or both mitral leaflets in mesosystole ≥2 mm can be observed or, alternatively, "hammock" holosystolic movement >3 mm. Bi-dimensional (2D) echocardiography confirms the diagnosis with the following findings: (1) systolic movement of one or both mitral leaflets towards the left atrium over to coaptation plane of the mitral valve, firstly in long-axis parasternal view (gold standard) and successively in four-chamber apical view; (2) thickening and/or redundancy of leaflets: thickness >5 mm in diastolic phase.

27.5.3 Elongated Tendinous Cords

This condition involves possible dilation and distortion of the valvular annulus. Finally, the use of color Doppler allows classification of the severity of mitral valve regurgitation associated with the MVP on the basis of qualitative and quantitative parameters into mild, moderate, or severe. By Doppler study it is also possible to observe any alteration in the flow of trans-mitral and trans-tricuspid ventricular refilling, which are very similar to those reported in constrictive pericarditis. Moreover, as the MVP associated with pectus excavatum is functional and acquired, the thickening and/or redundancy of the mitral leaflets is not necessarily present as in the primary forms in which specific pathological processes involve the valvular apparatus.

27.6 Pectus Excavatum and Marfan Syndrome

Sixty-six percent (66%) of patients with Marfan syndrome also have deformities of the chest wall due to the excessive growth of the ribs (Pyeritz and McKusick 1979). Marfan syndrome is a disease of the connective tissue that affects different organs and systems such as the eyes, skeleton, heart, aorta, central nervous system, lungs and skin. It is relatively common (2–3 people in 10,000) and can be found in all races and ethnic groups. It is an autosomically transmitted disease with high penetration, but in 25–30% of patients it is seen as a sporadic form. This disease is caused by the mutation of the gene that encodes for fibrillin-1 positioned on chromosome 15, causing the formation of abnormal microfibrils. The microfibrils connect the elastic lamina both to endothelial cells and to smooth muscle cells, contributing to the integrity of the vessel walls.

Dysfunction of the microfibrils causes fragmentation of the elastic fibers, causing the structural disintegration of connective and vascular tissue and leading to the formation of aneurisms and dissection of the vessel walls, particularly those of the aorta. The mutation of the fibrillin alters the regulation of growth factor signal, which induces excessive growth of bone, pulmonary alterations, aortic dilation and alterations of the cardiac valves. Subjects are unusually tall and consequently have very long bones in the arms, legs, hands and feet. These patients also present an ogival palate, partial dislocation of the lens and a predisposition to emphysema.

The most common cardiovascular manifestations are mitral valve prolapse (MVP) and dilatation of the sinuses of Valsalva, which is associated with mitral insufficiency, aortic insufficiency, and aortic dissection. If such cardiac pathologies remain untreated, they will, in most cases, result in premature mortality.

27.6.1 Cardiovascular Manifestations

The annulus of the aortic root is a fibrous band that surrounds the aorta and the valvular leaflets. Annular aortic ectasia, in particular the dilatation of the proximal part of ascending aorta, is found in 60–80% of adults affected by Marfan syndrome. Beginning as dilatation of the sinuses of Valsalva, it progresses to the sino-tubular junction, eventually affecting also the aortic annulus.

Dilation of the aortic root is the main cause of aortic insufficiency in Marfan syndrome, which, if serious, leads to degenerative dissection of the elastic tissue of the media with cystic necrosis in the muscle cells. Annular aortic ectasia causes varying levels of dilation of the aortic root, easily visible at CTA, which allows multi-planar and three-dimensional reconstructions from which it is possible to measure with extreme precision the diameters of the ascending aorta, of the sino-tubular junction and of the dilated aortic root.

In order to study the valvular apparatus, it is necessary to acquire images using ECG-gated CTA and then to reconstruct the images according to the various phases of the cardiac cycle. At the moment, corresponding to 10% of the R-R (mesodiastolic) interval, it is possible to see clearly the valvular aperture, while at that corresponding to 70% of the R-R (in systole) interval, the valvular closure can be documented. In mesodiastole the valvular cuspids are rigid and tethered: a consequence of the dilatation of the sinuses of Valsalva. In the mesosystole images, aortic valvular regurgitation is represented by the triangular defect of coaptation of the aortic leaflets. The ECG-gated CTA images provide a clear and detailed picture of the structural characteristics of the aortic root and the origins of the coronary arteries. When performed accurately, such radiological tests are of great use in the planning of corrective surgery.

The fusiform aortic aneurism is well documented with chest CTA; the speed of its progression is variable, and a series of evaluations with transthoracic echocardiography over a period of time is necessary as, in the absence of dissection, dilatation is limited to the part nearest to the ascending aorta, while growth speed is slow: only a few millimeters per year (Ha et al. 2007).

27.6.2 Aortic Dissection

This complication generally originates above the ostia of the coronary arteries (type A in Stanford's scheme) and extends over the entire aortic length (type IB); 10% of the cases begin distally of the left subclavian artery (type IIIB) and are rarely limited to the abdominal aorta. Aortic dissection is due to an intimal tear that allows blood to enter the middle layer of the aorta, creating a false lumen. MDCT, with its high sensitivity and specificity, is the most frequently used imaging modality for the diagnosis of aortic dissection. It allows clear documentation of the extension of the dissection, of the relationship between real and false lumen and involvement of the large vessels. It also allows exploration of the pericardial and pleural cavities.

Aortic dissection is defined as highly probable when a progressive aortic enlargement is observed over time or when there is a double border of the aortic arch with dislocation of the intimal calcifications greater than 6 mm. The sudden appearance of a pleural or pericardial effusion suggests the onset of an aortic dissection. A documented endarterial flap is, however, symptomatic of aortic dissection.

25.6.3 Mitral Valve Prolapse (MVP) in Marfan Syndrome

In Marfan syndrome the prolapse of the mitral valve is age-dependent and is more frequent in women. Incidence reaches 60–80% of cases when patients are evaluated by means of transthoracic color Doppler echocardiography. The mitral leaflets appear generally elongated, thickened and redundant. A progression of the prolapse, evaluated by the appearance or worsening of mitral insufficiency through clinical criteria and echocardiography, is verified in at least a quarter of patients with Marfan syndrome, a much larger portion than for MVP present in the general population, whose natural history is generally benign. The mitral valve annulus dilates and contributes to the insufficiency, like stretching and the occasional breakage of the cords that are abnormally elongated. For the study of mitral valve prolapse, see the corresponding preceding paragraph.

27.7 Pectus Excavatum and Congenital Heart Diseases

Pectus excavatum is almost always an isolated malformation, but can, however, coexist with a congenital cardiopathy (Shamberger et al. 1988; Lees and Caldicott 1975; Hasegawa et al. 2002). In an extensive case study involving 20,860 children who had undergone congenital cardiopathic surgery, the author. (Shamberger et al. 1988) found only 36 patients with a deformity of the anterior chest wall, almost all of whom also had PE. The most frequently seen congenital heart diseases were: six transpositions of the large vessels, six interventricular defects, five interatrial defects, three complete atrio-ventricular channels, one Ebstein anomaly and various other single cases.

MDCT, which allows a simultaneous study of the heart and chest in patients with PE, is an even more frequently used modality in the study of congenital cardiopathies. The fundamental advantages of MDCT in diagnosis of congenital heart diseases are high spatial resolution, which permits the study of small structures, and high temporal resolution, which reduces to a minimum the artifacts of cardiac and respiratory movement.

27.8 Pectus Excavatum and Compression of the Inferior Vena Cava

A further mechanism through which PE compromises cardiac function is the compression of the inferior vena cava (Yalamanchili et al. 2005). Patients with PE, as explained above, sometimes present paradoxical breathing characterized by inspirational re-entry of the sternum, different from that occurring in healthy children where the thoracic cage is expanded during inspiration. Paradoxical breathing itself can determine a series of alterations in cardiac function different from pulsus paradoxus (as in constrictive pericarditis), reduced resistance to exercise, a reduced amount of oxygen that can be transported and utilized at the muscular level (VO2max), reduced anaerobic threshold and reduced concentration of oxygen when monitored with pulse oximeter.

The presence of paradoxical breathing is one of the causes of a worsening defect during the years of puberty and adolescence. Adolescents, in fact, begin intensive sports activity, encouraged by parents and family doctors in the false hope that practicing a sport will improve thoracic muscular structure and thus the appearance of the malformation. In reality, the greater metabolic demand produced by effort causes an increase in both frequency and depth of respiration, triggering a vicious circle that significantly accentuates the phenomenon of paradoxical breathing and, with the compression of the inferior vena cava, worsens the depression of the chest, the mechanical compression of the heart and/or, indirectly, the obstacle to venous return.

At echocardiography, in such a condition, a reduction of transmitral and transcuspidal blood flow and a reduction of stroke volume during inspiration have been reported. All of the above could be caused by compression of the inferior vena cava produced by the diaphragm, in its turn compressed by the paradoxical depression of the sternum. This other consequence of PE causes a decreased venous return and consequent reduced stroke volume. The deformity of the thoracic wall thus contributes to the reduced venous return and to the decreased stroke volume with a different mechanism from that seen in the previous paragraphs.

References

Barauskas V (2003) Indications for the surgical treatment of the funnel chest. Medicina (Kaunas) 39:555–561

Beiser GD, Epstein SE, Stampfer M et al. (1972) Impairment of cardiac function in patients with pectus excavatum, with improvement after operative correction. N Engl J Med 287:267–272

Bevegard S, Holmgren A, Jonsson B (1960) The effect of body position on the circulation at rest and during exercise, with special reference to the influence on the stroke volume. Acta Physiol Scand 49:279–298

Brodkin HA (1953) Congenital anterior chest wall deformities of diaphragmatic origin. Dis Chest 24:259–277

Cartoski MJ, Nuss D, Goretsky MJ et al. (2006) Classification of the dysmorphology of pectus excavatum. J Pediatr Surg 41:1573–1581

Clausner A, Clausner G, Basche M et al. (1991) Importance of morphological findings in the progress and treatment of chest wall deformities with special reference to the value of computed tomography, echocardiography and stereophotogrammetry. Eur J Pediatr Surg 1:291–297

Coln E, Carrasco J, Coln D (2006) Demonstrating relief of cardiac compression with the Nuss minimally invasive repair for pectus excavatum. Pediatr Surg 41:683–686

Creswick HA, Stacey MW, Kelly RE Jr et al. (2006) Family study of the inheritance of pectus excavatum. J Pediatr Surg 41:1699–1703

Crossland DS, Auldist AW, Davis AM (2006) Malignant pectus excavatum. Heart 92:1511

Daunt SW, Cohen JH, Miller SF (2004) Age-related normal ranges for the Haller index in children. Pediatr Radiol 34:326–330

Derveaux L, Clarysse I, Ivanoff I et al. (1989) Preoperative and postoperative abnormalities in chest X-ray indices and in lung function in pectus deformities. Chest 95:850–856

Fonkalsrud EW (2003) Current management of pectus excavatum. World J Surg 27:502–508

Guller B, Hable K (1974) Cardiac findings in pectus excavatum in children: review and differential diagnosis. Chest 66:165–171

Ha HI, Seo JB, Lee SH et al. (2007) Imaging of Marfan syndrome: multisystemic manifestations. Radiographics 27:989–1004

Haller JA Jr, Kramer SS, Lietman SA (1987) Use of CT scans in selection of patients for pectus excavatum surgery: a preliminary report. J Pediatr Surg 22:904–906

Hasegawa T, Yamaguchi M, Ohshima Y et al. (2002) Simultaneous repair of pectus excavatum and congenital heart disease over the past 30 years. Eur J Cardiothorac Surg 22:874–878

Hoeffel JC, Bernard C, Marçon F (2000) Pseudo stenosis of the tricuspid valve ring caused by pectus excavatum. Presse Med 29:1913

Howard R (1959) Funnel chest: its effect on cardiac function. Arch Dis Child 34:5–7

Kilda A, Basevicius A, Barauskas V et al. (2007) Radiological assessment of children with pectus excavatum. Indian J Pediatr 74:143–147

Kowalewski J, Brocki M, Dryjanski T et al. (1999) Pectus excavatum: increase of right ventricular systolic, diastolic, and stroke volumes after surgical repair. J Thorac Cardiovasc Surg 118:87–92

Lawson ML, Mellins RB, Tabangin M et al. (2005) Impact of pectus excavatum on pulmonary function before and after repair with the Nuss procedure. J Pediatr Surg 40:174–180

Lawson ML, Barnes-Eley M, Burke BL et al. (2006) Reliability of a standardized protocol to calculate cross-sectional chest area and severity indices to evaluate pectus excavatum. J Pediatr Surg 41:1219–1225

Lees RF, Caldicott JH (1975) Sternal anomalies and congenital heart disease. Am J Roentgenol Radium Ther Nucl Med 124:423–427

Malek MH, Fonkalsrud EW, Cooper CB (2003) Ventilatory and cardiovascular responses to exercise in patients with pectus excavatum. Chest 124:870–882

Mansour KA, Thourani VH, Odessey EA et al. (2003) Thirty-year experience with repair of pectus deformities in adults. Ann Thorac Surg 76:391–395

Mocchegiani R, Badano L, Lestuzzi C (1995) Relation of right ventricular morphology and function in pectus excavatum to the severity of the chest wall deformity. Am J Cardiol 76:941–946

Nakahara K, Ohno K, Miyoshi S (1987) An evaluation of operative outcome in patients with funnel chest diagnosed by means of the computed tomogram. J Thorac Cardiovasc Surg 93:577–582

Nuss D, Kelly RE Jr, Croitoru DP et al. (1998a) A 10-year review of a minimally invasive technique for the correction of pectus excavatum. J Pediatr Surg 33:545–552

Nuss D, Kelly RE, Croitoru DP et al. (1998b) Repair of pectus excavatum. Pediatric Endosurg Innov Tech 2:205–221

Nuss D, Croitoru DP, Kelly RE Jr et al. (2002) Review and discussion of the complications of minimally invasive pectus excavatum repair. Eur J Pediatr Surg 12:230–234

Ohno K, Nakahira M, Takeuchi S et al. (2001) Indications for surgical treatment of funnel chest by chest radiograph. Pediatr Surg Int 17:591–595

Paterson A, Frush DP (2007) Dose reduction in paediatric MDCT: general principles. Clin Radiol 62:507–517

Pyeritz RE, McKusick VA (1979) The Marfan syndrome diagnosis and management. N Engl J Med 300:772–777

Raggi P, Callister TQ, Lippolis NJ et al. (2000) Is mitral valve prolapse due to cardiac entrapment in the chest cavity? A CT view. Chest 117:636–642

Ravitch MM (1961) Operative treatment of congenital deformities of the chest. Am J Surg 101:588–597

Saint-Mézard G, Chanudet X, Duret JC et al. (1986) Mitral valve prolapse and pectus excavatum. Expressions of connective tissue dystrophy? Arch Mal Coeur Vaiss 79:431–434

Shamberger RC, Welch KJ, Sanders SP (1987) Mitral valve prolapse associated with pectus excavatum. J Pediatr 111:404–407

Shamberger RC, Welch KJ, Castaneda AR et al. (1988) Anterior chest wall deformities and congenital heart disease. J Thorac Cardiovasc Surg 96:427–432

Sidden CR, Katz ME, Swoveland BC et al. (2001) Radiologic considerations in patients undergoing the Nuss procedure for correction of pectus excavatum. Pediatr Radiol 31:429–434

Soteropoulos GC, Cigtay OS, Schellinger D (1979) Pectus excavatum deformities simulating mediastinal masses. J Comput Assist Tomogr 3:596–600

Takahashi K, Sugimoto H, Ohsawa T (1992) Obliteration of the descending aortic interface in pectus excavatum: correlation with clockwise rotation of the heart. Radiology 182:825–828

Udoshi MB, Shah A, Fisher VJ et al. (1979) Incidence of mitral valve prolapse in subjects with thoracic skeletal abnormalities–a prospective study. Am Heart J 97:303–311

Williams AM, Crabbe DC (2003) Pectus deformities of the anterior chest wall. Paediatr Respir Rev 4:237–242

Yalamanchili K, Summer W, Valentine V (2005) Pectus excavatum with inspiratory inferior vena cava compression: a new presentation of pulsus paradoxus. Am J Med Sci 329:45–47

Zhao L, Feinberg MS, Gaides M et al. (2000) Why is exercise capacity reduced in subjects with pectus excavatum? J Pediatr 136:163–167

Thoracic Surgery and Asymptomatic Coronary Artery Disease

28

Jean-Pierre Laissy

CONTENTS

The diagnostic and therapeutic management of patients with coronary artery disease (CAD), either symptomatic or asymptomatic, who are scheduled for thoracic surgery has not yet clearly been defined and remains controversial (Carbajal 1998).

Cardiovascular preoperative evaluation in non-cardiac surgery aims to assess the patient's current cardiovascular status, to detect unknown diseases, to make recommendations concerning the medical management of the patient in the peri- and postoperative period, to plan the surgical strategy or, in some cases, to postpone non-cardiac surgery until the cardiac condition is corrected or stabilized; rarely, cardiovascular evaluation may result in an absolute contraindication for non-cardiac surgery (Hollenberg 1999). It is acknowledged that the major two risk factors for perioperative cardiac morbidity are recent myocardial infarction and current congestive heart failure (Mangano and Goldman 1995). Additional risk factors must be considered, such as cardiac arrhythmias and severe valvular disease, in particular aortic stenosis (Mangano and Goldman 1995; Potyk and Raudaskoski 1998).

28.1 Risk Stratification

The basic clinical evaluation obtained by history, physical examination and review of the ECG usually provides enough data to estimate the cardiac risk (Chassot et al. 2002). Patient's risk factors (unstable coronary syndromes, congestive heart failure, life-threatening arrhythmias and severe valvular heart diseases) and the type and setting of surgery are to be considered together with the clinical evaluation, along with other risk factors, such as a history of cerebrovascular events, diabetes mellitus and renal dysfunction. Additional non-invasive tests may be recommended to evaluate left ventricular function and the presence of myocardial ischemia only if expected data will eventually result in changing the surgical procedure or perioperative management (Hollenberg 1999). Echocardiography is particularly useful in patients with major risk factors, whereas the exercise stress test is able to assess the patient's functional capacity or to identify silent myocardial ischemia or significant arrhythmias. The overall goal of cardiac assessment should be a consideration of both the impending surgery and the long-term cardiac risk independent of the decision to go to surgery. It is almost never appropriate to recommend coronary bypass surgery or other invasive interventions, such as coronary angioplasty in

J.-P. Laissy, MD
Professor, Department of Radiology, Imagerie Médicale, Hôpital Bichat, 46 rue Henri Huchard, 75018 Paris, France

an attempt to reduce the risk of non-cardiac surgery when they would not otherwise be indicated. Ideas have indeed evolved since the results of the CASS trial published 10 years ago (Eagle et al. 1997).

28.2 CAD and Thoracic Surgery: Medical, Interventional or Surgical Management?

The major results of the CASS study showed that the risk of cardiac events in the periprocedural period was significantly higher in the CAD group without prior coronary arterial bypass graft (CABG) than in the CAD group with prior CABG and the nonCAD group. However, the risk of CABG itself exceeded the risk of noncardiac surgery (Hollenberg 1999; Eagle et al. 1997).

Approximately 5% of patients treated by coronary artery stenting undergo a noncardiac surgical procedure within 1 year after stenting. The two major acute and severe adverse events occurring after surgery are thrombosis on one hand and hemorrhage on the other hand.

Surgery might induce hypercoagulability. Early noncardiac surgery after coronary stenting markedly increases the risk of postoperative cardiac events (McFalls et al. 2004). Interruption of antiplatelet therapy seems to play an important role in this increased event rate. Prophylactic coronary revascularization in cardiac stable, but high-risk patients does not seem to improve outcome. On the other hand, patients with multiple cardiac risk factors are at high risk for postoperative adverse cardiac events and might even benefit from preoperative prophylactic coronary revascularization (Schouten et al. 2007a).

In a series of 40 patients operated on 1 to 39 days after coronary stent placement, 11 major bleedings and 7 myocardial infarcts (MIs) were observed in the early postoperative period, resulting in 8 deaths (Kałuza et al. 2000). All the major adverse events occurred in patients undergoing surgery within 14 days of stent implantation. The interruption or withdrawal of the antiplatelet regimen within these 2 weeks corresponds to the maximal occurrence of stent thrombosis. Of the seven MIs, four occurred within 24 h of the surgical procedure, while the other three were observed between 6 and 11 days after procedure. Overall, 8 of the 25 patients undergoing surgery within 14 days of stent placement died within 11 days of the surgical procedure after suffering an MI or significant bleeding episode (Kałuza et al. 2000).

Similar outcomes have been observed in another study. Eight patients among the 168 patients undergoing surgery 6 weeks after stent placement (4.0%) died or suffered a myocardial infarction or stent thrombosis. The frequency of these events ranged from 3.8% to 7.1% per week during each of the 6 weeks. Contrarily, no events occurred in the 39 patients undergoing surgery 7 to 9 weeks after stent placement. These data suggest that, whenever possible, non-cardiac surgery should be delayed 6 weeks after stent placement, by which time stents are generally endothelialized, and a course of antiplatelet therapy to prevent stent thrombosis has been completed (Wilson et al. 2003). The same complication rate was observed in a prospective study of 103 patients undergoing surgery within 1 year of coronary stent placement (Vicenzi et al. 2006), indicating that patients with coronary stents are at increased risk for perioperative stent-related complications, particularly if surgery is performed early after stenting.

Furthermore, with the use of drug-eluting stents, it is necessary to maintain double antiplatelet medication without interruption for at least 6 months. Any planned or unplanned surgery results in a real threat to this strategy (Sigwart 2007).

In a recent study, including both bare metal stents and drug-eluting stents (192 patients), early surgery and antiplatelet discontinuation were associated with an increased risk of perioperative cardiac events (Schouten et al. 2007b). Conversely, the risk of major cardiac complications in patients undergoing noncardiac surgery after coronary drug-eluting stent implantation seem to decrease significantly after 6 months (Compton et al. 2006).

These data corroborate those of other studies. No benefit was found from preoperative prophylactic coronary revascularization in a randomized trial in very high cardiac risk patients. Revascularization did not improve 30-day outcome; the incidence of the composite end point was 43% versus 33% (odds ratio 1.4, 95% confidence interval 0.7 to 2.8; P=0.30). Furthermore, no benefit during 1-year follow-up was observed after coronary revascularization (49% vs. 44%, odds ratio 1.2, 95% confidence interval 0.7 to 2.3; P=0.48) (Poldermans et al. 2007).

Numerous similar outcomes between patients with recent PTCA and those with nonrevascularized CAD have been described, such as in this large retrospective study of 686 patients. The patients with recent PTCA did not evolve better than nonrevascularized patients with CAD, with more than one fourth of each group having some adverse cardiac outcome after noncardiac surgery (Posner et al. 1999).

A recent review of medical literature has summarized the main principles of minimizing the risks of complications. This review reminds that any event in the coronary circulation, such as recent ischemia, infarction, or revascularization, induces a high-risk period of 6 weeks and an intermediate-risk period of 3 months. A 3-month minimum delay is therefore indicated before performing non-cardiac surgery after myocardial infarction or revascularization. However, if an urgent surgical procedure is requested, this delay may be too long, and it is then appropriate to use perioperative b-blockers, which reduce the cardiac complication rate in patients with, or at risk of, coronary artery disease (Chassot et al. 2002).

Administration of b-blockers associated with statin regimen has shown significant reduction of occurrence of perioperative ischemic events (Karthikeyan and Bhargava 2006; Noordzij et al. 2007). Several controlled studies (meta-analysis of 16 observational cohort studies and 2 randomized trials) suggest that the use of statins during the perioperative period in patients undergoing high-risk surgery may confer substantial benefits. Statin users exhibit perioperative rates of death or acute coronary syndromes that are 30% to 42% lower than those observed in patients who are not taking statins at the time of surgery (Kapoor et al. 2006).

28.2.1 Heart Failure

An other group of patients scheduled for noncardiac surgery is at significant risk of cardiovascular morbidity and mortality due to underlying symptomatic or asymptomatic cardiac disease. However, the majority of patients studied were not referred to thoracic surgery, but vascular surgery. Patients with heart failure (HF) scheduled for vascular surgery have indeed an increased risk of adverse postoperative outcome. Clinical cardiac risk scores are useful tools for the simple identification of patients with an increased perioperative cardiac risk. As in CAD, these risk scores include factors such as age, history of myocardial infarction, angina pectoris, congestive heart failure, cerebrovascular events, diabetes mellitus and renal dysfunction. Based on these cardiac risk scores, further cardiac testing might be warranted in patients at increased risk. In a recent study, a quantitative prognostic model for patients with HF was developed using wall motion patterns during dobutamine stress echocardiography (DSE). Multivariate independent predictors of late cardiac events were age and ischemia. Sustained improvement was associated with improved survival. The conclusions of this echocardiographic study are that DSE provides accurate risk stratification of patients with HF undergoing vascular surgery (Karagiannis et al. 2007).

Similar data have been reported in another large, randomized cohort study of 4,414 patients (McFalls et al. 2007). Using a Cox regression analysis, it was shown that patients without multiple cardiac risks or co-morbid conditions have a good outcome following elective vascular surgery; on the opposite, urgent surgery, congestive heart failure, ventricular arrhythmias and creatinine >3.5 mg/dl were significantly associated with long-term postoperative mortality.

28.3 Currently Available Preoperative Cardiac Imaging Assessment

Transthoracic echocardiography at rest does not predict ischemic complications in cardiac patients and merely assesses valves and left ventricular (LV) function. A decreased LV ejection fraction predicts only postoperative LV dysfunction and correlates better with late than early postoperative cardiac events (Chassot et al. 2002). Dobutamine stress echocardiography is likely to provide more precise predictors on cardiac outcome: in a series of patients who had positive stress echocardiograms after the administration of dobutamine with supplemental atropine, cardiac complications occurred in one-third (Karagiannis et al. 2007; McFalls et al. 2007; Poldermans et al. 1995).

Moreover, patients showing extensive ischemia under dobutamine stimulation (>5/16 left ventricular segments involved) experience ten times more cardiac events than patients with limited stress-induced ischemia (<4 segments involved) (Boersma et al. 2001).

In a recent study, a quantitative prognostic model for patients with HF was developed using wall motion patterns during dobutamine stress echocardiography (DSE). A total of 295 consecutive patients (mean age 67±12 years) with ejection fraction ≤35% was studied. During DSE, wall motion patterns of dysfunctional segments were scored as scar, ischemia, or sustained improvement. Cardiac death and myocardial infarction were noted perioperatively and during 5 years of follow-up. Of 4,572 dysfunctional segments, 1,783 (39%) had ischemia, 1,280 (28%) had sustained improvement, and 1,509 (33%) had scar. In 212 patients, ≥1 ischemic segment was present; 83 had only sustained improvement. Perioperative and late cardiac event rates were 20% and 30%, respectively. Using multivariate analysis, the number of ischemic segments was associated with perioperative cardiac events (odds ratio per segment 1.6, 95% confidence interval 1.05 to 1.8), whereas the number of segments with sustained improvement was associated with improved outcome (odds ratio per segment 0.2, 95% confidence interval 0.04 to 0.7) (Karagiannis et al. 2007).

Radionuclide scintigraphy has not demonstrated a real screening value when applied to a large unselected vascular or non-vascular population, or among patients already classified clinically as low- or high-risk candidates for surgery. Indeed, pharmacological-stress thallium scintigraphy associated with thallium redistribution does not seem to be significantly associated with the incidence of perioperative myocardial infarction, prolonged ischemia or other adverse outcomes (Mangano and Goldman 1995).

Coronary angiography is indicated only in cases of unstable coronary syndromes, of uncertain stress tests in high-risk patients undergoing major surgery or when there is a possible indication for coronary revascularization (Eagle et al. 2002). Coronary angiography should therefore be performed before a noncardiac operation only in high-risk patients who warrant coronary revascularization for medical reasons, irrespective of the preoperative context (Chassot et al. 2002).

28.4 Is There a Place for Cardiac MR and Cardiac CT?

There are no data available upon the usefulness of these techniques in this particular setting. Cardiac MR should be useful to assess cardiac function and myocardial viability in a selected population of patients. Cardiac CT does not seem to be recommended routinely. However, patients receiving effective chronic beta-blockers are difficult to evaluate with stress tests because they have a limited increase in heart rate and cardiac output on exercise. The sensitivity of stress tests for diagnosing a coronary lesion is significantly lowered under these circumstances (Chassot et al. 2002); these patients should benefit from the use of cardiac CT. Other indications are uncertain stress tests in high risk patients, but this needs to be confirmed.

28.4.1 Unresolved Questions

Some issues remain without responses and need to be further studied. Thoracic surgery, in particular pneumonectomy and lobectomy, results in axial shift and rotation (Smulders et al. 2007) of the major vessels (i.e., pulmonary artery and aorta). An aberrant course of the left coronary artery should have adverse consequences in the postoperative period, inducing myocardial ischemia and possibly infarction. So does mediastinal radiotherapy.

Oncologic patients undergoing thoracic surgery have frequently cardiovascular comorbidities associated to chronic obstructive pulmonary disease, independently of tobacco (McAllister et al. 2007; Graham Barr et al. 2007). In these patients, cardiac and coronary involvement should be sought in order to start appropriate medical treatment before surgery.

The future of thoracic imaging relies undoubtedly on increased acquisition speed. Associated with improvements in temporal resolution and volume coverage of CT systems, the next step probably will no longer require ECG-gated acquisitions. Thoracic imaging will hence be able to include high resolution, high quality images of the coronary tree.

28.5 Conclusion

Evaluation of patients with cardiovascular disease before thoracic surgery relies on a standard, simple, but thorough history and physical examination associated with adequate laboratory studies. The value of imaging techniques has little impact on the preoperative management of patients since there is no evidence that revascularization strategies before thoracic surgery improve patient status in the perioperative period as well as for the outcome. A reassessment after surgery can be useful for a better management of cardiac disease, as these patients at high risk for perioperative complications also tend to have worse long-term outcomes.

28.6 Take-Home Points

1) Perioperative statins are associated with lower rates of acute coronary syndromes and mortality; associated with b-blockers, they do as well or better than coronary revascularization before noncardiac surgery.
2) If coronary revascularization is mandatory, noncardiac surgery should be performed at least 6 weeks after the procedure.
3) Routine preoperative cardiovascular tests do not include imaging procedures, except dobutamine stress echocardiography.

References

Boersma E, Poldermans D, Bax JJ, Steyerberg EW, Thomson IR, Banga JD, van De Ven LL, van Urk H, Roelandt JR; DECREASE Study Group (Dutch Echocardiographic Cardiac Risk Evaluation Applying Stress Echocardiography) (2001) Predictors of cardiac events after major vascular surgery: Role of clinical characteristics, dobutamine echocardiography, and beta-blocker therapy. JAMA 285:1865–1873

Carbajal EV (1998) Noncardiac surgery in CAD patients. Circulation 98:823–824

Chassot PG, Delabays A, Spahn DR (2002) Preoperative evaluation of patients with, or at risk of, coronary artery disease undergoing non-cardiac surgery. Br J Anaesth 89:747–759

Compton PA, Zankar AA, Adesanya AO, Banerjee S, Brilakis ES (2006) Risk of noncardiac surgery after coronary drug-eluting stent implantation. Am J Cardiol 98:1212–1213

Eagle KA, Rihal CS, Mickel MC, Holmes DR, Foster ED, Gersh BJ (1997) Cardiac risk of noncardiac surgery: influence of coronary disease and type of surgery in 3,368 operations. CASS Investigators and University of Michigan Heart Care Program. Coronary Artery Surgery Study. Circulation 96:1882–1887

Eagle KA, Berger PB, Calkins H, Chaitman BR, Ewy GA, Fleischmann KE, Fleisher LA, Froehlich JB, Gusberg RJ, Leppo JA, Ryan T, Schlant RC, Winters WL Jr, Gibbons RJ, Antman EM, Alpert JS, Faxon DP, Fuster V, Gregoratos G, Jacobs AK, Hiratzka LF, Russell RO, Smith SC Jr; American College of Cardiology/American Heart Association Task Force on Practice Guidelines (Committee to Update the 1996 Guidelines on Perioperative Cardiovascular Evaluation for Noncardiac Surgery) (2002) ACC/AHA guideline update for perioperative cardiovascular evaluation for noncardiac surgery–executive summary. A report of the American College of Cardiology/American Heart Association Task Force on practice guidelines (Committee to update 1996 guidelines on perioperative cardiovascular evaluation for noncardiac surgery). Circulation 105:1257–1267

Graham Barr R, Mesia-Vela S, Austin JH, Basner RC, Keller BM, Reeves AP, Shimbo D, Stevenson L (2007) Impaired flow-mediated dilation is associated with low pulmonary function and emphysema in ex-smokers: The Emphysema and Cancer Action Project (EMCAP) Study. Am J Respir Crit Care Med 176:1200–1207

Hollenberg SM (1999) Preoperative cardiac risk assessment. Chest 115:51–57

Kałuza GL, Joseph J, Lee JR, Raizner ME, Raizner AE (2000) Catastrophic outcomes of noncardiac surgery soon after coronary stenting. J Am Coll Cardiol 35:1288–1294

Kapoor AS, Kanji H, Buckingham J, Devereaux PJ, McAlister FA (2006) Strength of evidence for perioperative use of statins to reduce cardiovascular risk: systematic review of controlled studies. BMJ 333:1149–1155

Karagiannis SE, Feringa HH, Vidakovic R, van Domburg R, Schouten O, Bax JJ, Karatasakis G, Cokkinos DV, Poldermans D (2007) Value of myocardial viability estimation using dobutamine stress echocardiography in assessing risk preoperatively before noncardiac vascular surgery in patients with left ventricular ejection fraction <35%. Am J Cardiol 99:1555–1559

Karthikeyan G, Bhargava B (2006) Managing patients undergoing non-cardiac surgery: need to shift emphasis from risk stratification to risk modification. Heart 92:17–20

Mangano DT, Goldman L (1995) Preoperative assessment of patients with known or suspected coronary disease. N Eng J Med 333:1750–1756

McAllister DA, Maclay JD, Mills NL, Mair G, Miller J, Anderson D, Newby DE, Murchison JT, Macnee W (2007) Arterial stiffness is independently associated with emphysema severity in patients with chronic obstructive pulmonary disease. Am J Respir Crit Care Med 15;176:1208–1214

McFalls EO, Ward HB, Moritz TE, Goldman S, Krupski WC, Littooy F, Pierpont G, Santilli S, Rapp J, Hattler B, Shunk K, Jaenicke C, Thottapurathu L, Ellis N, Reda DJ, Henderson WG (2004) Coronary-artery revascularization before elective major vascular surgery. N Engl J Med 351:2795–2804

McFalls EO, Ward HB, Moritz TE, Littooy F, Santilli S, Rapp J, Larsen G, Reda DJ (2007) Clinical factors associated with long-term mortality following vascular surgery: outcomes from the Coronary Artery Revascularization Prophylaxis (CARP) Trial. J Vasc Surg 46:694–700

Noordzij PG, Poldermans D, Schouten O, Schreiner F, Feringa HH, Dunkelgrun M, Kertai MD, Boersma E (2007) Beta-blockers and statins are individually associated with reduced mortality in patients undergoing noncardiac, nonvascular surgery. Coron Artery Dis 18:67–72

Poldermans D, Arnese M, Fioretti PM, Salustri A, Boersma E, Thomson IR, Roelandt JR, van Urk H (1995) Improved cardiac risk stratification in major vascular surgery with dobutamine atropine stress echocardiography. J Am Coll Cardiol 26:648–53

Poldermans D, Schouten O, Vidakovic R, Bax JJ, Thomson IR, Hoeks SE, Feringa HH, Dunkelgrün M, de Jaegere P, Maat A, van Sambeek MR, Kertai MD, Boersma E; DECREASE Study Group (2007) A clinical randomized trial to evaluate the safety of a noninvasive approach in high-risk patients undergoing major vascular surgery: the DECREASE-V Pilot Study. J Am Coll Cardiol 49:1763–1769

Posner KL, Van Norman GA, Chan V (1999) Adverse cardiac outcomes after noncardiac surgery in patients with prior percutaneous transluminal coronary angioplasty. Anesth Analg 89:553–560

Potyk D, Raudaskoski P (1998) Preoperative cardiac evaluation for elective noncardiac surgery. Arch Fam Med 7:164–173

Schouten O, Bax JJ, Poldermans D (2007a) Management of patients with cardiac stents undergoing noncardiac surgery. Curr Opin Anaesthesiol 20:274–278

Schouten O, van Domburg RT, Bax JJ, de Jaegere PJ, Dunkelgrun M, Feringa HH, Hoeks SE, Poldermans D (2007b) Noncardiac surgery after coronary stenting: early surgery and interruption of antiplatelet therapy are associated with an increase in major adverse cardiac events. J Am Coll Cardiol 49:122–124

Sigwart U (2007) Drug-eluting stents: some thoughts from old Europe. Am Heart Hosp J 5:135–137

Smulders SA, Holverda S, Vonk-Noordegraaf A, van den Bosch HC, Post JC, Marcus JT, Smeenk FW, Postmus PE (2007) Cardiac function and position more than 5 years after pneumonectomy. Ann Thorac Surg 83:1986–1892

Vicenzi MN, Meislitzer T, Heitzinger B, Halaj M, Fleisher LA, Metzler H (2006) Coronary artery stenting and noncardiac surgery–a prospective outcome study. Br J Anaesth 96:686–693

Wilson SH, Fasseas P, Orford JL, Lennon RJ, Horlocker T, Charnoff NE, Melby S, Berger PB (2003) Clinical outcome of patients undergoing non-cardiac surgery in the 2 months following coronary stenting. J Am Coll Cardiol 42:234–240

Diseases Developing Coronaro-Bronchial Anastomoses

29

Jean-Pierre Laissy

CONTENTS

Coronary-to-bronchial anastomoses are seen anecdotally, and their entity remains controversial (Angelini et al. 1999; Iwasaki et al. 1997; Bjork 1966; Moberg 1967; White et al. 1992). Several types of vascular anastomoses exist in the normal human heart, but they are not functional. When these normal anastomoses develop, they mainly represent the increase in caliber of pre-existing vessels in response to certain stimuli, such as generalized hypoxia, anemia, sustained exercise, total or partial occlusion of the coronary arteries or drugs (Esperanca and Goncalves 1981). Conversely, abnormal vascular connections are the result of various diseases, such as congenital disorders, total or partial occlusion of the coronary arteries, infection or degenerative vascular disorders. They can result in congestive heart failure, myocardial ischemia, infective endocarditis, atrial fibrillation, pulmonary hypertension and rupture.

Until recently, the diagnosis was usually made incidentally on the basis of invasive cardiac catheterization and coronary angiography (Smith et al. 1972), or bronchial artery angiography (Bjork 1966). Many patients can now be correctly diagnosed with this condition using transthoracic Doppler echocardiography (Chee et al. 2007) and multidetector CT (MDCT), the latter being able to demonstrate the vascular connections between these vessels. ECG-gated MDCT can delineate the origin, entire course, length and drainage of the fistula; furthermore, MDCT easily identifies the spatial relationship of the fistula with the coronary arteries, main pulmonary artery and right atrium without cardiac motion non-invasively (Funabashi and Komuro 2006). The comprehension of pathogenesis of collateral pathway development helps to understand the different patterns of these abnormalities.

29.1 Anatomy

The coronary tree is constituted of two coronary arteries arising from the root of the aorta and tapering progressively as they branch to supply the myocardium. A coronary artery fistula (CAF) exists if a substantive communication develops that bypasses the myocardial capillary bed and communicates with a

J.-P. Laissy, MD
Professor, Department of Radiology, Imagerie Médicale, Hôpital Bichat, 46 rue Henri Huchard, 75018 Paris, France

low-pressure cardiac cavity (atria or ventricle) or a branch of the systemic or pulmonary systems.

Normal thin-walled, small vessels exist at the arteriolar level that may drain into the cardiac cavity; these vessels do not steal significant flow and do not constitute fistulous connections. Fistulae usually are large (>250 microns) and dilated or ectatic, and they tend to enlarge over time. The limits of what constitutes a fistula and what constitutes a normal vessel are often debated.

Vascular anastomoses between coronary arteries and extracardiac vessels are commonly called fistulae despite the fact that few of them feature fistulous flow patterns (Angelini 2000). In fact, there are big differences between abnormal connections between two vascular structures without fistulous flow (e.g., coronary artery to left ventricle or circumflex artery to right coronary artery) and abnormal connections between two vascular structures with fistulous flow. A true fistula of the circulatory system is characterized by a clearly ectatic vascular segment that exhibits fistulous flow (Angelini 2000). Most fistulae arise from the right coronary artery (60%) and terminate in the right side of the heart (90%). The most frequent sites of termination, in descending order, are the right ventricle, right atrium, coronary sinus and pulmonary vasculature. Coronary fistula communications often appear in the context of other congenital cardiac anomalies, most frequently in critical pulmonary stenosis or atresia with an intact interventricular septum, but also in pulmonary artery branch stenosis, coarctation of the aorta and aortic atresia. Although most often congenital, a coronary fistula rarely may be acquired, such as after surgical resection of obstructing right ventricular muscle bundles (as in tetralogy of Fallot), endomyocardial biopsy, or penetrating or blunt trauma. CAF differ from coronary arteriovenous fistulae in the absence of outflow obstruction, in which coronary steal is the primary pathophysiologic problem.

29.2 Coronary to Bronchial Anastomoses

The porcine animal model seems to be the most representative of human coronary and bronchial arterial systems (Kotoulas et al. 2006). Experimental studies in such porcine models have shown that these connections resulted mainly in a bronchial to coronary network. Several studies have shown communications between the bronchial and coronary systems (Kotoulas et al. 2006; Gade et al. 1999). This communication is mainly located at the left atrial wall and the posterior and anterior wall of the left ventricle.

Owing to underlying diseases, it is likely that primary bronchopulmonay diseases will induce bronchial to coronary fistula, such as in chronic bronchial disease and after pulmonary transplantation where the bronchial arteries of the transplant are not reimplanted on the aorta and that ischemic coronary disease will induce coronary to bronchial fistula in order to rehabilitate better coronary artery flow beyond the site of obstruction.

In humans, coronary-to-bronchial anastomosis is perhaps not such a rare anomaly. This vascular abnormality may be subclinical or be responsible for several pathophysiological events and symptoms involving the respiratory and/or the coronary system. A study of bronchial arteries (BA) and their anastomoses with coronary arteries was performed in 53 adult subjects. In 6 cases BAs vascularized the left auricle; more than half of all cases had an anastomosis with the coronary arteries: 11 with the right coronary artery and 9 with the left one. These anastomoses could be useful to preserve the vascularization of the carina after a cardio-pulmonary transplantation. They should also play a role in the vascular supply of some coronary artery disease patients; in this study, associated coronary pathology was present in one fourth of the cases (Dupont et al. 1992).

29.2.1 Congenital

Several case reports are available in the literature. Some of them illustrate well the various presentations of these connections. Cyanotic congenital heart disease is one of the most frequent abnormalities. For instance, selective coronary arteriography was performed in 67 patients with congenital heart disease aged 1 to 33 years. Five of the 23 patients with cyanotic congenital heart disease had collateral vessels between the coronary and bronchial arteries; none of the 44 patients with noncyanotic congenital heart disease had such vessels. Each of the five patients with collateral vessels had severe obstruction of the right ventricular outflow tract or the pulmonary valve plus a ventricular septal defect and a right to left shunt. It appears that such collateral vessels from the coronary arteries provide an increment to pulmonary blood flow in patients with cyanotic congenital heart disease and diminished pulmonary flow (Zureikat 1980).

29.2.2 Acquired Cardiac Disease

The communication may be seen in patients with noncyanotic, acquired cardiac diseases (Iwasaki et al. 1997). In a huge cohort of 6,045 patients with various cardiopulmonary diseases who underwent coronary angiography, an angiographically visible coronary to bronchial artery anastomosis was found in seven (0.12%) patients. Aortitis syndrome was associated with four patients, whereas pulmonary embolism, aortic regurgitation and vasospastic angina were the diagnoses in the others. Coronary stenotic lesions were not observed in any patients. In five of six patients who underwent pulmonary perfusion scintigraphy, perfusion defect was observed in the area supplied by the bronchial artery, which had the anastomosis to the coronary artery. In each patient this anastomosis seemed to function as collateral circulation, compensating for decreased perfusion in either the lung or the heart. Such coronary to bronchial artery anastomosis is found likely to result in ischemic conditions affecting either the lung or the heart (Iwasaki et al. 1997).

The case of a patient with hemoptysis caused by an anomalous coronary-to-bronchial communication, who was concomitantly affected by aortic stenosis and coronary artery disease requiring surgical treatment, has been recently reported. A coronary angiogram clearly demonstrated the abnormal vascular connection between the proximal right coronary artery and the bronchial arteries of the left inferior right lobe. Hemoptysis resolved after aortic valve replacement, ligation of the coronary branch and coronary artery bypass (Lorusso et al. 2007). Previously, a case of extracardiac left coronary artery fistula connecting the circumflex branch and left bronchial artery with inferior wall myocardial insufficiency attributable to the right coronary artery atherosclerosis had been reported (Wandwi et al. 1996).

Another case of bronchial to coronary artery fistula was incidentally diagnosed during bronchial artery embolization. Embolization was performed successfully without complication, and an underlying important coronary artery stenosis was subsequently found at coronary CT angiography (Peynircioglu et al. 2007).

29.2.3 Chronic Bronchial Disease

The role of chronic bronchial disease has been advanced. In a patient with acute coronary syndrome, coronary angiography revealed severe double-vessel disease, as well as a coronary-bronchial artery fistula that arose from the left circumflex artery. Percutaneous coronary intervention was performed on the culprit lesion in the left anterior descending artery. A subsequent high-resolution CT of the thorax revealed mild bronchiectatic changes in the corresponding area supplied by the coronaro-bronchial artery fistula (Jim et al. 2003).

In a similar way, two cases of coronary-to-bronchial artery communication responsible for coronary steal were reported several years ago. In both cases the anastomosis originated from the proximal circumflex artery and developed because of bronchiectasis. In both cases closure of the anastomosis was achieved successfully by embolization, with the patients remaining free of symptoms at follow-up (Jarry et al. 1999).

29.3 Are There Different Underlying Causes with Coronary-Pulmonary Artery Fistula? Controversies with Hypertrophic Coronary-to-Bronchial Anastomosis

The case of localized congenital pulmonary dysplasia (Cijan et al. 2000), which is commonly accompanied by an abnormal vascular supply that originates from the thoracic or abdominal aorta, was recently reported. When the arterial supply comes from the coronary arteries, the abnormal vessels were variously labeled in the literature as coronary fistulae, as coronary-pulmonary collaterals or (erroneously) as coronary-bronchial fistulae (Angelini et al. 1999). Typically, such abnormal vessels are long channels with high vascular resistance, which carry limited blood flow to the lung parenchyma, while they empty into a branch of the pulmonary artery, but unlikely or never into a bronchial artery.

Other previous observations, both in cardiac and extracardiac fistulae, showed that coronary fistulae frequently have multiple supplying sources (Angelini et al. 1999). In the case reported above, the vascular malformation within the dysplastic left pulmonary segment was fed by a bronchial artery and two coronary arteries. Like in pulmonary sequestration, the dysplastic portion of the lung received an aberrant blood supply from arteries originating from the thoracic or abdominal aorta.

29.3.1
Coronary Steal

Although the pathogenesis of acquired coronary to pulmonary artery fistulae is not clear, it seems important to recognize that connections are always established with the arterial (and not venous) pulmonary circulation, a fact that supports a neovascularization mechanism that has been described in postoperative states (Funabashi and Komuro 2006). This mechanism can result in a steal from the supplying vessel, specifically from the coronary arteries. The long and thin neoformed vessels must indeed have much higher vascular resistance than does the coronary bed with which they must compete. Moreover, during exercise, coronary arterial resistances decrease more than pulmonary ones.

This hypothesis relies on several previous observations, such as two cases of coronary-pulmonary artery fistulae arising distal to obstructive coronary artery disease. The fistula in the first patient resulted in a tortuous dilatation of the distal portion of the right coronary artery flowing into the right pulmonary artery. In the second case, the fistula consisted in a plexus of vessels, which arose from the left anterior descending artery and entered the left pulmonary artery. Both the fistulae were successfully ligated at the time of concurrent coronary artery bypass graft surgery (Sathe et al. 1992). In another patient, a large coronary artery to bronchial artery anastomosis caused angina by coronary steal. Angina was refractory to medical treatment, but successfully relieved by surgical ligation of the anastomosis (St John Sutton et al. 1980).

29.3.2
Potential Cardiac Consequences

The consequences are not well known and yet polemic. In one instance, a patient with bronchiectasis had an inferolateral myocardial infarction. Coronary angiography revealed a large anastomosis from the left circumflex artery to the left lower lobe bronchial arteries. The relationship between the patient's myocardial infarction and possible coronary steal was very likely in this patient (Aupetit et al. 1988).

Other authors reported the case of a 44-year-old woman in whom a bronchial-to-coronary artery communication via the conus branch was discovered after distal bronchial artery embolization with gelatin sponge for hemoptysis. If this bronchial-to-coronary artery anastomosis, not visible prior to embolization, had been inadvertently embolized, the patient could have developed a myocardial infarction. To reduce the likelihood of a serious complication, the possibility of this anastomosis should be kept in mind, and angiography should be repeated before attempting proximal bronchial artery embolization (Miyazono et al. 1994).

Communications between coronary and bronchial vessels can hence be seen both on coronary angiography and bronchial artery angiography. A similar case of a bronchial to coronary artery anastomosis diagnosed prior to embolization in a patient with hemoptysis was reported. These anastomoses must be sought carefully during bronchial angiography and, contrary to coronary to bronchial anastomoses opacified via coronary angiography (Jarry et al. 1999), contraindicate embolization (Van den Berg et al. 1996).

29.4
Other Acquired Disease

29.4.1
Endocarditis and Infection

Coronary mycotic aneurysms, pseudoaneurysms and abscesses have been previously reported in both bare-metal and drug-eluting stent infections (Jang et al. 2007). However, no coronary-to-bronchial anastomoses have been described in this disease.

29.4.2
Takayasu Arteritis

The incidence of coronary lesions complicating Takayasu arteritis is relatively low; however, ischemia caused by coronary lesions is one of the major causes of death. Cardiac lesions have been found in 91.5% of 82 autopsy cases, including cardiomegaly in 81.7%, aortic regurgitation in 14.6% and myocardial infarction in 12.2%, but no coronary fistula (NAGATA 1990).

However, during life, Takayasu arteritis is associated with a low incidence of coronary artery involvement, such as stenosis, obstruction, aneurysm and coronary steal syndrome. In a study of 81 patients with Takayasu arteritis who underwent selective coronary angiography, 31 patients had abnormal coronary angiographic findings consisting of 24 coronary artery stenoses of greater than 75%, 3 coronary artery-bronchial artery anastomoses, 3 aneurysmal coronary ectasias and 1 combined coronary ectasia and anastomosis. Coronary steal phenomenon was always associated with occluded pulmonary arteries and pulmonary hypertension (ENDO et al. 2003).

One additional case of aortitis syndrome with development of a coronary to bronchial anastomosis has been reported with in a 44-year-old female patient suffering from cardiac failure. The angiogram revealed the presence of aortic regurgitation, pulmonary vascular lesions, anastomosis from left coronary artery to bronchial artery and hypervascularity of bronchial artery. The anastomosis from the left coronary artery to bronchial artery was considered as a collateral blood flow for the ischemic lesions of the lung (KAGURAOKA et al. 1989).

29.4.3 Trauma

Traumatic coronary artery fistulas are rare, but 80% are secondary to penetrating injuries. Although the left coronary artery is involved in 46% of cases, these are usually associated with fistulas to the right ventricle (JEGANATHAN et al. 2007).

29.4.4 Surgery

At the present time, acquired coronary fistulas can be seen after cardiac surgery, mostly coronary-to-pulmonary fistulas (ANGELINI 2000). Although the pathogenesis of acquired coronary to pulmonary artery fistulae is not clear, connections are always established with the arterial (and not venous) pulmonary circulation.

Fistulae originating from coronary arteries (typically from the left anterior descending or diagonal system) to the pulmonary artery have also been reported in post cardiac-transplantation patients (ANGELINI 2000). Collaterals may develop between coronary and pulmonary arteries after orthotopic heart transplantation, likely as a result of adhesions in the pericardial space (BALFOUR et al. 1999). It is also likely that coronary to bronchial fistulae develop spontaneously after lung transplantation when no bypass graft has been performed, but there are no data in the literature on the subject. Contrarily, several studies have shown the benefit of internal mammary to bronchial artery anastomosis (SUNDSET et al. 1997; HYYTINEN et al. 2000).

29.5 Imaging Studies, Treatment and Prognosis

Two-dimensional echocardiograms may reveal left atrial and left ventricular enlargement as a consequence of significant shunt flow or decreased regional or global dysfunction as a consequence of myocardial ischemia. The feeding coronary artery often appears enlarged, ectatic and tortuous. High-volume flow may be detected by color-flow imaging at the origin or along the length of the vessel (SMITH et al. 1972). Cardiac catheterization remains the modality of choice for defining coronary artery patterns of structure and flow. Most frequently, intracardiac pressures are normal and shunt flow is modest.

Aortography or selective coronary arteriography has long been the imaging technique required to manage the condition. In addition, therapeutic embolization using occlusive coils or devices may be performed via catheterization (JARRY et al. 1999). Owing to flow direction, bronchial artery angiography can reveal the bronchial to coronary communication. Spontaneous closure is rare, but may occur in small fistulae. Small fistulous connections in the asymptomatic patient may be monitored. Most lesions enlarge progressively and warrant surgical repair, either by transcatheter or surgical techniques.

Cardiac catheterization (transcatheter embolization) may be performed as intervention. Initial diagnostic catheterization should both define hemodynamic significance of the lesion and provide detailed angiographic assessment of the anatomy of the abnormality. Surgical options can be delineated by careful identification of the number of fistulous connections, nature of feeding vessel(s) and sites of drainage (St John Sutton et al. 1980). Indications for surgical intervention are the same as for embolization (see above). Some fistulae are unsuitable for the transcatheter approach and preferably are addressed surgically. These CAFs may include fistulae with multiple connections, circuitous routes and acute angulations that make catheter positioning difficult or impossible. Complications of surgery include myocardial ischemia and/or infarction (reported in 3% of patients) and recurrence of the fistula (4% of patients).

Major complications associated with transcatheter embolization relate to manipulation of stabilizing catheters and wires in the coronary vasculature and may include coronary artery spasm, ventricular dysrhythmias and perforation. Inappropriate positioning or proximal extension of occlusive coils or devices may result in obstruction of side branches and muscle loss. Intimal dissection of the coronary artery or thrombosis also may occur. However, morbidity and mortality rates generally are considered to be low.

29.6 Conclusions

The great majority of coronary-to-bronchial anastomoses, whether congenital or acquired, have little effect on coronary physiology and can be considered benign. It is likely that such abnormal vascular connections are caused either by congenital malformations, such as pulmonary dysplasia, or by acquired diseases, such as chronic pulmonary disease, lung transplantation on one hand, and more controversial, by chronic coronary occlusion on the other hand.

29.7 Take-Home Points

Coronary-to-bronchial anastomoses can be easily seen on coronary angiograms. They can induce ischemia via a steal phenomenon.

Bronchial to coronary anastomoses must be sought carefully at bronchial angiography and contraindicate a priori embolization in patients presenting with hemoptysis.

References

Angelini P (2000) Coronary-to-pulmonary fistulae. What are they? What are their causes? What are their functional consequences? Tex Heart Inst J 27:327–329

Angelini P, Villason S, Chan AV Jr, Diez JG (1999) Normal and anomalous coronary arteries in humans. In: Angelini P (ed) Coronary artery anomalies: a comprehensive approach.Lippincott Williams & Wilkins, Philadelphia, pp 27–150

Aupetit JF, Gallet M, Boutarin J (1988) Coronary-to-bronchial artery anastomosis complicated with myocardial infarction. Int J Cardiol 18:93–97

Balfour IC, Tinker K, Singh G, Fiore AC, Jureidini SB (1999) Coronary artery to pulmonary artery collaterals after heart transplantation. J Heart Lung Transplant 18:1027–1029

Bjork L (1966) Angiographic demonstration of extracardial anastomoses to the coronary arteries. Radiology 87:274–277

Chee TS, Tan PJ, Koh SK, Jayaram L (2007) Coronary artery fistula diagnosed by transthoracic Doppler echocardiography. Singapore Med J 48:e262–e264

Cijan A, Zorc-Pleskovic R, Zorc M, Klokocovnik T (2000) Local pulmonary malformation caused by bilateral coronary artery and bronchial artery fistulae to the left pulmonary artery in a patient with coronary artery disease. Tex Heart Inst J 27:390–394

Dupont P, Riquet M, Briere J, Weber S, Debesse B, Hidden G (1992) The bronchial arteries and their anastomoses with the coronary arteries (article in French). Bull Assoc Anat (Nancy) 76:5–12

Endo M, Tomizawa Y, Nishida H, Aomi S, Nakazawa M, Tsurumi Y, Kawana M, Kasanuki H (2003) Angiographic findings and surgical treatments of coronary artery involvement in Takayasu arteritis. J Thorac Cardiovasc Surg. 125:570–577

Esperanca Pina JA, Goncalves Pina J (1981) The vascular anastomoses of the human heart. Prog Clin Biol Res 59B:89–99

Funabashi N, Komuro I (2006) Aberrant fistula arteries from the left main branch and right coronary artery to the left pulmonary arterial sinus demonstrated by multislice computed tomography. Int J Cardiol 106:428–430

Gade J, Nørgaard MA, Andersen CB, Jakobsen H, Breitowicz B, Svendsen UG, Olsen PS (1999) The porcine bronchial artery. Anastomoses with oesophageal, coronary and intercostal arteries. J Anat. 195 (Pt 1):65–73

Hyytinen TA, Heikkilä LJ, Verkkala KA, Sipponen JT, Vainikka TL, Halme M, Hekali PE, Keto PE, Mattila SP (2000) Bronchial artery revascularization improves tracheal anastomotic healing after lung transplantation. Scand Cardiovasc J 34:213–218

Iwasaki K, Kusachi S, Hina K, Murakami M, Matano S, Ohnishi N, Kondo N, Kita T, Sakakibara N (1997) Coronary to bronchial artery anastomosis in patients with noncyanotic cardiopulmonary disease: report of seven cases. Can J Cardiol 13:898–900

Jang JJ, Krishnaswami A, Fang J, Go M, Ben VC (2007) Images in cardiovascular medicine. Pseudoaneurysm and intracardiac fistula caused by an infected paclitaxel-eluting coronary stent. Circulation 116:e364–365

Jarry G, Bruaire JP, Commeau P, Hermida JS, Leborgne L, Auquier MA, Delonca J, Quiret JC, Remond A (1999) Coronary-to-bronchial artery communication: report of two patients successfully treated by embolization. Cardiovasc Intervent Radiol 22:251–254

Jeganathan R, Irwin G, Johnston PW, Jones JM (2007) Traumatic left anterior descending artery-to-pulmonary artery fistula with delayed pericardial tamponade. Ann Thorac Surg 84:276–278

Jim MH, Lee SW, Lam L (2003) Localized bronchiectasis is a definite association of coronaro-bronchial artery fistula. J Invasive Cardiol 15:554–556

Kaguraoka H, Itaoka T, Itou H, Ono K, Yokonyama M, Nitta S (1989) [A case of aortitis syndrome with anastomoses from left coronary artery to bronchial artery.] Kokyu To Junkan 37:569–572 (article in Japanese)

Kotoulas C, Karnabatidis D, Kalogeropoulou C, Kokkinis K, Petsas T, Dougenis D (2006) Anastomoses between bronchial and coronary circulation in a porcine model: computed tomographic and angiographic demonstration. Hellenic J Cardiol 47:206–210

Lorusso R, De Cicco G, Faggiano P, Chiari E, Nardi M, Curello S, Ettori F, Niccoli L (2007) Coronary-to-bronchial anastomosis: an unusual cause of hemoptysis. J Cardiovasc Med (Hagerstown) 8:642–644

Miyazono N, Inoue H, Hori A, Kanetsuki I, Shimada J, Nakajo M (1994) Visualization of left bronchial-to-coronary artery communication after distal bronchial artery embolization for bronchiectasis. Cardiovasc Intervent Radiol 17:36–37

Moberg A (1967) Anastomoses between extracardiac vessels and coronary arteries. I. Via bronchial arteries. Postmortem angiographic study in adults and newborn infants. Acta Rad Diagn (Stockholm) 6:177–192

Nagata S (1990) Present state of autopsy cases of Takayasu's arteritis (aortitis syndrome) in Japan. J Jpn Coll Angiol 30:1303–1308

Peynircioglu B, Ergun O, Hazirolan T, Cil BE, Aytemir K (2007) Bronchial to coronary artery fistulas: an important sign of silent coronary artery disease and potential complication during bronchial artery embolization. Acta Radiol 48:171–172

Sathe S, Warren R, Vohra J, Skillington P, Hunt D (1992) Coronary-pulmonary artery fistula arising distal to obstructive coronary lesions. Cardiology 80:77–80

Smith SC, Adams DF, Herman MV, Paulin S (1972) Coronary-to-bronchial anastomoses: an in vivo demonstration by selective coronary arteriography. Radiology 104:289–290

St John Sutton MG, Miller GA, Kerr IH, Traill TA (1980) Coronary artery steal via large coronary artery to bronchial artery anastomosis successfully treated by operation. Br Heart J 44:460–463

Sundset A, Tadjkarimi S, Khaghani A, Kvernebo K, Yacoub MH (1997) Human en bloc double-lung transplantation: bronchial artery revascularization improves airway perfusion. Ann Thorac Surg 63:790–795

Van den Berg JC, Overtoom TT, De Valois JC (1996) Case report: bronchial to coronary artery anastomosis – a potential hazard in bronchial artery embolization. Br J Radiol 69:570–572

Wandwi WB, Mitsui N, Sueda T, Orihashi K, Sueshiro M, Azuma K, Matsuura Y (1996) Coronary artery fistula to bronchial artery on contralateral side of coronary atherosclerosis and myocardial insufficiency. A case report. Angiology 47:211–213

White FC, Carroll SM, Magnet A et al. (1992) Coronary collateral development in swine after coronary artery occlusion. Circ Res 71:1490–1500

Zureikat HY (1980) Collateral vessels between the coronary and bronchial arteries in patients with cyanotic congenital heart disease. Am J Cardiol. 45:599–603

Subject Index

A

B

C

D

E

F

G

H

I

K

L

M

Q

R

S

T

X

Z

List of Contributors

John Aldrich, PhD
Professor of Radiology
Department of Radiology
University of British Columbia
899 W 12th Avenue
Vancouver BC V5Z 1M9
Canada

Email: john.aldrich@vch.ca

Hatem Alkadhi, MD
PD, Institute of Diagnostic Radiology
University Hospital Zurich
Raemisstrasse 100
8091 Zurich
Switzerland

Email: hatem.alkadhi@usz.ch

Christoph R. Becker, MD
Department of Clinical Radiology
Ludwig-Maximilians-University
Großhadern Hospital
Marchioninistrasse 15
81377 Munich
Germany

Email: christoph.becker@med.uni-muenchen.de

Lorenzo Bonomo, MD
Professor, Department of Bioimaging and Radiological Sciences
Catholic University
Largo Agostino Gemelli 8
00168 Rome
Italy

Email: lbonomo@rm.unicatt.it

Kahimano Boroto, MD
Department of Thoracic Imaging
University Center of Lille
Boulevard du Prof. J. Leclercq
59037 Lille Cédex
France

Loic Boussel, MD
Service de Radiologie
Hôpital Louis Pradel
28 Avenue du Doyen Lépine
69677 Bron Cédex
France

Email: loic.boussel@libertysurf.fr

Erik Bouvier, MD
Centre Cardiologique du Nord
32–36 Avenue des Moulins Gémeaux
93200 Saint Denis
France

Filippo Cademartiri, MD, PhD
Department of Radiology
Azienda Ospedaliero
Universiy of Parma
Via Gramsci 14
43100 Parma
Italy
and
Department of Radiology and Cardiology
Eramus Medical Center
Dr. Molewaterplein 60
3015 GD Rotterdam
The Netherlands

Email: filippocademartiri@hotmail.com

Clio Camus, MD
Department of Pulmonary and Critical Care Medicine
Hôspital Universitaire du Bocage
2100 Dijon
France

Philippe Camus, MD
Department of Pulmonary and Critical Care Medicine
Hôspital Universitaire du Bocage
2100 Dijon
France

Email: aude.dumel@chu-dijon.fr

Andrea Caulo, MD
Department of Bioimaging and
Radiological Sciences
Catholic University
Largo Agostino Gemelli 8
00168 Rome
Italy

Thierry Couvreur, MD
Department of Medical Imaging
University Hospital of Liege
4000 Liege 1
Belgium
Email: T.couvreur@student.ulg.ac.be

Philippe Douek, MD
Professor, Service de Radiologie
Hôpital Louis Pradel
28 Avenue du Doyen Lépine
69677 Bron Cédex
France
Email: philippe.douek@creatis.univ-lyon1.fr

Michaël Dupont, MD
Department of Radiology
UCL Cliniques Universitaires Saint Luc
Avenue Hippocrate 10
1200 Brussels
Belgium

Brett Elicker, MD
Assistant Professor, Department of Radiology
University of California
505 Parnassus Avenue
San Francisco, CA 94122
USA

Jean-Baptiste Faivre, MD
Department of Thoracic Imaging
C.H.R.U. de Lille
Hôspital Calmette
Boulevard du Prof. J. Leclercq
59037 Lille Cédex
France

Jacques Feignoux, MD
Centre Cardiologique du Nord
32–36 Avenue des Moulins Gémeaux
93200 Saint Denis
France

Dominik Fleischmann, MD
Associate Professor of Radiology
Cardiovascular and Thoracic Imaging Sections
Department of Radiology
Stanford University Medical Center
300 Pasteur Drive, Room S-068B
Stanford, CA 94305–5105
USA
Email: d.fleischmann@stanford.edu

Thomas Flohr, PhD
Siemens Healthcare
Computed Tomography
Siemensstrasse 1
91301 Forchheim
Germany
Email: thomas.flohr@siemens.com

Pascal Foucher, MD
Department of Pulmonary and Critical Care Medicine
Hôspital Universitaire du Bocage
2100 Dijon
France
Email: aude.dumel@chu-dijon.fr

Delphine Gamondès, MD
Department of Thoracic and Cardiovascular Radiology
University Hospital Louis Pradel
69006 Lyon
France

Benoît Ghaye, MD
Department of Medical Imaging
University Hospital of Liege
4000 Liege 1
Belgium
Email: bghaya@chu.ulg.ac.be

Andrei-Bogdan Gorgos,
Department of Thoracic Imaging
C.H.R.U. de Lille
Hôpital Calmette
Boulevard du Prof. J. Leclercq
59037 Lille Cédex
France

Anne-Lise Hachulla, MD
Department of Thoracic Imaging
University Center of Lille
Boulevard du Prof. J. Leclercq
59037 Lille Cédex
France

Xavier Hamoir, MD
Department of Radiology
Clinique Notre Dame
Avenue Delmée 9
7500 Tournai
Belgium
Email: xavier.hamoir@skynet.be

David M. Hansell, MD, FRCP, FRCR
Department of Radiology
Royal Brompton Hospital
Sydney Street
London SW3 6NP
UK
Email: d.hansell@rbht.nhs.uk

Jacques Kirsch, MD
Department of Radiology
Clinique Notre Dame
Avenue Delmée 9
7500 Tournai
Belgium
Email: jacques.kirsch@radiologie.net

Ernst Klotz, Dipl. Phys.
Computer Tomography Division
Siemens Healthcare Sector
Siemensstrasse 1
91301 Forchheim
Germany

Ludovico La Grutta, MD
Department of Radiology and Cardiology
Eramus Medical Center
Dr. Molewaterplein 60
3015 GD Rotterdam
The Netherlands
and
Department of Radiology
University of Palermo
Italy

Jean-Pierre Laissy, MD
Professor, Department of Radiology
Imagerie Médicale
Hôpital Bichat
46 rue Henri Huchard
75018 Paris
France
Email: jean-pierre.laissy@bch.ap-hop-paris.fr

Anna Rita Larici, MD
Department of Bioimaging and Radiological Sciences
Catholic University
Largo Agostino Gemelli 8
00168 Rome
Italy

Francois Laurent, MD
Unité d'Imagerie Thoracique et Cardiovasculaire
Hôpital Cardiologique du Haut Lévèque
Avenue de Magellan
33604 Pessac
France
Email: francois.laurent@chu-bordeaux.fr

Margaret C. C. Lin, MD
Assistant Professor of Radiology
Thoracic Imaging Section
Department of Radiology
Stanford University Medical Center
300 Pasteur Drive, Room S-068B
Stanford, CA 94305–5105
USA

Guiseppe Macis, MD
Department of Bioimaging and Radiological Sciences
Chatolic University
Largo Agostino Gemelli, 8
00168 Rome
Italy

Erica Maffei, MD
Department of Radiology
Azienda Ospedaliero
Universiy of Parma
Via Gramsci 14
43100 Parma
Italy

Fabio Maggi, MD
Department of Bioimaging and Radiological Sciences
Catholic University
Largo Agostino Gemelli 8
00168 Rome
Italy

Borut Marincek, MD
Professor, Institute of Diagnostic Radiology
University Hospital Zurich
Raemistrasse 100
8091 Zurich
Switzerland
Email: borut.marincek@usz.ch

John R. Mayo, MD
Professor of Radiology and Cardiology
Department of Radiology
University of British Columbia
899 W 12th Avenue
Vancouver BC V5Z 1M9
Canada

Email: John.Mayo@vch.ca

Laura Menchini, MD
Department of Bioimaging and Radiological Sciences
Catholic University
Largo Agostino Gemelli 8
00168 Rome
Italy

Nico R. Mollet, MD, PhD
Department of Radiology and Cardiology
Eramus Medical Center
Dr. Molewaterplein 60
3015 GD Rotterdam
The Netherlands

Michel Montaudon, MD
Unité d'Imagerie Thoracique et Cardiovasculaire
Hôpital Cardiologique du Haut Lévèque
Avenue de Magellan
33604 Pessac
France

Bernd Ohnesorge, PhD
Siemens Limited China, Healthcare
Siemens International Medical Park
278 Zhou Zhu Road
SIMZ, Nanhui District
Shanghai 201318
P. R. China

Email: bernd.ohnesorge@siemens.com

Anselmo Alessandro Palumbo, MD
Department of Radiology
Azienda Ospedaliero
Universiy of Parma
Via Gramsci 14
43100 Parma
Italy
and
Department of Radiology and Cardiology
Eramus Medical Center
Dr. Molewaterplein 60
3015 GD Rotterdam
The Netherlands

Vittorio Pansini, MD
Department of Thoracic Imaging
C.H.R.U. de Lille
Hôpital Calmette
Boulevard du Prof. J. Leclercq
59037 Lille Cédex
France

François Pontana, MD
Department of Thoracic Imaging
C.H.R.U. de Lille
Hôpital Calmette
Boulevard du Prof. J. Leclercq
59037 Lille Cédex
France

Mathias Prokop, MD, PhD
Department of Radiology
University Medical Center Utrecht
Room E 01.123
P.O. Box 85500
3508 GA Utrecht
The Netherlands

Email: m.prokop@azu.nl

Salah D. Qanadli, MD
Service de Radiologie
CHU Vaudois
1011 Lausanne
Switzerland

Email: Salah.Qanadli@chuv.ch

Jacques Rémy, MD
Professor, Department of Thoracic Imaging
C.H.R.U. de Lille
Hôpital Calmette
Boulevard du Prof. J. Leclercq
59037 Lille Cédex
France

Email: j-remy@chru-lille.fr

Martine Rémy-Jardin, MD, PhD
Professor, Department of Thoracic Imaging
C.H.R.U. de Lille
Hôpital Calmette
Boulevard du Prof. J. Leclercq
59037 Lille Cédex
France

Email: mremy-jardin@chru-lille.fr

Didier Revel, MD
Department of Radiology
Hôspital Cardio-vasculaire, Louis Pradel
28 Avenue Doyen Lépine
69677 Bron Cédex
France
Email: didier.revel@creatis.univ-lyon1.fr

Elena Rizzo, MD
Service de Radiologie
CHU Vaudois
1011 Lausanne
Switzerland

Annemarieke Rutten, MD, PhD
Department of Radiology
University Medical Center Utrecht
Room E 01.123
P.O. Box 85500
3508 GA Utrecht
The Netherlands
Email: a.rutten@umcutrecht.nl

Jean-Louis Sablayrolles, MD
Centre Cardiologique du Nord
32–36 Avenue des Moulins Gémeaux
93200 Saint Denis
France
Email: jl.sablayrolles@ccncardio.com

Paul Stolzmann, MD
Institute of Diagnostic Radiology
University Hospital Zurich
Raemistrasse 100
8091 Zurich
Switzerland
Email: paul.stolzmann@usz.ch

Maria Luigia Storto, MD
Professor, Department of Radiology
University of Chieti
Via dei Vestini
66100 Chieti
Italy

Nicola Sverzellati, MD
Department of Clinical Sciences
Institute of Radiology
University of Parma
Via Gramsci 14
43100 Parma
Italy
Email: nicolasve@tiscali.it

Nunzia Tacelli, MD
C.H.R.U. de Lille
Hôspital Calmette
Boulevard du Prof. J. Leclercq
59037 Lille Cédex
France

Jean Marc Trautenaere, MD
Centre Cardiologique du Nord
32–36 Avenue des Moulins Gémeaux
93200 Saint Denis
France

Charles S. White, MD
Department of Diagnostic Radiology
University of Maryland Medical Center
22 S. Greene Street
Baltimore, MD 21201
USA
Email: cwhite@umm.edu

Seung Min Yoo, MD, PhD
Department of Diagnostic Radiology
University of Maryland Medical Center
22 S. Greene Street
Baltimore, MD 21201
USA
Email: syoo@umm.edu

Medical Radiology Diagnostic Imaging and Radiation Oncology

Titles in the series already published

Diagnostic Imaging

Innovations in Diagnostic Imaging
Edited by J. H. Anderson

Radiology of the Upper Urinary Tract
Edited by E. K. Lang

The Thymus - Diagnostic Imaging, Functions, and Pathologic Anatomy
Edited by E. Walter, E. Willich, and W. R. Webb

Interventional Neuroradiology
Edited by A. Valavanis

Radiology of the Lower Urinary Tract
Edited by E. K. Lang

Contrast-Enhanced MRI of the Breast
S. Heywang-Köbrunner and R. Beck

Spiral CT of the Chest
Edited by M. Rémy-Jardin and J. Rémy

Radiological Diagnosis of Breast Diseases
Edited by M. Friedrich and E. A. Sickles

Radiology of Trauma
Edited by M. Heller and A. Fink

Biliary Tract Radiology
Edited by P. Rossi. Co-edited by M. Brezi

Radiological Imaging of Sports Injuries
Edited by C. Masciocchi

Modern Imaging of the Alimentary Tube
Edited by A. R. Margulis

Diagnosis and Therapy of Spinal Tumors
Edited by P. R. Algra, J. Valk and J. J. Heimans

Interventional Magnetic Resonance Imaging
Edited by J. F. Debatin and G. Adam

Abdominal and Pelvic MRI
Edited by A. Heuck and M. Reiser

Orthopedic Imaging
Techniques and Applications
Edited by A. M. Davies and H. Pettersson

Radiology of the Female Pelvic Organs
Edited by E. K. Lang

Magnetic Resonance of the Heart and Great Vessels
Clinical Applications
Edited by J. Bogaert, A. J. Duerinckx, and F. E. Rademakers

Modern Head and Neck Imaging
Edited by S. K. Mukherji and J. A. Castelijns

Radiological Imaging of Endocrine Diseases
Edited by J. N. Bruneton
in collaboration with B. Padovani and M.-Y. Mourou

Radiology of the Pancreas
2nd Revised Edition
Edited by A. L. Baert. Co-edited by G. Delorme and L. Van Hoe

Trends in Contrast Media
Edited by H. S. Thomsen, R. N. Muller, and R. F. Mattrey

Functional MRI
Edited by C. T. W. Moonen and P. A. Bandettini

Emergency Pediatric Radiology
Edited by H. Carty

Liver Malignancies
Diagnostic and Interventional Radiology
Edited by C. Bartolozzi and R. Lencioni

Spiral CT of the Abdomen
Edited by F. Terrier, M. Grossholz, and C. D. Becker

Medical Imaging of the Spleen
Edited by A. M. De Schepper and F. Vanhoenacker

Radiology of Peripheral Vascular Diseases
Edited by E. Zeitler

Radiology of Blunt Trauma of the Chest
P. Schnyder and M. Wintermark

Portal Hypertension
Diagnostic Imaging and Imaging-Guided Therapy
Edited by P. Rossi.
Co-edited by P. Ricci and L. Broglia

Virtual Endoscopy and Related 3D Techniques
Edited by P. Rogalla, J. Terwisscha van Scheltinga and B. Hamm

Recent Advances in Diagnostic Neuroradiology
Edited by Ph. Demaerel

Transfontanellar Doppler Imaging in Neonates
A. Couture, C. Veyrac

Radiology of AIDS
A Practical Approach
Edited by J. W. A. J. Reeders and P. C. Goodman

CT of the Peritoneum
A. Rossi, G. Rossi

Magnetic Resonance Angiography
2nd Revised Edition
Edited by I. P. Arlart, G. M. Bongartz, and G. Marchal

Applications of Sonography in Head and Neck Pathology
Edited by J. N. Bruneton
in collaboration with C. Raffaelli, O. Dassonville

3D Image Processing
Techniques and Clinical Applications
Edited by D. Caramella and C. Bartolozzi

Imaging of the Larynx
Edited by R. Hermans

Pediatric ENT Radiology
Edited by S. J. King and A. E. Boothroyd

Imaging of Orbital and Visual Pathway Pathology
Edited by W. S. Müller-Forell

Radiological Imaging of the Small Intestine
Edited by N. C. Gourtsoyiannis

Imaging of the Knee
Techniques and Applications
Edited by A. M. Davies and V. N. Cassar-Pullicino

Perinatal Imaging
From Ultrasound to MR Imaging
Edited by F. E. Avni

Diagnostic and Interventional Radiology in Liver Transplantation
Edited by E. Bücheler, V. Nicolas, C. E. Broelsch, X. Rogiers and G. Krupski

Imaging of the Pancreas
Cystic and Rare Tumors
Edited by C. Procacci and A. J. Megibow

Imaging of the Foot & Ankle
Techniques and Applications
Edited by A. M. Davies, R. W. Whitehouse and J. P. R. Jenkins

Radiological Imaging of the Ureter
Edited by F. Joffre, Ph. Otal and M. Soulie

Radiology of the Petrous Bone
Edited by M. Lemmerling and S. S. Kollias

Imaging of the Shoulder
Techniques and Applications
Edited by A. M. Davies and J. Hodler

Interventional Radiology in Cancer
Edited by A. Adam, R. F. Dondelinger, and P. R. Mueller

Imaging and Intervention in Abdominal Trauma
Edited by R. F. Dondelinger

Radiology of the Pharynx and the Esophagus
Edited by O. Ekberg

Radiological Imaging in Hematological Malignancies
Edited by A. Guermazi

Functional Imaging of the Chest
Edited by H.-U. Kauczor

Duplex and Color Doppler Imaging of the Venous System
Edited by G. H. Mostbeck

Multidetector-Row CT of the Thorax
Edited by U. J. Schoepf

Radiology and Imaging of the Colon
Edited by A. H. Chapman

Multidetector-Row CT Angiography
Edited by C. Catalano and R. Passariello

Focal Liver Lesions
Detection, Characterization, Ablation
Edited by R. Lencioni, D. Cioni, and C. Bartolozzi

Imaging in Treatment Planning for Sinonasal Diseases
Edited by R. Maroldi and P. Nicolai

Clinical Cardiac MRI
With Interactive CD-ROM
Edited by J. Bogaert, S. Dymarkowski, and A. M. Taylor

Dynamic Contrast-Enhanced Magnetic Resonance Imaging in Oncology
Edited by A. Jackson, D. L. Buckley, and G. J. M. Parker

Contrast Media in Ultrasonography
Basic Principles and Clinical Applications
Edited by E. Quaia

Paediatric Musculoskeletal Disease
With an Emphasis on Ultrasound
Edited by D. Wilson

MR Imaging in White Matter Diseases of the Brain and Spinal Cord
Edited by M. Filippi, N. De Stefano, V. Dousset, and J. C. McGowan

Imaging of the Hip & Bony Pelvis
Techniques and Applications
Edited by A. M. Davies, K. Johnson, and R. W. Whitehouse

Imaging of Kidney Cancer
Edited by A. Guermazi

Magnetic Resonance Imaging in Ischemic Stroke
Edited by R. von Kummer and T. Back

Diagnostic Nuclear Medicine
2nd Revised Edition
Edited by C. Schiepers

Imaging of Occupational and Environmental Disorders of the Chest
Edited by P. A. Gevenois and P. De Vuyst

Virtual Colonoscopy
A Practical Guide
Edited by P. Lefere and S. Gryspeerdt

Contrast Media
Safety Issues and ESUR Guidelines
Edited by H. S. Thomsen

Head and Neck Cancer Imaging
Edited by R. Hermans

Vascular Embolotherapy
A Comprehensive Approach
Volume 1: *General Principles, Chest, Abdomen, and Great Vessels*
Edited by J. Golzarian. Co-edited by S. Sun and M. J. Sharafuddin

Vascular Embolotherapy
A Comprehensive Approach
Volume 2: *Oncology, Trauma, Gene Therapy, Vascular Malformations, and Neck*
Edited by J. Golzarian. Co-edited by S. Sun and M. J. Sharafuddin

Vascular Interventional Radiology
Current Evidence in Endovascular Surgery
Edited by M. G. Cowling

Ultrasound of the Gastrointestinal Tract
Edited by G. Maconi and G. Bianchi Porro

Parallel Imaging in Clinical MR Applications
Edited by S. O. Schoenberg, O. Dietrich, and M. F. Reiser

MRI and CT of the Female Pelvis
Edited by B. Hamm and R. Forstner

Imaging of Orthopedic Sports Injuries
Edited by F. M. Vanhoenacker, M. Maas and J. L. Gielen

Ultrasound of the Musculoskeletal System
S. Bianchi and C. Martinoli

Clinical Functional MRI
Presurgical Functional Neuroimaging
Edited by C. Stippich

Radiation Dose from Adult and Pediatric Multidetector Computed Tomography
Edited by D. Tack and P. A. Gevenois

Spinal Imaging
Diagnostic Imaging of the Spine and Spinal Cord
Edited by J. Van Goethem, L. van den Hauwe and P. M. Parizel

Computed Tomography of the Lung
A Pattern Approach
J. A. Verschakelen and W. De Wever

Imaging in Transplantation
Edited by A. Bankier

Radiological Imaging of the Neonatal Chest
2nd Revised Edition
Edited by V. Donoghue

Radiological Imaging of the Digestive Tract in Infants and Children
Edited by A. S. Devos and J. G. Blickman

Pediatric Chest Imaging
Chest Imaging in Infants and Children
2nd Revised Edition
Edited by J. Lucaya and J. L. Strife

Color Doppler US of the Penis
Edited by M. Bertolotto

Radiology of the Stomach and Duodenum
Edited by A. H. Freeman and E. Sala

Imaging in Pediatric Skeletal Trauma
Techniques and Applications
Edited by K. J. Johnson and E. Bache

Image Processing in Radiology
Current Applications
Edited by E. Neri, D. Caramella, C. Bartolozzi

Screening and Preventive Diagnosis with Radiological Imaging
Edited by M. F. Reiser, G. van Kaick, C. Fink, S. O. Schoenberg

Percutaneous Tumor Ablation in Medical Radiology
Edited by T. J. Vogl, T. K. Helmberger, M. G. Mack, M. F. Reiser

Liver Radioembolization with ^{90}Y Microspheres
Edited by J. I. Bilbao, M. F. Reiser

Pediatric Uroradiology
2nd Revised Edition
Edited by R. Fotter

Radiology of Osteoporosis
2nd Revised Edition
Edited by S. Grampp

Gastrointestinal Tract Sonography in Fetuses and Children
A. Couture, C. Baud, J. L. Ferran, M. Saguintaah and C. Veyrac

Intracranial Vascular Malformations and Aneurysms
2nd Revised Edition
Edited by M. Forsting and I. Wanke

High-Resolution Sonography of the Peripheral Nervous System
2nd Revised Edition
Edited by S. Peer and G. Bodner

Imaging Pelvic Floor Disorders
2nd Revised Edition
Edited by J. Stoker, S. A. Taylor, and J. O. L. DeLancey

Coronary Radiology
2nd Revised Edition
Edited by M. Oudkerk and M. F. Reiser

Integrated Cardiothoracic Imaging with MDCT
Edited by M. Rémy-Jardin and J. Rémy

Multislice CT
3rd Revised Edition
Edited by M. F. Reiser, C. R. Becker, K. Nikolaou, G. Glazer

MRI of the Lung
Edited by H.-U. Kauczor

Imaging in Percutaneous Musculoskeletal Interventions
Edited by A. Gangi, S. Guth, and A. Guermazi

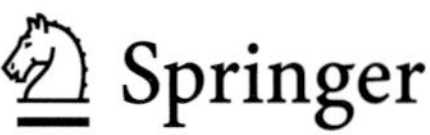

Medical Radiology Diagnostic Imaging and Radiation Oncology

Titles in the series already published

Radiation Oncology

Lung Cancer
Edited by C. W. Scarantino

Innovations in Radiation Oncology
Edited by H. R. Withers and L. J. Peters

Radiation Therapy of Head and Neck Cancer
Edited by G. E. Laramore

Gastrointestinal Cancer – Radiation Therapy
Edited by R. R. Dobelbower, Jr.

Radiation Exposure and Occupational Risks
Edited by E. Scherer, C. Streffer, and K.-R. Trott

Interventional Radiation
Therapy Techniques – Brachytherapy
Edited by R. Sauer

Radiopathology of Organs and Tissues
Edited by E. Scherer, C. Streffer, and K.-R. Trott

Concomitant Continuous Infusion
Chemotherapy and Radiation
Edited by M. Rotman and C. J. Rosenthal

Intraoperative Radiotherapy – Clinical Experiences and Results
Edited by F. A. Calvo, M. Santos, and L. W. Brady

Interstitial and Intracavitary Thermoradiotherapy
Edited by M. H. Seegenschmiedt and R. Sauer

Non-Disseminated Breast Cancer
Controversial Issues in Management
Edited by G. H. Fletcher and S. H. Levitt

Current Topics in Clinical Radiobiology of Tumors
Edited by H.-P. Beck-Bornholdt

Practical Approaches to Cancer Invasion and Metastases
A Compendium of Radiation Oncologists' Responses to 40 Histories
Edited by A. R. Kagan with the Assistance of R. J. Steckel

Radiation Therapy in Pediatric Oncology
Edited by J. R. Cassady

Radiation Therapy Physics
Edited by A. R. Smith

Late Sequelae in Oncology
Edited by J. Dunst, R. Sauer

Mediastinal Tumors. Update 1995
Edited by D. E. Wood, C. R. Thomas, Jr.

Thermoradiotherapy and Thermochemotherapy
Volume 1:
Biology, Physiology, and Physics
Volume 2:
Clinical Applications
Edited by M. H. Seegenschmiedt, P. Fessenden and C. C. Vernon

Carcinoma of the Prostate
Innovations in Management
Edited by Z. Petrovich, L. Baert, and L. W. Brady

Radiation Oncology of Gynecological Cancers
Edited by H. W. Vahrson

Carcinoma of the Bladder
Innovations in Management
Edited by Z. Petrovich, L. Baert, and L. W. Brady

Blood Perfusion and Microenvironment of Human Tumors
Implications for Clinical Radiooncology
Edited by M. Molls and P. Vaupel

Radiation Therapy of Benign Diseases
A Clinical Guide
2nd Revised Edition
S. E. Order and S. S. Donaldson

Carcinoma of the Kidney and Testis, and Rare Urologic Malignancies
Innovations in Management
Edited by Z. Petrovich, L. Baert, and L. W. Brady

Progress and Perspectives in the Treatment of Lung Cancer
Edited by P. Van Houtte, J. Klastersky, and P. Rocmans

Combined Modality Therapy of Central Nervous System Tumors
Edited by Z. Petrovich, L. W. Brady, M. L. Apuzzo, and M. Bamberg

Age-Related Macular Degeneration
Current Treatment Concepts
Edited by W. E. Alberti, G. Richard, and R. H. Sagerman

Radiotherapy of Intraocular and Orbital Tumors
2nd Revised Edition
Edited by R. H. Sagerman and W. E. Alberti

Modification of Radiation Response
Cytokines, Growth Factors, and Other Biolgical Targets
Edited by C. Nieder, L. Milas and K. K. Ang

Radiation Oncology for Cure and Palliation
R. G. Parker, N. A. Janjan and M. T. Selch

Clinical Target Volumes in Conformal and Intensity Modulated Radiation Therapy
A Clinical Guide to Cancer Treatment
Edited by V. Grégoire, P. Scalliet, and K. K. Ang

Advances in Radiation Oncology in Lung Cancer
Edited by B. Jeremić

New Technologies in Radiation Oncology
Edited by W. Schlegel, T. Bortfeld, and A.-L. Grosu

Multimodal Concepts for Integration of Cytotoxic Drugs and Radiation Therapy
Edited by J. M. Brown, M. P. Mehta, and C. Nieder

Technical Basis of Radiation Therapy
Practical Clinical Applications
4th Revised Edition
Edited by S. H. Levitt, J. A. Purdy, C. A. Perez, and S. Vijayakumar

CURED I • LENT
Late Effects of Cancer Treatment on Normal Tissues
Edited by P. Rubin, L. S. Constine, L. B. Marks, and P. Okunieff

Radiotherapy for Non-Malignant Disorders
Contemporary Concepts and Clinical Results
Edited by M. H. Seegenschmiedt, H.-B. Makoski, K.-R. Trott, and L. W. Brady

CURED II • LENT
Cancer Survivorship Research and Education
Late Effects on Normal Tissues
Edited by P. Rubin, L. S. Constine, L. B. Marks, and P. Okunieff

Radiation Oncology
An Evidence-Based Approach
Edited by J. J. Lu and L. W. Brady

Primary Optic Nerve Sheath Meningioma
Edited by B. Jeremić, and S. Pitz

Springer